The Oxford Handbook of Dimensional Models of Psychopathology

The Oxford Handbook of Dimensional Models of Psychopathology

Edited by

CHRISTOPHER C. CONWAY

and

ROBERT F. KRUEGER

OXFORD
UNIVERSITY PRESS

OXFORD
UNIVERSITY PRESS

Oxford University Press is a department of the University of Oxford. It furthers the University's objective of excellence in research, scholarship, and education by publishing worldwide. Oxford is a registered trade mark of Oxford University Press in the UK and in certain other countries.

Published in the United States of America by Oxford University Press
198 Madison Avenue, New York, NY 10016, United States of America.

CIP data is on file at the Library of Congress

ISBN 9780197769645

DOI: 10.1093/9780197769676.001.0001

Printed by Integrated Books International, United States of America

The manufacturer's authorized representative in the EU for product safety is Oxford University Press España S.A. of Parque Empresarial San Fernando de Henares, Avenida de Castilla, 2 – 28830 Madrid (www.oup.es/en or product.safety@oup.com). OUP España S.A. also acts as importer into Spain of products made by the manufacturer.

MIX
Paper
FSC FSC® C183721

CONTENTS

CONTRIBUTORS

Awais Aftab, MD is Clinical Associate Professor, Department of Psychiatry, Case Western Reserve University School of Medicine, Cleveland, US.

Timothy Allen, PhD is Assistant Professor of Psychiatry, University of Pittsburgh, US.

Paul S. Appelbaum, MD is Dollard Professor of Psychiatry, Medicine & Law, Department of Psychiatry, Columbia University, New York, US; New York State Psychiatric Institute, New York, US.

Shayan Asadi, MS is PhD Candidate, Department of Psychology, University of Michigan, Ann Arbor, US.

Thomas A. Bart, MS is Clinical Psychology PhD Candidate, University of North Texas, Denton, US.

Rebecca Berman, PhD is Program Official, Division of Translational Research; Scientific Program Manager, Research Domain Criteria Unit, National Institute of Mental Health, Bethesda, US.

Kiran Boone, BA is Doctoral Student in Clinical Psychology, Department of Psychology, University of Houston, US.

Marina Bornovalova, PhD is Associate Professor, Department of Psychology, University of South Florida, Tampa, US.

Erin Elisa Carsten is Psychology Graduate Student, Department of Psychology, University of South Florida, Tampa, US.

David C. Cicero, PhD is Professor, Director of Clinical Training, Director of the Center for Psychosocial Health Disparities Research, Department of Psychology, University of North Texas, Denton, US.

Christopher C. Conway, PhD is Associate Professor of Psychology, Fordham University, New York, US.

William Copeland, PhD is Professor of Psychiatry, University of Vermont, Burlington, US.

Bruce N. Cuthbert, PhD is Emeritus Senior Advisor to the Director (resigned February 21, 2025), Research Domain Criteria Unit, at the National Institute of Health.

Alexandre Dombrovski, MD is Professor, Department of Psychiatry, University of Pittsburgh School of Medicine, Pittsburgh, US.

Dominic Dwyer, PhD is Associate Professor of Youth Mental Health, Centre for Youth Mental Health, University of Melbourne, Parkville, AU; Associate Professor of Computer Science, AIM for Health, Monash University, Melbourne, AU; Head of Clinical Artificial Intelligence, Orygen, The National Centre of Excellence in Youth Mental Health, Parkville, AU.

Haya Fatimah is Assistant Professor in Psychology, University of Notre Dame, Notre Dame, US.

Michael B. First, MD is Professor of Clinical Psychiatry, Psychiatry, Columbia University.

Peter Fonagy, PhD is Director of the Division of Psychology and Language Sciences and Professor of Contemporary Psychoanalysis and Developmental Science, University College London, UK.

Miriam K. Forbes, PhD is Associate Professor, School of Psychological Sciences, Macquarie University, AU.

Lindsay N. Gabel, MSc is PhD Candidate, Department of Psychology, Western University, London, CA.

Haley E. Green, MSc is PhD Candidate, Clinical Science and Psychopathology, Western University, London, CA.

Michael Hallquist, PhD is Professor, Department of Psychology and Neuroscience, University of North Carolina at Chapel Hill, Chapel Hill, US.

Nick Haslam, PhD is Professor of Psychology, Melbourne School of Psychological Sciences, University of Melbourne, Parkville, AU.

Elizabeth P. Hayden, PhD is Professor, Department of Psychology, Centre for Brain and Mind, University of Western Ontario, London, CA.

Teague R. Henry, PhD is Assistant Professor, Department of Psychology and School of Data Science, University of Virginia, Charlottesville, US.

Alexandra Hines, MS is Clinical Psychology Doctoral Student, University of Kentucky, Lexington, US.

Christopher Hopwood, PhD is Professor of Psychology, University of Zurich, CH.

Masha Ivanova, PhD is Associate Professor, Psychiatry, University of Vermont, US.

Jared W. Keeley, PhD is Associate Professor of Psychology, Virginia Commonwealth University, Richmond, US.

Christopher Samuel Kleva is Doctoral Candidate, Virginia Commonwealth University, Richmond, US.

Robert F. Krueger, PhD is Distinguished Professor of Psychology, University of Minnesota, Minneapolis, US.

Eun-Sun Lee, MA is Doctoral Student in Clinical Psychology, Department of Psychology, University of South Florida, Tampa, US.

Julia M. Levitan, MA is Doctoral Student in Clinical Psychology, University of North Carolina at Chapel Hill, US.

Rae Lutz, MS is Clinical Psychology Doctoral Student, Virginia Commonwealth University, Richmond, US.

Patrick Luyten is Professor of Clinical Psychology, University of Leuven, BE, University College London, UK.

Patrick D. McGorry, MD, PhD is Professor and Head of the Centre for Youth Mental Health, University of Melbourne, Parkville, AU; Executive Director, Orygen, The National Centre of Excellence in Youth Mental Health, Parkville, AU.

Cristina Mei, PhD is Research Fellow, Orygen, The National Centre of Excellence in Youth Mental Health, Parkville, AU; Centre for Youth Mental Health, University of Melbourne, Parkville, AU.

Gabrielle R. Messner, MA is Graduate Student, Department of Psychology and Neuroscience, University of North Carolina at Chapel Hill, US.

Michael C. Neale, PhD is Banks Distinguished Professor of Psychiatry, Virginia Commonwealth University, US.

Barnaby Nelson, PhD is Professor of Youth Mental Health, University of Melbourne, Parkville, AU; Orygen, The National Centre of Excellence in Youth Mental Health, Parkville, AU.

Sienna Nielsen, MS is Doctoral Candidate in Clinical Science, Psychology Department, University of Michigan, Ann Arbor, US.

Aysenur Okan, MA is Doctoral Candidate, The University of North Carolina at Chapel Hill, Chapel Hill, US.

Thomas Olino, PhD is Professor of Psychology and Neuroscience, Temple University, Philadelphia, US.

Joshua R. Oltmanns, PhD is Assistant Professor of Psychological & Brain Sciences, Washington University in St. Louis, St. Louis, US.

Jennifer Pacheco, PhD is Program Official, Division of Translational Research; Scientific Program Manager, Research Domain Criteria Unit, National Institute of Mental Health, Bethesda, US.

Sophie Paolizzi, MA is Doctoral Candidate, University of North Carolina at Chapel Hill, Chapel Hill, US; Harvard Medical School/McLean Hospital, Cambridge, US.

Bailey Pascuzzi is Graduate Student, Psychology Department, Virginia Commonwealth University, Richmond, US.

Zheyue Peng is Graduate Student of Clinical Science Program, Vanderbilt University, Nashville, US.

Tam Pham is Clinical Psychology Doctorate Student, Macquarie University, AU.

Aaron Pincus, PhD is Professor, Department of Psychology, Pennsylvania State University, University Park, US.

Thomas Rodebaugh, PhD is Professor of Psychology and Neuroscience, Department of Psychology and Neuroscience, University of North Carolina at Chapel Hill, Chapel Hill, US.

Craig Rodriguez-Seijas, PhD is Assistant Professor of Psychology, Department of Psychology, University of Michigan.

Charles A. Sanislow, PhD is Professor of Psychology, Professor and Chair, Neuroscience and Behavior, Wesleyan University, Middletown, US.

Carla Sharp, PhD is John and Rebecca Moores Professor of Psychology and Associate Dean for Faculty and Research, University of Houston, Houston, US.

Lindley R. Slipetz is Quantitative Psychology PhD Student, Department of Psychology, University of Virginia, Charlottesville, US.

Charlie Chung-Yih Su, MS is Psychology Intern, Washington DC; VA Medical Center, University of North Texas, Denton, TX, US.

Ashley Watts, PhD is Assistant Professor of Psychology, Vanderbilt University, Nashville, US.

Thomas Widiger is Professor, Psychology, University of Kentucky, Lexington, US.

Sylia Wilson, PhD is Associate Professor, Institute of Child Development, University of Minnesota, Minneapolis, US.

Aidan Wright, PhD is Professor, Department of Psychology, University of Michigan, Ann Arbor, US.

Asif Zaarur is Clinical Psychology PhD Student, University of South Florida, Tampa, US.

Peter Zachar, PhD is Professor, Department of Psychology, Auburn University Montgomery, Montgomery, US.

CHAPTER 1

Overview of Dimensional Perspectives on Psychopathology

CHRISTOPHER C. CONWAY AND ROBERT F. KRUEGER

Overview

The way we diagnose mental health problems affects nearly every aspect of clinical science and practice. What we include in official nomenclatures determines what the field, and society at large, deem pathological, and what is worth studying and treating. There are reverberations in legal, economic, and public health sectors, as well.

Nosology, the classification of disorder, has always been controversial in the mental health field. Nevertheless, since at least the 1980s, there has been one dominant model, which assigns people to diagnostic categories defined by lists of observable signs and symptoms. This *categorical* system is embodied in two official taxonomies, the International Classification of Diseases (ICD) and *Diagnostic and Statistical Manual of Mental Disorders* (DSM). The constituent diagnostic categories, such as generalized anxiety disorder, bipolar disorder, and attention-deficit/hyperactivity disorder, have been for many years the common language for clinical communication, study design, and dissemination of research findings.

Today, however, we are in an era of paradigm shift. Alternative diagnostic rubrics have real traction, including support from major governmental and funding bodies. Most of them challenge the assumption that mental health problems are categorically separate from one another and from mental health. Despite this common theme, the alternatives are diverse in terms of motivation, structure, and application. They represent a wide array of intellectual and professional backgrounds, and, politically, they tend to be promoted by different camps. Often these alternatives are portrayed as competitors, even if they are generally compatible substantively.

This Handbook brings together classification systems that represent *dimensional* models of psychopathology, a (re)emerging paradigm for diagnosis. Broadly speaking, dimensional diagnosis involves conceptualizing mental health problems as existing on one or more continua of psychopathology. Dimensional approaches posit that the information relevant to diagnosing, explaining, and treating psychopathology is distributed continuously in the population. In other words, individual differences in mental health are a matter of degree, not kind. In contrast, traditional nosologies, descendants of early medical classifications, generally assume that people are either members or non-members of a diagnostic category, with no gray area in between.

In this volume, our goal is to organize current scholarship on the conceptual and empirical bases for dimensional perspectives on psychopathology. We contrast dimensional and categorical views, and we compare the diverse dimensional systems to one another, probing for conceptual compatibility versus divergence. We cover aspects of the systems' theoretical background, structure, research support and applications, and clinical utility. Ultimately, we hope that bringing these perspectives together can advance our thinking about how dimensional systems can improve diagnosis; accumulation of knowledge of the origins, correlates, and treatment of psychopathology; and intervention and prevention strategies for mental health problems.

Categorical Diagnosis

For millennia, mental health professionals have described mental distress with discrete disease categories. Hippocrates may have developed one of the earliest typologies, which linked bodily fluids (humors) to temperamental differences (e.g., phlegmatic, choleric). Textbooks tend to cite humorism as a forerunner to contemporary mental health taxonomies. Categorical nomenclatures—now considerably more advanced, albeit largely based on "clinical observation" like Hippocrates' model—remain the dominant model today, because they are enshrined in ICD and DSM. These manuals, in turn, are adopted by training programs to teach the next generations of mental health clinicians and investigators. ICD and DSM, therefore, have become the default map of the psychopathology space. In the rest of this section, we very briefly describe these two manuals' structure, use, and limitations so that readers can juxtapose them with dimensional perspectives.

Basic Features

The World Health Organization (WHO) publishes the ICD, which is the authoritative nosology for mental health *and medical* conditions worldwide. All WHO member states adopt ICD's framework to enable a common statistical system and language for communication about mental health. The most recent update, ICD-11, went into effect in 2022 (WHO, 2022). The ICD generally represents mental health problems as binary categories that someone either belongs to or doesn't, just as it does for medical diseases. There are some exceptions, however, including ICD-11's dimensional classification for personality disorders, which we return to below.

The DSM, published by the American Psychiatric Association (APA), is ICD's counterpart in the United States. Whereas ICD is the most common diagnostic system for clinical practice internationally, DSM tends to be more popular for academic research. It is also the primary clinical tool for diagnosis in the United States. Its latest iteration, a text revision to DSM-5, was released in 2022 (APA, 2022). There are important points of divergence, currently and historically, across ICD and DSM, but for the purposes of this introduction, we treat the categorical approaches represented in both classifications as largely the same, given their joint emphasis on diagnostic categories. For simplicity, we refer to DSM (instead of ICD and DSM) in this chapter to represent the categorical approach.

Reification

DSM is not the only possible approach to diagnosis. It is not even the only viable perspective on categorical diagnosis (cf. Psychodynamic Diagnostic Manual; Lingiardi & McWilliams, 2017). However, in practice, it has had a monopoly on the concept of diagnosis in clinical and, to a smaller degree, research communities in the United States for the better part of 50 years. Therefore, people in the mental health field tend to conflate DSM's lists of operational diagnostic criteria with the phenomena that the criteria are intended to represent. Zachar (2014) calls this assumption *diagnostic literalism*. From this perspective, DSM-5's definition of panic disorder *is* clinically significant panic and vice versa.

Mental health problems are actually "open concepts," not reducible to any one operational definition (Meehl, 1986). They are fundamentally latent entities that diagnosticians aim to connect to observable features. Much like "love" or "the economy," any form of psychopathology might have thousands of plausible operational definitions, and these might differ across culture, time, theoretical orientation, and so on. Kendler (2016a) offers a thought experiment to bring this point into sharper relief: if we turned back the clock thousands of years and waited for human civilization to develop a mental health discipline and eventually write a diagnostic manual, what would it look like? What if we repeated this experiment 100 times? The answer, according to Kendler, is that many of the modern-day DSM categories would not replicate very consistently (see also Kendler [2016b]).

Limitations

The point is that DSM, while ubiquitous, is a fallible heuristic. The question is *how* fallible? And how does it compare, in terms of validity and utility, to alternative models that are waiting in the wings? There has been extensive empirical research on DSM's performance as a diagnostic system, and its shortcomings are well cataloged in the literature. We summarize some of the primary limitations—many of which are points of departure for alternative systems—in this section.

Binarizing natural continua. DSM's categorical diagnoses, such as panic disorder, schizophrenia, and oppositional defiant disorder, imply a discontinuity between health and disorder. Someone is either in or out, they have the condition or they do not. This model is a poor fit to a great deal of psychometric data that indicate people can vary to many different degrees on psychopathological phenomena (e.g., panic, delusions, and oppositionality) (e.g., Haslam et al. 2020). Artificially grouping people who fall above versus below a certain cutoff can throw away clinically useful information. For example, someone meeting four out of nine DSM-5 criteria for major depressive disorder (MDD) might not look so different clinically (e.g., impairment, need for treatment) from someone meeting five out of nine, but DSM-5's diagnostic algorithm for MDD would classify these two people as having qualitatively different mental health statuses.

Unreliability. It can be hard to measure categorical diagnoses consistently across time and raters. Repeated assessments of conditions that should be fairly stable over short periods of time often yield different results. Extending the example above, if someone meets four criteria for MDD on one occasion and then five criteria a short time later, they will cross the categorical threshold from health to disorder, even as overall symptom severity has not changed substantially. Difficulty judging whether someone's symptoms fall just above or below a diagnostic threshold also puts a ceiling on consistency across raters. In DSM-5 field trials, 40% of diagnoses did not meet standards for acceptable inter-rater reliability (Regier et al., 2013), meaning that clinicians often could not independently agree on whether patients were members or non-members of diagnostic categories.

Blind spots. Clinicians encounter an incredible diversity of symptom presentations in routine practice, many of which cannot be shoehorned into any DSM category. These presentations that fall into interstitial spaces end up being classified using DSM's "other specified" and "unspecified" designations. Such "residual" diagnoses are fairly prevalent. Research suggests that they represent a particularly big share of personality (Verheul & Widiger, 2004), eating (Smink, van Hoeken, & Hoek, 2013), and dissociative (Johnson, Cohen, Kasen, & Brook, 2006) diagnoses assigned with DSM.

Comorbidity. Categorically different conditions are supposed to be qualitatively distinct from one another and from health. Yet empirically there is rampant comorbidity—a synonym for co-occurrence—between DSM diagnoses. In epidemiological studies, people who qualify for a diagnosis are more likely than not to have two or more (Kessler et al., 1994). In clinical settings, comorbidity rates tend to be even higher (e.g., Brown et al., 2001).

This overlap creates a problem for researchers. Take the case-control design, the workhorse of traditional psychopathology research, where the objective is to compare clinical and control groups on some outcome variable. If the, say, social phobia group has a higher average outcome score than the healthy-control group, we would like to be able to attribute the group difference to social phobia. However, comorbidity clouds the picture, because it may be the case that some condition that tends to present alongside social phobia (e.g., other anxiety disorders, MDD) is responsible for (some of) the group difference. Investigators might look for a way around this confound by recruiting people who qualify for only one categorical diagnosis. But this maneuver undercuts generalizability, because, as we just noted, such a sample would not be representative of the population of people with social phobia.

Comorbidity is equally problematic in the clinic. Although most patients have multiple diagnoses, we have very little data on how to intervene on comorbid conditions. Should the different conditions be addressed simultaneously or sequentially? If sequentially, in what order? Practitioners currently lack solid guidance on how to handle these common scenarios.

Intra-category heterogeneity. Many DSM diagnoses bring together a diverse constellation of signs and symptoms. Borderline personality disorder (BPD), for example, includes features related to abandonment fear, recklessness, dysphoria, suicidality, paranoia, and more. DSM's BPD unites this range of pathology under a single diagnostic umbrella. On the one hand, this consolidation reduces complexity and, in theory, streamlines communication. On the other hand, the label itself has unclear meaning. Some patients with that diagnosis will struggle primarily with interpersonal problems and others primarily with emotion-driven impulsivity, for example. Thus it is hard to generalize what we learn about one patient to other patients.

Little etiological and treatment specificity. There are no known causes of one and only one categorical disorder (Hyman, 2010; Insel, 2014). To the contrary, we consistently see that potent risk factors for psychopathology cut across DSM boundaries. This "multifinality" implies that traditional diagnostic categories are not etiologically distinct (Lahey et al., 2017). A very similar pattern characterizes mental health interventions. Evidence-based pharmacological and psychological treatments generally are not specifically effective for any one categorical disorder, even if they are marketed that way. Instead, they tend to have an impact on many related conditions. Selective serotonin reuptake inhibitors are a case in point. They are prescribed for myriad mental health conditions, ranging from depression to insomnia to nicotine dependence (Waszczuk et al., 2017). Together, these observations undermine the idea that categorical diagnoses represent discrete entities with independent etiological profiles and recommended clinical approaches.

Dimensional Models of Psychopathology

Categorical nosologies might have significant limitations, but what are the alternatives? Here we describe contemporary dimensional approaches that have made breakthroughs in the literature. Some are in fact *re*-emerging, because they—or at least their fundamental ideas—preceded or were contemporaries of early DSMs, and they are now experiencing a renaissance. In this section, we provide just a brief introduction to the dimensional rubrics that will be described in more detail in later Handbook chapters.

Some dimensional frameworks reconfigure the same signs and symptoms that compose DSM diagnoses. The Achenbach System of Empirically Based Assessment (ASEBA) and Hierarchical Taxonomy of Psychopathology (HiTOP) are part of this group. Based on factor analytic results, these models organize mental health problems into a hierarchy of psychopathology dimensions. Narrower constructs, such as tight-knit symptom clusters (e.g., insomnia), are aggregated into higher-order constructs (e.g., fear, internalizing) based on empirical patterns of covariance. When allowed to aggregate according to trends in the data, DSM's basic units (signs and symptoms) often form constellations that transcend DSM boundaries, which were devised via clinical consensus and/or tradition (Forbes et al., 2024).

DSM-5's Alternative Model for Personality Disorders and ICD 11's personality disorder chapter also feature hierarchical models of individual differences. Synthesizing factor analytic findings from the normal- and maladaptive-range personality literatures, they articulate how finer-grain personality dimensions (e.g., callousness) are nested in broader ones (e.g., antagonism). At the same time, they both include a "personality dysfunction" dimension that is meant to describe, primarily in psychodynamic terms, the core features of all personality disorders, cutting across all possible expressions or styles of personality pathology. These newer personality disorder models are, therefore, an interesting hybrid of data-driven approaches, like ASEBA and HiTOP, and theory-driven approaches.

Network theory is another system that reorganizes the same basic psychopathology features that compose DSM diagnoses. Network models conceptualize mental health problems as a complex system of causal interactions among symptoms. A classic example in the network literature is that insomnia causes fatigue, which in turn causes difficulty concentrating (e.g., Fried & Cramer, 2017). From the network perspective, it is more useful to conceptualize depression as emerging out of this dynamic of symptom activation over time than to posit that any latent (categorical or dimensional) depression entity accounts for how and when insomnia, fatigue, concentration problems, and other depression symptoms are expressed (e.g., Borsboom & Cramer, 2013).

Other dimensional models define psychopathology with an entirely different set of building blocks. They pull from different data sources and conceptual backgrounds (e.g., Kent et al., 2023). Psychodynamic theory is one of these systems. DSM's early editions actually framed psychopathology in terms of psychodynamic theory, but, starting in 1980 with DSM-III, psychodynamic concepts have given way to more descriptive (versus inferential), theoretically neutral features in most respects (albeit the categorical DSM-defined PDs contain more inferential criteria compared to other DSM-defined mental disorders). There is much to learn about how dynamic factors (e.g., nonconscious motives, defense mechanisms, object relations) might support *dimensional* thinking about personality and psychopathology (e.g., Luyten & Fonagy, 2022; Remmers et al., 2023).

Contemporary Integrative Interpersonal Theory (CIIT), not unlike psychodynamic models, recasts psychopathology as a social process. It defines the spectrum of mental health versus disorder in terms of recurrent (dys)regulation in interpersonal interactions (Wright et al., 2023). Built on empirically validated models of social-cognitive and affective processes, CIIT offers a method of interpersonal case conceptualization that articulates the interpersonal antecedents and consequences of psychopathology, as well as a set of interpersonal disorders.

Other dimensional systems represent the social, biological, and psychological *contexts* for mental health versus illness, as compared to psychopathology symptoms per se. The Research Domain Criteria (RDoC), a U.S. National Institute of Mental Health initiative (Insel et al., 2010), aims to articulate the "underlying" machinery of psychopathology, ranging from genetic and cellular levels up through social, environmental, and developmental forces. It is oriented around the basic functions of psychobiological systems, such as threat sensitivity and working memory, that contribute to health and illness. RDoC presumes that these systems are dimensional, operating to some degree across all members of a population.

Temperament and personality models describe the psychobiological foundations of mental disorder. (Although the boundaries between temperament/personality and psychopathology are fuzzy [e.g., Wright & Hopwood, 2022].) Here, too, factor analysis has been the primary tool for outlining the hierarchical structure of temperament dimensions. However, theory-based biological models of the origins of temperament also play a prominent role, and they connect to RDoC's focus on neurobiology.

Clinical staging models include the familiar signs and symptoms of DSM-defined psychopathology, but they incorporate other data. They refer to indicators of social/self functioning and neurocognition to determine the stage of a mental health condition. Stages range from asymptomatic presentations all the way through severe and refractory conditions. Clinical staging, more than other models (with the possible exception of network theory), foregrounds time. It attends to how symptom presentations can morph over time, often crossing DSM diagnostic boundaries, in style and severity.

Structure of This Handbook

In formulating this Handbook, we organized chapters into four sections, plus this introductory section, dedicated to different aspects of the dimensional landscape. The first section, "Categorical Psychopathology Diagnosis: History, Politics, and Use," covers the origin story and current structure of official categorical rubrics. In chapter 2, Keeley et al. present the evolution of DSM and ICD, highlighting how shifting organizational principles over the decades have produced very different manuals from edition to edition. In chapter 3, Widiger et al. describe the co-development of DSM and ICD after World War II. They point to the difficulty in balancing innovation—in response to research developments—with compatibility across manuals, a tension very relevant to proposals for novel dimensional diagnostic systems that break from the status quo. In chapter 4, Aftab provides a historical and conceptual analysis of the "medical model" of psychopathology, including how mental health diagnosis traces its roots to general medicine. Aftab points out misunderstandings of the medical model, and contends that it is compatible with both categorical and dimensional diagnosis. In chapter 5, Zachar et al. outline the political, philosophical, and scientific challenges in creating a diagnostic model that responds to competing interests from various communities and users. They primarily analyze DSM and ICD, but also consider what lessons learned from categorical models mean for the potential development and dissemination of dimensional rubrics.

The Handbook's second section is called "Dimensional Approaches to Psychopathology: Origins, Research Advances, and Clinical Applications." Here we cover some of the most promising and popular dimensional frameworks for understanding mental health problems. In chapter 6, Pham and Forbes outline the HiTOP's origins and structure. They detail the various ways HiTOP can be applied as a research and clinical tool, and also comment on current limitations and procedures for refining the model. In chapter 7, Sanislow et al. present RDoC, including its current value as a research framework and potential future role as a clinical tool. In chapter 8, Rodebaugh et al. examine network theory. They emphasize that network theory's compatibility with dynamic and idiographic perspectives positions it to make discoveries that other models might miss. In chapter 9, Sharp and Boone examine the dimensionalization of personality pathology, and they focus on the scientific status of "personality dysfunction," a conceptual innovation in DSM-5 and ICD-11.

In chapter 10, Gabel et al. differentiate temperament and personality, and they evaluate various conceptual models—and associated empirical results—that link dimensions of temperament and personality to psychopathology over the life course. In chapter 11, Copeland presents the history and use of ASEBA, one of the first data-driven models of psychopathology. He spotlights ASEBA's multi-informant assessment format, rich normative databases, and multicultural validation. In chapter 12, Mei et al. explain the clinical staging model and illustrate how it supports clinical decision-making, particularly for early-stage clinical presentations that fall below categorical thresholds in DSM and ICD. In chapter 13, Pincus et al. define CIIT, demonstrating how it functions both as a diagnostic system and case conceptualization method. In chapter 14, Luyten and Fonagy observe how dimensional thinking has characterized various psychodynamic approaches to personality development and psychopathology. They make the case for a hybrid dimensional-prototype model that incorporates psychodynamic data (e.g., defenses).

The Handbook's third section covers "Methodologies for Creating and Evaluating Dimensional Models." In chapter 15, Watts and Peng review the basic concepts of factor analysis and explain why this method partners so effectively with hierarchical and dimensional diagnostic conceptual models. Watts and Peng also call attention to various misunderstandings and misapplications of factor analysis that can lead to shaky inferences about the structure and utility of dimensional models. In chapter 16, Haslam summarizes the field of taxometrics, which evaluates to what degree measurements of psychopathology are consistent with a taxonic, as opposed to a dimensional, latent structure. In chapter 17, Bornovalova et al. review the major paradigms in behavior genetics, including quantitative and molecular genetic methods, and how these have informed substantive theory about the dimensional nature of psychopathology. In chapter 18, Hallquist et al. describe the emerging field of computational psychiatry and connect it to efforts to use "big data" and other alternative data sources to construct models of personality and psychopathology. In chapter 19, Slipetz and Henry outline network analysis, the set of quantitative approaches designed to model temporal associations in repeated measures data that supports network theories of mental disorder. Related, in chapter 20, Olino and Wilson present longitudinal data analysis models relevant to evaluating and advancing dimensional diagnosis from a developmental perspective.

The Handbook's fourth section is titled "Mechanics and Sociology of Paradigm Change in Diagnosis." This group of chapters considers some of the pressing social, political, and logistical challenges facing dimensional diagnosis, paralleling the first section's historical analysis of how DSM and ICD have grappled with these same issues. In chapter 21, Su et al. review the literature on the clinical utility of dimensional versus categorical classification. They show that, to be valuable in clinical practice, diagnostic systems must not only be valid representations of psychopathology, but also be easy to use, aid clinical decision-making, and ultimately improve patient outcomes. In chapter 22, Nielsen et al. address to what extent alternative diagnostic systems function as intended for—and could potentially disadvantage—people from diverse, underrepresented, and epistemically excluded populations. In chapter 23, Hopwood assesses the potential for consensus among different dimensional rubrics. Could the approaches covered in this Handbook be integrated, conceptually or even quantitatively, or do differences in underlying epistemologies make consensus a nonstarter? This chapter also looks ahead to the next generation of theory, research, and clinical application using dimensional models of psychopathology.

References

American Psychiatric Association. (2022). *Diagnostic and statistical manual of mental disorders* (5th ed., text rev.). https://doi.org/10.1176/appi.books.9780890425787

Borsboom, D., & Cramer, A. O. (2013). Network analysis: an integrative approach to the structure of psychopathology. *Annual Review of Clinical Psychology*, *9*(1), 91–121.

Brown, T. A., Campbell, L. A., Lehman, C. L., Grisham, J. R., & Mancill, R. B. (2001). Current and lifetime comorbidity of the DSM-IV anxiety and mood disorders in a large clinical sample. *Journal of Abnormal Psychology*, *110*(4), 585.

Forbes, M. K., Baillie, A., Batterham, P. J., Calear, A., Kotov, R., Krueger, R. F., Markon, K. E., Mewton, L., Pellicano, E., Roberts, M., Rodriguez-Seijas, C., Sunderland, M., Watson, D., Watts, A. L., Wright, A. G. C., & Clark, L. A. (2024). Reconstructing psychopathology: A data-driven reorganization of the symptoms in the Diagnostic and Statistical Manual of Mental Disorders. *Clinical Psychological Science, 13*(3), 462–488. https://doi.org/10.1177/21677026241268345 (Original work published 2025).

Fried, E. I., & Cramer, A. O. (2017). Moving forward: Challenges and directions for psychopathological network theory and methodology. *Perspectives on Psychological Science, 12*(6), 999–1020.

Haslam, N., McGrath, M. J., Viechtbauer, W., & Kuppens, P. (2020). Dimensions over categories: A meta-analysis of taxometric research. *Psychological Medicine, 50*(9), 1418–1432.

Hyman, S. E. (2010). The diagnosis of mental disorders: The problem of reification. *Annual Review of Clinical Psychology, 6*, 155–179.

Insel, T. R. (2014). The NIMH research domain criteria (RDoC) project: Precision medicine for psychiatry. *American Journal of Psychiatry, 171*, 395–397.

Insel, T., Cuthbert, B., Garvey, M., Heinssen, R., Pine, D. S., Quinn, K., Sanislow, C., & Wang, P. (2010). Research domain criteria (RDoC): Toward a new classification framework for research on mental disorders. *American Journal of Psychiatry, 167*(7), 748–751. https://doi-org.avoserv2.library.fordham.edu/10.1176/appi.ajp.2010.09091379

Johnson, J. G., Cohen, P., Kasen, S., & Brook, J. S. (2006). Dissociative disorders among adults in the community, impaired functioning, and axis I and II comorbidity. *Journal of Psychiatric Research, 40*(2), 131–140.

Kendler, K. S. (2016a). The nature of psychiatric disorders. *World Psychiatry, 15*(1), 5–12.

Kendler, K. S. (2016b). The phenomenology of major depression and the representativeness and nature of DSM criteria. *American Journal of Psychiatry, 173*(8), 771–780.

Kent, J. S., Markon, K., & MacDonald, A. W. III. (2023). Theories of psychopathology: Introduction to a special section. *Journal of Psychopathology and Clinical Science, 132*(3), 223–227. https://doi.org/10.1037/abn0000824

Kessler, R. C., McGonagle, K. A., Zhao, S., Nelson, C. B., Hughes, M., Eshleman, S., Wittchen, H.-U., & Kendler, K. S. (1994). Lifetime and 12-month prevalence of DSM-III-R psychiatric disorders in the United States: Results from the National Comorbidity Survey. *Archives of General Psychiatry, 51*(1), 8–19. https://doi-org.avoserv2.library.fordham.edu/10.1001/archpsyc.1994.03950010008002

Lahey, B. B., Krueger, R. F., Rathouz, P. J., Waldman, I. D., & Zald, D. H. (2017). A hierarchical causal taxonomy of psychopathology across the life span. *Psychological Bulletin, 143*(2), 142.

Lingiardi, V., & McWilliams, N. (Eds.). (2017). *Psychodynamic diagnostic manual (PDM-2)* (2nd ed.). Guilford.

Luyten, P., & Fonagy, P. (2022). Integrating and differentiating personality and psychopathology: A psychodynamic perspective. *Journal of Personality, 90*(1), 75–88.

Meehl, P. E. (1986). Diagnostic taxa as open concepts: Metatheoretical and statistical questions about reliability and construct validity in the grand strategy of nosological revision. In T. Millon & G. Klerman (Eds.), *Contemporary directions in psychopathology* (pp. 215–231). Guilford Press.

Regier, D. A., Narrow, W. E., Clarke, D. E., Kraemer, H. C., Kuramoto, S. J., Kuhl, E. A., & Kupfer, D. J. (2013). DSM-5 field trials in the United States and Canada, Part II: test-retest reliability of selected categorical diagnoses. *American Journal of Psychiatry, 170*(1), 59–70.

Remmers, C., Wester, R., Repnik, L. G., Plumbohm, M., Unger, S., & Jauk, E. (2023). Psychodynamic theory meets HiTOP: The nomological network between motivational conflicts and dimensions of the hierarchical taxonomy of psychopathology (HiTOP). *Journal of Research in Personality, 106*, 104418.

Smink, F. R., van Hoeken, D., & Hoek, H. W. (2013). Epidemiology, course, and outcome of eating disorders. *Current Opinion in Psychiatry, 26*(6), 543–548.

Verheul, R., & Widiger, T. A. (2004). A meta-analysis of the prevalence and usage of the personality disorder not otherwise specified (PDNOS) diagnosis. *Journal of Personality Disorders, 18*(4), 309–319.

Waszczuk, M. A., Zimmerman, M., Ruggero, C., Li, K., MacNamara, A., Weinberg, A., . . . & Kotov, R. (2017). What do clinicians treat: Diagnoses or symptoms? The incremental validity of a symptom-based, dimensional characterization of emotional disorders in predicting medication prescription patterns. *Comprehensive Psychiatry, 79*, 80–88.

WHO. (2022). International statistical classification of diseases and related health problems (ICD) (11th rev.). WHO. https://www.who.int/standards/classifications/classification-of-diseases

Wright, A. G., & Hopwood, C. J. (2022). Integrating and distinguishing personality and psychopathology. *Journal of Personality*, *90*(1), 5–19.

Wright, A. G., Pincus, A. L., & Hopwood, C. J. (2023). Contemporary integrative interpersonal theory: Integrating structure, dynamics, temporal scale, and levels of analysis. *Journal of Psychopathology and Clinical Science*, *132*(3), 263.

Zachar, P. (2014). *A metaphysics of psychopathology*. MIT press.

PART I

Categorical Psychopathology Diagnosis

History, Politics, and Use

CHAPTER 2

A Brief History of the ICD and DSM Classifications of Mental Disorders

JARED W. KEELEY, CHRISTOPHER SAMUEL KLEVA,
RAE LUTZ, AND BAILEY PASCUZZI

Introduction

It may seem odd that a chapter on diagnostic classification systems typically presumed to be categorical would be present in a book on dimensional understandings of psychopathology. Understanding the development of these systems, which have predominated use for research and practice (First et al., 2018), is necessary to understand the context for dimensional alternatives, many of which were direct reactions to categorical classification systems (Kotov et al., 2017; Kozak & Cuthbert, 2016; Widiger & Samuel, 2005). Further, these systems are not purely categorical; they incorporate a number of dimensional ideas in a variety of ways. The purpose of this chapter is to provide a conceptual overview of the various editions of two of the most important classification systems of psychopathology: the *International Classification of Diseases and Related Health Problems* (ICD) and the *Diagnostic and Statistical Manual of Mental Disorders* (DSM).

This chapter will be structured around a set of four theoretical dichotomies that can be used to characterize these classifications. It is important to note that we do not assume that these theoretical dichotomies are true dichotomies; as we will see, most classification systems will exhibit some characteristics of both sides. Rather, they are just a convenient way of describing some features of these classification systems that are important to unpack. The first dichotomy is to what extent the development of the concepts in the classification system was based on rational definition versus empirical definition. A rationally defined concept is one whose features are derived primarily from theory, whereas an empirically defined concept is based on observations. The second dichotomy is to what extent the classification is descriptive versus etiological. A descriptive classification makes no claims about how the concepts in the classification come to be; it just summarizes features that tend to go together. An etiological classification makes claims about the causes of the concepts under discussion. The third dichotomy regards the preference for biological versus psychological descriptions and explanations of the disorders in the classification. While these approaches are certainly not mutually exclusive, there does seem to be a dynamic tension between people who place higher priority on biological factors in the description and explanation of a disorder relative to psychosocial factors. The last dichotomy concerns preferences the creators of the classification have for the granularity of the concepts. Some have termed this distinction "lumpers" versus "splitters" to refer to a differential preference for combining similar presentations into larger concepts versus dividing unique presentations into smaller concepts (Havens, 1985).

As an example of these dichotomies, take the early Greek humoral theory as a description of mental and physical health concerns. This theory posited that health within the human body was maintained by creating a balance among four vital fluids, termed humors. Prior to the humoral theory, the primary explanation for unusual behavior was the supernatural influence of the gods, such as being struck "mad" by the furies or being inspired by one of the muses. Instead, the humoral theory was grounded solely in the natural world, reflecting a preference for the level of biological as opposed to psychological explanation. The identification of the humors came from observations made by early Greek physicians, thus giving the theory a degree of empirical development. However, why only four humors? The number and balance of the humors was driven largely by philosophical assumptions prevalent at the time about symmetry in nature paralleling four fundamental elements (air, earth, water, fire), thus also placing a rational lens on its development. The theory was also inherently etiological; it sought to offer an explanation for the pattern of signs and symptoms the patient exhibited. Humoral theory might also be considered leaning toward "lumping," as it took various syndromes that had previously been considered separate and linked them via an explanation stemming from the excess, lack, or interaction of four bodily fluids.

Two Important Pre-ICD and DSM Perspectives

There is a substantial history of the classification of mental disorders, but much of that may be better covered elsewhere (Reed, Robles, & Dominguez-Martinez, 2016). For the purpose of this chapter, we will begin with two figures who exerted a substantial influence on the development of the ICD-6 and DSM-I. The first is Emil Kraepelin (b. 1856–d. 1926). Kraepelin was a German psychiatrist who had trained under the famous neurologist Wilhelm Griesinger, whose other students, like Paul Broca, Carl Wernicke, and Theodor Meynert, were responsible for identifying localized functions of behavior in the brain (Berrios & Hauser, 1988). For example, Broca gathered patients who had lost the ability to speak and, following autopsies after their deaths, identified a region of the brain responsible for speech production now termed "Broca's area." Griesinger was credited with saying "all mental diseases are physical diseases"; specifically, he believed that any unusual behavior could eventually be identified and explained through the study of the brain. This influence clearly falls on the biological end of the spectrum, but Kraepelin's later theories would not be so exclusive (Heckers & Kendler, 2020).

Kraepelin's first job was as the director of a psychiatric hospital in modern-day Estonia. This fact was very influential on the development of Kraepelin's classifications of psychopathology, because he did not speak the same language as his patients. Rather, he had to rely either on indirect reports from his nurses (some of whom spoke German) or behavioral observations. This hospital also influenced his theories via another fortuitous accident; it was next to a train station, which enabled patients to easily return after their discharge for follow-up appointments. As such, Kraepelin was able to track the course of an individual's illness better than was the norm for the time. As a mechanism for keeping track of his observations, Kraepelin kept note cards (*Zählkarten* in German) on which he recorded information like demographics, symptomatology, course, and treatments he attempted (Weber & Engstrom, 1997). Kraepelin's classifications came from him literally sorting these cards into piles, based on similarities in presentation, course, and response to treatment. These piles then became the disorders in his classification, which he disseminated by writing textbooks on psychopathology. Each pile became the heading of a chapter, which morphed and grew over the course of his career and eight editions of his textbook.

Kraepelin's classification was solidly grounded in empiricism, as his categories were the product of systematic observations of patients over time. The disorders in his classifications started as descriptive concepts, just identifying a common pattern. However, Kraepelin held the goal that these concepts would identify specific causes, so we might call his system aspirationally etiological. Kraepelin did not rule out psychological causes of disorders per se, but his training definitely biased him toward preferring biological causes. Last, Kraepelin was one of the most successful splitters. Some of his most famous and long-lasting ideas came from distinguishing cases that were believed to be the same. For example, he made a distinction between what would today be termed bipolar disorder and unipolar depression. By tracking individuals over time, he noticed that some people cycled between manic and depressive episodes, while others only experienced depressive episodes.

Another influential figure during the same period was Sigmund Freud (b. 1856–d. 1939). It is worth noting that he and Kraepelin were born in the same year and both were German. That said, it seems that they had relatively little awareness of each other and their stories developed along separate tracks. Many readers are probably already familiar with Freud as the founder of psychoanalysis. Nonetheless, there are several facts of the development of psychoanalysis that serve as important counterpoints to Kraepelin's classification. First, Kraepelin worked in a psychiatric hospital, which inherently focused his efforts on the more severe end of psychopathology. The individuals he saw necessitated a level of care that justified their hospitalization. In contrast, Freud primarily worked with individuals whose cases would not be considered as severe; he worked in the modern equivalent of an outpatient setting. As such, these two men saw different kinds of problems in the individuals with whom they worked.

Interestingly, psychoanalysis also was couched within neurology as the discipline that led to its birth. Specifically, there was an interest among neurologists regarding the practice of hypnotism. Hypnosis was initially popularized by Franz Anton Mesmer, who theorized that the magnetic fields of humans (and other animals) could be manipulated with magnets to produce various effects. However, Mesmer's demonstrations of hypnotism were more like a circus sideshow than a serious academic pursuit. A neurologist named Jean-Martin Charcot happened to attend one of Mesmer's shows and recognized the potential medical application of hypnotism, particularly for surgery, as modern anesthetics had yet to be developed. Freud studied with Charcot for a three-month fellowship, and both recognized the potential for hypnotism to be applied to so-called hysteria, which was the presentation of symptoms that looked neurological but lacked an identifiable neurological cause (Aguayo, 1986). Another neurologist from Vienna named Josef Breuer attempted applying hypnotism to a case given the pseudonym Anna O. and found that her symptoms lessened in severity after talking about them while under hypnosis. Freud and Breuer collaborated to write up these findings, leading to Freud's "talking cure" (Breuer & Freud, 1895).

The development of Freud's theory of psychoanalysis did start from his interactions with various patients, but the bulk of the theory can be better characterized as rational rather than empirical, as once Freud developed his explanations for how the mind worked, particularly the interplay between the conscious and unconscious mind and his theory of psychosexual development, the theory drove the definition of what was considered a disorder. His theory is also more psychological than biological, prioritizing the interplay of various psychological factors to produce psychopathology. His theory is also strongly etiological, positing the mechanisms whereby psychological problems arise via conflicts between unconscious desires and the demands of society. Last, Freud's theory of psychoanalysis was neutral regarding lumping and splitting. In some ways it produced more fine-grained distinctions among some kinds of problems and combined other sorts of problems, based on how the theory played out.

Establishment of ICD-6 and DSM-I

In the late 1800s and early 1900s, the classification of medical conditions, including psychopathology, was chaotic (Grob, 1991). There was little to no agreement within and across countries regarding diagnostic terminology or procedures. At the extreme, individual hospitals were like an island onto their own regarding what diagnostic concepts were used and how they were applied. At the same time, academic medicine was fascinated with developing elaborate classification systems of the kinds of diseases, inspired in part by biology's success in classifying species (Kendell, 1990). The first International Statistical Congress was held in Brussels in 1853, at which William Farr—the first medical statistician in the General Register Office of England—was tasked with creating an international classification of causes of death. His list of causes of death was then adapted by Jacques Bertillon and adopted by the Institute of International Statistics in 1899 as what is generally considered the first ICD. This list was revised roughly every ten years until the establishment of the World Health Organization (WHO) following World War II, which formally took over responsibility for managing the ICD (Reed et al., 2016).

The WHO was established at the same time as the United Nations as a mechanism for overseeing the health of all individuals in the world. Part of the WHO's constitutional responsibilities is the development and maintenance of a classification of diseases for the purpose of tracking health conditions. From its outset, the WHO's definition of health was inclusive of mental health, and so its development of the ICD incorporated a section on mental disorders. The first version of the ICD produced by the WHO (ICD-6) expanded the list from mortality to morbidity, that is, any cause of illness (Reed et al., 2016). Every member country of the WHO has agreed by treaty to report health statistics using the ICD.

In the United States, the development of medical classifications was not well integrated with what was happening in Europe with the ICD. Prior to 1900, there was no formalized classification system for mental health. In 1908, the U.S. Bureau of the Census asked the American Medico-Psychological Association (the precursor of the American Psychiatric Association) to remedy this situation by developing a system for gathering statistics on the number of people in the population affected by a mental disorder. It established a group called the Committee on the Nomenclature of Diseases that generated a list of medical conditions that could cause psychiatric symptoms (e.g., psychosis due to tumor, psychosis due to an infection). Its list included categories with an identified medical pathogenesis, a miscellaneous category called psychosis not otherwise specified, or a person could be labeled not insane (Grob, 1991). Notably, there was no mention of less severe forms of psychopathology or any descriptive categories without an identified etiology. One individual on the committee, Adolf Meyer, deserves particular mention, because he was a German national who was familiar with the work of both Kraepelin and Freud (Lidz, 1966). In subsequent editions of the classification, he was able to infuse some of their ideas into the list. In particular, he preferred to refer to mental health conditions as "reactions," implying an interaction between the individual and the environment. He was, however, unsuccessful in advocating for these ideas in the initial version.

During World War II, psychiatrists achieved a new degree of prominence in the American military. Karl Menninger was the first psychiatrist to reach the rank of general, due to the success of psychiatrists treating casualties during the war. Specifically, psychiatrists found a high rate of success working with individuals experiencing acute traumatic reactions who were then able to return to the front lines and continue fighting. American psychiatrists recognized that extreme environmental circumstances could produce psychopathological symptoms (i.e., a psychological "reaction") in the absence of a medical condition. The psychiatrists in

World War II recognized that their existing classification system was all but useless for these circumstances, and so they drafted a new classification system termed *War Department Technical Bulletin, Medical 203* (Houts, 2000), which included psychologically oriented descriptive categories. After the war, Menninger and others began lobbying within the American Psychiatric Association to include a broader definition of mental disorder beyond conditions with a clear medical etiology. For the first time, American psychiatrists were also interested in outpatient work, and they needed a new set of diagnoses to pursue that work.

Thus, at the same time that Menninger and colleagues were lobbying for change, the WHO released the ICD-6, which incorporated both biologically and psychologically defined conditions (WHO, 1949). The United States, as a member of the newly formed WHO, recognized that it needed its classifications to be compatible with the ICD-6, which created additional pressure for the American Psychiatric Association to revise its classification. The resulting new product was the first DSM (Grob, 1991).

The committee that developed the first DSM worked very deliberately to harmonize it with the ICD-6 (Reed et al., 2016; see Widiger et al., this volume). The two manuals had very similar hierarchical organizations. There was a primary distinction between "organic" and "functional" conditions, whereby the first had an identifiable biological origin and the other was undefined or psychological in nature (APA, 1952). The organization of both manuals mirrored the decision-making process of clinicians. Specifically, one would first determine if the condition had an identifiable medical cause (landing one in the organic half of the manual). If none was found, then one would work through a hierarchy of symptoms in descending severity until one landed on a diagnosis. Working through the manual, one could finish with one and only one diagnosis (in contrast to modern ICDs and DSMs, where comorbidity—or the diagnosis of multiple conditions—is common; Kessler et al., 2005), with more severe diagnoses trumping less severe ones (e.g., a diagnosis of schizophrenia would take precedence over a diagnosis of an anxiety disorder).

It is clear that the ICD and DSM found a balance between biological and psychological explanations for disorders. They also included some conditions that were defined by their etiologies, and others that were purely descriptive with no presumed etiology. Many of the disorders in the functional portion of the DSM included Meyer's term "reaction" in the name. However, despite some claims to the contrary (Houts, 2000), neither the ICD-6 nor DSM-I were particularly psychoanalytic in nature (Aragona, 2015; Cooper & Blashfield, 2016). Some psychoanalytic concepts certainly were represented, but only insofar as they were the only available theoretical framework at the time for discussing psychologically derived symptoms.

The disorders in the DSM-I were defined in prose paragraphs. These paragraphs would list common symptoms or features, but they rarely indicated which of those features needed to be present for a diagnosis. Rather, these descriptions functioned more like prototypes, whereby a clinician would match the presentation of a patient with the description that provided the closest fit.

The WHO allowed each member country to create a local adaptation of the ICD for its particular circumstances. Many countries followed a similar path to that of the United States and created their own classification that they then harmonized with the ICD system. Generally, the ICD-6 was not popular. Only five countries adopted the ICD-6 without adaptation: Finland, New Zealand, Peru, Thailand, and the United Kingdom. To understand why, the WHO asked British psychiatrist Erwin Stengel to review the classification systems in place around the world. The result was that the classifications were widely disparate, often with inconsistent terminology intended to refer to the same concept and varied beliefs about the etiology of the conditions (Stengel, 1959). Stengel's recommendation was to create operational definitions of the terms used in the ICD (both symptoms and disorders) so that they could be applied consistently across countries and to remove any reference to etiology, which seemed to at least partially result in local professionals' unwillingness to use the ICD system.

ICD-8 and DSM-II

Following Stengel's (1959) review, it became apparent that the international psychiatric community needed a cohesive diagnostic system that would be universally adopted. The result was the ICD-8 (World Health Organization, 1968) and its American counterpart, DSM-II (APA, 1968). Although the two diagnostic systems were nearly identical, several important differences existed. First, the ICD-8 attempted to bypass some of the linguistic confusion across countries by incorporating code numbers for diagnoses. Regardless of language or translation, the codes, written in decimal form, would be consistent. Second, the DSM-II shifted from labeling mental disorders as "reactions" to disorders (e.g., "depressive reaction" became "depressive disorder"). The removal of the term "reaction" can be explained as an initial step away from implied assumptions of causality and toward an atheoretical etiologic orientation (Fischer, 2012; Suris et al., 2016). While the DSM-I still had a very inpatient psychiatric focus, the DSM-II enhanced the needs of outpatient mental health by expanding anxiety disorders, depressive disorders, personality disorders, and including disorders of childhood and adolescence. The DSM-II and ICD-8 also slightly varied on the inclusion of two diagnostic categories: hysterical psychosis and passive-aggressive personality disorder. While the ICD-8 included hysterical psychosis, U.S. mental health professionals believed it was "an oxymoron" due to hysteria being conceptualized as a neurotic disorder within psychoanalysis. Conversely, the DSM-II included passive-aggressive personality disorder, which the international psychiatric community found to be "pejorative and disingenuous." Another major difference was that DSM-II, similar to DSM-I, included a brief prose description of each diagnostic category, while ICD-8 only provided diagnostic terms without any clarification or description for mental health professionals (Blashfield et al., 2014). Although Stengel had recommended creating a glossary of terms for ICD-8, it was not ultimately published.

Despite the improvements in both ICD-8 and DSM-II, a number of individuals—both inside and outside of the field—continued to express dissatisfaction with mental health diagnosis and classification. The so-called antipsychiatry movement consisted of scholars and practitioners who did not necessarily form a unitary community but all held skeptical positions regarding psychiatry's hegemony on the definition and description of mental disorders. Over time, the antipsychiatry movement evolved to fight against all authoritarian psychiatric practices including coercive hospitalizations and pharmacological treatment (Rissmiller & Rissmiller, 2006). Unfortunately, growing research did not assist by providing evidence for the legitimacy of psychiatry but, rather, findings consistently showed low rates of diagnostic reliability and, therefore, validated the concerns of the antipsychiatry movement (Shorter, 1997).

Studies in the 1960s and 1970s suggested that clinicians faced difficulties in achieving high levels of agreement across various areas of psychopathology. One prominent example was the U.K./U.S. Diagnostic Project, which uncovered significant variations in diagnostic practices between Britain and the United States (Cooper et al., 1972; Kendell et al., 1971). These studies indicated that Americans exhibited a broader interpretation of schizophrenia, often applying the diagnosis to any patient with psychotic symptoms. Conversely, British psychiatrists demonstrated greater precision in diagnosing schizophrenia. These disparities likely arose from variations in the conceptualization and application of schizophrenia by individual psychiatrists, as well as differences in its definition across regions.

Another influential paper was Rosenhan's (1973) study "On Being Sane in Insane Places," which sought to examine the validity of psychiatric diagnosis. The two-part study began with eight "pseudo patients" claiming auditory hallucination in which a voice said "thud," "empty," or "hollow" in order to be admitted to psychiatric hospitals across the United States. Once admitted, the pseudo patients were to no longer report any hallucinations and to behave "normally." All patients recorded meticulous notes during their stay, which hospital staff never questioned but rather viewed the behavior as pathological, related to their illness. Overall, the pseudo patients were confined for an excessive period of time, an average of 19 days but as many as 52 days. Seven of the eight pseudo patients were discharged with a diagnosis of "Schizophrenia in remission." The second part of the study consisted of notifying several hospitals that over the upcoming three-month period, Rosenhan would be sending pseudo patients to attempt to be admitted into their hospitals. During that duration, the hospital identified 41 patients as being pseudo patients; however, Rosenhan had never sent a single pseudo patient during that time. Despite some key methodological problems with Rosenhan's conclusions (e.g., Millon, 1975; Spitzer, 1975), and claims that Rosenhan falsified portions of the results (Scull, 2023), the paper nonetheless was regularly cited as a challenge to the very concept of psychiatric disorders, questioning professionals' ability to detect the boundary between normal and pathological behavior.

Throughout the 1960s, the antipsychiatry movement had grown stronger, in part due to forming alliances with activist groups rebelling against all forms of political, sexual, and racial injustice. In May 1970, members of the antipsychiatry movement collaborated with gay activists to create a human chain obstructing psychiatrists from accessing the American Psychiatric Association's 124th annual meeting. This action was repeated the following year, with gay activist Frank Kameny taking control of the podium to denounce psychiatry's classification of homosexuality as a psychiatric disorder in the DSM. In response to these protests, the American Psychiatric Association established a task force. In 1973, following a vote in which 58% were in favor, homosexuality was officially removed from the list of mental illnesses in the DSM (Rissmiller & Rissmiller, 2006).

Two of the most prominent voices of the antipsychiatry movement were the Hungarian-American psychiatrist Thomas Szasz and the French philosopher Michel Foucault. Szasz's (1961) influential work, "The Myth of Mental Illness" and Foucault's seminal writings on the history of psychiatry (see Foucault, 1988), significantly contributed to the antipsychiatry movement and influenced the transformation of psychiatric diagnoses in the DSM and ICD. Szasz challenged the medicalization of behaviors and experiences deemed deviant from societal norms, arguing that mental illness was a myth perpetuated by psychiatry as a means of social control. His critique of the medical model of psychiatry sparked skepticism about the validity and reliability of psychiatric diagnoses, highlighting the subjective nature of psychiatric classification. Similarly, Foucault's examination of the power dynamics within psychiatric institutions shed light on the coercive and disciplinary nature of psychiatric practices, fueling discontent with traditional psychiatric approaches. These perspectives influenced a shift toward more nuanced understandings of psychiatric disorders, emphasizing the social, cultural, and historical context in which they are constructed. As a result, subsequent editions of the DSM and ICD incorporated more comprehensive and multidimensional diagnostic criteria, shifting from a heavy psychoanalytic lens to reflecting a broader understanding of mental health and illness that considers the complex interplay of biological, psychological, and social factors (i.e., the biopsychosocial model).

In reaction to the antipsychiatry movement, a group of biologically oriented psychiatrists at Washington University in St. Louis emerged in the mid-20th century who became known as the Neo-Kraepelinians (North et al., 2010). The name came from a recognition that the basic principles they valued reflected a similar approach to that of Kraepelin, that is, a focus on identifying the biological causal mechanisms of mental disorders via the systematic description of groups of patients displaying similar symptoms. Similar to the supporters of the antipsychiatry movement, the Neo-Kraepelinians recognized the inherent flaws of the current diagnostic classification in psychiatry. In response, they sought to revitalize psychiatric diagnosis and research by applying rigorous scientific methods and establishing clear diagnostic criteria. Within the Neo-Kraepelinian movement, an "invisible college" formed—the term describes a network of scholars and researchers united by a shared interest and commitment to advancing a particular field of study (Blashfield, 1984). This network at Washington University consisted of prominent figures such as Eli Robins, Samuel Guze, and George Winokur, among others. Together, they worked to develop a more systematic approach to psychiatric diagnosis and classification.

In 1970, Robins and Guze published a landmark manifesto outlining their vision for validating psychiatric disorders. Their approach emphasized the importance of establishing clear diagnostic criteria based on empirical evidence, including biological, psychological, and social factors. They advocated for a multi-method approach to validation, incorporating longitudinal studies, family studies, and laboratory research to support the existence and distinctiveness of psychiatric disorders. Following Robins and Guze's manifesto, Feighner et al. (1972) proposed a set of diagnostic criteria for several psychiatric disorders (Kendler et al., 2010), which laid the groundwork for the Research Diagnostic Criteria (RDC; Spitzer et al., 1978) developed by Robert Spitzer, John Endicott, and Eli Robins. These criteria aimed to standardize psychiatric diagnosis by providing clear operational definitions for each disorder, facilitating greater reliability and consistency across clinicians and research studies (Shorter, 2015).

One of the key objectives of these efforts was to increase reliability in psychiatric diagnosis by creating more homogeneous diagnostic groups. By operationalizing diagnostic criteria, researchers hoped to reduce variability in diagnosis and increase the reproducibility of research findings. Moreover, standardized diagnostic criteria were seen as essential for securing funding and enhancing the perceived legitimacy and "medicalness" of the psychiatric profession. Through these initiatives, the Neo-Kraepelinians at Washington University played a pivotal role in shaping modern psychiatric diagnosis and research practices.

DSM-III and ICD-9

The rise in popularity of the Neo-Kraepelinians resulted in a shift in power within the American Psychiatric Association. A psychiatrist by the name of Robert Spitzer was appointed chair of the third revision of the DSM, partially because of his success negotiating a compromise regarding the removal of homosexuality from the DSM-II and his development of the RDC (Drescher, 2013). Spitzer's alignment with the Neo-Kraepelinian approach is clear in the resulting classification.

Spitzer organized the process by creating "workgroups" that were responsible for revising the disorders in a particular domain of psychopathology. Each workgroup faced substantial responsibilities, requiring rigorous analysis of information and collaboration with other experts in the field. The division of labor among workgroups likely contributed to the acceptance of the resulting classifications. Nonetheless, challenges were also evident in the process. When committees were formed, personal and professional conflicts arose. Trying to divide psychopathology into distinct areas proved challenging, resulting in overlapping responsibilities among committees and disputes. Once a committee received a specific assignment, it hesitated to give up areas of psychopathology that might have been more appropriately classified elsewhere.

Resolving these disputes was difficult when political processes in and between workgroups affected the solutions. The researchers with more publications and higher reputations typically were favored. Still, to this day, practicing clinicians have seldom been chosen, and individuals with relevant diagnoses have never been included, even though their perspectives could be valuable in assessing the usability and acceptability of the resulting product (Kamens et al., 2019). The workgroups were filled with members who shared similar research interests and who often collaborated, resulting in a shared thought process (Blashfield & Reynolds, 2012). Experts tend to hold strong beliefs, which usually results in the loudest voices being the ones who win (Frances & Widiger, 2012). Spitzer had a particularly loud voice and was often directly involved in the meetings of various workgroups, inserting his particular opinions.

Spitzer, along with the committee overseeing DSM-III, recognized the growing divide between psychoanalytic and biological explanations. As a result, they determined that maintaining a theory-neutral stance for DSM-III would improve accessibility for mental health professionals across various disciplines (which is the same conclusion Stengel reached nearly 20 years earlier). This approach received negative feedback for the lack of a well-defined guiding theory but continues to persist in the DSM and ICD (Castiglioni & Laudisa, 2014; Harkness et al., 2014). However, most experts agree that the DSM-III is implicitly based on the biological or medical model rather than being truly theory-neutral (Harkness et al., 2014; Sedler, 2016). Nonetheless, this edition of the DSM was touted to be purely descriptive, moving away from any claims about the causal nature of the diagnoses.

Spitzer recognized that it would be necessary to directly address the antipsychiatry concern about delimiting "normal" behavior from psychopathology to legitimize the conditions in the DSM-III, and thus attempted to establish a definition of mental disorder. In 1978, Spitzer and Endicott published a direct attempt to define both mental disorders and medical disorders, with mental disorders being a subset of medical disorders. It is valuable to present their definitions in their entirety, as they are still echoed in each DSM since.

> A medical disorder is a relatively distinct condition resulting from an organismic dysfunction which in its fully developed or extreme form is directly and intrinsically associated with distress, disability, or certain other types of disadvantage. The disadvantage may be of physical, perceptual, sexual, or interpersonal nature. Implicitly there is a call for action on the part of the person who has the condition, the medical or its allied professions, and society.
>
> A mental disorder is a medical disorder whose manifestations are primarily signs or symptoms of a psychological (behavioral) nature, or if physical, can be understood only using psychological concepts. (Spitzer & Endicott, 1978, p. 18)

Controversy arose when Spitzer proclaimed that "mental disorders are a subset of medical disorders" (Spitzer et al., 1977, p. 4), leading many to perceive this statement as an attempt to establish exclusive control over mental disorder treatment for psychiatry versus allied disciplines. As unpacked further by later work (Lilienfeld & Marino, 1995; Wakefield, 1992), this definition attempted to provide an "objective" definition of mental disorder that scholars could use to independently determine if a condition rose to the level of a mental disorder versus being nonpathological.

DSM-III was different from other DSMs in that it was more specific and detailed with its diagnostic criteria. Prior to the DSM-III, descriptions of each of the mental disorders were typically conveyed in a narrative or written form. These descriptions implicitly conveyed the disorder's fundamental nature or core characteristics rather than adhering to a more structured or standardized format seen post-DSM-III publication. Individuals were more likely to fit a diagnostic category when they endorsed more characteristics from the list, leading to the comparison of the DSM-III's diagnostic criteria structure to a prototype from cognitive psychology (Cantor et al., 1980).

DSM-III was also the first manual to use a multiaxial system to classify disorders, such that clinicians were to categorize patients along five axes: (I) symptom picture, (II) personality style, (III) medical disorder, (IV) environmental stressors, and (V) role impairment (APA, 1980). Additionally, DSM-III significantly restructured the hierarchical organization of mental disorder categories into 17 major headings (e.g., "mood disorder" or "personality disorder"). This organization was essentially "flat" such that disorder groups were all at the same level of the hierarchy, and the decision-tree structure of the DSM-I and II was removed. The DSM-III and subsequent editions also relaxed the stipulation that an individual could not meet the requirements for more than one disorder, introducing diagnostic comorbidity (which we discuss more in the next section). Lastly, DSM-III was a larger manual than the previous editions, with 256 categories and 494 pages, almost double the number of categories as DSM-I and four times the length (Blashfield et al., 2014), placing this work clearly in the "splitters" camp.

The DSM-III was a financial success, resulting in the American Psychiatric Association publishing a large number of copies along with other companion books. Despite being American, the DSM-III gained substantial popularity among academics and researchers in Europe, especially for its clear operational definitions via diagnostic criteria. The ICD-9 (WHO, 1979) received little attention despite its concurrent development to the DSM-III, which may be, in part, due to its limited change from its predecessor, the ICD-8.

Due to the influx of research, the American Psychiatric Association revised the DSM-III (DSM-III-R; APA, 1987) only seven years later with the goal of revising the categories based on recent publications. However, the changes from DSM-III and DSM-III-R were not only to the diagnostic criteria, but new categories were also added. Many categories were also altered (e.g., subtypes of schizophrenia were dropped, and categories by course were added), dropped (e.g., attention deficit disorder without hyperactivity), or added (e.g., premenstrual syndrome, which had a name change and was added to the appendix).

DSM-IV and ICD-10

One year after the release of DSM-III-R, a DSM-IV task force was appointed and Allen Frances, a psychoanalyst from New York who had been assigned to the personality disorders section of DSM-III, was appointed chair of the next revision. Similar to the timing of previous revisions, the development of the DSM-IV was in response to the upcoming release of ICD-10 in 1993 (Fischer, 2012; Frances et al., 1989). The release of the DSM-IV and ICD-10 marked a significant return to harmonization between these two influential diagnostic manuals. Efforts were made to align the criteria and terminology used in both manuals, aiming for consistency and coherence in psychiatric diagnosis worldwide. This shift reflected a priority on stability rather than radical change, emphasizing the need for reliability and continuity in diagnostic practices (Millon & Klerman, 1986). Arguably, the most radical change made to the DSM-IV was the systematic addition of "clinically significant distress or impairment" across all diagnostic categories (Suris et al., 2016) which was an attempt to help delimit pathological presentations from "normal" states.

To ensure transparency and rigor in the development of diagnostic criteria, explicit rules were established for literature searches and the review of evidence. Frances created thirteen workgroups representing the various subsections of the DSM-IV. Each workgroup was tasked with identifying and reviewing databases that existed in the United States on mental disorders to determine which diagnostic categories needed updating (Blashfield et al., 2014). Widiger et al. (1990) extensively documented this process, outlining the criteria for selecting and evaluating studies to inform changes to the diagnoses. This systematic approach aimed to enhance the credibility and validity of the diagnostic criteria (Frances et al., 1989). As a result, the DSM-IV grew to 383 categories, swinging the pendulum even further in favor of "splitters." In addition, the appendix for "Categories Needing Further Review" expanded from three in the DSM-III-R to seventeen distinct categories (Blashfield et al., 2014).

In the time surrounding the DSM-IV, there was a growing dissatisfaction with the categorical/medical models of psychiatric diagnosis. It became increasingly more apparent that traditional diagnostic systems tended to pigeonhole individuals into discrete categories based on predefined symptom clusters, often oversimplifying the complexity of human experience and behavior. As a result, there was a notable increase in the popularity of dimensional models, which offered a more nuanced understanding of disorders. Specific to personality disorders, dimensional approaches acknowledged the continuous variation in personality traits and emphasized the importance of considering the degree and severity of dysfunction rather than rigidly classifying individuals into distinct diagnostic categories. By embracing dimensional models, clinicians could better capture the subtleties and nuances of personality pathology, leading to more accurate and comprehensive assessments and ultimately enhancing treatment planning and outcomes. A dimensional model of personality disorders was proposed for the DSM-IV; however, it was ultimately rejected for being too radical of a shift (Gunderson, 1992; Widiger, 2007).

One notable aspect of the emphasis on stability was exemplified by a "text-revision" version, the DSM-IV-TR (APA, 2000), which aimed to maintain consistency with the previous edition while addressing any shortcomings or updates based on new research and clinical insights. By and large, the purpose of the revision was simply to provide more details in the text of the manual—not the criteria—based on the research conducted since the release of DSM-IV (Fischer, 2012). This approach provided a sense of familiarity and continuity for clinicians while still allowing for necessary revisions and improvements.

Relatedly, there was recognition that comorbidity posed a challenge for traditional categorical/medical models of psychiatric diagnosis. After relaxing the exclusion rules of the earlier manuals, prevalence studies of mental disorders noted that individuals often met the diagnostic requirements for multiple disorders (Boyd et al., 1984; Kessler et al., 1994, 2005). Indeed, the rates at which this diagnostic overlap occurred greatly exceeded what would be expected by chance. One interpretation of this pattern of comorbidity was that it indicated a larger dimensional structure across mental disorder categories (Krueger & Markon, 2006). As a result, there was a notable increase in structural studies of psychopathology, seeking to understand the complex relationships between different psychiatric disorders and their underlying mechanisms (e.g., Kotov et al., 2017; Krueger et al., 2005). This shift reflected a growing acknowledgment of the interconnected nature of mental health conditions and the limitations of rigid diagnostic categories.

The release of ICD-10 (WHO, 1992) acknowledged the need for flexibility in diagnostic systems, recognizing that one size does not fit all. This led to the development of various versions tailored to different contexts, including statistical, clinical, research, and primary care versions. Briefly, the statistical version included the code numbers and names for the various disorders in the classification along with a brief one- or two-sentence description. This version was intended for use by medical coders, administrative staff, and policymakers. The WHO Department of Mental Health and Substance Abuse also developed a version for the mental and behavioral disorders chapter of the ICD-10 that mirrored the scope and content of the DSM, including elaborated diagnostic guidance, associated features, etc. The diagnostic guidance in this clinical version was deliberately flexible, with the understanding that clinicians from various cultures working in various settings would need some leeway when applying the diagnostic concepts. They also produced a separate version for researchers that had more strictly operationalized rules to satisfy the internal validity requirements for research studies. Last, they also developed a version for primary care settings that had a reduced number of the most common mental health conditions, recognizing that treatment in this setting is targeted at broad, general concerns and that specific diagnostic distinctions would require referral to a mental health specialist. This multiplicity of versions aimed to cater to the diverse needs of clinicians, researchers, and healthcare practitioners, reflecting a commitment to adaptability and inclusivity in psychiatric diagnosis and classification.

DSM-5 and ICD-11

Early in the revision process for DSM-5, a series of conferences and white papers were published establishing an optimistic agenda for the scope of possible changes (Kupfer et al., 2002). The chairs of the DSM-5 taskforce—and much of the field generally—carried a hope that the next edition would revolutionize mental health diagnoses, including incorporating dimensionality explicitly in various places throughout the classification (Regier et al., 2012). Sadly, those hopes were tempered by forces pulling for stability, and changes were much more incremental in nature.

One way dimensionality was reflected in the DSM-5 was the reorganization of the order of disorder groupings across the manual based on structural studies of psychopathology (Regier et al., 2012). Reflecting the advances in thinking about comorbidity as non-random indicators of structure to the nature of psychopathological symptoms, the order of disorder groups was explicitly arranged to reflect higher levels of similarity (and diagnostic overlap) among near neighbors. For example, internalizing spectrum disorders, such as depressive disorders, anxiety disorders, and somatic symptom disorders, were placed together.

Similar to the DSM-III and DSM-IV, the DSM-5 also utilized a workgroup structure during the revision process. This included 13 content-based groups (e.g., neurodevelopmental disorders) and six "study groups" that reflected considerations that cut across diagnostic boundaries (e.g., lifespan developmental approaches; APA, 2013). There were some notable departures from the development process of DSM-IV. For example, the DSM-5 included scientific guidance regarding best-practices for conducting literature searches, documenting thresholds of evidence for a change, and systematic inclusion of relevant datasets much like the DSM-IV, but there was less consistency in how the workgroups applied those procedures or documented their efforts. There was also a dynamic tension between wanting to appear transparent regarding decisions, manifested by a public comment period whereby proposals were posted on the internet, and pressures to preserve privileged information, manifested by controversial non-disclosure agreements that workgroup members were required to sign. Allen Frances, the chair of the DSM-IV revision, was quite vocal about concerns regarding these practices (Frances, 2009; Frances & Widiger, 2012), which were echoed by many others in public discourse.

Another interesting departure regarded the timing of DSM-5's release relative to the ICD-11. Heretofore, every edition of the DSM was released slightly after the corresponding edition of the ICD to allow for harmonization between the manuals (Reed et al., 2016). Initially, the workgroup assigned to facilitate harmonization with the ICD-11 worked closely with representatives from the WHO. However, the DSM-5 was published in 2013, six years before the release of the statistical version of the ICD-11, and a full decade before the release of the Clinical Descriptions and Diagnostic Requirements of the mental and behavioral disorders chapter, which contains the detailed diagnostic guidance that is equivalent to the material included in the DSM. Some authors speculated that the push to jump ahead of the release of the ICD was motivated by the publishing branch of the American Psychiatric Association (Roy et al., 2019). The result was that some proposals for changes to the ICD-11 did not receive full consideration in the DSM-5, and there were inevitable departures between the two manuals. Some differences reflected genuine disagreements regarding the best approach to diagnose some conditions. For example, in trauma-related research, there has been a recognition that some individuals experience additional symptoms beyond the traditional three symptom domains of PTSD (i.e., re-experiencing, avoidance, and hyperarousal). The DSM-5 committee opted to expand the definition of PTSD to include those additional symptoms, considering the difference to be one of severity rather than kind, where the ICD-11 opted to add a diagnosis called Complex PTSD (Maercker et al., 2013; Resick et al., 2012).

Other differences reflected a shared intent but resulted in discrepancies because of political forces. A key example of this type of difference between the DSM-5 and ICD-11 is their treatment of personality disorders. The DSM-5 workgroup on personality and personality disorders started their work with the ambition of developing a dimensional model for personality disorder diagnosis, reflecting the current research in this domain (Krueger et al., 2012). However, as their process evolved, concerns arose from various interests that it would be too radical a change that was not well-enough supported by existing research, and there were internal disagreements among the workgroup regarding the shift as well (Zachar et al., 2016). The end result was that the personality disorders in the regular section of the manual were simply copied from the DSM-IV and the alternative model was listed in an appendix for further research. In contrast, the ICD-11 has moved to a fully dimensional model of personality disorder, removing any personality disorder types excepting a "borderline pattern" specifier. Instead, there is a single diagnosis of personality disorder, graded across severity and characterized by a profile of maladaptive personality traits (Tyrer et al., 2011).

Part of the DSM-5's rush to completion was mitigated by the promise that it would undergo regular intra-edition revisions. Indeed, the major impetus for shifting to using Arabic rather than Roman numerals to denote the edition had been the idea of denoting subrevisions (e.g., DSM-5.1, DSM-5.2; First et al., 2017). Thus, there was an implicit understanding that these revisions could be a mechanism to later harmonize the DSM-5 with the ICD-11 once its work was complete. However, that promise was not realized. While the DSM-5 leadership did propose a mechanism for how these intra-edition revisions would occur and they established a committee to oversee the process, it quickly became clear that the work involved in doing so was too extensive. Instead, in 2022, they released a text revision (DSM-5-TR) similar to what had been done for the DSM-IV that incorporated some selected changes to the text and the addition of a few diagnostic categories (First et al., 2023). One category that was added was prolonged grief disorder. This category was originally rejected from DSM-5 as not having sufficient evidence for its inclusion. However, prolonged grief disorder was added to the ICD-11, and thus this text revision was an opportunity to bring the manuals into closer alignment on this issue.

The previously mentioned delay in the release of ICD-11 was partially due to the extensive amount of work that went into its revision. The ICD-10 was well used in many parts of the world (First et al., 2018), but there were notable limitations to the quality and consistency of the text in the clinical version. There was also a recognition that despite being a product of the WHO intended for use in all the world, it was a product of almost exclusively European design. Thus, the ICD-11 International Advisory Group (2011) was intentional about including professionals in the revision process across world regions, languages, income levels, gender identities, racial identities, and professions. While the DSM-5 made significant strides as well regarding including more international perspectives, it is still largely the product of a high-income country reflecting the primacy of one mental health discipline (i.e., psychiatry). Notably, both manuals lacked deliberate recruitment of individuals with lived experience of the disorders or individuals who cared for them (Kamens et al., 2019).

The revision of the ICD-11 had an explicit goal of focusing on the clinical utility of the manual. There was a recognition that a hypothetical most reliable and valid diagnostic category would be meaningless if practicing clinicians are unable to apply it. Thus, explicit attention was paid to the usability of the diagnostic concepts, including ease of application, understandability, fit with the clinical population, usefulness for communicating with other professionals and the public, etc. (Reed, 2010). This focus led to some intentional differences in the wording and structure of diagnostic guidance relative to the DSM. The wording tended to reflect a degree of flexibility not present in the DSM-5 criteria. For example, a duration requirement of "2 weeks" in the DSM is usually interpreted as a hard cutoff of 14 days, whereas corresponding wording in the ICD-11 might be "about 2 weeks," allowing a degree of flexibility in its interpretation. While a shift of 13 to 14 days might have a substantial impact on prevalence estimates in an epidemiological study, it likely has less meaning when applied in a treatment setting where the individual is describing how long they have felt sad. Indeed, when an individual is describing their mood, they may not be able to make meaningful distinctions at the level of granularity required by the diagnostic criteria. Put differently, a person's experience of their symptoms might be less specific than the definition professionals have made to operationalize it for the sake of scientific precision. The overprecision of diagnostic definitions for the purpose of enhancing reliability might be termed "pseudospecificity," as it is more specific than the concept it is intending to capture.

Somewhat ironically, the move to create more specific diagnostic definitions in DSM-III following the concerns about clinical reliability from the 1960s and 1970s may have led to lower reliability. The field trials of the ICD-11 found substantially higher inter-clinician reliability for a number of diagnostic categories than the corresponding DSM-5 field trials (Reed et al., 2018; Regier et al., 2013). For example, the DSM-5 field trial found a kappa of .28 for major depressive disorder (Regier et al., 2013), whereas the ICD-11 field trial kappa was .64 for single episode depressive disorder and .74 for recurrent depressive disorder (Reed et al., 2018). This difference is partially due to methodological considerations as well, as the DSM-5 field trial estimate also included variance regarding how the clinician gathered information; the DSM-5 design had clinicians independently assess the same person, whereas the ICD-11 design had clinicians assess the same person simultaneously.

The ICD-11 also moved toward incorporating more dimensionality during its revision. In addition to the example of personality disorders given previously, the description of psychotic symptoms in schizophrenia and schizoaffective disorder moved toward a dimensional measurement model in ICD-11. For context, in ICD-10 varieties in presentation of these two disorders were captured categorically via subtypes, for example, a paranoid type reflecting a predominance of hallucinations and delusions in the symptom profile. However, these subtypes did not capture the heterogeneity of individuals' symptoms very well and had been rarely investigated in the scientific literature (Keeley et al., 2018). ICD-11 removed the subtypes and replaced them with a series of dimensional ratings of various symptom domains: positive symptoms, negative symptoms, depressive symptoms, manic symptoms, psychomotor symptoms, and cognitive symptoms (Keeley & Gaebel, 2018). Interestingly, a field study of how clinicians would apply these symptom domains found that clinicians were able to accurately apply mild and severe descriptors, but struggled with moderate ratings (Keeley et al., 2018). As such, the authors argued that certain purposes and settings may benefit from collapsing the dimensional rating into a presence/absence indication to increase clinician agreement.

Conclusions

The history of the ICD and DSM has reflected an ebb and flow of various priorities and strategies (Blashfield et al., 2014). A common model of science across many disciplines is for observations of patterns to lead to systematic investigations that elucidate causal principles. For example, careful study of the properties of elements in chemistry helped establish the theory of atom structure (Needham, 2004). In psychopathology, it is interesting that early classifications started by assuming various etiologies, and as the field progressed, it backed away from these claims toward more neutral descriptions. Following the model of Kraepelin, the description of a pattern of symptoms among a group of individuals is believed to hold the promise that scientific study will eventually identify causal mechanisms for these symptoms. After well over 100 years of attempting this model, a number of scientists are ready to abandon this assumption. The most widescale instantiation of this paradigm shift is the National Institute of Mental Health's (NIMH) Research Domain Criteria (RDoC) project (Kozak & Cuthbert, 2016). The impetus for the RDoC project is to move away from relying on broad syndromal definitions of constructs for study, because these constructs are too heterogenous to likely elucidate individual causal mechanisms, especially those linked to neural circuitry or genetics. Additionally, the RDoC prioritizes examining the full range of human variability on relevant constructs, not just the variability once someone passes a threshold, for that construct to be considered disordered. In that sense, it is also a move toward a more dimensionalized understanding of psychopathology.

Nonetheless, the descriptive categories used in clinical practice may still have a purpose even if they are not tied to identifying etiology. These concepts do still seem to hold some heuristic value for practicing professionals. One reason these categories persist is their ease of use. Human beings are categorical thinkers. One of the earliest ways children organize information about the world is via categories (Murphy, 2002). Categories feel "natural" to clinicians, even if these concepts are socially constructed and have little if any reflection in nature (Zachar, 2000). Categories exist as a way of summarizing complex information. Human lives are complex, and attempting to aid a person in a clinical context can be entirely overwhelming unless the clinician is able to somehow summarize the nearly infinite information about the person's life into a usable unit.

The classifications described in this chapter also varied regarding to what degree they were rationally versus empirically derived. The modern ethos surrounding this dichotomy certainly seems to prioritize empirically defined diagnostic concepts. However, there are glimpses of how top-down processes are still at play. Take the previously mentioned example of Complex PTSD. Based on the same data (the empirical derivation), the DSM-5 and ICD-11 came to different conclusions about what those data meant. We would argue that rational definition has not taken a back seat in the definition of classification systems; instead it has become hidden or implicit. The authors of these systems have background assumptions about how this process should go and preferences about what the end result should be; these beliefs almost certainly shape the resulting classifications in a confirmatory way (Sadler, 2005).

Along those same lines, the psychological and biological have been prioritized in different ways across these classifications. The modern DSMs and ICDs would claim a degree of neutrality if not synthesis on this point. Nonetheless, many have argued that the underlying assumptions of the DSMs have been largely biomedical (Deacon, 2013). A fine-grained analysis of the categories in both manuals would find that some concepts are more biologically minded (e.g., dementia is typically tied to specific biological etiologies) and others are much more psychologically minded (e.g., adjustment disorder is defined by one's psychological reaction to an event or circumstance). Interestingly, in a study where clinicians were asked to sort disorders based on their similarity, a dimension of psychological versus biological definition emerged as one factor influencing their choices (Roberts et al., 2012).

The DSMs and ICDs have almost exclusively instantiated biases toward splitting rather than lumping. Each edition has been larger than the last (Blashfield et al., 2014). There are relatively few examples of groups of disorders being combined (such as the combination of autism spectrum disorder from autism, Asperger's disorder, and other developmental disorders). It is much more common to find examples of more fine-grained distinctions, or new disorders being proposed to capture some heretofore uncaptured aspect of psychopathology. However, a move toward dimensional models may represent the pendulum swinging toward lumping. Dimensional models inherently represent the similarity across concepts rather than the differences. The most salient example of a dimensionalized approach to psychopathology is the Hierarchical Taxonomy of Psychopathology (HiTOP) model (Kotov et al., 2017), which across varying hierarchical levels summarizes existing diagnostic categories by a reduced number of more generalized dimensions.

The history of the DSMs and ICDs elucidates several lessons. First, the target is ever moving. As society shifts and with it the values of its people, the ways in which one might violate those values shift and necessitate new diagnoses or the removal of irrelevant ones. A belief that there will be a "final" version of either manual is naïve, as they will always have to adapt to the changing nature of human needs. Second, a move in one direction usually precipitates a move in the opposite direction in the next generation. The advancement of the study of psychopathology (and most everything else) relies on reactions to the problems of the current mode of operating. The solutions to those problems create new problems for others to react against. A move away from categorical models and toward dimensional models will almost certainly create a new set of problems for a future generation to react against.

References

Aguayo, J. (1986). Charcot and Freud: Some implications of late 19th-century French psychiatry and politics for the origins of psychoanalysis. *Psychoanalysis and Contemporary Thought*, 9, 223–260.

American Psychiatric Association (1952). *Diagnostic and statistical manual of mental disorders*. Author.

American Psychiatric Association. (1968). *Diagnostic and statistical manual of mental disorders* (2nd ed.). American Psychiatric Publishers.

American Psychiatric Association. (1980). *Diagnostic and statistical manual of mental disorders* (3rd ed.). Author.

American Psychiatric Association. (1987). *Diagnostic and statistical manual of mental disorders* (3rd ed., rev.). Author.

American Psychiatric Association. (1994). *Diagnostic and statistical manual of mental disorders* (4th ed.). American Psychiatric Publishers.

American Psychiatric Association. (2000). *Diagnostic and statistical manual of mental disorders* (4th ed., text revision). American Psychiatric Publishers.

American Psychiatric Association. (2013). *Diagnostic and statistical manual of mental disorders* (5th ed.). American Psychiatric Publishers.

Aragona, M. (2015). Rethinking received views on the history of psychiatric nosology: Minor shifts, major continuities. In. P. Zachar, D. Stoyanov, M. Aragona, & A. Jablensky (Eds.), *Alternative perspectives on psychiatric validation* (pp. 27–46). Oxford University Press.

Berrios, G. E., & Hauser, R. (1988). The early development of Kraepelin's ideas on classification: A conceptual history. *Psychological Medicine*, *18*, 813–821.

Blashfield, R. K. (1984). *The classification of psychopathology: Neo-Kraepelinian and quantitative approaches*. Plenum Press.

Blashfield, R. K., Keeley, J. W., Flanagan, E. H., & Miles, S. R. (2014). The cycle of classification: DSM-I through DSM-5. *Annual Review of Clinical Psychology, 10*, 25–51. https://doi-org.proxy.library.vcu.edu/10.1146/annurev-clinpsy-032813-153639

Blashfield, R. K., & Reynolds, S. M. (2012). An invisible college view of the DSM-5 personality disorder classification. *Journal of Personality Disorders, 26*, 821–829.

Boyd, J. H., Burke, J. D., Gruenberg, E., Holzer, C. E., Rae, D. S., George, L. K., Karno, M., Stoltzman, R., McEvoy, L., & Nestadt, G. (1984). Exclusion criteria of DSM-III: A study of cooccurrence of hierarchy-free syndromes. *Archives of General Psychiatry, 41*, 983–989.

Breuer, J., & Freud, S. (1895). *Studies in hysteria* (J. Strachey, Trans.).Hogarth Press.

Cantor, N., Smith, E. E., French, R., & Mezzich, J. (1980). Psychiatric diagnosis as prototype categorization. *Journal of Abnormal Psychology, 89*, 181–193.

Castiglioni, M., & Laudisa, F. (2014). Toward psychiatry as a "human" science of mind. The case of depressive disorders in DSM-5. *Frontiers in Psychology, 5*, 1517.

Cooper, J. E., Kendell, R. E., Gurland, B. J., Sharpe, L., Copeland, J. R. M., & Simon, R. (1972). *Psychiatric diagnosis in New York and London* [Maudsley Monograph No. 20]. Oxford University Press.

Cooper, R., & Blashfield, R. K. (2016). Re-evaluating DSM-I. *Psychological Medicine, 46*, 449–456. https://doi.org/10.1017/S0033291715002093

Deacon, B. J. (2013). The biomedical model of mental disorder: A critical analysis of its validity, utility, and effects on psychotherapy research. *Clinical Psychology Review, 33*, 846–861. https://doi.org/10.1016/j.cpr.2012.09.007

Drescher, J. (2013). An interview with Robert L. Spitzer, MD. In *Ex-Gay Research* (pp. 323–339). Routledge.

Feighner, J. P., Robins, E., Guze, S. B., Woodruff, R. A., Winokur, G., & Munoz, R. (1972). Diagnostic criteria for use in psychiatric research. *Archives of General Psychiatry, 26*(1), 57–63. https://doi.org/10.1001/archpsyc.1972.01750190059011

First, M. B., Clarke, D. E., Yousif, L., Eng, A. M., Gogtay, N., & Appelbaum, P. S. (2023). DSM-5-TR: Rationale, process, and overview of changes. *Psychiatric Services, 74*, 869–875.

First, M. B., Kendler, K. S., & Leibenluft, E. (2017). The future of the DSM: Implementing a continuous improvement model. *JAMA Psychiatry, 74*, 115–116. doi:10.1001/jamapsychiatry.2016.3004

First, M. B., Rebello, T. J., Keeley, J. W., Bhargava, R., Dai, Y., Kulygina, M., . . . Reed, G. M., (2018). Do mental health professionals use diagnostic classifications the way we think they do? A global survey. *World Psychiatry, 17*(2), 187–195. doi:10.1002/wps.20525

Fischer, B. A. (2012). A review of American psychiatry through its diagnoses: The history and development of the Diagnostic and Statistical Manual of Mental Disorders. *The Journal of Nervous and Mental Disease, 200*(12), 1022–1030. https://doi.org/10.1097/NMD.0b013e318275cf19

Foucault, M. (1988). *Madness and civilization: A history of insanity in the Age of Reason.* Vintage Books.

Frances, A. J. (2009). A warning sign on the road to DSM-V: Beware of its unintended consequences. *Psychiatric Times, 26*, 1.

Frances, A. J., & Widiger, T. (2012). Psychiatric diagnosis: Lessons from the DSM-IV past and cautions for the DSM-5 future. *Annual Review of Clinical Psychology, 8*, 109–130.

Frances, A. J., Widiger, T. A., & Pincus, H. A. (1989). The development of DSM-IV. *Archives of General Psychiatry, 46*(4), 373–375. https://doi.org/10.1001/archpsyc.1989.01810040079012

Grob, G. (1991). Origins of DSM–I: A study in appearance and reality. *American Journal of Psychiatry, 148*, 421–431.

Gunderson, J. G. (1992). Diagnostic controversies. In A. Tasman & M. B. Riba (Eds.), *Review of Psychiatry.* Vol. 11 (pp. 9–24). American Psychiatric Publishing.

Harkness, A., Reynolds, S., & Lilienfeld, S. (2014). A review of systems for psychology and psychiatry: Adaptive Systems, Personality Psychopathology Five (PSY-5), and the DSM-5. *Journal of Personality Assessment, 96*, 121–139.

Havens, L. (1985). Historical perspectives on diagnosis in psychiatry. *Comprehensive Psychiatry, 26*, 326–336.

Hester, S., & Kendler, K. S. (2020). The evolution of Kraepelin's nosological principles. *World Psychiatry, 19*, 381–388.

Houts, A. C. (2000). Fifty years of psychiatric nomenclature: Reflections on the 1943 War Department Technical Bulletin, Medical 203. *Journal of Clinical Psychology, 56*, 935–967.

International Advisory Group for the Revision of ICD-10 Mental and Behavioral Disorders (2011). A conceptual framework for the revision of the ICD-10 classification of mental and behavioral disorders. *World Psychiatry, 10*, 86–92.

Kamens, S. R., Cosgrove, L., Peters, S. M., Jones, N., Flanagan, E., Longden, E., Schulz, S., Robbins, B. D., Olsen, S., Miller, R., & Lichtenberg, P. (2019). Standards and guidelines for the development of diagnostic nomenclatures and alternatives in mental health research and practice. *Journal of Humanistic Psychology, 59*, 401–427. https://doi.org/10.1177/0022167818763862

Keeley, J. W., & Gaebel, W. (2018). Symptom rating scales for schizophrenia and other primary psychotic disorders in ICD-11. *Epidemiology and Psychiatric Sciences, 27*, 219–224. https://doi.org/10.1017/S2045796017000270

Keeley, J. W., Gaebel, W., First, M. B., Peterson, D. L., Rebello, T., Sharan, P., & Reed, G. M. (2018). Psychotic disorder symptom rating scales: Are dichotomous or multi-point scales more clinically useful?—An ICD-11 field study. *Schizophrenia Research, 202*, 254–259. https://doi.org/10.1016/j.schres.2018.07.006

Kendell, R. E. (1990). A brief history of psychiatric classification in Britain. In N. Sartorius, A. Jablensky, D. A. Regier, J. D. Burke, Jr., & R. M. A. Hirschfeld (Eds.), *Sources and traditions of psychiatric classification* (pp. 139–151). Hogrefe & Huber.

Kendell, R. E., Cooper, J. E., Gourlay, A. J., Sharpe, L., & Gurland, B. J. (1971). Diagnostic criteria of American and British psychiatrists. *Archives of General Psychiatry, 25*, 123–130.

Kendler, K. S., Muñoz, R. A., & Murphy, G. (2010). The development of the Feighner criteria: A historical perspective. *American Journal of Psychiatry, 167*(2), 134–142. https://doi.org/10.1176/appi.ajp.2009.09081155

Kessler, R. C., Chiu, W. T., Demler, O., & Walters, E. E. (2005). Prevalence, severity, and comorbidity of 12-month DSM-IV disorders in the National Comorbidity Survey Replication. *Archives of General Psychiatry, 62*(6), 617–627. https://doi.org/10.1001/archpsyc.62.6.617

Kessler, R. C., McGonagle, K. A., Zhao, S., Nelson, C. B., Hughes, M., Eschlman, S., Wittchen, H-U., & Kendler, K. S. (1994). Lifetime and 12-month prevalence of *DSM-III-R* psychiatric disorders in the United States: Results from the National Comorbidity Survey. *Archives of General Psychiatry, 51*, 8–19.

Kotov, R., Krueger, R. F., Watson, D., Achenbach, T. M., Althoff, R. R., Bagby, R. M., . . . Zimmerman, M. (2017). The Hierarchical Taxonomy of Psychopathology (HiTOP): A dimensional alternative to traditional nosologies. *Journal of Abnormal Psychology, 126*, 454–477. http://dx.doi.org/10.1037/abn0000258

Kozak, M. J., & Cuthbert, B. N. (2016). The NIMH research domain criteria initiative: Background, issues, and pragmatics. *Psychophysiology, 53*, 286–297.

Krueger, R. F., Derringer, J., Markon, K. E., Watson, D., & Skodol, A. E. (2012). Initial construction of a maladaptive personality trait model and inventory for DSM-5. *Psychological Medicine, 42*, 1879–1890. https://doi.org/10.1017/S0033291711002674

Krueger, R. F., & Markon, K. E. (2006). Reinterpreting comorbidity: A model-based approach to understanding and classifying psychopathology. *Annual Review of Clinical Psychology, 2*, 111–133.

Krueger, R. F., Markon, K. E., Patrick, C. J., & Iacono, W. G. (2005). Externalizing psychopathology in adulthood: A dimensional-spectrum conceptualization and its implications for DSM–V. *Journal of Abnormal Psychology, 114*, 537–550.

Kupfer, D. J., First, M. B., & Regier, D. E. (2002). *A research agenda for DSM–V*. Washington, DC: American Psychiatric Association.

Lidz, T. (1966). Adolf Meyer and the development of American psychiatry. *American Journal of Psychiatry, 123*, 320–332.

Lilienfeld, S. O., & Marino, L. (1995). Mental disorder as a Roschian concept: A critique of Wakefield's "harmful dysfunction" analysis. *Journal of Abnormal Psychology, 104*, 411–420.

Maercker, A., Brewin, C. R., Bryant, R. A., Cloitre, M., Ommeren, M., Jones, L. M., Humayan, A., Kagee, A., Llosa, A. E., Rousseau, C., Somasundaram, D. J., Souza, R., Suzuki, Y.,Weissbecker, I.,

Wessely, S. C., First, M. B., & Reed, G. M. (2013). Diagnosis and classification of disorders specifically associated with stress: Proposals for ICD11. *World Psychiatry, 12*(3), 198–206. https://doi.org/10.1002/wps.20057
Millon, T. (1975). Reflections on Rosenhan's "On being sane in insane places." *Journal of Abnormal Psychology, 84*, 456–461.
Millon, T., & Klerman, G. L. (Eds.). (1986). *Contemporary directions in psychopathology: Toward the DSM-IV.* The Guilford Press.
Murphy, G. (2002). *The big book of concepts*. MIT Press.
Needham, P. (2004). When did atoms begin to do any explanatory work in chemistry? *International Studies in the Philosophy of Science, 18*, 199–219. https://doi.org/10.1080/0269859042000296521
North, C., Yutzy, S., & Goodwin, D. W. (2010). Evolution of psychiatric diagnosis. In *Goodwin and Guze's psychiatric diagnosis* (pp. 1–14). Oxford University Press.
Reed, G. M. (2010). Toward ICD-11: Improving the clinical utility of WHO's international classification of mental disorders. *Professional Psychology: Research and Practice, 41*, 457–464.
Reed, G. M., Robles, R., & Dominguez-Martinez, T. (2016). Classification of mental and behavioral disorders. In J. C. Norcross, G. R. VandenBos, & D. K. Freedheim (Eds.), *APA handbook of clinical psychology*. American Psychological Association.
Reed, G. M., Sharan, P., Rebello, T. J., Keeley, J. W., Elena Medina-Mora, M., Gureje, O., . . . Pike, K. M. (2018). The ICD-11 developmental field study of reliability of diagnoses of high-burden mental disorders: Results among adult patients in mental health settings of 13 countries. *World Psychiatry, 17*, 174–186. https://doi.org/10.1002/wps.20524
Regier, D. A., Kuhl, E. A., Narrow, W. E., & Kupfer, D. J. (2012). Research planning for the future of psychiatric diagnosis. *European Psychiatry, 27*, 553–556.
Regier, D. A., Narrow, W. E., Clarke, D. E., Kraemer, H. C., Kuramoto, S. J., Kuhl, E. A., & Kupfer, D. J. (2013). DSM-5 field trials in the United States and Canada, part II: Test-retest reliability of selected categorical diagnoses. *American Journal of Psychiatry, 170*, 59–70.
Resick, P. A., Bovin, M. J., Calloway, A. L., Dick, A. M., King, M. W., Mitchell, K. S., Suvak, M. K., Wells, S. Y., Stirman, S. W., & Wolf, E. J. (2012). A critical evaluation of the complex PTSD literature: Implications for DSM-5. *Journal of Traumatic Stress, 25*(3), 241–251. https://doi.org/10.1002/jts.21699
Rissmiller, D. J., & Rissmiller, J. H. (2006). Evolution of the antipsychiatry movement into mental health consumerism. *Psychiatric Services, 57*(8), 1216.
Roberts, M., Medina-Mora, M., Reed, G., Keeley, J., Sharan, P., Johnson, D., Mari, J., Ayuso-Mateos, J., Gureje, O., Xiao, Z., Maruta, T., Khoury, B., Robles, R., & Saxena, S. (2012). A global clinicians' map of mental disorders to improve ICD-11. *International Review of Psychiatry, 24*, 578–590.
Robins, E., & Guze, S. B. (1970). Establishment of diagnostic validity in psychiatric illness: Its application to schizophrenia. *American Journal of Psychiatry, 126*, 983–987.
Rosenhan, D. (1973). On being sane in insane places. *Science, 114*, 316–322.
Roy, M., Rivest, M.-P., Namian, D., & Moreau, N. (2019). The critical reception of the DSM-5: Towards a typology of audiences. *Public Understanding of Science, 28*(8), 932–948. https://doi.org/10.1177/0963662519868969
Sadler, J. Z. (2005). *Values and psychiatric diagnosis*. Oxford University Press.
Scull, A. (2023). Rosenhan revisited: Successful scientific fraud. *History of Psychiatry, 34*, 180–195. https://doi-org/10.1177/0957154X221150878
Sedler, M. (2016). Medicalization in psychiatry: The medical model, descriptive diagnosis, and lost knowledge. *Medicine, Health Care, and Philosophy, 19*(2), 247–252.
Shorter, E. (2015). The history of nosology and the rise of the Diagnostic and Statistical Manual of Mental Disorders. *Dialogues in Clinical Neuroscience, 17*(1), 59–67. https://doi.org/10.31887/DCNS.2015.17.1/eshorter
Shorter, E. (1997). *A history of psychiatry: From the era of the asylum to the age of Prozac.* John Wiley & Sons.
Spitzer, R. L. (1975). On pseudoscience in science, logic in remission and psychiatric diagnosis: A critique of Rosenhan's "On being sane in insane places." *Journal of Abnormal Psychology, 84*, 442–452.

Spitzer, R., & Endicott, J. (1978). Medical and mental disorder: Proposed definition and criteria. In R. Spitzer & D. Klein (Eds.), *Critical issues in psychiatric diagnosis* (pp. 15–40). Raven Press.
Spitzer, R. L., Endicott, J., & Robins, E. (1978). Research diagnostic criteria: Rationale and reliability. *Archives of General Psychiatry, 35*(6), 773–782. https://doi.org/10.1001/archpsyc.1978.01770300115013
Spitzer, R., Sheehy, M., & Endicott, J. (1977). *DSM–III*: Guiding principles. In V. Rakoff, H. Stancer, & H. Kedward (Eds.), *Psychiatric diagnosis* (pp. 1–24). Brunner/Mazel.
Stengel, E. (1959). Classification of mental disorders. *Bulletin of the World Health Organization, 21*, 601–663.
Surís, A., Holliday, R., & North, C. (2016). The evolution of the classification of psychiatric disorders. *Behavioral Sciences, 6*(1), 5. https://doi.org/10.3390/bs6010005
Szasz, T. S. (1961). *The myth of mental illness*. Hoeber-Harper.
Tyrer, P., Crawford, M., Mulder, R., Blashfield, R., Farnam, A., . . . Reed, G. M. (2011). The rationale for the reclassification of personality disorder in the 11th revision of the International Classification of Diseases (ICD-11). *Personality and Mental Health, 5*, 246–259.
Weber, M. M., & Engstrom, E. J. (1997). Kraepelin's "diagnostic cards": The confluence of clinical research and preconceived categories. *History of Psychiatry, 8*, 375– 85.
Wakefield, J. (1992). Disorder as harmful dysfunction: A conceptual critique of *DSM–III–R*'s definition of mental disorder. *Psychological Review, 99*, 232–247.
Widiger, T. A. (2007). Dimensional models of personality disorder. *World Psychiatry, 6*(2), 79–83.
Widiger, T. A., Frances, A. J., Pincus, H. A., & Davis, W. W. (1990). DSM-IV literature reviews: Rationale, process, and limitations. *Journal of Psychopathology and Behavioral Assessment, 12*(3), 189–202. https://doi.org/10.1007/BF00960617
Widiger, T. A., & Samuel, D. B. (2005). Diagnostic categories or dimensions? A question for the Diagnostic and Statistical Manual of Mental Disorders—Fifth Edition. *Journal of Abnormal Psychology, 114*, 494–504.
World Health Organization (1949). *International statistical classification of diseases, injuries, and causes of death* (6th rev.). Author.
World Health Organization. (1968). *Manual of international statistical classification of diseases, injuries, and causes of death* (8th rev.). Author.
World Health Organization (1979). *International statistical classification of diseases, injuries, and causes of death*, (9th rev.). Author.
World Health Organization. (1992). *ICD-10 Classification of Mental and Behavioural Disorders: Clinical Descriptions and Diagnostic Guidelines*. World Health Organization.
Zachar, P. (2000). Psychiatric disorders are not natural kinds. *Philosophy, Psychiatry, and Psychology, 7*, 167–182.
Zachar, P., Krueger, R. F., & Kendler, K. S. (2016). Personality disorder in DSM-5: An oral history. *Psychological Medicine, 46*, 1–10.

CHAPTER 3

Co-Development and Evolution of DSM and ICD

THOMAS A. WIDIGER*, ALEXANDRA HINES, AND JOSHUA R. OLTMANNS

Introduction

THE purpose of this chapter is to provide a history and overview of the co-development and evolution of the American Psychiatric Association's (APA) *Diagnostic and Statistical Manual of Mental Disorders* (DSM) and the World Health Organization's (WHO) International Classification of Diseases (ICD), with particular attention regarding dimensional versus categorical classification. The ICD provides the authoritative diagnostic nomenclature for all member countries of the WHO (including the United States); the DSM is the United States' version of the ICD and provides the authoritative diagnostic nomenclature for the country.

It is perhaps self-evident that a common language for the classification of psychopathology is necessary for clinical practice. Imagine the confusion, if not chaos, if clinicians used whatever classification they preferred. Even if they used the same diagnostic term, they would surely apply different criteria for its assessment. The primary purpose of a diagnostic manual is to facilitate reliable (and valid) diagnostic practice for clinicians and professional agencies through the provision of a uniform nomenclature.

A common language is also advantageous to scientific research (Widiger, 2012). It would be quite difficult to accumulate a body of knowledge concerning psychopathology if each researcher used his or her own idiosyncratic nomenclature. Of course, an authoritative nomenclature, such as the APA DSM, might in principle hinder creativity, innovation, and progress if it stifled alternative conceptualizations (Lilienfeld & Treadway, 2016). Some have even suggested that clinical psychology and psychiatry would be better off without any official nomenclature (e.g., Markon, 2013). Hyman (2010) and Insel (2014), past Directors of the National Institute of Mental Health (NIMH), argued against the predominance of the APA DSM for research purposes. This is now somewhat ironic, given that the NIMH has since indicated that researchers should adhere to their own diagnostic system to obtain funding (i.e., the Research Domain Criteria; Insel, 2014; Insel & Quirion, 2005).

In any case, it is debatable if the APA and ICD nomenclatures have actually stifled scientific research. Even when researchers disagree with or are critical of the DSM, the APA nomenclature has served as a useful foil, a common point of comparison. Researchers have been free to assert through argument and empirical research their own version of a diagnostic construct, including fundamental paradigm shifts to a dimensional rather than categorical model

* Correspondence concerning this chapter should be addressed to Thomas A. Widiger, PhD, 115 Kastle Hall, Department of Psychology, University of Kentucky, Lexington, KY, 40506-0044; phone: 859-967-6320; email: widiger@uky.edu.

of classification (First, 2003; Keeley, Chung, & Kleva, 2023; Krueger, Watson, & Barlow, 2005; Widiger & Clark, 2000).

Classification Premorbid to ICD-6

Prior to ICD-6, each country, and to some extent each medical center within the United States, had developed its own nomenclature (Widiger, 2001). It was suggested that the production of a new system for classifying psychopathology was a rite of passage for the young, aspiring psychiatrist.

> To produce a well-ordered classification almost seems to have become the unspoken ambition of every psychiatrist of industry and promise, as it is the ambition of a good tenor to strike a high C. This classificatory ambition was so conspicuous that the composer Berlioz was prompted to remark that after their studies have been completed a rhetorician writes a tragedy and a psychiatrist a classification. (Zilboorg, 1941, p. 450)

Initial efforts to develop a uniform language did not meet with much success (Widiger, 2012). The Statistical Committee of the British Royal Medico-Psychological Association produced a classification in 1892, and conducted formal revisions in 1904, 1905, and 1906. However, "the Association finally accepted the unpalatable fact that most of its members were not prepared to restrict themselves to diagnoses listed in any official nomenclature" (Kendell, 1975, p. 88). The Association of Medical Superintendents of American Institutions for the Insane (a forerunner to the American Psychiatric Association) adopted a slightly modified version of the British nomenclature, but it was not any more successful in getting its members to use it.

The American Bureau of the Census struggled to obtain national statistics for the prevalence of mental disorders in the absence of an officially recognized nomenclature (Grob, 1991). In 1908, the Bureau asked the American Medico-Psychological Association (which revised its name to the American Psychiatric Association in 1921) to appoint a Committee on Nomenclature of Diseases to develop a standard nosology. This committee affirmed the need for a uniform system.

> The importance and need of some system whereby uniformity in reports would be secured have been repeatedly emphasized by officers and members of this Association, by statisticians of the United States Census Bureau, by editors of psychiatric journals. . . . The present condition with respect to the classification of mental diseases is chaotic. Some states use no well-defined classification. In others the classifications used are similar in many respects but differ enough to prevent accurate comparisons. Some states have adopted a uniform system, while others leave the matter entirely to the individual hospitals. This condition of affairs discredits the science of psychiatry. (Salmon, Copp, May, Abbot, & Cotton, 1917, pp. 255–256)

The American Medico-Psychological Association, in collaboration with the National Committee for Mental Hygiene, issued a nosology in 1918 titled the *Statistical Manual for the Use of Institutions for the Insane* (Grob, 1991; Menninger, 1963). The National Committee for Mental Hygiene published and distributed this nosology. This nomenclature was of use to the census, but many hospitals failed to adopt the system for clinical practice, in part because of its narrow representation. The diagnoses were confined largely to psychoses with a presumably neurochemical pathology (Salmon et al., 1917). Confusion continued to be the norm.

> In the late twenties, each large teaching center employed a system of its own origination, no one of which met more than the immediate needs of the local institution. . . . There resulted

a polyglot of diagnostic labels and systems, effectively blocking communication. (APA, 1952, p. v)

A conference was held at the New York Academy of Medicine in 1928 with representatives from various government agencies and professional associations. A trial edition of a proposed nomenclature (modeled after the *Statistical Manual*) was distributed to hospitals in 1932 within the American Medical Association's Standard Classified Nomenclature of Disease. Most hospitals and teaching centers used this system, or at least a modified version that was compatible with the perspectives of the clinicians at that particular center. However, the Standard Classified Nomenclature proved to be grossly inadequate when the attention of mental health clinicians expanded beyond the severe "organic" psychopathologies that had been the predominant concern of inpatient hospitals to consider the less severe disorders within outpatient psychiatry.

ICD-6 and DSM-I

The United States Navy, Army, and Veterans Administration had each developed its own, largely independent nomenclatures during World War II, due in large part to the inadequacies of the Standard Classified Nomenclature. "Military psychiatrists, induction station psychiatrists, and Veterans Administration psychiatrists, found themselves operating within the limits of a nomenclature specifically not designed for 90% of the cases handled" (APA, 1952, p. vi). World War II indeed was instrumental in convincing the profession that a common language of psychopathology was necessary. Effective communication on the battlefield regarding the many psychological casualties of the war was sorely handicapped by the absence of a uniform nomenclature.

Two medical statisticians, William Farr in London and Jacques Bertillon in Paris, had convinced the International Statistical Congress back in 1853 of the value of producing a uniform classification of causes of death (Widiger, 2001). A classification system was eventually developed by Farr, Bertillon, and Marc d'Espine (of Geneva). The Bertillon Classification of Causes of Death, which included some mental disorders, was of substantial benefit and interest to many governments and public health agencies. In 1889 the International Statistical Institute urged that the task of sponsoring and revising the nomenclature be accepted by a more official governing body. The French government therefore convened a series of international conferences in 1900, 1920, 1929, and 1938, producing successive revisions of the International List of Causes of Death (Kendell, 1975).

The WHO accepted the authority in 1948 to produce the sixth edition of the renamed International Classification of Diseases (ICD), due in large part to the inability of clinicians from different countries to communicate effectively when treating the psychological casualties of the Second World War (Kendell, 1975). Note that this nomenclature included all medical disorders; mental disorders were covered in one of its many chapters.

The United States, as a member of the WHO, is required to use the ICD. The code numbers used in all clinics and hospitals within the United States (and included within DSM-5) are the ICD code numbers. However, each member country of the WHO can modify the diagnostic criteria for a respective disorder as long as this modification does not result in a distinctly different disorder. Each country can also decline to include a particular disorder within its version of the ICD if the existence of this disorder is not recognized within a respective country. Finally, each country can also add a disorder to its own version of the ICD that is not included in the official WHO ICD, as long as that country does not use a code number that is already in use.

For example, the ICD-9 code number in DSM-IV for hypochondriasis and body dysmorphic disorder was precisely the same (i.e., 300.7), yet in the United States these are considered to be very different disorders (APA, 1994, 2000). The same code number had to be used because the ICD-9 did not recognize any distinction between these syndromes, considering body dysmorphia to be a variant of hypochondriasis (WHO, 1992). Little has changed in DSM-5. In DSM-IV hypochondriasis and body dysmorphic disorder were at least included in the same section of the manual (for somatoform disorders). However, for DSM-5, the APA shifted body dysmorphic disorder out of the somatoform section and into an obsessive-compulsive disorders section, and hypochondriasis was largely folded into a broader condition of illness anxiety disorder (but remaining within the somatic symptom disorders). Nevertheless, although again clearly very different disorders, at least from the perspective of American psychiatry, their ICD-10 code numbers remained largely the same (i.e., F45.21 and F45.22, respectively), because from the perspective of the ICD-10, both continue to be variants of hypochondriasis. It was proposed for ICD-11 that hypochondriasis (rather than body dysmorphia) leave the somatoform section to join the anxiety and obsessive-compulsive disorders (Gureje, 2015), although body dysmorphia would follow suit (remaining a variant of hypochondriasis).

The United States Public Health Service commissioned a committee, chaired by George Raines, with representation from a variety of professional and public health associations, to develop a variant of ICD-6 for use within the United States. Responsibility for publishing and distributing the nosology was provided to the American Psychiatric Association (1952) under the title, "Diagnostic and Statistical Manual. Mental Disorders" (hereafter referred to as DSM-I). Subsequent editions of the DSM were developed under the sole authority of the APA. DSM-I was very congruent with ICD-6, although there were some notable differences. For example, DSM-I included a diagnosis of passive-aggressive personality disorder that was not included in ICD-6, which, curiously, might have even been the most frequently diagnosed personality disorder by American psychiatrists during the war, accounting for 6% of all admissions to U.S. Army hospitals (Malinow, 1981).

Pertinent to the focus of this text, DSM-I and ICD-6 diagnosed mental disorders categorically, with one notable exception: mental retardation (whose title was subsequently changed to intellectual disability and currently titled intellectual developmental disorder). Intellectual developmental disorder is diagnosed along a continuum of cognitive and social functioning. Intelligence, or intellectual functioning, is distributed as a hierarchical, multifactorial continuous variable concerning the ability to reason, plan, solve problems, think abstractly, comprehend complex ideas, learn quickly, and learn from experience (Schalock, Luckasson, & Tassé, 2021). Level of intelligence is often measured with respect to the intelligence quotient, or IQ. Most persons' levels of intelligence, including most of those with an intellectual disability, are the result of a complex interaction of multiple genetic, fetal, and infant development, and environmental influences (Deary, Spinath, & Bates, 2006). There are no discrete breaks in its distribution that would provide an absolute distinction between normal and abnormal intelligence (Roy & Kogan, 2024). The point of demarcation for the diagnosis of an intellectual developmental disorder is an arbitrary, quantitative distinction along the normally distributed levels of hierarchically and multifactorially defined intelligence (Patel, Cabral, Ho, & Merrick, 2020). This point of demarcation is arbitrary in the sense that it does not carve nature at a discrete joint, but it was not, of course, randomly or mindlessly chosen. It is a defensible selection that was informed by the impairments in adaptive functioning considered necessary for independent living (Schalock et al., 2021). In DSM-I the cutoff point was an intellectual quotient (IQ) of 85 (APA, 1952), although lowered in subsequent editions when it became recognized that persons with an IQ lower than 85 can function independently. The current cutoff point is an IQ of 70 with an emphasis on a concurrent documentation of impairment in functioning (APA, 2013, 2022).

Many instances of intellectual developmental disorder are due in large part to specific etiologies, such as tuberous sclerosis, microcephaly, von Recklinghausen's disease, Trisomy 21, Mosaicism, and Prader Willi syndrome (Schalock et al., 2021). Nevertheless, the disorders that result from these specific etiologies are generally understood as medical conditions, an associated feature of which is an intellectual disability that would be diagnosed concurrently and independently as a mental disorder. The intellectual disability that is diagnosed as a mental disorder within ICD 6 and DSM I is itself a multifactorially determined and heterogeneous dimensional construct falling along the broad continuum of intellectual functioning. "The causes of intellectual disabilities are typically complex interactions of biological, behavioral/psychological, and sociocultural factors" (Naglieri, Salter, & Rojahn, 2008, p. 409). An important postnatal cause for intellectual developmental disorder is "simply" psychosocial deprivation, resulting from poverty, chaotic living environment, and/or child abuse or neglect. No clear etiology will be evident in up to 40% of cases (APA, 2022). In sum, the initial editions of the ICD and DSM included a compelling model for the rest of the diagnostic manual for a dimensional classification.

DSM-I was largely successful in providing a common, authoritative nomenclature for American psychiatry (Grob, 1991; Kendell, 1975). However, fundamental objections and criticisms regarding the reliability and validity of psychiatric diagnoses were being raised at this time, and much of this objection was directed at inadequacies of the diagnostic manual (e.g., Zigler & Phillips, 1961). A widely cited reliability study by Ward, Beck, Mendelson, Mock, and Erbaugh (1962) concluded that most of the poor agreement among psychiatrists' diagnoses was due largely to inadequacies of DSM-I rather than to idiosyncracies of the clinical interview or inconsistent patient reporting. "Two thirds of the disagreements were charged to inadequacies of the nosological system itself" (Ward et al., 1962, p. 205). The largest single disagreement was determining "whether the neurotic symptomatology or the characterological pathology is more extensive or 'basic'" (Ward et al., 1962, p. 202). Ward et al. criticized the DSM-I requirement that the clinician choose between a neurotic condition or a personality disorder when both appeared to be present. The second-most-frequent cause of disagreement was unclear diagnostic criteria.

The WHO was also concerned with the failure of all of its member countries to adopt the mental disorders section of ICD-6 and therefore commissioned a review by the English psychiatrist Erwin Stengel. Stengel (1959) reiterated the importance of establishing an official diagnostic nomenclature.

> A . . . serious obstacle to progress in psychiatry is difficulty of communication. Everybody who has followed the literature and listened to discussions concerning mental illness soon discovers that psychiatrists, even those apparently sharing the same basic orientation, often do not speak the same language. They either use different terms for the same concepts, or the same term for different concepts, usually without being aware of it. (Stengel, 1959, p. 601)

Stengel recommended that future nomenclatures be shorn of theoretical and etiological assumptions and provide instead behaviorally specific descriptions. DSM-I and ICD-6 were heavily influenced by a psychodynamic perspective, which actually placed little interest in diagnosis given that the same form of psychoanalysis was applied to most cases (Spitzer, Williams, & Skodol, 1980).

DSM-II and ICD-8

ICD-6 was revised to ICD-7 in 1955, but there were no revisions to the mental disorders section. In 1965, the APA appointed the Committee on Nomenclature and Statistics to revise DSM-I to be compatible with ICD-8 and yet also be suitable for use within the United States (Spitzer & Wilson, 1968). Mental disorder diagnosis, though, remained fundamentally controversial (e.g., Rosenhan, 1973). A significant problem continued to be the absence of support for reliability, let alone validity.

The modern effort to demarcate a taxonomy of distinct clinical conditions is often traced to Kraepelin (Kendell, 1975; Spitzer et al., 1980). Considerable interest in diagnosis and classification was developing among neurobiologically oriented researchers, often referred to as "Neo-Kraepelinian," given their emphasis on careful and systematic diagnosis. One research team in particular, from Washington University in St. Louis, spearheaded the effort to develop well validated psychiatric diagnoses. A principal model for mental disorder diagnostic categories was provided by Robins and Guze (1970), from Washington University, who articulated five fundamental phases of validation: clinical description, laboratory study, delimitation from other disorders, follow-up, and family studies. With respect to the delimitation from other disorders, the diagnostic "criteria should . . . permit exclusion of borderline cases and doubtful cases (an undiagnosed group) so that the index group may be as homogeneous as possible" (Robins & Guze, 1970, p. 108), embracing the spirit that each diagnostic category would have a unique etiology, pathology, and treatment. The most influential effort in the construction of mental disorder diagnostic categories was the widely cited Feighner et al. (1972) specific and explicit criterion sets for 14 disorders (as well as secondary depression), which followed the spirit of Stengel's (1959) recommendations for the ICD and became the role model for DSM-III (APA, 1980; Kendell & Jablensky, 2003; Spitzer et al., 1980). Feighner et al. (1972) became the most widely cited article in psychiatry.

DSM-III and ICD-9

The authors of ICD-9 had decided to include a glossary that would provide relatively more precise descriptions of each disorder, consistent with Stengel (1959), but it was apparent that ICD-9 would not include the more specific and explicit criterion sets developed by the Neo-Kraepelinian researchers (Kendell, 1975; Kramer, Sartorius, Jablensky, & Gulbinat, 1979). In 1974, the APA appointed a task force, chaired by Robert Spitzer, to revise DSM-II in a manner that would be compatible with ICD-9 but would also incorporate many of the current innovations in diagnosis. Robert Spitzer was a technical consultant for DSM-II, but he became a predominant expert on diagnosis and classification through his effort to address the controversy over the inclusion of homosexuality in DSM-II (Spitzer, 1973), his expansion of the specific and explicit criterion sets of Feighner et al. (1972), and his development of a structured interview for their assessment (Spitzer & Robins, 1978).

Dr. Spitzer was not only the Chair of the DSM-III Task Force; he also chaired each of the individual DSM-III work groups. DSM-III was published in 1980 and was remarkably innovative, including: (1) specific and explicit criterion sets for all but one of the disorders (schizoaffective); (2) a substantially expanded text discussion of each disorder to facilitate diagnosis (e.g., age at onset, course, complications, sex ratio, and familial pattern); and (3) removal of terms (e.g., "neurosis") that appeared to favor a particular theoretical model (APA, 1980; Spitzer et al., 1980). Dr. Spitzer was the APA representative to ICD-9 and attempted to convince the WHO to include specific and explicit criterion sets. However, his repeated efforts were rebuffed given that the ICD-9 was being constructed primarily for the benefit of clinicians in settings in which the assessment of the lengthy criterion sets of DSM-III would not be particularly realistic (Reed, 2010). The ICD had to be acceptable to psychiatrists around the world—a very daunting task when one recognizes the variation in culture, values, and clinical practice across such diverse countries as China, Russia, Japan, Korea, India, and Germany. Obtaining agreement on behaviorally specific diagnostic criteria under these circumstances would be rather difficult. In frustration, Dr. Spitzer eventually stopped attending ICD-9 meetings.

DSM-III-R

A difficulty for DSM-III was an absence of much research to guide the construction of many of the criterion sets beyond Feighner et al. (1972). Subsequent research with the DSM-III criterion sets quickly revealed a number of errors and problems (e.g., panic disorder could not be diagnosed in the presence of a major depression). Dr. Spitzer therefore convinced the APA to develop DSM-III-R to address the problems that had been identified. It was not titled DSM-IV, because it was not a new edition in coordination with a fundamental revision of the ICD. DSM-III was to be revised only "for consistency, clarity, and conceptual accuracy" (APA, 1987, p. xvii).

However, it was perhaps unrealistic to expect the authors of DSM-III-R to confine their efforts to simply refinement, given the success of DSM-III and the acclaim given to its authors (Frances & Widiger, 2012). It was not difficult to find persons who wanted to be involved in DSM-III-R, and everyone involved wanted to have a significant impact. There were in fact many more persons involved in constructing DSM-III-R than had been involved in the construction of DSM-III. Not surprisingly, there were many proposals for significant revisions and even new diagnostic categories, despite the limited mandate.

The threshold for the inclusion of new diagnoses in DSM-III and DSM-III-R was also quite liberal. As expressed by Spitzer, Sheehy, and Endicott (1977), "if there is general agreement among clinicians, who would be expected to encounter the condition, that there are a significant number of patients who have it and that its identification is important in their clinical work, it is included in the classification" (p. 3). No actual research in the spirit of Robins and Guze (1970) was required. Four of the proposals approved by the task force for inclusion (i.e., sadistic personality disorder, self-defeating [or masochistic] personality disorder, premenstrual dysphoric disorder, and paraphiliac rapism) generated so much controversy that a special ad hoc committee was appointed by the Board of Trustees of the APA to reconsider their inclusion. A concern common to all four was that their inclusion might be harmful to women. For example, paraphiliac rapism might be used to mitigate the criminal responsibility of a serial rapist and self-defeating personality disorder might be used to blame female victims for having been abused. Another concern was the lack of sufficient empirical support to address or offset these concerns. A compromise was eventually reached in which the two personality disorders and premenstrual dysphoric disorder were included in an appendix (APA, 1987; Endicott, 2000; Widiger, 1995); paraphiliac rapism was deleted entirely.

DSM-IV and ICD-10

DSM-III-R was supposed to be completed in 1985 but was behind schedule. By the time work was completed on DSM-III-R, work had already begun on ICD-10 (WHO, 1992). Dr. Spitzer suggested that the DSM-III-R Task Force become the DSM-IV Task Force and simply continue their meetings and deliberations with the new directive to construct DSM-IV, but this proposal was rejected, in part because of the controversy over some of the proposals for DSM-III-R, his effort to expand the DSM-III-R beyond its original mandate, as well as the problematic relationship with the WHO that had developed during the construction of DSM-III.

In May 1988, the year after DSM-III-R was published (APA, 1987), the APA Board of Trustees appointed a DSM-IV Task Force, chaired by Allen Frances. Mandates for DSM-IV were to be more compatible with ICD-10, more user-friendly for the clinician, and more explicitly empirically based (Frances, Widiger, & Pincus, 1989). With respect to the third mandate, one of the more common concerns regarding DSM-III and DSM-III-R was the lack of compelling empirical support for the revisions and new diagnoses. It was often suggested that the decisions were more consistent with a priori wishes of work group members than with the published research (Gunderson, 1983). The primary authors of DSM-IV suggested that "the major innovation . . . will not be in its having surprising new content but rather will reside in the systematic and explicit method by which DSM-IV will be constructed and documented" (Frances et al., 1989, p. 375). Proposals for additions, deletions, and revisions were guided by 175 literature reviews that used a required format that maximized the potential for critical review, containing (for example) a method section that detailed explicitly the criteria for including and excluding studies and the process by which the literature had been reviewed (Frances et al., 1989). It was emphasized that the intention and focus of the literature reviews was not simply to make the best case for a respective proposal (Widiger, Frances, Pincus, Davis, & First, 1991). The authors were also required to acknowledge and address findings inconsistent with their proposals (Frances & Widiger, 2012). An explicit method of literature search was required to maximize the likelihood that it would be objective and systematic, including the specification of the criteria for study inclusion and exclusion, thereby making it difficult to confine the review to a limited set of studies that were most consistent with the viewpoints of the authors (Widiger et al., 1991). The reviews were published within a three-volume DSM-IV Sourcebook (e.g., Widiger et al., 1994). Testable questions that could be addressed with existing data sets were explored in 36 studies funded by the MacArthur Foundation, which emphasized the aggregation of multiple data sets from independent researchers. Twelve field trials, funded by the NIMH, were conducted to provide reliability and validity data on proposed revisions. Each field trial had to compare a proposal with the respective DSM-III-R diagnosis (if such was available). The results of the 36 studies and 12 field trials were published in the fourth volume of the DSM-IV Sourcebook (Widiger et al., 1998). Critical reviews of these 223 projects were obtained by sending initial drafts to advisors or consultants to a respective work group, by presenting drafts at relevant conferences, and by submitting drafts to peer-reviewed journals (Widiger et al., 1991).

Dr. Frances had for some time advocated a shift to a dimensional model of classification, particularly for the personality disorders, his own area of specialty (Frances, 1980, 1982; Widiger & Frances, 1985). However, DSM-IV continued with the categorical diagnoses, including for the personality disorders (APA, 1994). A problem at the time of DSM-IV was the presence of many alternative dimensional models of personality disorder, with no apparent common ground. Providing only one model would be quite narrow, if not biased; providing all of them would be unduly complex and confusing. Therefore, a model that provided a good-faith effort to represent the primary alternatives was proposed. "The proposal [consisted] of extraversion, neuroticism, constraint, antagonism (versus agreeableness), openness, reward dependence, and cognitive disorganization (developed in consultation with Drs. Cloninger, Costa, Eysenck, McCrae, Siever, Tellegen, and Wiggins)" (Widiger, 1996, p. 795). The proposal was ultimately rejected, as it was considered to be too complex (Gunderson, 1996). Frances et al. (1995) also suggested that the dimensional trait proponents were too much in disagreement with one another and could not therefore settle on one unifying model.

The decision of the authors of DSM-III to develop an alternative to ICD-9 was instrumental in developing a highly innovative manual (Kendell, 1991; Spitzer et al., 1980). However, its innovations were also at the cost of decreasing compatibility with the ICD-9 nomenclature that was used throughout the rest of the world, which is problematic to the stated purpose of providing a common language for psychiatry. As noted earlier, one of the mandates for DSM-IV was to increase compatibility with the ICD. Dr. Frances required each DSM-IV work group to include at least one feature from a respective ICD-10 proposal as an explicit gesture of improving coordination (Widiger, Mangine, Corbitt, Ellis, & Thomas, 1995).

The authors of ICD-10 again considered replacing the narrative descriptions of each disorder with the specific and explicit criterion sets that were instrumental in the success of DSM-III. However, they retained the narrative paragraph format of ICD-9. Researchers can devote more than two hours to assess the personality disorder diagnostic criteria, but this is unrealistic for the general practitioner (Mullins-Sweatt & Widiger, 2009). The WHO did provide separate versions of ICD-10 for the researcher and for the clinician (Sartorius, 1988; Sartorius et al., 1993). The researcher's version included relatively more specific and explicit criterion sets (although not to the extent of DSM-III or DSM-IV), whereas the clinician's version included only the narrative descriptions. The DSM-IV Task Force in turn considered this option of different versions for the researcher and the clinician but decided that it would complicate the generalization of research findings to clinical practice, and vice versa (Frances et al., 1990). The DSM-IV Task Force also questioned the implication of providing more reliable criterion sets for researchers, and simpler, less reliable criterion sets for clinical decisions, as if diagnoses in clinical practice did not need to be as reliable or valid as the diagnoses obtained for research.

DSM-IV-TR

One of the innovations of DSM-III was the inclusion of a relatively detailed text discussion of each disorder, including information on age of onset, gender, course, and familial pattern (Spitzer et al., 1980). This text was expanded in DSM-IV to include cultural and ethnic group variation, variation across age, and laboratory and physical exam findings (Frances et al., 1995). No such information was provided within the ICD. Largely excluded from the text was information concerning etiology, pathology, and treatment, as this material was considered to be too theoretically specific and more suitable for academic texts. Nevertheless, it had also become apparent that DSM-IV was being used as a textbook, and the material on age, course, prevalence, and family history was quickly becoming outdated as new information was obtained.

Therefore, in 1997, the APA appointed a DSM-IV Text Revision Work Group, chaired by Michael First (Editor of the Text and Criterion Sets for DSM-IV) and Harold Pincus (Vice-Chair for DSM-IV) to update the text material. No substantive changes in the criterion sets were to be considered, nor were any new additions, subtypes, deletions, or other changes in the status of any diagnosis to be implemented. In addition, each of the proposed revisions to the text had to be supported by a systematic literature review (including citations and a reference list) that was critiqued by external advisors. The DSM-IV Text Revision (DSM-IV-TR) was published in 2000 (APA, 2000).

The outcome, however, was not entirely consistent with the original intentions. Significant revisions were made to the criterion sets for the tic disorders and for the paraphilias that involved a nonconsenting victim (First & Pincus, 2002), albeit no acknowledgments of these revisions were provided within the manual. In addition, no documentation of the scientific support for the text revisions was provided, due to the inconsistency in the quality of the work (e.g., some authors clearly emphasized their own work rather than provide a fair and balanced summary of the research literature). Rather than have inconsistent and/or inadequate documentation, it was decided to have none at all.

DSM-5 and ICD-11

The development of DSM-5 was preceded by a series of preparatory conferences, much of which was concerned with shifting the nomenclature to a dimensional model. The first "DSM-V Research Planning Conference" was held in October 1999. The Nomenclature Work Group of this conference concluded that it would be "important that consideration be given to advantages and disadvantages of basing part or all of DSM-V on dimensions rather than categories" (Rounsaville et al., 2002, p. 13). This work group suggested that this shift was most clearly suited for the personality disorders. "If a dimensional system of personality performs well and is acceptable to clinicians, it might then be appropriate to explore dimensional approaches in other domains" (Rounsaville et al., 2002, p. 13).

The Personality Disorders and Relational Disorders Work Group summarized the research in support of shifting the personality disorders to a dimensional trait model and identified the primary alternatives (First et al., 2002). They recommended that DSM-5 revise "the classification of personality disorders using a dimensional approach that avoids the artificiality of the current categorical approach and facilitates the identification and communication of the patient's clinically relevant personality traits" (First et al., 2002, p. 179).

This initial DSM-5 preparatory conference was followed by a series of international conferences, which included some of the future authors of ICD-11. The first, "Dimensional Models of Personality Disorder: Etiology, Pathology, Phenomenology, & Treatment," was held in December 2004. Its purpose was to review the literature and set a research agenda "that would be most effective in leading the field toward a dimensional classification of personality disorder" (Widiger, Simonsen, Krueger, Livesley, & Verheul, 2005, p. 315). An integration of existing models was proposed, consisting of the four domains of emotional dysregulation versus emotional stability, extraversion versus introversion, antagonism versus compliance, and constraint versus impulsivity. It was suggested, though, that a fifth broad domain, unconventionality versus closed to experience, would be necessary to be fully comprehensive in its coverage of maladaptive personality traits. Unconventionality versus closedness was not within the integrative model because it is was not included within some of the predominant systems, such as Livesley's four-dimensional model, assessed by the Dimensional Assessment of Personality Pathology-Basic Questionnaire (DAPP-BQ; Livesley & Jackson, 2009), and Clark's three-factor model, assessed by the Schedule for Nonadaptive and Adaptive Personality (SNAP; Clark, Simms, Wu, & Casillas, in press). However, unconventionality versus closedness was included within the five-factor model of general personality structure (Widiger & Trull, 2007).

The seventh and final of the international conferences series was devoted to redefining much of the entire manual, including the mood, anxiety, and other disorders, to fundamental dimensions (Helzer et al., 2008). It should be noted that the authors of these chapters would not necessarily be appointed to a respective DSM-5 work group (although many were eventually appointed); their proposals therefore should be understood as suggestions or speculations with respect to what might occur. For example, Helzer, Bucholz, and Gossup (2008) recommended that each of the diagnostic criteria for substance use disorders be scored on a dimensional scale. Andrews et al. (2008) recommended that DSM-5 include a supplemental scale for assessing major depressive episodes quantitatively. Shear, Bjelland, Beesdo, Glostor, and Wittchen (2008) provided a comparable recommendation for the anxiety disorders, along with a proposal to include a higher-order cross-cutting dimension (comparable to internalization) that would cover both the anxiety and mood disorders. Krueger, Skodol, Livesley,

Shrout, and Huang (2008) recommended that the DSM-5 shift the personality disorders to a dimensional trait model, and presented Livesley's DAPP-BQ (Livesley & Jackson, 2009) as an illustrative example.

The principal authors of DSM-5 intended this next revision to provide a "paradigm shift" (Kupfer, First, & Regier, 2002, p. xix); more specifically, toward a dimensional classification of psychopathology. "We have decided that one, if not the major difference, between DSM-IV and DSM-V will be the more prominent use of dimensional measures" (Regier et al., 2009, p. 649). However, in the end, it was acknowledged in the introduction to the diagnostic manual that "DSM-5 remains a categorical classification of separate disorders" (APA, 2013, p. xii). Note that Regier et al. (2009) had referred to the inclusion of dimensional "measures," not a shift to dimensional constructs. "What is being proposed for DSM-V is not to substitute dimensional scales for categorical diagnoses, but to add a dimensional option to the usual categorical diagnoses for DSM-V" (Kraemer, 2008, p. 9).

However, some revisions did reflect shifts toward a dimensional model of classification (APA, 2013, 2022). Autism and schizophrenia were explicitly conceptualized as spectrum disorders, with different variants existing along a common dimension of underlying pathology. The problematic distinction between substance abuse and dependence was eliminated and replaced by a level of severity. The DSM-IV disorders of hypochondriasis, somatization, and pain disorder were collapsed into one category of somatic symptom disorder with three levels of severity (APA, 2013). Within the introductory text of DSM-5, some disorders were reorganized within internalizing (anxiety, depressive, and somatic) and externalizing (impulsive, disruptive, and substance use) domains (APA, 2013), consistent with research conducted on disorders of childhood (Achenbach & Edelbrock, 1984) and adulthood (Krueger, McGue, & Iacono, 2001).

The most dramatic shift was proposed for the personality disorders, consistent with Rounsaville et al. (2002). Proposed for DSM-5 was an Alternative Model for Personality Disorders (AMPD), which included a level of personality functioning scale describing self and interpersonal pathology from psychodynamic theory (Kernberg, 2012; Sharp & Wall, 2021) and a five-domain 25-trait dimensional model of maladaptive personality functioning, consisting of negative affectivity, detachment, antagonism, disinhibition, and psychoticism that was aligned with the five-factor model of general personality structure (Krueger et al., 2011). These two components served as the basis for the criterion sets for six diagnostic categories retained from DSM-IV (i.e., antisocial, borderline, schizotypal, obsessive-compulsive, avoidant, and narcissistic).

Two of the Personality Disorder Work Group members resigned in the final year of its deliberation, in part because they felt the process with which it was being constructed was not well grounded in the research, but also because they felt that the proposed revisions were too conservative (i.e., Livesley, 2012; Verheul, 2012). The proposals for DSM-5 were ultimately rejected by the DSM-5 oversight committees and the APA Board of Trustees (Krueger, 2013; Skodol, Morey, Bender, & Oldham, 2013; Widiger, 2013). The proposals were relegated to Section III of DSM-5 for emerging measures and models (APA, 2013). The official personality disorder section was essentially unchanged from DSM-IV.

It is also worth noting that Frances, the Chair of DSM-IV and a longtime advocate of shifting the personality disorders to a dimensional trait model (Frances, 1980, 1982), was actually strongly critical of the DSM-5 AMPD. In a rather unbridled critique of the proposal, he characterized it as "unreliable, untested, and impossibly complicated" (Frances, 2023, p. 21).

The personality disorders section was not the only problem for DSM-5. The development of DSM-5 was beset by a number of controversies. The development of DSM-5 may have gotten off on the wrong foot with the requirement that work group and task force members sign confidentiality agreements (Greenburg, 2013; Wakefield, 2016). No such requirement had previously been imposed on the authors of DSM-IV or any prior edition. It is perhaps understandable for a work group not to want to have preliminary ideas disseminated prematurely. Work group members will float ideas that might be outrageously flawed and rejected fairly quickly. However, significant concerns with respect to the process with which DSM-5 was being constructed were raised by Robert Spitzer, Chair of DSM-III and DSM-III-R, after being denied minutes of DSM-5 Work Group meetings (Greenburg, 2013). Drs. Frances and Spitzer (Chairs of DSM-IV and DSM-III, respectively) eventually submitted a joint letter to the Board of Trustees of the APA on July 7, 2009, expressing concerns with respect to the process with which DSM-5 was being constructed (particularly the absence of compelling empirical support), including the confidentiality agreements (Greenburg, 2013).

The letter by Frances and Spitzer was initiated by the fact that the field trial for DSM-5 was about to begin before the proposals had received any critical review and before some had even been revealed. Frances followed this joint letter with additional letters of his own and a series of articles and blog posts that eventually led to the decision of the DSM-5 Task Force to postpone the field trial until after all of the proposals had been posted on a website in February 2010, thereby allowing for public awareness and external review. The website posting, though, resulted in considerable objection and opposition to many of the proposals, vindicating the concerns raised by Spitzer and Frances.

There was also considerable interest in shifting ICD-11 (WHO, 2023) to a more dimensional model of classification (Maercker, Rebellow, Ritchie, & Reed, 2024). In their summary of the changes that occurred for ICD-11, Reed et al. (2019) stated that a "major innovation in the ICD-11 classification has been the incorporation of dimensional approaches" (p. 5). However, the shifts for ICD-11 were, for the most part, minor. As acknowledged by Reed (2023), "the innovation is the integration of dimensional approaches *within the categorical structure of ICD-11*" (p. 12, our emphasis). The schizophrenia subtypes of ICD-10 were replaced by underlying dimensions of "positive symptoms (delusions, hallucinations, disorganized thinking and behaviour, experiences of passivity and control); negative symptoms (constricted, blunted or flat affect, alogia or paucity of speech, avolition, anhedonia); depressive mood symptoms; manic mood symptoms; psychomotor symptoms (psychomotor agitation, psychomotor retardation, catatonic symptoms); and cognitive symptoms (particularly deficits in speed of processing attention/concentration, orientation, judgment, abstraction, verbal or visual learning, and working memory)" (Reed et al., 2019, p. 11). The personality disorders section of ICD-11 was substantially shifted toward a dimensional trait model (Reed, 2018).

Work on the DSM-5 AMPD was well underway when work began on the ICD-11 personality disorders (Tyrer, Mulder, Kim, & Crawford, 2019). Lee Anna Clark was the DSM-5 representative to the ICD-11 Personality and Personality Disorders Working Group. The ICD-11 did not initially receive much opposition, despite the fact that the proposal for the personality disorders provided a much more radical shift than did the DSM-5 AMPD (Widiger, Tyrer, McCabe, & Kim, in press). The ICD-11 personality disorders section consists of largely three components: a level of personality disorder severity; a dimensional trait model (negative affectivity, detachment, dissociality, disinhibition, and anankastia [compulsivity]); and a borderline pattern specifier (Swales, Clark, & Farnam, 2024). The original ICD-11 level of severity was confined to a relatively small set of maladaptive traits, obtained from the dimensional trait model, along with impairments secondary to these traits. As stated by Tyrer (2014), the Chair of the ICD-11 Personality Disorders Working Group, "the ICD-11 classification contains no assessment of self-pathology" (p. 723). However, in the final year of its consideration, the ICD-11 proposal received substantial external opposition (i.e:, Herpertz et al., 2017). In an effort to address the opposition, the ICD-11 level of severity was substantially revised to emphasize the self-interpersonal impairments, comparable to those provided in the DSM-5 AMPD (Tyrer, Mulder, Kim, & Crawford, 2019), while still retaining some aspects from the original level of severity (Bach et al., 2021; Reed, 2018). The ICD-11 level of severity concerns "a) the degree and pervasiveness of disturbances in functioning of aspects of the self (e.g., stability and coherence of identity, self-worth, accuracy of self-view, capacity for self direction); b) the degree and pervasiveness of interpersonal dysfunction (e.g., understanding others' perspectives, developing and maintaining close relationships, managing conflict) across various contexts and relationships; c) the pervasiveness, severity and chronicity of emotional, cognitive and behavioural manifestations of personality dysfunction; and d) the extent to which these patterns are associated with distress or psychosocial impairment" (Reed et al., 2019, p. 16; see also Bach et al., 2021).

It is again worth noting that Frances (2023) was also critical of the ICD-11 shift to a dimensional trait model. He did not mince words. "The ICD-11 approach is entirely new, disturbingly radical, completely unfamiliar and totally untested" (Frances, 2023, p. 21). He characterized it as "half-baked and not ready for prime time" (p. 21). This appears to have been rather disconcerting for the editor of the text in which Frances' chapter appears. The editor was Peter Tyrer, who was the principal author of the ICD-11 personality disorders. In a rather unusual move, Tyrer (2023) included editorial remarks in the chapter by Frances, indicating where he felt that Frances was not providing an accurate summary of the process with which ICD-11 was developed or its empirical support. Mulder (2023) provided a summary of the extensive empirical support for the ICD-11 personality disorders in a subsequent chapter within the same edited text.

The DSM-5 AMPD was said to be providing a paradigm shift in the classification of personality disorder (Skodol, 2012; Skodol, Morey, Bender, & Oldham, 2013). However, this status is perhaps more appropriately awarded to the ICD-11 (Krueger, 2016; Tyrer, 2014). The DSM-5 AMPD proposal retained six of the DSM-IV personality disorder syndromes. If DSM-5 AMPD had been adopted, it is quite possible that there would have been little change in clinical practice, as clinicians would still be focused on the six diagnostic categories rather than the level of personality functioning or the dimensional trait model. The ICD-11 retains only one of the prior diagnostic categories (borderline) and, perhaps of most significance, it was officially approved by the WHO, whereas the DSM-5 AMPD was rejected. However, the DSM-5 AMPD has generated a considerable amount of research attention (Garcia, Gutierrez, Garcia, & Aluja, in press; Sharp & Wall, 2021; Widiger & Hines, 2022; Zimmermann, Kerber, Rek, Hopwood, & Krueger, 2019).

Conclusions

As noted earlier, the modern effort to demarcate a taxonomy of distinct clinical conditions is often traced to Kraepelin (Kendell, 1975; Spitzer et al., 1980). Kraepelin (1917), however, had himself acknowledged, "wherever we try to mark out the frontier between mental health and disease, we find a neutral territory, in which the imperceptible change from the realm of normal life to that of obvious derangement takes place" (p. 295).

In 1989, L. Robins and Barrett (1989) edited a text in honor of the historical contribution of Robins and Guze (1970), who had formulated the predominant model for the validation of psychopathology diagnostic categories. Kendell (1989) provided the final word in his closing chapter. His conclusions, however, were curiously negative. "Ninety years have now elapsed since Kraepelin first provided the framework of a plausible classification of mental disorders. Why then, with so many potential validators available, have we made so little progress since that time?" (Kendell, 1989, p. 313). He answered his rhetorical question in the next paragraph:

"One important possibility is that the discrete clusters of psychiatric symptoms we are trying to delineate do not actually exist but are as much a mirage as discrete personality types" (Kendell, 1989, p. 313).

In the future, neither the DSM nor the ICD is likely to undergo major revisions at one particular time. The WHO is more interested in helping member countries around the world to implement more effective medical services, rather than spending a considerable amount of money, time, and effort in revising diagnostic nomenclatures. A singular overhaul of the entire diagnostic manual also encourages substantial and unnecessary revisions (i.e., work group members are not going to spend four to six years on a committee that implements no change at all; Frances & Widiger, 2012). The APA as well is shifting away from conducting massive, singular overhauls of the DSM in favor of simply having a standing committee, the DSM-5 Revision Steering Committee (initially chaired by Paul Appelbaum), to which persons can submit proposals at any time it is believed that a revision or addition has become suitable. Indeed, this APA committee has been considering a proposal to shift the personality disorders section toward a dimensional model that would be consistent with ICD-11.

References

Achenbach, T. M., & Edelbrock, C. S. (1984). Psychopathology of childhood. *Annual Review of Psychology, 35*, 227–256.

American Psychiatric Association. (1952). *Diagnostic and statistical manual. Mental Disorders*. Author.

American Psychiatric Association. (1980). *Diagnostic and statistical manual of mental disorders* (3rd ed.).Author.

American Psychiatric Association. (1987). *Diagnostic and statistical manual of mental disorders* (3rd ed., rev. ed.).Author.

American Psychiatric Association. (1994). *Diagnostic and statistical manual of mental disorders* (4th ed.).Author.

American Psychiatric Association. (2000). *Diagnostic and statistical manual of mental disorders. Text revision* (4th ed., rev. ed.).Author.

American Psychiatric Association. (2013). *Diagnostic and statistical manual of mental disorders* (5th ed.).Author.

American Psychiatric Association. (2022). *Diagnostic and statistical manual of mental disorders. Text revision* (5th ed., rev. ed.).Author.

Andrews, G., Bruggha, T., Thase, M. E., Duffy, F. F., Rucci, P. and Slade, T. (2008). Dimensionality and the category of major depressive episode. In J. E. Helzer, H. C. Kraemer, R. F. Krueger, H-U Wittchen, P. J., Sirovatka, & D. Regier (Eds.), *Dimensional approaches in diagnostic classification* (pp. 35–51).American Psychiatric Association.

Bach, B., Brown, T. A., Mulder, R. T., Newton-Howes, G., Simonsen, E., & Sellbom, M. (2021). Development and initial evaluation of the ICD-11 personality disorder severity scale: PDS-ICD-11. *Personality and Mental Health, 15*, 223–236.

Clark, L. A., Simms, L. J., Wu, K. D., & Casillas, A. (in press). *Manual for the schedule for nonadaptive and adaptive personality (SNAP-2)*.University of Minnesota Press.

Deary, I. J., Spinath, F. M., & Bates, T. C. (2006). Genetics of intelligence. *European Journal of Human Genetics, 14*, 690–700.

Endicott, J. (2000). History, evolution, and diagnosis of premenstrual dysphoric disorder. *Journal of Clinical Psychiatry, 62* (suppl. 24), 5–8.

Feighner, J. P., Robins, E., Guze, S. B., Woodruff, R. A., Winokur, G., & Munoz, R. (1972). Diagnostic criteria for use in psychiatric research. *Archives of General Psychiatry, 26*, 57–63.

First, M. B. (2003). Psychiatric classification. In A. Tasman, J. Kay, & J. Lieberman (Eds.), *Psychiatry* (2nd ed., Vol. 1, pp. 659–676).Wiley.

First, M. B., Bell, C. B., Cuthbert, B., Krystal, J. H., Malison, R., Offord, D. R., Reiss, D., Shea, M. T., Widiger, T. A., & Wisner, K. L. (2002). Personality disorders and relational disorders: A research agenda for addressing crucial gaps in DSM. In D. J. Kupfer, M. B. First, & D. A. Regier (Eds.), *A research agenda for DSM-V* (pp. 123–199)American Psychiatric Association.
First, M. B., & Pincus, H. A. (2002). The DSM-IV text revision: Rationale and potential impact on clinical practice. *Psychiatric Services, 53*, 288–292.
Frances, A. J. (1980). The DSM-III personality disorders section: A commentary. *American Journal of Psychiatry, 137*, 1050–1054.
Frances, A. J. (1982). Categorical and dimensional systems of personality diagnosis: A comparison. *Comprehensive Psychiatry, 23*, 516–527.
Frances, A. J. (2023). ICD-11 + DSM-5 = a diagnostic babel. In P. Tyrer (Ed.), *Making sense of the ICD-11 for mental health professionals* (pp. 17–24). Cambridge University Press.
Frances, A. J., First, M. B., & Pincus, H. A. (1995). *DSM-IV guidebook*.American Psychiatric Press.
Frances, A. J., Pincus, H. A., Widiger, T. A., Davis, W. W., & First, M. B. (1990). DSM-IV: Work in progress. *American Journal of Psychiatry, 147*, 1439–1448.
Frances, A. J., & Widiger, T. A. (2012). Psychiatric diagnosis: Lessons from the DSM-IV past and cautions for the DSM-5 future. *Annual Review of Clinical Psychology, 8*, 109–130.
Frances, A. J., Widiger, T. A., & Pincus, H. A. (1989). The development of DSM-IV. *Archives of General Psychiatry, 46*, 373–375.
Garcia, L. F., Gutierrez, F., Garcia, O., & Aluja, A. (in press). The Alternative Model of Personality Disorders: Assessment, convergent and discriminant validity, and a look to the future. *Annual Review of Clinical Psychology*.
Greenberg, G. (2013). *The book of woe: The DSM and the unmaking of psychiatry*. Blue Rider Press.
Grob, G. N. (1991). Origins of DSM-I: A study in appearance and reality. *American Journal of Psychiatry, 148*, 421–431.
Gunderson, J. G. (1983). DSM-III diagnoses of personality disorders. In J. Frosch (Ed.), *Current perspectives on personality disorders* (pp. 20–39).American Psychiatric Press.
Gunderson, J. G. (1996). Personality disorders. In T. A. Widiger, A. J. Frances, H. A. Pincus, R. Ross, M. B. First, & W. W. Davis (Eds.), *DSM-IV source*book (Vol. 2, pp. 647–664).American Psychiatric Association.
Gureje, O. (2015). Classification of somatic syndromes in ICD-11. *Current Opinion in Psychiatry, 28*, 345–349.
Helzer, J. E., Bucholz, K. K., & Gossop, M. (2008). A dimensional option for the diagnosis of substance dependence in DSM-V. In J. E. Helzer, H. C. Kraemer, R. F. Krueger; H-U Wittchen, P. J., Sirovatka, & D. Regier (Eds.), *Dimensional approaches in diagnostic classification* (pp. 19–34).American Psychiatric Association.
Helzer, J. E., Kraemer, H. C. Krueger, R. F., Wittchen, H-U., Sirovatka, P. J., & Regier, D. (Eds.). (2008). *Dimensional approaches in diagnostic classification*. American Psychiatric Association.
Herpertz, S. C., Huprich, S. K., Bohus, M., Chanen, A., Goodman, M., Mehlum, L., Moran, P., Newton-Howes, G., Scott, L., & Sharp, C. (2017). The challenge of transforming the diagnostic system of personality disorders. *Journal of Personality Disorders, 31*, 577–589.
Hyman, S. E. (2010). The diagnosis of mental disorders: The problem of reification. *Annual Review of Clinical Psychology, 6*, 155–179.
Insel, T. R. (2014). The NIMH research domain criteria (RDoC) project: Precision medicine for psychiatry. *American Journal of Psychiatry, 171*, 395–397.
Insel, T. R., & Quirion, R. (2005). Psychiatry as a clinical neuroscience discipline. *Journal of the American Medical Association, 294*, 2221–2224.
Keeley, J. W., Chung, L., & Kleva, C. (2023). Classification in traditional nosologies. In R. F. Krueger & P. H. Blaney (Eds.), *Oxford handbook of psychopathology* (4th ed., pp. 3–32). Oxford University Press.
Kendell, R. E. (1975). *The role of diagnosis in psychiatry*. Blackwell Scientific Publications.
Kendell, R. E. (1989). Clinical validity. In L. N. Robins & J. E. Barrett (Eds.), *The validity of psychiatric diagnosis* (pp. 305–321). Raven Press.

Kendell, R. E. (1991). Relationship between the DSM-IV and the ICD-10. *Journal of Abnormal Psychology, 100*, 297–301.

Kendell, R. E., & Jablensky, A. (2003). Distinguishing between the validity and utility of psychiatric diagnosis. *American Journal of Psychiatry, 160*, 4–12.

Kernberg, O. F. (2012). Overview and critique of the classification of personality disorders proposed for DSM-V. *Swiss Archives of Neurology and Psychiatry, 163*, 234–238.

Kraemer, H. C. (2008). DSM categories and dimensions in clinical and research contexts. In J. E. Helzer, H. C. Kraemer, R. F. Krueger, H-U. Wittchen, P. J. Sirovatka, & D. A. Regier (Eds.), *Dimensional approaches to diagnostic classification. Refining the research agenda for DSM-V* (pp. 5–17).American Psychiatric Association.

Kraepelin, E. (1917). *Lectures on clinical psych*iatry (3rd ed.). William Wood.

Kramer, M., Sartorius, N., Jablensky, A., & Gulbinat, W. (1979). The ICD-9 classification of mental disorders. A review of its development and contents. *Acta Psychiatrica Scandinavika, 59*, 241–262.

Krueger, R. F. (2013). Personality disorders are the vanguard of the post-DSM-5.0 era. *Personality Disorders: Theory, Research, and Treatment, 4*, 355–362.

Krueger, R. F. (2016). The future is now: Personality disorder and the ICD-11. *Personality and Mental Health, 10*(2), 118–119.

Krueger, R. F., Eaton, N. R., Clark, L. A., Watson, D., Markon, K. E., Derringer, J., Skodol, A., & Livesley, W. J. (2011). Deriving an empirical structure of personality pathology for DSM-5. *Journal of Personality Disorders, 25*, 170–191.

Krueger, R. F., McGue, M., & Iacono, W. G. (2001). The higher-order structure of common DSM mental disorders: Internalization, externalization, and their connections to personality. *Personality and Individual Differences, 30*, 1245–1259.

Krueger, R. F., Skodol, A. E., Livesley, W. J., Shrout, P. E., & Huang, Y. (2008). Synthesizing dimensional and categorical approaches to personality disorders: Refining the research agenda for DSM-V Axis II. In J. E. Helzer, H. C. Kraemer, R. F. Krueger, H-U Wittchen, P. J., Sirovatka, & D. Regier (Eds.). (2008). *Dimensional approaches in diagnostic classification* (pp. 19–34).American Psychiatric Association.

Krueger, R. F., Watson, D., & Barlow, D. H. (2005). Introduction to the special section: Toward a dimensionally based taxonomy of psychopathology. *Journal of Abnormal Psychology, 114*, 491–493.

Kupfer, D. J., First, M. B., & Regier, D. A. (2002). Introduction. In D. J. Kupfer, M. B. First, & D. A. Regier (Eds.), *A research agenda for DSM-V* (pp. xv–xxiii). American Psychiatric Association.

Lilienfeld, S. O., & Treadway, M. T. (2016). Clashing diagnostic approaches: DSM-ICD versus RDoC. *Annual Review of Clinical Psychology, 12*, 435–463.

Livesley, W. J. (2012). Tradition versus empiricism in the current DSM-5 proposal for revising the classification of personality disorders. *Criminal Behavior and Mental Health*, 22, 81–90.

Livesley, W. J., & Jackson, D. (2009). *Manual for the dimensional assessment of personality pathology—Basic questionnaire*. Sigma Press.

Maercker, A., Rebellow, T. J., Ritchie, P, L-J., & Reed, G. M. (2024). A psychological approach to diagnosis. In G. M. Reed, P-J Ritchie, & A. Maercker (Eds.), *A psychological approach to diagnosis using the ICD-11 as a framework* (pp. 3–22).American Psychological Association and the International Union of Psychological Science.

Malinow, K. (1981). Passive-aggressive personality. In J. Lion (Ed.), *Personality disorders* (2nd ed., pp. 121–132).Williams & Wilkins.

Markon, K. (2013). Epistemological pluralism and scientific development: An argument against authoritative nosologies. *Journal of Personality Disorders, 27*, 554–579.

Menninger, K. (1963). *The vital balance*. Viking Press.

Mulder, R. (2023). Personality disorders. In P. Tyrer (Ed.), *Making sense of the ICD-11 for mental health professionals* (pp. 110–121). Cambridge University Press.

Mullins-Sweatt, S. N., & Widiger, T. A. (2009). Clinical utility and DSM-V. *Psychological Assessment, 21*, 302–312.

Naglieri, J., Salter, C., & Rojahn, J. (2008). Cognitive disorders of childhood: Specific learning and intellectual disabilities. In J. E. Maddux & B. A. Winstead (Eds.), *Psychopathology: Foundations for a contemporary understanding* (2nd ed., pp. 401–416). Routledge/Taylor & Francis Group.

Patel, D. R., Cabral, M. D., Ho, A., & Merrick, J. (2020). A clinical primer on intellectual disability. *Translational Pediatrics*, 9(Suppl 1), S23.
Reed, G. M. (2010). Toward ICD-11: Improving the clinical utility of WHO's International Classification of Mental Disorders. *Professional Psychology: Research and Practice*, *41*, 457–464.
Reed, G. M. (2018). Progress in developing a classification of personality disorders for ICD-11. *World Psychiatry*, *17*, 227–229.
Reed, G. M. (2023). Development and innovation in the ICD-11 chapter on mental, behavioural, and neurodevelopmental disorders. In P. Tyrer (Ed.), *Making sense of the ICD- 11 for mental health professionals* (pp. 5–16). Cambridge University Press.
Reed, G. M., First, M. B., Kogan, C. S., Hyman, S. E., Gureje, C., Gaebel, W., Maj, M., Stein, D. J., Maercker, A., Tyrer, P., & Saxena, S. (2019). Innovations and changes in the ICD-11 classification of mental, behavioural and neurodevelopmental disorders. *World Psychiatry*, *18*, 3–19.
Regier, D. A., Narrow, W. E., Kuhl, E. A., & Kupfer, D. J. (2009). The conceptual development of DSM-V. *American Journal of Psychiatry*, *166*, 645–655.
Robins, E., & Guze, S. B. (1970). Establishment of diagnostic validity in psychiatric illness: Its application to schizophrenia. *American Journal of Psychiatry*, *126*, 107–111.
Robins, L. N., & Barrett, J. E. (Eds.). (1989). *The validity of psychiatric diagnosis*. Raven Press.
Rosenhan, D. L. (1973). On being sane in insane places. *Science*, *179*, 250–258.
Rounsaville, B. J., Alarcon, R. D., Andrews, G., Jackson, J. S., Kendell, R. E., Kendler, K. S., & Kirmayer, L. J. (2002). Toward DSM-V: Basic nomenclature issues. In D. J. Kupfer, M. B. First, & D. A. Regier (Eds.), *A research agenda for DSM-V* (pp. 1–30). American Psychiatric Press.
Roy, A., & Kogan, C. S. (2024). Disorders of intellectual development and developmental learning disorders. In G. M. Reed, P-J Ritchie, & A. Maercker (Eds.), *A psychological approach to diagnosis using the ICD-11 as a framework* (pp. 41–59).American Psychological Association and the International Union of Psychological Science.
Salmon, T. W., Copp, O., May, J. V., Abbot, E. S., & Cotton, H. A. (1917). Report of the committee on statistics of the American Medico-Psychological Association. *American Journal of Insanity*, *74*, 255–260.
Sartorius, N. (1988). International perspectives of psychiatric classification. *British Journal of Psychiatry*, *152* (supplement), 9–14.
Sartorius, N., Kaelber, C. T., Cooper, J .E., Roper, M., Rae, D. S., Gulbinat, W., Ustun, T. B., & Regier, D. A. (1993). Progress toward achieving a common language in psychiatry. *Archives of General Psychiatry*, *50*, 115–124.
Schalock, R. L., Luckasson, R., & Tassé, M. J. (2021). An overview of intellectual disability: Definition, diagnosis, classification, and systems of supports (12th ed.). *American Journal on Intellectual and Developmental Disabilities*, *126*(6), 439–442.
Sharp, C., & Wall, K. (2021). DSM-5 level of personality functioning: Refocusing personality disorder on what it means to be human. *Annual Review of Clinical Psychology*, *17*, 313–337.
Shear, M. K., Bjelland, I., Beesdo, K., Glostor, A. T., & Wittchen, H-U. (2008). Supplemental dimensional assessment in anxiety disorders. In J. E. Helzer, H. C. Kraemer, R. F. Krueger, H-U Wittchen, P. J. Sirovatka, & D. Regier (Eds.), (2008). *Dimensional approaches in diagnostic classification* (pp. 85–100).American Psychiatric Association.
Skodol, A. (2012). Diagnosis and DSM-5: Work in progress. In T. A. Widiger (Ed.), *The Oxford handbook of personality disorders* (pp. 35–57). Oxford University Press.
Skodol, A. E., Morey, L. C., Bender, D. S., & Oldham, J. M. (2013). The ironic fate of the personality disorders in DSM-5. *Personality Disorders: Theory, Research, & Treatment*, *4*, 342–349.
Spitzer, R. L. (1973). A proposal about homosexuality and the APA nomenclature: Homosexuality as an irregular form of sexual behavior and sexual orientation disturbance as a psychiatric disorder. *American Journal of Psychiatry*, *130*, 1214–1216.
Spitzer, R. L., & Robins, E. (1978). Research diagnostic criteria: Rationale and reliability. *Archives of General Psychiatry*, *35*, 773–782.
Spitzer, R. L., Sheehy, M., & Endicott, J. (1977). DSM-III: Guiding principles. In V. Rakoff, H. Stancer, & H. Kedward (Eds.), *Psychiatric diagnosis* (pp. 1–24). Brunner/Mazel.

Spitzer, R. L., Williams, J. B. W., & Skodol, A. E. (1980). DSM-III: The major achievements and an overview. *American Journal of Psychiatry*, *137*, 151–164.

Spitzer, R. L., & Wilson, P. T. (1968). A guide to the American Psychiatric Association's new diagnostic nomenclature. *American Journal of Psychiatry*, *124*, 1619–1629.

Stengel, E. (1959). Classification of mental disorders. *Bulletin of the World Health Organization*, *21*, 601–663.

Swales, M. A., Clark, L. A., & Farnam, A. (2024). Personality disorder. In G. M. Reed, P-J Ritchie, & A. Maercker (Eds.), *A psychological approach to diagnosis using the ICD-11 as a framework* (pp. 311–326).American Psychological Association and the International Union of Psychological Science.

Tyrer, P. (2014). The likely classification of borderline personality disorder in adolescents in ICD-11. In C. Sharp & J. Tackett (Eds.), *Handbook of borderline personality disorder in children and adolescents* (pp. 451–457). Springer.

Tyrer, P. (Ed.). (2023). *Making sense of the ICD-11 for mental health professionals*. Cambridge University Press.

Tyrer, P., Mulder, R., Kim, Y. R., & Crawford, M. J. (2019). The development of the ICD-11 classification of personality disorders: An amalgam of science, pragmatism, and politics. *Annual Review of Clinical Psychology*, *15*, 481–502.

Verheul, R. (2012). Personality disorder proposal for DSM-5: A heroic and innovative but nevertheless fundamentally flawed attempt to improve DSM-IV. *Clinical Psychology and Psychotherapy*, *19*, 369–371.

Wakefield, J. C. (2016). Diagnostic issues and controversies in DSM-5: Return of the false positives problem. *Annual Review of Clinical Psychology*, *12*, 105–132.

Ward, C. H., Beck, A. T., Mendelson, M., Mock, J. E., & Erbaugh, J. K. (1962). The psychiatric nomenclature. Reasons for diagnostic disagreement. *Archives of General Psychiatry*, *7*, 198–205.

Widiger, T. A. (1995). Deletion of the self-defeating and sadistic personality disorder diagnoses. In W. J. Livesley (Ed.), *The DSM-IV personality disorders* (pp. 359–373). Guilford.

Widiger, T. A. (1996). Personality disorder dimensional models. In T. A. Widiger, A. J. Frances, H. A. Pincus, R. Ross, M. B. First, & W. W. Davis (Eds.), *DSM-IV sourcebook* (Vol. 2, pp. 789–798).American Psychiatric Association.

Widiger, T. A. (2001). Official classification systems. In W. J. Livesley (Ed.), *Handbook of personality disorders* (pp. 60–83).Guilford.

Widiger, T. A. (2012). Historical developments and current issues. In T. A. Widiger (Ed.), *The Oxford handbook of personality disorders* (pp. 13–34). Oxford University Press.

Widiger, T. A. (2013). A postmortem and future look at the personality disorders in DSM-5. *Personality Disorders: Theory, Research, and Treatment*, *4*, 382–387.

Widiger, T. A., & Clark, L. A. (2000). Toward DSM-V and the classification of psychopathology. *Psychological Bulletin*, *126*, 946–963.

Widiger, T. A., & Frances, A. J. (1985). The DSM-III personality disorders. Perspectives from psychology. *Archives of General Psychiatry*, *42*, 615–623.

Widiger, T. A., Frances, A. J., Pincus, H., Davis, W., & First, M. B. (1991). Toward an empirical classification for DSM-IV. *Journal of Abnormal Psychology*, *100*, 280–288.

Widiger, T. A., Frances, A. J., Pincus, H., Ross, R., First, M. B., Davis, W. W., & Kline, M. (Eds.). (1998). *DSM-IV sourcebook* (Vol. 4).American Psychiatric Association.

Widiger, T. A., & Hines, A. (2022). The DSM-5 Alternative Model of Personality Disorder. *Personality Disorders: Theory, Research, and Treatment*, *13*, 347–355.

Widiger, T. A., Mangine, S., Corbitt, E. M., Ellis, C. G., & Thomas, G. V. (1995). *Personality disorder interview-IV. A semistructured interview for the assessment of personality disorders*. Psychological Assessment Resources.

Widiger, T. A., Simonsen, E., Krueger, R., Livesley, W. J., & Verheul, R. (2005). Personality disorder research agenda for the DSM-V. *Journal of Personality Disorders*, *19*, 315–338.

Widiger, T. A., & Trull, T. J. (2007). Plate tectonics in the classification of personality disorder: Shifting to a dimensional model. *American Psychologist*, *62*, 71–83.

Widiger, T. A., Tyrer, P., McCabe, G. A., & Kim, Y-R. (in press). Personality disorders: The ICD-11 and DSM-5 alternative models of personality disorder. In A. Tasman (Ed.), *Psychiatry* (5th edition).John Wiley & Sons.

World Health Organization. (1992). *The ICD-10 classification of mental and behavioural disorders. Clinical descriptions and diagnostic guidelines*. Author.

World Health Organization. (2023). *Clinical descriptions and diagnostic requirements for ICD-11 mental, behavioural, and neurodevelopmental disorders*. Author.

Zigler, E., & Phillips, L. (1961). Psychiatric diagnosis: A critique. *Journal of Abnormal and Social Psychology*, *63*, 607–618.

Zilboorg, G. (1941). *A history of medical psychology*. W.W. Norton & Company.

Zimmermann, J., Kerber, A., Rek, K., Hopwood, C. J., & Krueger, R. F. (2019). A brief but comprehensive review of research on the Alternative DSM-5 Model for Personality Disorders. *Current Psychiatry Reports*, *21*(9), 1–19.

CHAPTER 4

The Medical Model of Psychopathology

AWAIS AFTAB

What Is the "Medical Model"?

> As the issues have become caught up in interprofessional disputes and public controversies, the term "medical model" has taken on different meanings. Like "law and order" and "neighborhood schools," "medical model" has become a slogan for use in public debate—more an epithet for attacking one's enemies or a rallying cry for gathering one's followers than a term of precision for furthering intellectual discussion or scientific discovery.
>
> —Gerald L. Klerman, 1977

ALREADY in the 1970s, "medical model" was a fraught term in the context of mental health care. The psychiatrist Gerald Klerman noted in 1977 that the term had evolved into a slogan used more for rhetorical impact than scientific clarification. As Klerman described it, for psychiatrists it symbolized a unifying concept essential for defending the medical identity of psychiatry as a profession and the existence and accessibility of mental health services within the broader healthcare apparatus of medicine. Cognitive and behavioral therapists used it to contrast their focus on observable behaviors with the psychoanalytic emphasis on unconscious conflicts. For public activists, the term was a reminder of the superficial efforts of the medical community to address problems that were fundamentally social in nature. For psychologists and social workers, it represented efforts at gatekeeping professional prestige and privilege. Sociologists saw the application of the medical model to psychopathology as a form of control of socially deviant behaviors. For many within and outside the profession at that time, it stood for biological treatments like electroconvulsive therapy and psychosurgery. Finally, for biologically oriented psychiatrists of the 1970s and 1980s, it encapsulated a rallying cry for a return to the roots of scientific medicine and mainstream medical practices, bolstered by the development of new pharmaceutical treatments (Klerman, 1977).

These contradictory connotations of the term persist to this day. Little has changed in these intervening decades, and the term "medical model" remains charged as ever, serving as a vehicle for critique as well as defense. Shah and Mountain note, "The term 'medical model' is frequently used in psychiatry with denigration, suggesting that its methods are paternalistic, inhumane and reductionist. This view has influenced mental health organisations, which in certain areas advocate a departure from the medical model, and contributes to the difficulties in leadership being played out between politicians, professionals and patients" (Shah and Mountain, 2007).

In contrast, proponents have used the concept of medical model as a way of establishing psychiatry's medical identity. For them, the fundamental idea behind the medical model in psychopathology is the value—and even necessity—of extending the concepts of general medicine to the study and treatment of mental disorders. The sentiment is expressed by Guze (1993) as follows: ". . . psychiatry will most likely thrive and progress if it follows the general strategy, and uses the concepts, of general medicine, in clinical practice and in research. Diagnosis, pathogenesis, etiology, natural history, treatment, and epidemiology are all medical concepts and suggest clinical strategies and research for psychiatric disorders."

This aspiration to mimic general medicine is important, because our notion of medical model for psychopathology will depend on our understanding of the medical model as it applies to the rest of medicine (Nesse & Stein, 2012; Huda, 2019, 2021). Arguably, many in the psychiatric community have understood the framework used within general medicine in an overly narrow manner—one that implicitly takes psychiatric disorders to be etiologically similar to conditions such as infectious diseases and autosomal dominant genetic disorders rather than multifactorial complex medical syndromes (Kendler, 2019).

Many limitations of the medical model of psychopathology, as commonly understood, spring from this overly narrow understanding and can be remedied by appreciating the complexity involved across medicine. Furthermore, medicine is conceptually and scientifically dynamic. "Medical model" is not a static conceptual framework but is itself evolving and adapting in response to developments within medicine as well as critiques from outside. Consider, for instance, the American Psychological Association dictionary definition of the medical model: "the concept that mental and emotional problems are analogous to biological problems—that is, they have detectable, specific, physiological causes (e.g., an abnormal gene or damaged cell) and are amenable to cure or improvement by specific treatment" (APA, 2018). This definition is highly inadequate. Instead of "biological problems," it would be more accurate to say that the medical model considers mental and emotional problems to be analogous to problems encountered in general medicine. The second, and more serious, error here is that it immediately restricts the range of possible options to "detectable, specific, physiological causes," when, in reality, medicine deals with a very wide range of problems including situations where physiological changes are not always detectable, and changes are not always specific. Causes in medicine are often environmental or traumatic, and highly influenced by social factors, which is why public health interventions can be so effective.

Due to the current dominance of DSM and ICD, it may be tempting to use "medical model" to refer to a model that privileges *categorical* classifications, and this may be contrasted with dimensional and idiographic approaches. As we will discuss subsequently in this chapter, however, there is no reason to think that the medical model of psychopathology is unable to accommodate dimensionality, given how common dimensional phenomena are in general medicine.

Shah and Mountain (2007) propose that the medical model should simply be understood as "a process whereby, informed by the best available evidence, doctors advise on, coordinate or deliver interventions for health improvement." Klerman (1977) identified three components of the medical model: the application of the sick role to the mentally ill, the concept of disease in mental illness, and the expansion of mental health care to non-institutionalized individuals. He argued for the role of societal negotiation in defining and managing mental illness. Among contemporary commentators, Huda (2019) uses the term "medical model" to refer to a system that physicians use in clinical or research practice to identify clinical problems and to make predictions as to outcomes and responses to treatment of these clinical problems.

For our purposes, it would be reasonable to understand the medical model as referring to a model of practice that is analogous to the practice of general medicine in the following ways:

1. Classification and diagnosis play a central role in the assessment and treatment of mental disorders.
2. The notion of "mental disorder" is thought to legitimately (but not exclusively) fall under the category of "medical disorder."
3. Causal explanations posit a crucial role for physiological and neuroscientific mechanisms, while recognizing multi-level causality.
4. Treatment modalities such as pharmacotherapies and neuromodulation are considered to be a vital part of the clinical armamentarium.

Understanding "medical model" in this manner allows us to avoid the denigratory connotations discussed previously, while at the same time recognizing distinctive areas of emphasis.

The boundaries of "medical model" are fuzzy, and its contents overlap with those of adjacent disciplines such as psychology and social work. This fuzziness of boundaries is to be expected given the historical development of the mental health professions. In the 18th and 19th centuries, the oversight of asylums was primarily assigned to physicians, a decision influenced significantly by the professional absence of other disciplines that could've assumed that responsibility. Burns (2006), Bynum (2008), and Huda (2019) suggest that since professional alternatives such as psychologists or social workers did not exist in the 1800s, this led to physicians assuming the role of asylum superintendents by default, leading to the subsequent dominance of the medical perspective on psychopathology. Later in the 20th century, psychological treatments such as psychoanalysis and cognitive therapy were also initially developed by physicians given their dominance in the clinical role. This historical context is critical in understanding why our clinical and scientific understanding of psychopathology is inevitably enmeshed with the medical approach. The prominence of the medical approach in the study and treatment of psychopathology is arguably a product of historical circumstances and not something that arises intrinsically from the nature of psychiatric conditions. In most healthcare systems, at least in the Western world, mental health services currently exist as part of the broader medical system. Primary care physicians (and allied professionals, such as nurse practitioners) often assume the responsibility of providing medical care for common disorders such as depressive and anxiety disorders, co-existing with psychiatrists as well as non-medical specialists such as psychologists and psychotherapists. Reimbursement for psychological assessments and treatments is also typically governed by health-related compensation through private insurance or government programs. In order to meaningfully talk about the "medical model," the discussion in this chapter will focus on aspects that are comparatively more specific to psychiatry, but this should not be misunderstood to imply that medicine and psychology do not overlap or that psychotherapies are excluded from the medical model.

Historical Roots of Medical Classification of Psychopathology

The classification of mental disorders has been a part of the broader efforts within medicine to classify diseases from the earliest days. Psychiatric conditions feature prominently in medical classifications of ancient physicians such as Hippocrates and Avicenna. Thomas Sydenham in the 17th century had a profound influence on medical classification with his view that diseases, including mental illnesses, could be systematically categorized based on their symptoms and course of illness. Sydenham's approach, grounded in empirical observations and the belief in nature's consistency in disease production, led him to classify mental illnesses into categories like "hysteria," "mania," and "melancholia" (Koutouvidis, Marketos, & Beveridge 1995). This methodology mirrored his work in general medicine and was influenced by humoral theories of the time. The 18th century marked further progress in medical classifications, epitomized by figures such as Carolus Linnaeus, François Boissier de Sauvages, and Rudolph Vogel, who created symptom-based classifications of disease (Munsche & Whitaker 2012). These classifications included various psychiatric conditions, signaling early efforts to define mental disturbances based on observable symptoms. William Cullen, another pivotal figure, grouped certain psychiatric disorders with neurological disorders under the category of "neuroses"—afflictions of the nervous system (Munsche & Whitaker 2012; Pichot 1994).

Throughout the 18th and 19th centuries, psychiatric nosologies were often the works of individual psychiatrists or neurologists and reflected their theoretical understandings and clinical observations. This era saw the creation of various classifications based on different principles, including etiology, phenomenology, course of illness, and treatment response (Berrios, 1999). In particular, psychiatrists began to recognize that different psychiatric presentations had distinct trajectories over time that could be used to understand and categorize them.

In 1801, Phillipe Pinel classified alienation into the four categories of melancholia, mania, dementia, and idiotism. He viewed mental illnesses as modes of expression of a broader underlying condition of insanity. This view, subsequently named "unitary psychosis," became the dominant view in the mid-19th century (Aftab & Ryznar, 2021). This early modern period also saw the differentiation between acute conditions caused by intoxication or identifiable brain lesions and chronic conditions that lacked visible lesions but were nonetheless believed to be brain-related (Brown 1994).

The Kahlbaum-Hecker-Kraepelin Tradition

Emil Kraepelin is the father of modern psychiatric nosology, and he was heavily influenced by the earlier foundational work of Karl Kahlbaum and Ewald Hecker. Kraepelin's textbooks marked a critical turning point in the understanding and classification of mental disorders. Kahlbaum and Hecker, deeply aware of the heterogeneous nature of symptoms in conditions like melancholia, mania, and dementia, compared them to general symptoms like abdominal pain or headache, which lack specificity in diagnosis (Kendler & Engstrom, 2017). They argued that traditional diagnoses were fostering confusion rather than clarity, particularly with regards to the neuroanatomical and neuropathological study of mental illness that was then predominant in 19th-century European psychiatry. They posited that effective etiological research in psychiatry could only be conducted with a more nuanced understanding of diseases, one that encompassed not only symptoms but the entire trajectory of the illness.

Emblematic of their approach was the case of general paresis of the insane, a manifestation of neurosyphilis (Kendler & Engstrom, 2017). Its etiology was unknown at the time, yet its symptomatic pattern and progression were well established. Observing patients longitudinally, particularly adolescents and young adults, Kahlbaum and Hecker proposed categories like hebephrenia, catatonia, and cyclic insanity.

Emil Kraepelin, dissatisfied with the stagnation in neuroanatomical and neuropathological approaches, embraced and expanded upon Kahlbaum and Hecker's framework. Kraepelin meticulously observed and documented clinical features, pursuing a methodical and iterative process to discern "proto-disease entities." His extensive clinical experience and diligent record-keeping for a vast number of patients laid the foundation for his classification system (Aftab & Csernansky, 2020).

Central to Kraepelin's nosology of psychoses without identifiable brain pathology (discernible by technology at the time) was the distinction between "dementia praecox" and "manic-depressive insanity." This bifurcation was based on the course of the disorders: dementia praecox was associated with a progressive decline in mental functioning, while manic-depressive insanity was not. He observed that conditions like hebephrenia, catatonia, and dementia paranoides, despite their unique features, shared a fundamental pattern of cognitive and psychological decline, leading him to categorize them collectively under dementia praecox. In contrast, manic-depressive insanity was defined by the absence of such cognitive and personality deterioration despite recurrent episodes of psychosis. Kraepelin recognized that some symptoms could be present in both dementia praecox and manic-depressive insanity, with the progression of the illness often being the key differentiator. While he emphasized clinical course and outcome as primary validators of diagnoses, he also acknowledged other distinctive aspects, such as the characteristic disruption in inner psychic associations in dementia praecox (Heckers & Kendler, 2020).

Kraepelin's nosology provided a starting point for subsequent psychiatric classification efforts, and later psychiatrists such as Eugen Bleuler and Kurt Schneider modified Kraepelinian concepts for their purposes (Aftab & Ryznar, 2021). Bleuler, for instance, transformed Kraepelin's dementia praecox into the broader concept of "schizophrenia," focusing on the disruption of psychic associations rather than the progression of the illness into cognitive deterioration (Pichot, 1994).

The Jasperian Tradition

Karl Jaspers, a pivotal figure in the 20th-century field of psychopathology, endeavored to bridge the scientific and humanistic aspects of psychiatry. He advocated for methodological pluralism, a stance that acknowledges the validity of employing multiple methodological perspectives (Ghaemi, 2007). Central to Jaspers' approach was the application of the distinction between *Erklären* (explanation) and *Verstehen* (understanding), originally posited by Wilhelm Dilthey, and the concept of ideal types, as developed by sociologist Max Weber (Zachar et al., 2023).

Explanation, in this context, refers to identifying causal, law-like connections in clinical phenomena, which are discoverable through inductive methods based on repeated experiences. In contrast, understanding relates to recognizing meaningful connections through empathy, envisaging the mental life of another. It involves grasping how individual experiences and personal contexts contribute to a patient's condition, like understanding the impact of personal history on a person's depressive episode. This form of comprehension is more individualistic and less general than causal explanations.

Jaspers also integrated Weber's idea of ideal types into psychopathology (Zachar et al., 2023). Ideal types, abstracted from specific observations, focus on the most striking or unique aspects of a phenomenon, providing a means to understand a particular case without reducing it to mere generalizations. The notion of ideal types is closely related to the contemporary notion of prototypes, and this is important, as many advocates of the medical model—particularly Huda (2019)—consider the medical model to be primarily a prototypical model in clinical application.

Jaspers posited that psychiatric conditions could be categorized into three distinct groups: somatic entities (like brain tumors and Alzheimer's disease), psychological and developmental syndromes (including major psychoses like bipolar disorder and schizophrenia), and psychopathies (encompassing personality disorders and neuroses like anxiety and depression). He saw these groups as fundamentally different, each presenting unique methodological considerations (Zachar et al., 2023).

In Jaspers' view, somatic entities, with their identifiable etiology and pathology, did not pose significant methodological challenges. Psychological and developmental syndromes, although their etiology and pathology might not be fully understood, resembled disease forms. However, for personality disorders and neuroses, he suggested that conceptualizing them as disease forms was inappropriate and advocated for the use of ideal types in understanding these categories. These conditions are often so intertwined with an individual's personality that labeling them as disease entities was a recipe for misunderstanding the nature of the phenomenon.

Modern Psychiatric Nosologies: DSM and ICD

The evolution of contemporary psychiatric nosology is entangled with the increasing use of medical statistics in psychopathology. Throughout the 19th century, there was an increasing need for precise recording of hospitalizations and mortality causes. The *Diagnostic and Statistical Manual of Mental Disorders* (DSM) and the International Classification of Diseases (ICD) are the end products of these developments. These systems, unlike their predecessors, were the result of collaborative efforts by large organizations in various countries, aiming for practical application and consensus among diverse stakeholders (Aftab & Ryznar, 2021).

Development of ICD

In 1946 the World Health Organization (WHO) assumed responsibility for international medical statistical classification. Two years later, WHO published the ICD, referred to as ICD-6 because it was the sixth revision of earlier international statistical classification, but this was the first time the system was referred to by this name. ICD-6 opened a new chapter in medical statistics by introducing a combined classification of morbidity and mortality, intended for international cooperation and standardized reporting. Notably, it was the first edition to feature a dedicated section for mental disorders, offering divisions for psychoses; psychoneurotic disorders; and disorders of character, behavior, and intelligence.

ICD-6 and ICD-7 contained mainly lists of psychiatric conditions with assigned code numbers, lacking detailed descriptions. The transformation of ICD's psychiatric classifications began with the eighth edition (ICD-8), which, influenced by Sir Aubrey Lewis, adopted a predominantly descriptive approach (Fulford & Sartorius, 2009). ICD-8 consolidated all psychiatric disorders into a single section; expanded several diagnostic categories, including personality disorders and addictions; and achieved international adoption.

DSM-I and DSM-II

The period during and following World War II saw a shift in psychiatric classification needs, particularly within the armed forces and the Veterans Affairs in the United States. The existing nomenclatures were considered inadequate at meeting these needs, and in response, William Menninger developed a classification document known as Medical 203, which was adopted by the military. This nomenclature was heavily influenced by Freudian and Meyerian principles, focused on psychiatric problems as psychological reactions and including a smaller section on mental deficiencies, psychotic disorders, and affective disorders.

By the late 1940s, the existence of multiple, distinct psychiatric nomenclature systems prompted the American Psychiatric Association to introduce a new, comprehensive catalog—the DSM. This manual categorized mental disorders into two broad groups, based on their etiological origins—neurological versus primary psychiatric—while still retaining a descriptive approach to diagnosis. The first group encompassed neuropsychiatric manifestations of neurological conditions, including dementias and intellectual disabilities. The second group consisted of psychiatric disorders, conceptualized as reactions in the Meyerian tradition of psychobiology. This categorization covered a spectrum of psychotic disorders, such as involutional psychosis, manic-depressive illness, depressive illness, various subtypes of schizophrenia, and paranoia, framing them as reactions to the environment. The DSM-II, released in 1968, sought alignment with ICD-8 and adopted the general use of the term "disorder." DSM-II took an eclectic approach to classification and, although it was influenced by psychodynamic thinking in its general understanding of the concept of "neurosis," the definitions of specific neuroses were largely descriptive, similar to ICD-8 glossary definitions (Aragona, 2014).

During the mid-20th century, the field of psychiatric nosology was experiencing a significant period of change and uncertainty, concurrent with the dominance of psychoanalysis in American psychiatry. Attitudes among psychiatric practitioners varied widely, with many expressing skepticism or outright doubt regarding the prevailing methods of classification. In a report commissioned by the World Health Organization in 1959, Stengel observed that a growing number of psychiatrists were becoming ambivalent or even cynical toward conventional classification systems. This skepticism was partly due to a general mistrust in the accuracy of diagnoses, particularly those based on the Kraepelinian system, which, despite fierce criticisms, continued to be used around the world (Stengel, 1959). In countries such as the United States, ambivalent attitudes toward descriptive diagnoses were linked to the mid-20th-century rise of psychoanalysis. For psychoanalytic practitioners, descriptive diagnosis wasn't particularly useful, since greater importance was given to unconscious psychological dynamics and conflicts, and, as a result, the attitude toward Kraepelinian diagnoses was often one of indifference and neglect.

This period of doubt and questioning in psychiatric nosology was further intensified by a series of research studies that revealed significant issues with the reliability of psychiatric diagnoses (Aftab & Csernansky, 2020). These studies shed light on the concerning variability in diagnoses given by different practitioners, emphasizing the pressing need for a more consistent and stable approach in psychiatric classification. Notably, the U.S.-U.K. diagnostic project uncovered striking differences in diagnostic practices between the two countries. For instance, a study from this project found substantial discrepancies among trained psychiatrists in the United States and United Kingdom when they were tasked with diagnosing the same patients based on video recordings of diagnostic interviews (Kendell et al., 1971). In particular, patients given diagnoses of manic-depressive illness or personality disorder by British psychiatrists were given diagnoses of schizophrenia by American psychiatrists.

The results underscored the importance of achieving diagnostic reliability in psychiatry. These findings acted as a catalyst, driving the development of more standardized and operationalized diagnostic criteria. This shift aimed to address the inconsistencies in diagnosis and bring a greater degree of uniformity and reliability to the field, laying the groundwork for the advancements in psychiatric classification that would follow.

DSM-III and Beyond

The DSM-III, introduced in 1980, represented a dramatic shift in the standard approach to a classification of mental disorders. It emphasized descriptive and operationalized diagnosis as fundamental to both research and clinical practice. This approach was seen as a culmination of a long-standing movement advocating for operational definitions in psychiatry based on observable criteria. The revolutionary nature of the DSM-III lay in its reliance on descriptions of clinical presentations that could, it was hoped, be consistently recognized by psychiatrists, irrespective of their theoretical orientations regarding the causes of psychiatric disorders.

DSM-III's ostensibly neutral stance on theoretical underpinnings was aligned with a practical viewpoint that discouraged reliance on speculative theories about the origins of mental disorders for reasons of scientific rigor and operational feasibility. However, despite its ostensibly atheoretical approach, the DSM-III and its successors were still deeply entrenched in various theoretical assumptions. Building on the Feighner criteria (Feighner et al., 1972), DSM-III set out operational criteria for each diagnostic category to improve inter-rater reliability, which was empirically tested for major categories through field trials. DSM-III's method of targeting reliability through operationalized criteria marked a significant innovation. It was hoped that this focus on improving reliability would lead to greater validity in diagnoses.

A notable feature of DSM-III was the inclusion of a specific definition of mental disorder, defining it as a clinically significant behavioral or psychological syndrome or pattern associated with distress or disability. This definition was partly influenced by the controversy surrounding the declassification of homosexuality in the DSM-II, which was justified on the grounds of the absence of distress and disability. Despite its non-etiological stance, DSM-III's philosophical orientation was grounded in the medical model. Robert Spitzer, who led the DSM-III task force, had initially proposed defining mental disorders as a subset of medical disorders, a notion that faced significant opposition, particularly from the American Psychological Association. Following the neo-Kraepelinian approach (Blashfield, 1982), DSM-III implicitly assumed the existence of disease entities in psychopathology, which would be identified by convergence of etiological validators via iterative research (Robins and Guze, 1970).

In the early stages of the development of DSM-5, there was an expressed hope for a "paradigm shift" toward etiology-based diagnoses (Zachar et al., 2019). However, the limitations of scientific understanding at the time led to DSM-5 being a more conservative update. DSM-5 also attempted to incorporate dimensional aspects into its classification system, but this endeavor was met with considerable controversy over its implementation. Ultimately, DSM-5 introduced acknowledged dimensionality of psychopathology by recognizing that diagnostic categories exist along spectrums with varying levels of severity and added a dimensional classification of personality disorders—Alternative Model for Personality Disorders (AMPD)—in the "Emerging Measures and Models" section (Krueger & Hobbs, 2020).

Biomedical Model versus Biopsychosocial Model

It is almost axiomatic in contemporary psychiatric education that the medical model of psychopathology is "biopsychosocial" rather than "biomedical." The biopsychosocial model (BPSM) is itself subject to considerable debate and interpretation, but fundamentally, it reflects the aspirations of the medical community to avoid the pitfalls of biological reductionism. BPSM was developed by George Engel in the 1970s (Engel 1977, 1980). Rapid technological advances in medicine in the mid-20th century led to an increasing understanding of disorders in primarily biological terms, with the implicit inference that clinicians need not be concerned with the psychosocial aspects of a person's medical problem in a systematic and scientific manner.

Engel constructed the BPSM utilizing a basic framework provided by general systems theory. Systems theory posits that natural organization occurs in a hierarchical continuum of systems, or levels of organization, where larger and more complex units are dominant over smaller, less complex ones. Within this hierarchy, each system—ranging from a cell to an organ, an individual, or a family—exists at a specific level of complexity, characterized by unique attributes and interactions. Each level exists in dynamic interactions with other levels. Building on this theoretical foundation, Engel offered a framework that sought to account for multiple levels of organization involved in etiology, presentation, and care of medical problems.

The biomedical model, as Engel viewed it, assumed "disease to be fully accounted for by deviations from the norm of measurable biological (somatic) variables" (Engel, 1977). He argued that biological abnormalities at best constitute a necessary but not sufficient condition for illness and do not take into account the human experience of the illness and the social context that shape how the illness comes to attention and how it is optimally treated. Understanding the human experience of disease—encompassing self-perception or societal perception of illness, the manner of reporting sickness, and its effects on one's life—necessitates the inclusion of psychological, social, and cultural elements (Engel 1977, 1980).

Establishing a relationship between a clinical presentation and an underlying biological etiology requires a scientific understanding of behavior and psychosocial aspects, because that is how patients report their symptoms. Patients approach clinicians when they are either unsure of their medical condition or, even when aware, find themselves unable to manage it on their own. Engel emphasized the "psychobiological unity" of humans, advocating for clinicians to take on the responsibility of assessing and addressing any issues presented by patients, irrespective of their direct relation to biological disturbances in the body:

> To provide a basis for understanding the determinants of disease and arriving at rational treatments and patterns of health care, a medical model must also take into account the patient, the social context in which he lives, and the complementary system devised by society to deal with the disruptive effects of illness, that is, the physician role and the health care system. This requires a biopsychosocial model. (Engel, 1977)

Engel recognized the unique position of psychiatry within the medical profession as the only clinical discipline still concerned primarily with the study of the human condition. He considered it a lasting contribution of Freud and Meyer that they had provided frames of reference that led to the inclusion of psychological processes in the concept of disease.

The BPSM was imagined by Engel as "a blueprint for research, a framework for teaching, and a design for action in the real world of health care" (1977). From a philosophical standpoint, this approach highlights how suffering and illness are influenced by various organizational levels, spanning from social structures to molecular details. Practically, it underscores the significance of the patient's personal experience as a vital factor in achieving precise diagnoses, effective health outcomes, and compassionate care (Borrell-Carrió et al., 2004).

BPSM has been of tremendous influence in psychiatry as well as other areas of medicine as primary care. In the case of psychiatry, BPSM provided a practical common ground for the psychodynamic and biological camps and helped the field move toward a compromise. There is no doubt that BPSM is an advance over a biomedical perspective. Critics contend that the biopsychosocial model, as it is currently applied, has transformed into a confusing collection of suppositions regarding psychiatric conditions, resulting in a tendency among clinicians toward indiscriminate eclecticism. In the view of many mental health professionals today, this model merely states the obvious: that all illnesses encompass elements that are biological, psychological, and social (Ghaemi, 2009). In this sense, BPSM is excessively broad and provides no real guidance to clinicians or researchers. To address some of these critiques, Bolton & Gillett (2019) have sought to update BPSM by conceptualizing it as a philosophical account of causal interactions across levels of organization. Bolton and Gillett's attempt to update BPSM has had a mixed reception (Aftab & Nielsen, 2021; Maung, 2021; Tabb, 2021), and the practical impact of these theoretical developments on the clinical application of the medical model in psychiatry remains limited at best (Huda, 2021).

In one sense, BPSM is a manifestation of the philosophical outlook of scientific pluralism in psychiatry. According to pluralism, various perspectives to explain and comprehend phenomena are available to us, such that each perspective contributes a limited understanding of a particular aspect of a multifaceted phenomenon (Campaner, 2014). This notion of explanatory pluralism is frequently paired with a pragmatic approach that prioritizes different explanatory perspectives based on how well they achieve specific explanatory objectives and practical goals (Maung, 2020). One framework for such a pluralistic formulation, referred to as the "Perspectives" approach, utilizes the four perspectives of diseases, dimensions of personality, goal-directed behaviors, and life stories to understand psychopathology (McHugh & Slavney, 1998). In the enactive psychiatry framework (de Haan, 2020), psychopathology has four integrated dimensions: physiological, experiential, sociocultural, and existential. Such frameworks highlight that an approach that takes the psychosocial aspects of illness seriously need not sort phenomena into the three bins of "biological," "psychological," and "social" the way BPSM currently invites. Enactive approaches to multilevel causality also interface with conceptual approaches such as network theories and complex, dynamic systems, which tend to view psychiatric symptoms as existing in networks of relationships in which they cause one another through mutually reinforcing, self-sustaining feedback loops (Borsboom & Cramer, 2013; Borsboom, 2017).

The Concept of Disorder

Defining terms such as "health," "disease," and "illness" can be challenging, yet these concepts are often easily identifiable in clear-cut cases. The difficulties in definition become particularly pertinent when determining the scope of medical intervention. From a medical standpoint, the concept of disease involves identifying states of ill health that warrant medical attention, followed by uncovering the associated structural or functional abnormalities (Huda, 2021). Arthur Kleinman's influential work delineates "illness" as the subjective experience of symptoms and suffering from the individual's perspective, contrasting it with "disease," which refers to the medical practitioner's focus on biological structure and function (Kleinman, 1978). People interpret their illness experiences through personal and cultural beliefs about health and disease, and societal views on what conditions warrant professional healthcare intervention (Pendleton et al., 1984).

The term "disorder" has largely replaced "disease" as the preferred terminology, especially in psychiatry and psychology. Their technical meaning is generally the same in philosophical and scientific literature, but "disease" has strong connotations of biological dysfunction and discreteness that the term "disorder" strictly lacks. It has also been argued that the term "medical condition" may be a more suitable descriptor for states associated with distress, impaired functioning, or increased risk warranting healthcare attention (Huda, 2019).

Medical diagnoses are an eclectic mix of symptoms, injuries, syndromes with well-defined etiologies, and diagnoses in terms of pathological change (Huda, 2019). Physicians use diagnoses like "chronic low back pain," "dyspepsia," "tension headache," "urinary retention," as much as they use specific diagnoses referring to disease entities such as "glioblastoma multiforme." Medical and psychiatric diagnoses refer to a variety of problems and conditions, which include broad and heterogenous symptom presentations ("acute abdominal pain," "first episode psychosis," "chronic pain"), clearly defined syndromes (catatonia), syndromes with identified etiology (Down's syndrome, autoimmune encephalitis), fuzzy categories with operational definitions (generalized anxiety disorder), consequences of injuries and trauma (fractures, post-traumatic stress reactions), dimensional variations associated with risk or maladaptation (hypertension, personality disorders), and other conditions that are often managed by healthcare professionals but are not illnesses (pregnancy, grief).

The concept of "disorder" consists of two broad and nebulous elements:

1. judgments of harm (distress, disability, risk, etc.), and
2. judgments of "abnormality" (or "dysfunction"), which can be based on the subjective experience of illness; or sociocultural, value-laden judgments that *something* has gone wrong; or more precise notions of abnormality in terms of anatomical change, evolutionary function, or biostatistical comparisons.

The roots of contemporary judgments of psychopathology lie in ordinary, commonsensical judgments, such as whether the behaviors and experiences are unexpected, unfamiliar, not easily intelligible, disproportionate in reaction or excessive in some fashion, violating norms of shared rationality, etc. (Aftab & Rashed, 2021). These judgments are then subjected to further scientific scrutiny, operationalization, and refinement, but the folk character of these judgments persists in contemporary diagnostic manuals such as DSM and ICD. Problems arise because folk judgments that "something has gone wrong" (e.g., the judgment in the diagnosis of generalized anxiety disorder that the anxiety is "excessive") do not necessarily correspond to dysfunction defined in natural terms, for example, failure of a mechanism to perform its "natural" function.

Recognizing the value-laden nature of disorder concepts reorients our understanding of the medical model as a particular way to responding to certain forms of distress, disability, and deviation. The value-ladenness of medical concepts demands continuous examination of our diagnostic practices, the biases and social forces to which they are subject, and an ongoing democratic dialogue that involves all stakeholders (Aftab & Rashed, 2021; Bolton, 2008; Glackin, 2019). Medicine is unavoidably vulnerable to mirroring and reinforcing wider societal ideas, and this is particularly notable in psychiatry (Aftab, 2024).

Philosophical discussions of the concept of "disorder" (and "disease") have often been framed in terms of the "naturalism" versus "normativism" dichotomy (Murphy, 2020). At one pole, strong naturalism argues for an objective, value-free understanding of disorders, in line with the methodologies of natural sciences like chemistry and genetics. In the context of psychopathology, proponents believe psychiatric disorders arise from neurobiological dysfunctions and objectively abnormal brain functioning. The most notable philosophical advocate for a naturalist view of disease is Boorse (1977), who views health in biostatistical terms as a state of species-typical biological functioning.

On the opposite end, strong normativism asserts that disorder attributions are thoroughly value-laden, with biological processes that cannot be characterized as "dysfunctional" in an objective sense. Fulford (1989), for example, anchors the concept of disorder in the "illness experience," which is subjective and heavily shaped by sociocultural norms. An unusual position on this spectrum is taken by Szasz (1960), a prominent critic of medical psychiatry, who takes a naturalist view of "disease," understanding it in terms of cellular pathology, only to assert that conditions we call "mental illnesses" are thereby excluded from the definition of disease; the Szaszian view considers psychopathological judgments to be judgments of deviance without evidence of biological disease, and therefore medical treatment of psychopathology lacks scientific legitimacy (Stein et al., 2024).

In attempting to bridge the divide between naturalism and normativism, several integrative positions have emerged. Wakefield's "harmful dysfunction analysis" is the most prominent as a hybrid view that includes both naturalist and normative elements (Wakefield, 2007). Dysfunction is defined by Wakefield in evolutionary terms, whereas harm is considered through a normative lens, largely determined by social standards. Jon Tsou (2021) aims for integration by defining mental disorders as biological kinds with harmful effects. This approach sidesteps the debate on natural selection, focusing instead on the presence of regularities and predictable patterns due to stable sets of interacting biological mechanisms. Others, like Gagné-Julien (2024) and Nielsen and Ward (2020), propose frameworks that blend the naturalist and normativist views, suggesting that judgments about dysfunction are value-laden yet objective in other ways. They emphasize that disorders should be understood in relation to an individual's functioning within their social context. In addressing these controversies, it is increasingly argued that an approach that involves multiple stakeholders, inclusive of patients, is recommended to navigate value disagreements with regards to decisions such as expanding or restricting the domain of recognized disorders. DeYoung and Krueger (2018, 2023) have proposed that psychopathology is best understood as "cybernetic dysfunction," that is, persistent failure to move toward one's goals, due to failure to generate effective new goals, interpretations, or strategies when existing ones prove unsuccessful. They nonetheless endorse a hybrid account of mental disorder because in addition to a naturalistic account of psychopathology, mental disorder requires an additional value judgment about what level of severity is worthy of treatment. Cybernetic theory is particularly appealing, because it draws from empirical research in neuroscience, psychometrics, and personality theory, and has the potential to improve our scientific understanding of psychopathology, something that prior theoretical accounts of mental disorder have struggled to do.

Essentalism and the Medical Model

Historically, psychiatry has grappled with "essentialism," the belief that mental disorders possess inherent essences or defining features (Zachar, 2014). This view posits that psychiatric conditions, akin to infectious diseases in medicine, are caused by central neurobiological dysfunctions that can be discovered through scientific inquiry. This essentialist view was endorsed by Kraepelin at the end of the 19th century and later by neo-Kraepelinians in the 1960s and 1970s, with a belief in natural disease entities onto which pathological anatomy, etiology, and symptomatology would converge. However, scientific research in the late 20th century and early 21st century revealed that different validators do not appear to converge onto categorical disease entities, nor do they correspond to traditional psychiatric categories, challenging the view that diagnostic categories have unique neurobiological or neuropsychological essences. The complexity, dimensionality, and multifactorial nature of mental illnesses complicate the aspirations for a single, valid classification of psychopathology (Aftab & Ryznar, 2021).

The resulting debate oscillates between considering psychiatric classifications as "natural kinds," entities existing independently of human interests, and as "social kinds," almost entirely constructed by social processes. Both positions are inadequate when it comes to recognizing the transdiagnostic relationships identified between neurobiological processes and psychiatric symptoms. Offering a middle ground is the concept of "practical kinds," (Zachar, 2000) which contends that while psychiatric categories do not correspond to discrete categories, they are informed by symptom patterns and covariation that reflect scientific and clinical realities (Stein et al., 2024). In this view, boundaries and thresholds in psychiatric classification are influenced by both facts and values, serving as heuristic tools for scientific and clinical objectives.

Over the last few decades, the medical model of psychopathology has moved away from rigid, essentialist, and neo-Kraepelinian views toward a pragmatic understanding of diagnostic categories that accommodates the dimensionality of symptom clusters, the transdiagnostic nature of neurobiological associations, etiological heterogeneity, and individual developmental trajectories (Stein et al., 2024). For clinicians, this evolving understanding of psychiatric taxonomy highlights the importance of going beyond the symptom checklist approach to target comprehensive clinical characterization. Comprehensive evaluations should consider a variety of domains, including symptom severity, cognitive schemas, environmental factors, and an individualized understanding of each patient's unique circumstances.

Categories, Dimensions, and Prototypes in the Medical Model

Given the degree to which DSM and ICD are viewed as examples of the medical model of psychopathology, there is the temptation to assume that the medical model is uncomfortable with notions of dimensionality, but that is far from the case. Dimensional phenomena are common in medicine—physiological functioning of most organ systems lies on quantitative continua—and this dimensionality poses little nosological problems in general medicine.

The debate between categorical and dimensional approaches in psychiatry revolves around the most effective method for simplifying the complexity of clinical phenomena for clinical and research applications. This entails choosing between defining mental health issues as distinct classes (categories) or as a range of continuous, quantifiable traits (dimensions). Historically, categorical classification has been predominant in psychiatry and medicine, yet recent years have seen a significant growth in dimensional models. Psychiatric categories can be understood and measured in both ways, but whether their underlying structure is truly categorical or dimensional is a question for empirical investigation (Ruscio & Ruscio, 2008). Thus, the scientific inquiry into the intrinsic structure of psychopathology is distinct from the clinical application of categorical versus dimensional models.

In both medicine and clinical psychology, classifications are practical tools designed to organize and direct clinical practice. Since many clinical decisions are binary, categorical models often align well with clinical needs, whereas dimensional models might be more suitable for research, due to their ability to capture the full spectrum of physiological and psychological functioning. From a clinical point of view, the distinction between dimensions and categories can be misleading, as dimensions can be transformed into categories based on practical thresholds. In general medicine, conditions like blood pressure and body weight are dimensional, but categories such as hypertension and obesity are defined using specific thresholds. Similarly, psychiatric classifications can integrate dimensionality by recognizing conditions as spectra with varying severity levels (e.g., subthreshold, mild, moderate, severe).

Although the question of whether the latent structure of psychopathological conditions is categorical or dimensional remains without a conclusive resolution, the bulk of taxometric research supports the assertion that the majority of psychopathological differences between people are latently continuous (Haslam et al., 2020). At the same time, the perceived mutual exclusivity of categories and dimensions is increasingly being challenged by attention to psychopathological changes *within* people and differences *between* people (Borsboom et al., 2016; Aftab et al., 2024). Classical views of categories (like Kraepelinian disease entities) and dimensions (such as intelligence quotient) might not fully capture the nature of psychopathology. It is plausible that psychopathological conditions could be understood as "categorical" in terms of dynamic changes or phase shifts within individuals over time and as "dimensional" in terms of symptom distribution across a population (Eaton et al., 2023).

In clinical practice, categorization doesn't always strictly adhere to the concept of individually necessary and jointly sufficient conditions with discrete boundaries, as seen in classical categorical thinking. Instead, categories are often conceptualized as fuzzy kinds, ideal types, or prototypes (Zachar, 2000). In this approach, clinicians engage in a process of matching the key features of a patient's clinical presentation to prototypical diagnostic profiles to find the best fit. This initial assessment is then refined through further clinical evaluation (Huda, 2019; Aftab et al., 2024).

The prototype model is grounded in the idea of a typical example within a category, with members of the category resembling the prototype to varying degrees (Hampton, 2006). Unlike classical categories with clear-cut boundaries, prototypes have vague, overlapping borders. For example, in the prototype model, certain members are more representative of a category than others, much like a robin is more prototypically a bird than an ostrich is (Zachar, 2000). This model accommodates prototypical, atypical, and borderline examples without demanding strict criteria for inclusion. It aligns with the concept of "family resemblance," where members of a category share a set of overlapping features. The DSM's use of "polythetic" criteria reflects the prototype model. Instead of defining a single, precise disorder type, it allows for myriad symptom combinations, creating a spectrum of types (Zachar, 2000).

Updating the Medical Model

As noted earlier in the chapter, in an effort to emulate general medicine, the psychiatric profession in the 1970s adopted an overly narrow understanding of medical disorders and expected that we will be able to identify specific neurobiological causes and biomarkers for DSM-style descriptive categories. This scientific agenda has largely been a disappointment. In contrast to the narrow view, the explanatory approach taken by general medicine places disordered functioning within a physiological understanding of the normal functions of bodily systems. This wider perspective recognizes that symptoms can serve protective functions, and that syndromes can be reflections of failure and dysregulation of organ systems, with the dysregulated state being etiologically heterogenous, arising from a variety of causes. Congestive heart failure, for example, can be caused by ischemic heart disease, valvular heart disease, hypertension, infectious myocarditis, cardiac amyloidosis, peripartum cardiomyopathy, thyrotoxicosis, thiamine deficiency, etc. Neo-Kraepelinian psychiatry hoped that mental disorders would turn out to be more discrete and definable than is often the case in the rest of medicine.

Nesse and Stein (2012) outline three ways in which the medical model in psychiatry can be updated to reflect insights from general medicine:

1. A recognition that emotional response such as anxiety and low mood are evolved and adaptive responses, similar to pain and fever.
2. Many medical syndromes reflect system failures with diverse etiologies.
3. Many medical problems are disorders of feedback dysregulation.

Symptoms as Evolutionary Adaptations

Similar to how cough and pain serve as protective mechanisms in response to physical threats, emotions like anxiety and mood have likely evolved because of the selective advantages they confer to the organism (Nesse, 2023). Emotions regulate various aspects of physiology, cognition, behavior, and motivation, enhancing the ability to cope with a range of situations. Disorders arise when systems regulating emotional expression are perturbed and emotional experiences become maladaptive.

The challenge in psychiatry is distinguishing between "normal" and "abnormal" emotional responses. While some conditions like severe melancholic depression and mania are clearly abnormal, diagnosing an emotional expression as abnormal without considering the situational context is akin to diagnosing a pain disorder without identifying potential sources of ongoing tissue damage. Nesse and Stein (2012) suggest that emotional disturbances should be considered and understood in the context in which they exist and arise. Such an approach aligns with how symptoms are evaluated in the rest of medicine, where, for example, the presence of a symptom like a cough initiates a search for causes. Significant emotional distress experienced in an abusive marriage can impair psychological functions as profoundly as pneumonia can affect respiratory functions. In clinical practice, understanding a patient's emotional experiences requires a thorough exploration of their current life situation, including goals, strategies, opportunities, and obstacles, taking into account individual psychological characteristics and their developmental experiences.

Nesse and Stein (2012) acknowledge the difficulties involved in differentiating normal from abnormal in the psychological realm. Unlike more straightforward physical symptoms like cough or fever, emotions like anxiety, anger, and low mood are often triggered by complex, less easily identifiable situations. Emotional disorders in psychiatry cannot be adequately diagnosed with a focus only on the intensity and duration of emotions; diagnosis should also involve assessing the individual's trait vulnerabilities and the intensity of current situations that could trigger emotional responses.

Syndromes as System Failures

Many medical syndromes are defined by failures of functional systems with diverse etiologies, rather than a single cause. We have noted the example of Congestive Heart Failure earlier. Other examples include renal failure, liver failure, and neurocognitive disorders such as delirium and dementia. Again, psychiatric syndromes pose greater challenges than do physiological syndromes, because while functioning of organs such as the heart can be objectively measured and is underpinned by well-understood physiology, brain-behavior relationships are much more complex and less well understood.

Popular criticisms of the DSM diagnoses, such as comorbidity and heterogeneity, may stem from unrealistic expectations. Syndromes resulting from dysregulated systems are unlikely to have specific causes or clear boundaries. Thus, a brain-based diagnostic system may not adequately categorize them, and the comorbidity, heterogeneity, and blurry boundaries of many traditional psychiatric categories might actually reflect the complex reality of these conditions.

Disorders of Feedback Dysregulation

Many medical disorders are "functional" in the sense that they reflect abnormal functioning of an organ system despite no identifiable tissue abnormalities. These disorders, which include essential tremor, tinnitus, and chronic pain, might be caused by feedback dysregulation such that the system is either stuck in an abnormal state or the feedback loop results in a vicious cycle. In psychiatry, disorders like panic disorder can arise from a positive feedback loop where physiological changes fuel fear and fear fuels further physiological changes, escalating into a panic attack (Robinaugh et al., 2021). These disorders, often resulting from feedback spirals, may not have disorder-specific neurophysiological changes but are interconnected aspects of a feedback cycle (Nesse & Stein, 2012). Feedback cycles may also be involved in the genesis of depressive states—for example, low mood and social withdrawal—creating a vicious cycle, as well as other conditions such as eating disorders. Disorders arising from feedback dysregulation will not necessarily have common causes or consistent brain abnormalities, because the symptom clusters are better understood as end products of complex feedback cycles.

Conclusion

"Medical model" has a history fraught with varied connotations and interpretations. These controversies are reflective of the turbulent development of psychiatry as a medical discipline and the different stages through which it has evolved and is evolving. Medicine has struggled with the challenges and complexities involved in defining and categorizing mental disorders. Unlike many other areas of medicine, where classifications are based on an understanding of causal and etiological mechanisms, or based on physiological functioning of the organ system, medical classifications of psychopathology remain descriptive in nature. DSM and ICD, arising from the need for standardized nomenclatures, adopted descriptive and operationalized criteria in the second half of the 20th century to optimize clinical reliability and provide a research framework for validation. DSM-III implicitly adopted a neo-Kraepelinian view of psychopathology, with the assumption that descriptive and operationalized study of psychopathology would lead to the identification of distinct disease entities. This implicit theoretical worldview drove medical research in psychopathology for the next thirty years, yet the quest to define valid, categorical psychopathological diseases has largely been unfruitful.

Acknowledging and moving beyond neo-Kraepelinian assumptions reveals that DSM and ICD diagnostic categories are pragmatic in nature. The diagnostic categories are convenient ways of mapping a dynamic and dimensional landscape of psychopathology that allows for a shared language and serves as a guide for clinical decision-making. Although these manuals do identify significant group differences across various validators, they do not reflect the quantitative and formal structure of psychopathology as derived from statistical clustering techniques. It is increasingly recognized that etiological heterogeneity is inevitable when disorders are reflections of phenomena such as system failures and higher order feedback dysregulation. The medical model of psychopathology is not static; it is dynamic, continuously adapting in response to scientific advancements, societal shifts, and developments in adjacent disciplines such as neuroscience, psychology, and social work. The medical model of psychopathology at the current moment in the 21st century takes a pragmatic view of diagnostic categories (while searching for causal explanations and etiological mechanisms), recognizes the prototypicality inherent in clinical diagnosis, advocates for explanatory and methodological pluralism, approaches mental illnesses as complex, multi-level disorders, and incorporates insights from evolutionary biology and dynamical systems theory.

References

Aftab, A. (2024). Psychiatry and the critical landscape. In A. Aftab (Ed.), *Conversations in critical psychiatry*. Oxford University Press.

Aftab, A., Banicki, K., Ruffalo, M. L., & Frances, A. (2024). Psychiatric diagnosis: A clinical guide to navigating diagnostic pluralism. *Journal of Nervous and Mental Disease*, *212*(8), 445–454.

Aftab, A., & Csernansky, J. G. (2020). Diagnosis and conceptualization. In E. Ryznar, A. B. Pederson, M. A. Reinecke, and J. G Csernansky (Eds.), *Landmark papers in psychiatry*. Oxford University Press.

Aftab, A., & Nielsen, K. (2021). From Engel to enactivism: Contextualizing the biopsychosocial model. *European Journal of Analytic Philosophy*, *17*(2), M2–22.

Aftab, A., & Rashed, M. A. (2021). Mental disorder and social deviance. *International Review of Psychiatry*, *33*(5), 478–485.
Aftab, A., & Ryznar, E. (2021). Conceptual and historical evolution of psychiatric nosology. *International Review of Psychiatry*, *33*(5), 486–499.
American Psychological Association. (2018). APA Dictionary of Psychology. https://dictionary.apa.org/medical-model (accessed October 11, 2024).
Aragona, M. (2014). Rethinking received views on the history of psychiatric nosology: Minor shifts, major continuities. In P. Zachar, D. St. Stoyanov, M. Aragona, & A. Jablensky (Eds.), *Alternative perspectives on psychiatric validation: DSM, IDC, RDoC, and beyond* (pp. 27–46). Oxford University Press.
Berrios, G. E. (1999). Classifications in psychiatry: A conceptual history. *Australian & New Zealand Journal of Psychiatry*, *33*, 145–60.
Blashfield, R. K. (1982). Feighner et al., invisible colleges, and the Matthew effect. *Schizophrenia Bulletin*, *8*, 1–6.
Bolton, D. (2008). *What is mental disorder? An essay in philosophy, science, and values*. Oxford University Press.
Bolton, D., & Gillett, G. (2019). The biopsychosocial model of health and disease: New philosophical and scientific developments. Springer.
Boorse, C. (1977). Health as a theoretical concept. *Philosophy of Science*, *44*(4), 542–573.
Borrell-Carrió, F., Suchman, A. L., & Epstein, R. M. (2004). The biopsychosocial model 25 years later: Principles, practice, and scientific inquiry. *The Annals of Family Medicine*, *2*(6), 576–582.
Borsboom, D. (2017). A network theory of mental disorders. *World Psychiatry*, *16*(1), 5–13.
Borsboom, D., & Cramer, A. O. (2013). Network analysis: An integrative approach to the structure of psychopathology. *Annual Review of Clinical Psychology*, *9*, 91–121.
Borsboom D., Rhemtulla M., Cramer A. O., van der Maas H. L., Scheffer M., & Dolan C. V. (2016). Kinds versus continua: A review of psychometric approaches to uncover the structure of psychiatric constructs. *Psychological Medicine*, *46*, 1567–1579.
Brown, E. M. (1994). French psychiatry's initial reception of Bayle's discovery of general paresis of the insane. *Bulletin of the History of Medicine*, *68*(2), 235–253.
Burns T. (2006). *Psychiatry: A very short introduction*. Oxford University Press.
Bynum W. (2008). *The history of medicine: A very short introduction*. Oxford University Press.
Campaner, R. (2014). Explanatory pluralism in psychiatry: What are we pluralists about, and why? In Maria Carla Galavotti, Dennis Dieks, Wenceslao J. Gonzalez, Stephan Hartmann, Thomas Uebel, & Marcel Weber (Eds.), *New directions in the philosophy of science* (pp. 87–103). Springer.
de Haan, S. (2020). *Enactive psychiatry*. Cambridge University Press.
DeYoung, C. G., & Krueger, R. F. (2018). A cybernetic theory of psychopathology. *Psychological Inquiry*, *29*(3), 117–138.
DeYoung, C. G., & Krueger, R. F. (2023). A cybernetic perspective on the nature of psychopathology: Transcending conceptions of mental illness as statistical deviance and brain disease. *Journal of Psychopathology and Clinical Science*, *132*(3), 228.
Eaton, N. R., Bringmann, L. F., Elmer T., Fried, E. I., Forbes, M. K., Greene, A. L., Krueger, R. F., Kotov, R., McGorry, P. D., & Mei, C (2023). A review of approaches and models in psychopathology conceptualization research. *Nature Reviews Psychology*, 2, 622–636.
Engel, G. L. (1977). The need for a new medical model: A challenge for biomedicine. *Science*, *196*(4286), 129–136.
Engel, G. L. (1980). The clinical application of the biopsychosocial model. *American Journal of Psychiatry*, 137(5), 535–44.
Feighner, J. P., Robins, E., Guze, S. B., Woodruff, R. A., Winokur, G., & Munoz, R. (1972). Diagnostic criteria for use in psychiatric research. *Archives of General Psychiatry*, *26*(1), 57–63.
Fulford, K. W. M. (1989). *Moral theory and medical practice*. Cambridge University Press.
Fulford, K. W. M., & Sartorius, N. (2009). A secret history of ICD and the hidden future of DSM. In M. Broome & L. Bortolotti (Eds.), *Psychiatry as cognitive neuroscience* (pp. 29–48). Oxford University Press.
Gagné-Julien, A. M. (2024). Beyond conceptual analysis: Social objectivity and conceptual engineering to define disease. *The Journal of Medicine and Philosophy*, *49*(2), 147–159.

Ghaemi, S. N. (2007). Existence and pluralism: The rediscovery of Karl Jaspers. *Psychopathology, 40*(2), 75–82.
Ghaemi, S. N. (2009). The rise and fall of the biopsychosocial model. *The British Journal of Psychiatry, 195*(1), 3–4.
Glackin, S. N. (2019). Grounded disease: Constructing the social from the biological in medicine. *The Philosophical Quarterly, 69*(275), 258–276.
Guze, S. B. (1993). The future of psychiatry and the medical model. *The Journal of Nervous and Mental Disease, 181*(10), 593–594.
Hampton JA (2006). Concepts as prototypes. *Psychology of Learning and Motivation*, 46:79–113.
Haslam, N., McGrath, M. J., Viechtbauer, W., & Kuppens, P. (2020). Dimensions over categories: A meta-analysis of taxometric research. *Psychological Medicine*, 50:1418–1432.
Heckers, S., & Kendler, K. S. (2020). The evolution of Kraepelin's nosological principles. *World Psychiatry, 19*(3), 381–388.
Huda, A. S. (2019). *The medical model in mental health: An explanation and evaluation*. Oxford University Press.
Huda, A. S. (2021). The medical model and its application in mental health. *International Review of Psychiatry, 33*(5), 463–470.
Kendell, R. E., Cooper, J. E., Gourlay, A. J., Copeland, J. R., Sharpe, L., & Gurland, B. J. (1971). Diagnostic criteria of American and British psychiatrists. *Archives of General Psychiatry, 25*(2), 123–130.
Kendler, K. S. (2019). From many to one to many—The search for causes of psychiatric illness. *JAMA Psychiatry, 76*(10), 1085–1091.
Kendler, K. S., & Engstrom, E. J. (2017). Kahlbaum, Hecker, and Kraepelin and the transition from psychiatric symptom complexes to empirical disease forms. *American Journal of Psychiatry, 174*(2), 102–109.
Kleinman, A. (1978). Clinical relevance of anthropological and cross-cultural research: Concepts and strategies. *The American Journal of Psychiatry, 135*(4), 427–431.
Klerman, G. L. (1977). Mental illness, the medical model, and psychiatry. *The Journal of Medicine and Philosophy, 2*(3), 220–243.
Koutouvidis, N., Marketos, S. G., & Beveridge, A. (1995). The contribution of Thomas Sydenham (1624–1689) to the evolution of psychiatry. *History of Psychiatry, 6*(24), 513–520.
Krueger, R. F., & Hobbs, K. A. (2020). An overview of the DSM-5 alternative model of personality disorders. *Psychopathology, 53*(3–4), 126–132.
Maung, H. H. (2020). Pluralism and incommensurability in suicide research. *Studies in history and philosophy of science part C: Studies in history and philosophy of biological and biomedical sciences, 80*, 101247.
Maung, H. H. (2021). Causation and causal selection in the biopsychosocial model of health and disease. *European Journal of Analytic Philosophy, 17*(2), M5–27.
McHugh, P. R., & Slavney, P. R. (1998). The perspectives of psychiatry: Johns Hopkins University Press.
Munsche, H., & Whitaker, H. A. (2012). Eighteenth century classification of mental illness: Linnaeus, de Sauvages, Vogel, and Cullen. *Cognitive and Behavioral Neurology, 25*(4), 224–239.
Murphy, D. (2020). Concepts of disease and health. *The Stanford Encyclopedia of Philosophy* (Fall 2023 edition), Edward N. Zalta & Uri Nodelman (eds.), https://plato.stanford.edu/archives/fall2023/entries/health-disease/
Nesse, R. M. (2023). Evolutionary psychiatry: Foundations, progress and challenges. *World Psychiatry, 22*(2), 177–202.
Nesse, R. M., & Stein, D. J. (2012). Towards a genuinely medical model for psychiatric nosology. *BMC Medicine, 10*, 1–9.
Nielsen, K., & Ward, T. (2020). Mental disorder as both natural and normative: Developing the normative dimension of the 3e conceptual framework for psychopathology. *Journal of Theoretical and Philosophical Psychology, 40*(2), 107.
Pendleton D., Schofield T., Tate P., and Havelock P. (1984). *The Consultation: An Approach to Learning and Teaching*. Oxford University Press, UK.
Pichot, P. (1994). Nosological models in psychiatry. *The British Journal of Psychiatry, 164*(2), 232–240.

Robinaugh, D. J., Haslbeck, J. M., Ryan, O., Fried, E. I., & Waldorp, L. J. (2021). Invisible hands and fine calipers: A call to use formal theory as a toolkit for theory construction. *Perspectives on Psychological Science, 16*(4), 725–743.

Robins, E., & Guze, S. B. (1970). Establishment of diagnostic validity in psychiatric illness: Its application to schizophrenia. *American Journal of Psychiatry, 126*(7), 983–987.

Ruscio, J., & Ruscio, A. M. (2008). Categories and dimensions: Advancing psychological science through the study of latent structure. *Current Directions in Psychological Science, 17*(3), 203–207.

Shah, P., & Mountain, D. (2007). The medical model is dead–Long live the medical model. *The British Journal of Psychiatry, 191*(5), 375–377.

Stein, D. J., Nielsen K., Hartford, A., Gagne-Julien, A. M., Glackin, S., Friston, K., Maj, M., Zachar, P., Aftab, A. (2024) Philosophy of psychiatry: Theoretical advances and clinical implications. *World Psychiatry*. In Press.

Stengel, E. (1959). Classification of mental disorders. *Bulletin of the World Health Organization, 21*(4–5), 601.

Szasz, T. S. (1960). The myth of mental illness. *American Psychologist, 15*(2), 113.

Tabb, K. (2021). Centrifugal and centripetal thinking about the biopsychosocial model in psychiatry. *European Journal of Analytic Philosophy, 17*(2), M3–28.

Tsou, J. Y. (2021). *Philosophy of psychiatry*. Cambridge University Press.

Wakefield, J. C. (2007). The concept of mental disorder: Diagnostic implications of the harmful dysfunction analysis. *World Psychiatry, 6*(3), 149.

Zachar P (2000). Psychiatric disorders are not natural kinds. *Philosophy, Psychiatry, & Psychology, 7*(3), 167–182.

Zachar, P. (2014). *A metaphysics of psychopathology*. MIT Press.

Zachar, P., Banicki, K., & Aftab, A. (2023). Historical and philosophical considerations in studying psychopathology. In R. F. Krueger & P. H. Blaney (Eds.), *Oxford Textbook of Psychopathology (4th Edition)* (p. 33). Oxford University Press.

Zachar, P., Regier, D. A., & Kendler, K. S. (2019). The aspirations for a paradigm shift in DSM-5: An oral history. *The Journal of Nervous and Mental Disease, 207*(9), 778–784.

CHAPTER 5

Principles and Commitments Guiding the Construction of the ICD-DSM Classifications

A History

PETER ZACHAR, MICHAEL B. FIRST, AND PAUL S. APPELBAUM

Introduction

CLASSIFICATION is a fundamental human activity—for instance, distinguishing between poisonous versus edible, dangerous versus safe, and dead versus alive. Conceptual contrasts such as these are both shared and increasingly multiplied by language. The proliferation of concepts extends to the specialized languages of professional communities, including languages for psychopathology.

This chapter reviews the history and development of two prominent classification systems of mental disorders, namely, the mental, behavioral, and neurodevelopmental disorders section of the International Classification of Diseases (ICD), which is developed by the World Health Organization (WHO), and the *Diagnostic and Statistical Manual of Mental Disorders* (DSM), which is developed by the American Psychiatric Association (APA) (American Psychiatric Association, 2022; World Health Organization, 2022).

In this chapter we will explore a multiplicity of complications involved in constructing psychiatric classifications. Throughout this chapter we will also emphasize features of this history that have been neglected in previous accounts. The topics to be discussed are the development of the ICD and DSM in a shared international context, their descriptive focus, the importance placed on clinical utility, the role of expert judgment and curation in their development, and how the resulting classifications are often compromises among competing interests.

The Development of the ICD and DSM

In the 19th and early 20th centuries, psychiatric classification systems were developed by single individuals. Some of the better-known psychiatric taxonomists from this era were Cullen, Thomas Arnold, Pinel, David Skae, Thomas Clouston, Kraepelin, Wernicke, and Schneider. The downside to a "great professor" approach to classification is that it generates diverse, and sometimes contradictory, classifications—and professionals end up speaking different languages. The terminology of psychiatric classification becomes like a Tower of Babel.

Kramer (1968) notes that in 1880, Frederick Wines, who was working to develop a uniform classification of mental disorders, claimed that "it seems impossible for those best qualified to form an opinion to agree upon any scheme which can be devised" (p. xii). On one hand, the number of scientific and professional perspectives has likely increased over time, so the situation is still complicated. On the other, for the present at least, there are two primary classification systems (ICD-11 and DSM-5-TR), and they agree on many points.

International coordination was articulated as a goal for the collection of public health statistics after public health became more institutionalized in the 19th century. Hacking (1990) reports that a significant impetus for an increased interest in the collection and analysis of public health statistics was related to psychiatry. Jean-Étienne Esquirol, a famed French psychiatrist, claimed that suicide should be considered as a kind of madness and under the purview of medicine, not the clergy. He also believed that it was more rampant in England than in France. This led each country to increase their collection and analysis of statistical data on suicide.

Over a series of biennial international statistical conferences beginning in 1853, work on a uniform international classification for use in public health was conducted, but agreement was hard to reach (Moriyama et al., 2011). In 1893, however, a committee chaired by the French statistician Jacques Bertillon synthesized classifications from several countries to construct the first International List of Causes of Death (World Health Organization, 2021). Over the next 60 years, the Bertillon classification was revised five times.

In 1948, under the guidance of the recently formed World Health Organization, the sixth revision of the international classification sought to incorporate all diseases, not just those that resulted in death (i.e., it classified both mortality and morbidity) and was renamed the International Statistical Classification of Diseases, Injures, and Causes of Death (ICD-6). One section was devoted to the classification of mental disorders (Keeley et al., 2023). All WHO member nations were expected to use the ICD-6 in compiling national statistics, but professional organizations within countries could continue to develop and use their own classifications for clinical purposes.

American psychiatry was inclined to do exactly that—resulting in the publication of the DSM-I in 1952. Beginning in 1917, the APA contributed to the production of the *Statistical Manual for the Use of Hospitals for Mental Disease*. Its purpose was to support the national collection of morbidity data.[1] This "Statistical Manual" was replaced by the DSM-I, which revised several classifications that were in general use after World War II to create a single new system (see the fourth section, on the ICD and DSM seeking to include disorders important for clinicians, for more details). Table 5.1 lists all editions of the ICD and DSM.

In the construction of psychiatric classifications there is ongoing tension about whether their primary purpose is to promote the collection of statistical information or to be clinical nomenclatures. A statistical classification need only be a list of categories—often broad—used for counting. For example, "depression" is sufficient for statistical purposes. Adding melancholic depression, atypical depression, and postpartum depression would complicate data collection and coding. A nomenclature, however, should flexibly accommodate the variety of presentations encountered in clinical practice in more detail.

At the first planning meeting for the DSM-I revision, some members claimed that there should be separate committees, one for a nomenclature and a second for a statistical classification. The majority of the members believed that a statistical classification logically depends on a nomenclature rather than being separate from it (Menninger et al., 1963). As a result, the DSM-I did not merely name disorders for counting purposes but also provided qualifying

[1] At this time the APA was named the American Medico-Psychological Association. Its partner in developing the *Statistical Manual* was the U.S. Public Health Service's National Committee for Mental Hygiene.

TABLE 5.1 Editions of the ICD and DSM

Edition	Publication Date	Edition	Publication Date
ICD-6	1948	DSM-III-R	1987
DSM-1	1952	ICD-10	1990
ICD-7	1957	DSM-IV	1994
ICD-8	1967	DSM-IV-TR	2000
DSM-II	1968	DSM-5	2013
ICD-9	1978	ICD-11	2022
DSM-III	1980	DSM-5-TR	2022

phrases that allowed for more specificity in diagnosis. Like the *Statistical Manual*, it also included descriptions of clinical phenomenology.[2] For example, the definition of manic-depressive reaction, depressed type, was:

> Here will be classified those cases with outstanding depression of mood and with mental and motor retardation and inhibition; in some cases, there is much uneasiness and apprehension. Perplexity, stupor or agitation may be prominent symptoms and may be added to the diagnosis as manifestations. (American Psychiatric Association, 1952, p. 25)

According to Raines (1952), after the establishment of the National Institute of Mental Health in 1949, its Biometrics Branch was charged with reporting national statistics, removing the burden on the drafters of DSM-I to develop a typology primarily to support the collection of morbidity data. Thus, the manual was able to assume a more clinical form. The relative importance of each purpose was reflected in the new title: *Diagnostic and Statistical Manual.*

The ICD-6 list of mental disorders was adopted in very few countries, because, like in the United States, many countries preferred using their own local classifications (Stengel, 1959). Although ICD-7, published in 1955, included many updates, the mental disorders section was left unchanged from ICD-6 (Moriyama et al., 2011).

To address international dissatisfaction with the ICD classification of mental disorders, the WHO commissioned a report by Erwin Stengel (1959), who recommended that in addition to just listing disorders, the ICD should also include a glossary containing operational definitions for all mental disorders—with the goal of making it an acceptable classification across nations. For Stengel, an operational definition meant a description of key clinical features that are available to everyone through observation and stated in terms that mean the same thing to everyone who uses them. Stengel pointed to the descriptions in the DSM-I as an example of a "glossary."

The Mental Disorders section in ICD-8 began as a joint U.S. and U.K. proposal developed by a committee chaired by British psychiatrist Aubrey Lewis. This proposal was then integrated with proposals from seven other countries and then further revised as other member nations weighed in (Kramer, 1968). Once the ICD-8 was published in 1967, Spitzer and Wilson (1968) reported that the DSM-II revision was undertaken to make the DSM and the ICD-8

[2] A PDF of the original *Statistical Manual* is available from the HathiTrust, https://archive.org/details/statisticalmanuooassogoog/page/n2/mode/2up?ref=ol&view=theater.

compatible. Several features of the ICD-8 were modified in the DSM-II, but for the most part the disorders listed in the two classifications were in harmony.[3]

The ICD-8 classification did not include glossary descriptions of clinical phenomenology until a revision of a British glossary was appended to it in 1974. For the ICD-9, published in 1978, the glossary was integrated into the mental disorders section itself.

Once the ICD-9 revision began, it was time also to again revise the DSM. Rather than simply trying to coordinate with the committee working on the ICD-9, the APA made major changes for the DSM-III of 1980 that resulted in the ICD-9 and DSM-III diverging from one another.

Robert Spitzer (2001) reported that the DSM-III Task Force believed it was more important to be innovative than to be in complete harmony with the ICD-9. The most important innovation was the inclusion of diagnostic criteria modeled on the criteria proposed by Feighner et al. (1972) (the "Feigner criteria") and the *Research Diagnostic Criteria* (Spitzer et al., 1978), both of which were developed for use in research. These criteria consisted of lists of symptoms, a subset of which must be present to qualify for a diagnosis. For example, the Feighner criteria for mania required the following:

> A. euphoria or irritability; and B. at least three of the following six: (1) hyperactivity, (2) pressure to keep talking; (3) racing thoughts; (4) grandiosity; (5) decreased sleep; and (6) distractibility; and C. lasting at least two weeks.

In addition, the information included about each disorder in DSM-III is more extensive than those in previous versions, being almost textbook-like. For example, the DSM-II definitions for manic-depressive illness and its three types (manic type, depressed type, and circular type) could be contained on one page. In contrast, the DSM-III diagnostic criteria for a manic episode and bipolar disorder and its accompanying text (which included additional information such age-at-onset, course, prevalence, sex ratio, and familial pattern) occupied more than four pages.

The international consensus was further upended when countries in addition to the United States began using the DSM-III criteria, which had been translated into thirteen languages. Cooper (1982) reported that in order to avoid any further divergence between rival classifications, in 1979 the WHO in Geneva and the Alcohol, Drug Abuse, and Mental Health Administration (ADAMHA) in the United States cooperated to create nine joint working groups, which met to review recent research and define priorities for future collaborative efforts. This culminated in an international conference in 1982, held in Copenhagen, where the recommendations from the working groups were reviewed and further recommendations articulated.

Kendell (1991) claimed that this conference played an important role in the ICD-10's implementing diagnostic criteria following the model used in the DSM-III and its 1987 revision, the DSM-III-R. Kendell did not think that the WHO would have been able to implement diagnostic criteria without the American example. He reported that the ICD has to be acceptable to multiple countries and is translated for use by a diverse collection of hospitals, educational systems, legal systems, insurance companies, and public health departments—which, in Kendell's view, constrain the opportunities for innovation.

The development of the mental disorders chapter in ICD-10 was completed in 1990 on what Kendell (1991) described as a shoestring budget. There was a clinical diagnostic version, a version with diagnostic criteria for research, and a version for use in primary care. In contrast,

[3] In the United States the ICD-8 was modified to be more useful for indexing hospital records (ICDA-8). Later, the ICD-9 was also modified to be used for reimbursement in clinical settings (ICD-9-CM).

from DSM-III onward, one single manual was developed for use in both clinical and research settings. Moreover, the development of DSM-IV was bankrolled by the considerable proceeds the APA received from the sales of DSM-III and DSM-III-R. The APA had the financial resources to support an extensive revision effort, which included conducting extensive literature reviews, data re-analysis of existing diagnostic datasets, and diagnosis-focused field trials (Frances et al., 1989). The DSM work groups carefully studied ICD-10 drafts and used them continuously in all phases of the revision. Another part of the DSM-IV–ICD-10 harmonization effort was the convening of small conferences in the middle of the DSM-IV revision, at which the corresponding ICD-10 and DSM-IV work groups met to try to work out differences, if possible.

Despite these efforts, First (2009) reports that, once the DSM-IV was published in 1994, the criteria in DSM-IV and in the research diagnostic criteria version of the ICD-10 differed for nearly every disorder. In some cases, these differences were arbitrary variations in the wording of diagnostic criteria, but in others, there were intentional differences in how the disorders were conceptualized. For example, in the ICD-10, schizophrenia could be diagnosed after one month of symptoms, while the DSM-IV required six months.

A concerted attempt at harmonization was implemented for the ICD-11 and DSM-5. Early planning for both revisions occurred across several internationally focused "refining the research agenda" conferences and books (Kupfer et al., 2002; Regier et al., 2009). In addition, the leaders of both revisions attended each other's meetings, and the ICD-11 working groups and DSM-5 work groups shared members.

The DSM-5 was published in 2013. The ICD-11 working groups then evaluated the suitability of incorporating the DSM-5 changes into ICD-11, which was published in 2019. Once completed, the two systems continued to diverge. Each classification contains disorders that the other does not, and 70% of the shared disorders have major or minor differences (First et al., 2021). The two systems, however, are more similar to each other than they have been at any point since the ICD-8 and DSM-II.[4]

In a more recent development, ongoing changes to the DSM-5 criteria are managed by the DSM Steering Committee and five broad review committees (Appelbaum et al., 2021). Adhering to the *Guide to submitting proposals for changes to DSM-5* (APA DSM Team, 2021) the steering committee believes that conceptual and linguistic harmony with the ICD is desirable, when possible. There are currently no equivalent guidelines or processes in place for making changes to ICD-11.

ICD and DSM Classifications Are Descriptive, Not Etiological

Descriptive psychopathology is often contrasted by psychiatrists and philosophers with etiological classification (Hempel, 1961; Hyman, 2010). For example, tuberculosis can be classified based on observable features or on etiology and pathogenesis. In medicine, classification based on etiology and pathogenesis is considered ideal, because having knowledge about causal mechanisms reveals more avenues for preventing, ameliorating, and/or reversing morbid changes.

[4] Unlike the three ICD-10 versions, the ICD-11 has a single section named "clinical descriptions and diagnostic guidelines" that is more like DSM diagnostic criteria, but the ICD is not as strict as the DSM about diagnostic thresholds.

For psychiatric disorders, because both etiology and pathogenesis tend to be complex, the contrast between descriptive versus etiological approaches has historically also embodied a contrast between descriptive versus speculative formulations. In fact, the modern roots of descriptive classification reside in the natural history approach of the philosophical empiricists, who were suspicious of speculation about the ultimate causes and essences of diseases (Anstey, 2011; Zachar & Kendler, 2017).

Likewise, the German psychiatrist Emil Kraepelin's emphasis on description based on clinical observation followed from his opposition to speculation about both biological and psychological causes (Engstrom & Kendler, 2015). The speculative approach for Kraepelin was illustrated by the Viennese psychiatrist Theodor Meynert's approach to etiology, which freely combined inferences about biological and psychological causes. For example, according to Meynert, all behavior is activated either by aggressive emotion due to excessive blood flow in the brain or defensive emotion due to constricted blood flow (Marx, 1970).

The primary justification for a descriptive approach in the late 19th century was that conditions such as tuberculosis and general paresis of the insane were identified and described prior to the discovery of any valid information about etiology. In Kraepelin's view, they are recognizable *disease forms*. For Kraepelin, a disease form was more than a list of signs and symptoms, it also included course and outcome (Heckers & Kendler, 2020).

As noted in the second section, on the development of the ICD and DSM, Stengel recommended that the ICD incorporate observation-based operational definitions. In discussing operational definitions, Stengel credited the philosopher of science Carl Hempel, but recent scholarship indicates that his thinking on this matter was also reflective of a distinction between public and private classifications suggested in 1959 by Aubrey Lewis (Fulford & Sartorius, 2009). Public classifications are descriptive and operational. They should avoid categories based on theoretical concepts in order to be usable by those with different theoretical perspectives and assumptions—including clinicians, researchers, and governments. Private classifications, in contrast, are used by smaller groups for their own purposes and may even be suitable only for those purposes. Such purposes can include using agreed-upon theoretical assumptions. For example, defining borderline personality by a reliance on defense mechanisms such as splitting and projective identification would be what Lewis meant by a private classification.

Because the DSM-II defined neurosis as caused by conscious or unconscious anxiety, it is often seen as being psychodynamically oriented, but the APA Committee on Nomenclature intended to promote a more descriptive, less speculative approach to classification. In the forward to DSM-II, Gruenberg (1968) reported that the nomenclature committee attempted to avoid terms that carry implications about the nature of disorders or their causes. In the introduction to DSM-II, Kramer (1968) specifically stated that that the manual's descriptions of the disorders are "operational definitions."

The conventional story that descriptive psychopathology was introduced to American psychiatry in the DSM-III is thus not correct, although certainly the meaning of "operational definition" changed in the DSM-III.[5] Rather than referring to narrative clinical descriptions, operational definition referred to the use of explicit diagnostic criteria that were formulated at the lowest order of inference necessary to describe the characteristic features of the disorder. Wherever possible, the criteria were behavioral, but some criteria such as identity disturbance in borderline personality required a higher order of inference. In short, operational diagnostic

[5] The diagnostic criteria of the DSM-III are symptom checklists and would not count as operational definitions as originally proposed by the physicist Percy Bridgman as test conditions, that is, if you drop it and it breaks, it is fragile. Bridgman, P. W. (1927). *The logic of modern physics.* Macmillan.

criteria were included in DSM-III not only to increase reliability and to facilitate their use in research, but also to continue a previously initiated shift to a descriptive classification.

The ICD and DSM Seek to Include Disorders That Are Important for Clinicians (Clinical Utility)

In psychiatry, new disorders are periodically proposed to better represent what clinicians are encountering in practice. One of the most dramatic expansions of disorder constructs in psychiatry occurred in the middle of the 20th century in the United States. To explain this expansion, we will delve a little deeper into how classifications developed in the United States in particular. The classifications in use during this expansion and their relationships to each other are listed in Table 5.2.

Clinical Usefulness in the First DSM

In the early part of the century, psychiatry in the United States was a small specialty, with most psychiatrists working in institutional settings. The country's entry into World War II significantly changed American psychiatry by broadening its scope of practice. During the war, the number of physicians assigned to psychiatry units in the military increased from only 35 to over 2,000 (Grob, 1991).

After the attack on Pearl Harbor in December 1941, large numbers of men enlisted and were drafted into the military and sent to battle. Based on previous experience in World War I, military doctors knew that the stress of war would lead to many psychiatric casualties. In contrast to the prevailing notion that recovery required removing a person from the source of the troubling distress, the plan was to implement a triage model whereby an intervention occurred early on, with the goal of returning soldiers to active duty as soon as they were ready. In addition, rather than expecting that most cases would include people with pre-existing problems exacerbated by war, military physicians expected that the stress of war could precipitate psychiatric distress reactions in soldiers even if they did not have pre-existing conditions (Houts, 2000). This perspective normalized psychiatric distress and engendered increased hopefulness about recovery.

TABLE 5.2 Classification in use during and after World War II

Statistical Manual for the Use of Hospitals for Mental Disease (i.e. Statistical Manual), ten editions from 1917 to 1942 (after 1934 incorporated into the Standard Nomenclature)
Standard Nomenclature of Diseases and Operations, four editions between 1933 and 1952
U. S. Dept of Navy Classification, 1944
U. S. Dept of Army Classification, 1945
Armed Services Classification (Medical 203), 1946 (same as Army classification)
Veterans Administration (V. A.) Classification, 1946 (similar to Army classification)
ICD-6, (1948) (informed by Armed Forces and V.A. classifications)
DSM-I, (1952) (included in the 1952 Standard Nomenclature as Diseases of the Psychobiologic Unit)

The U.S. Armed Forces faced an increasing psychiatric caseload as the war continued. It soon became apparent that the psychiatric classification contained in the *Standard Nomenclature of Diseases*[6] developed primarily for use in public mental hospitals, did not account for the many kinds of problems that psychiatrists were encountering. Psychiatrists in the military found themselves operating within the limits of a nomenclature specifically not developed for a large majority of their cases (Raines, 1952). These included cases involving personality disturbances, psychosomatic conditions, and several types of reaction to stress. In response to these deficiencies, the U.S. Navy and U.S. Army each developed their own classifications. The army classification was more extensive and was eventually adopted by all the armed forces. It was also modified for use by the Veterans Administration (V.A.).

Many of the physicians who had been assigned to treating psychiatric patients in the war continued to practice psychiatry after the war ended, not just in institutions but also in private practice and outpatient clinics. Soldiers returning from the war had to re-adjust to civilian life, and the kinds of problems psychiatrists confronted expanded even further.

A few years after the end of the war, four nomenclatures (the prewar Standard Nomenclature, Armed Forces, Veterans Administration, and ICD-6) were in general use. A list of the disorders in most recent version of the APA's *Statistical Manual* was incorporated into the *Standard Nomenclature*. In addition, local teaching centers mixed and matched features from these various classifications.

With an eye on this chaotic situation, the American Psychiatric Association postponed an update of its *Statistical Manual* to study the new Armed Forces and V.A. classifications. The APA Committee on Nomenclature and Statistics discovered that these classifications were viewed positively by both clinicians and statisticians and were seen as being superior to the APA classification (Menninger et al., 1963). The APA then contacted psychiatrists to assess their level of support for constructing a new classification, with those in private practice and outpatient clinics being especially supportive—they viewed the armed forces and V.A. classifications to be more useful (Raines, 1952). As described in the second section, the result was the DSM-I.

We should also note that DSM-I was published around the time that psychoanalysis was becoming the dominant paradigm in American psychiatry. In an editorial promoting the importance of the DSM-I, Raines (1953) acknowledged that it had become popular to decry diagnosis in psychiatry. Many psychoanalysts did not view diagnosis and classification as useful, because, in their view, focusing on manifest clinical phenomenology diverted attention from the unconscious conflicts that were the primary causes of psychiatric distress (Horwitz, 2021). They considered these conflicts too grounded in individual histories to be captured by standard diagnostic labels.

DSM-III Makes Clinical Usefulness Paramount

In DSM-I, improving clinical usefulness meant expanding coverage and increasing specificity for diagnosing individual cases. As described in the second section, for DSM-II, improving clinical usefulness meant offering descriptions that reduce ambiguity and confusion about the meaning of terms. Although improving clinical usefulness was important to the first two DSMs, the DSM-III elevated its importance. This third revision had many goals, such as improving an embarrassingly low degree of inter-rater reliability, but according to Robert Spitzer (2001), the highest priority during the development of the DSM-III was that it be useful to clinicians. Indeed, first among the ten goals for DSM-III noted in its introduction

[6] Beginning in 1942 the nomenclature and the operations manual were separated.

was its "clinical usefulness for making treatment and management decisions in varied clinical settings" (American Psychiatric Association, 1980, p. 2).

A clinically useful classification/diagnosis (a) aids in communicating the nature of the problem to patients, other professionals, and third-party payers; (b) facilitates predictions about prognosis and treatment, and (c) offers a bridge between patients' problems and the scientific and professional literature. As noted by First (2010), a clinically useful diagnosis also is one that working professionals can apply in an accurate way.

Spitzer reports that the DSM-III Task Force adopted a principle of inclusiveness, by which they meant expanding coverage. The Task Force would add any diagnostic category that was considered important for clinical practice even in the absence of research demonstrating reliability or validity. Among the new categories added in the DSM-III were borderline and narcissistic personality disorders, panic disorder, generalized anxiety disorder, post-traumatic stress disorder (PTSD), and anorexia nervosa. Other than a practical consideration that new disorders should have clinical face validity, the only firm requirement for adding a new disorder was that it had to be operationally defined. This emphasis on clinical usefulness created a rift between Spitzer and the authors of the Feighner criteria, who asserted that diagnostic criteria for not-yet-validated disorders should be left out of the manual (Decker, 2013).

Clinical usefulness has been listed as the *most important* goal of every subsequent DSM revision.

> The first listed goal of both DSM-III and DSM-III-R is its "*clinical usefulness for making treatment and management decisions in varied clinical settings*" (DSM-III, p. 2; DSM-III-R p. xix).
>
> "*Our highest priority has been to provide a helpful guide to clinical practice*" (DSM-IV, p. xv and DSM-IV-TR, p. xxiii).
>
> "*. . . this edition of the DSM was designed first and foremost to be a useful guide to clinical practice*" (DSM-5, p. xii, DSM-5-TR, p. xxiii).

Improving clinical care is perhaps the most important reason to add a new disorder to a classification. The first step in treatment is successful recognition of the diagnosis. Thus, if a condition is not in the classification with reliable criteria, clinicians are likely to miss diagnosing it. Virtually all proposals to add new disorders to DSM have been based on this argument, especially if there are successful treatments.

The ICD classification serves as the framework for monitoring threats to public health and disease burden around the world which has had a unique impact on which disorders are included in ICD-11. For example, ICD-11 includes ten dissociative disorders, while the DSM-5 includes only four.[7] The inclusion of conditions such as trance disorder and possession trance disorder in ICD-11 reflects the clinical importance of these conditions in some non-Western populations.

Another example is the fact that internet gaming disorder was included as an official category in the ICD-11 chapter "Disorders Due to Substance Use or Addictive Behaviors," whereas it was relegated to the "Emerging Measures and Models" section in DSM-5 in order to facilitate future research. Although it had been shown to be a growing problem in China, the paucity of supporting research combined with this condition not being perceived to be a significant enough problem in the United States did not warrant its inclusion in the main section of DSM-5 (Petry et al., 2015). From the ICD-11 perspective, those diagnosable with "gaming disorder"

[7] We should note that the DSM-5 revision did not emphasize expanding coverage. In fact, the *Guidelines for Making Changes to the DSM-5* set a very high bar of evidence required for adding new disorders to the manual, and thus very few new disorders were added.

are a legitimate clinical group who can benefit from services. Furthermore, this condition has sufficient public health consequences in some WHO member states to justify the collection and reporting of epidemiological data (Reed et al., 2022).

Initial Decisions about Disorders in the ICD and DSM Are Made by Committees of Experts

Millon (1986) reports that as early visions for the DSM-III revision were being articulated, within the APA an ad hoc committee composed of members selected for being innovative was charged with evaluating current research data and theoretical proposals for the next DSM, but their work was rejected by the standing nomenclature committee. With an eye toward having an innovative committee that could actually implement changes, in 1974, the nomenclature committee was reconstituted with new members and Robert Spitzer as the Chair. As Decker (2013) notes, given that many psychiatrists did not view the DSM as important, this change was not particularly noticed. The new committee was renamed the Task Force and subcommittees for specific classes of disorders were named work groups.

Krueger et al. (2018) observe that the ICD-DSM committees rely on both (a) an authoritative approach to their work, one based on expertise, disciplinary background, and tradition, and (b) considerations of specific kinds of empirical evidence. We concur with them that a mix of factors including traditional clinical lore, clinical experience, and scientific expertise has informed DSM (and ICD) psychopathology. Writing about science in general, Kuhn (1977) referred to the back-and-forth struggle between commitment to accepted knowledge and the search for innovation as "the essential tension."

These committees of experts have, however, been critiqued by some for not being scientific enough. For example, Ghaemi (2023) asserts that the DSM is constructed on pragmatic grounds, relying on social, economic, and political considerations more than scientific considerations.

In our view, such critiques misrepresent the process. For example, consider the composition of the DSM-5 work groups. In 2022, for a conference presentation focusing on the substance-related disorders work group, one of us consulted Google Scholar to determine each work group member's then current h-index and number of publications (Zachar, 2022). The lowest h-index was 40, the highest was 103. An h-index of 40 means a researcher has at least 40 papers that have been cited at least 40 times. The smallest number of publications was 154, the highest was 620. If someone was not a productive researcher, they would not have been appointed to this work group. Given the composition of the DSM work groups, it is doubtful that scientific considerations do not inform the decisions made—although one's record of research might inform one's views about how to balance scientific, clinical, and practical considerations in a variety of possible ways.

Others have critiqued these committees of experts for being too scientific and not sufficiently clinically oriented. For example, Allen Frances (2011) criticized the DSM committee structure for being composed of inbred researchers and academics who did not understand the clinical world. The work groups, Frances believed, contained the wrong kind of expertise—one that did not appreciate how an idea that works well in a narrow research setting may not work in everyday clinical practice. He was very concerned about the harmful consequences of false positive diagnoses, but he also worried that researchers lack the experience to appreciate the ambiguities of making diagnoses in difficult clinical settings.

There is certainly room for legitimate disagreement about how to balance scientific and clinical considerations in constructing classifications, but some of the critiques may also be attributing too much influence to the committees of experts. For example, a committee's recommendations are advisory and, traditionally, extensive input from outside the committees has kept them from being insular. At the end of the day, the work groups do not make the final decisions. The final decision on the ICD as a whole is made by the World Health Assembly,[8] whereas for the DSM it is made by the Board of Trustees of the American Psychiatric Association.

The ICD and DSM Classifications Are Curated

Curation involves a person with expertise selecting and organizing content from a larger number of possibilitics—often with some goals or standards in mind. Selecting the great books of literature, influential film noir movies, or the key works of Van Gogh are typical examples of curation. The concept of curation indicates that *decisions* are involved, and the outcomes are *not inevitable*.

Chapters in undergraduate textbooks and topics covered in a course syllabus are also curated. In this vein, the microbiologist Ludwik Fleck (1935/1979) wrote about different repositories of scientific knowledge, including:

popular science—written for non-experts

textbook science—college textbooks and scholarly handbooks

journal science—articles in peer-reviewed journals

guidebook science (*vademecum* science)[9]—to be explained later in this section

These different types of repositories are not independent and can overlap. Every expert begins their exposure to the discipline with popular science and later textbook science. Textbook science is a guided introduction to the realm of expertise.

By journal science, Fleck means detailed, technical, and specialized articles. In journal science, the norms of scientific publishing promote a culture of tentativeness. This repository, therefore, will be full of conflicting, even contradictory information and may constitute a confusing array.

The vademecum is paradigm-like. In fact, Thomas Kuhn (1970) claimed that Fleck anticipated many of his ideas about scientific paradigms. A vademecum refers to thoughts about current, best knowledge and has an air of being institutional and legitimated. Like textbooks, a vademecum is often presented as communicating matters of settled fact and expert judgment. Unlike textbooks, a vademecum is more likely to serve as a guide for future research—in part by defining basic concepts and problems to work on. As Kuhn (1979) suggests, curation imparts "authority" to the vademecum. According to Fleck:

> The vademecum is therefore not simply the result of either a compilation or a collection of various journal contributions. . . . A vademecum is built up from individual contributions through selection and orderly arrangement like a mosaic from many colored stones. (p. 119)

In Fleck's view, research groups that are attempting to curate and transform their journal science into vademecum science occupy the role of vanguards. This implies that there will be differing judgments about what should be part of the vademecum.

The vademecum domain is where classification systems like the ICD and DSM reside. They trail journal science and put competing, detailed claims in the background. The authors of

[8] The World Health Assembly makes a yes or no decision on the entire ICD in a single vote.

[9] This is usually translated as "handbook science," but Oxford Handbooks and Cambridge Companions are versions of textbook science.

these systems, with an eye on journal science, typically acknowledge their provisional natures. Many users, however, either do not read or proceed to ignore such cautions—resulting in diagnostic literalism and notions such as the DSM is the psychiatric Bible. For instance, Hyman (2010) writes:

> Unfortunately, the disorders within these classifications are not generally treated as heuristic, but to a great degree have become reified. Disorders within the DSM-IV or ICD-10 are often treated as if they were natural kinds, real entities that exist independently of any particular rater. (p. 156)

For the design of classification systems, the choices involved in curation may have to adjudicate among competing empirical, theoretical, and practical claims. Competing empirical and theoretical claims are usually conceptualized as curating the science. Examples of curation include the implementation of operationalized diagnostic criteria in DSM-III and the elimination of some of the diagnostic hierarchies in DSM-III-R.

A recent example of curation from the DSM-5 was the substance-related disorders work group's argument for collapsing the putatively less-serious substance abuse category and the more-serious substance dependence category into a single substance use disorder category for each class of substance (Hasin et al., 2013). They showed that criteria for abuse and dependence are manifestations of a single unidimensional factor in which abuse and dependence criteria are intermixed, with some abuse criteria being more severe than some dependence criteria. Although it included the dimensional specifiers mild, moderate, and severe, the DSM-5 did not emphasize the psychometric unidimensionality of disordered substance use but instead presented substance use disorder as a polythetic category with a new diagnostic threshold, that is, someone must have 2 of 11 symptoms to be diagnosed. This decision was not inevitable.

Into this new category the work group also added a criterion for craving. The work group realized that adding craving did not improve the criterion set by increasing diagnostic accuracy, but a little over half the members decided to add it anyway, because craving is an important treatment target and may have clear biomarkers (Zachar et al., 2022). This also exemplifies curation.

In our view, curation is unavoidable, because facts rarely point to a single classificatory outcome. Facts are partial and incomplete and have to be selected and interpreted in the light of goals and commitments. When the experts cannot agree, decisions often come down to a "vote" or, if not a formal vote, some evaluation of what the majority can agree on. Whether a formal vote or a general consensus, such decisions are based on a mingling of competing scientific and practical considerations. The downside to the curation of classifications is not that decisions are a part of the process but that, when the curation is invisible, users may treat outcomes as inevitable matters of fact.

The ICD and DSM Classifications Are Compromises between Different Purposes and Perspectives

Classifications serve multiple purposes, and in constructing classifications, to a large extent, these purposes have to be balanced against one another. The practical need to balance use in research and use in clinical settings was evident in the DSM-III. There are also multiple purposes within research and practice, such as for use in epidemiological research versus neuroscientific research or for making decisions about need for treatment versus need for hospitalization in clinical practice. The DSM specifically notes that the thresholds should be treated flexibly for different uses. If we also include use in forensic settings or use in determining eligibility for social services, classifications serve public policy purposes as well.

In addition to balancing multiple goals and purposes, the process of constructing classifications sometimes involves attempts to reach some consensus among multiple stakeholders. For example, as stated in Appendix A of the DSM-I:

> The construction of a practical scheme of classification of disease and injury for general statistical use involves various compromises. . . . Adjustments must also be made to meet the varied requirements of vital statistics offices, hospitals of different types, medical services of the armed forces, social insurance organizations, sickness surveys, and numerous other agencies. (American Psychiatric Association, 1952, p. 88)

In theory, the possible stakeholders include specialist clinicians, non-specialists, primary care physicians, neighboring professionals like psychologists and social workers, and researchers. Other potential stakeholders include service users, professional organizations, insurance companies, government agencies, school systems, the pharmaceutical industry, other industries like publishers, and the legal system.

One consistent theme for the ICD and DSM has been the expectation of seeking advice from outside the committee, especially from clinicians. The DSM-I and DSM-II used surveys of practicing psychiatrists. Beginning with DSM-III, the APA Assembly, which includes representation of practicing psychiatrists from district and state branches across the United States, was consulted, and by the time of DSM-5, the Assembly was treated as one of the approval bodies. The field trials for both the ICD and the DSM also bring clinicians into the process.

In the United States, many of the controversies about classification during past revisions took the form of opposition from professionals not involved in the revision process. For the DSM-III, this included psychoanalysts upset at the elimination of neurosis as a distinct pathological process (Decker, 2013). For the DSM-III-R and DSM-IV, there were controversies about diagnoses that were seen as reflecting biases against women, such as masochistic personality disorder and premenstrual dysphoric disorder (Caplan, 1995). For the DSM-5, opposition to the diagnosis of attenuated psychosis, the elimination of the bereavement exclusion for depression, and implementing a dimensional model for personality disorder were spearheaded by other professionals (Shedler et al., 2010; Society for Humanistic Psychology, 2011; Wakefield, 2011). The public nature of the controversies is a good example of the DSM being the victim of its own success, because multiple stakeholders believe that what is in the DSM matters to them.

We close this section by discussing two recent trends with respect to the consideration of stakeholders. The first is an attempt to more systematically address potential conflicts of interest—especially financial conflicts of interest (FCOI). The second is a call to bring service users into the process of constructing classifications.

First, there was a long gap between the publication of DSM-IV in 1994 and the start of the DSM-5 process in 2010. During that time there was a sea change with respect to concerns about the influence of industry on academics. For example, the optics of the pharmaceutical industry's role in the development of the DSM was not helped when several prominent psychiatrists were discovered to have undisclosed income from pharmaceutical companies while at the same time advocating for new diagnoses that were of particular interest to those companies (Lenzer, 2008). This is problematic, because a new diagnosis allows for the potential expansion of FDA-approved indications for medication, such as for pediatric bipolar disorder, thus increasing the medication's use and expanding industry profits.

When work started on DSM-5, APA realized that it had better put into place stringent limits on pharmaceutical involvement. This led to the setting of limits on income, including investment income, that work group members can receive from industry. Transparency was increased by requiring work group members to disclose all sources of income. Furthermore, for revisions to the DSM-5 text that resulted in the DSM-5-TR, all recommended changes were reviewed by a COI Review Editor to assess whether committee members' outside interests could have influenced the recommendation (Appelbaum, 2024).

As with any new policy, there are also foreseen and unforeseen negative consequences. For the FCOI policy, once one becomes a recognized expert, among the opportunities that become available is to be a consultant to industry. Once the FCOI policy was implemented, one of its possibly unforeseen consequences was that many leading experts who would otherwise be considered for working on the DSM became ineligible to serve.

Second, as opposed to reducing the influence of some outside stakeholder groups, another trend seeks to increase the influence of other groups in the development process, specifically patients or service users. This is important for several reasons. Even minor changes to diagnostic criteria can have consequences for who is eligible for services. Kamens et al. (2019) argue that the primary purpose in revising any classification should be to minimize harm to those classified. They also argue that all changes should be made only for the benefit of those classified and not for any other group.

For the DSM, service users and related parties such as family members have the option of submitting feedback about proposed changes during the public commentary phase—and frequently do. Kamens et al. argue that they should also have representation on the actual work groups, because they possess expertise by experience. Kamens et al. do not claim that having a disorder provides one with expertise. As Friesen (2021) notes, the concept of "expertise" also implies that one's experience has been augmented by a process of critical reflection even if some aspects of experience in itself may be relevant to the diagnostic revision process—and hopefully they would be considered more than token members.

ICD-DSM Classifications and Future Innovation

A tension between a commitment to "current knowledge" and the search for innovation has been a running theme across the ICD and DSM revisions. For example, consider these quotes from Raines (1953) writing about the publication of the DSM-I.

> Resistance to change, especially in this field, is great, and nomenclature revisions frequently consist of only minor arrangements of terms with no major repair work being done. (p. 548)

> It is therefore necessary that psychiatric nomenclature, as well as other medical nomenclature, be revised from time to time to keep it in step with the moving body of psychiatric knowledge. (p. 548)

From the DSM-III onward (and arguably before), each revision of the manual was intended by its designers to reflect recent clinical and scientific advances, but there have also been occasional shifts in the degree of desire for innovation. The DSM-III revolution and the calls for a paradigm shift at the beginning of the DSM-5 revision could be considered high points in the quest for innovation. In response to these ambitious stances, the DSM-IV process and the latter part of the DSM-5 process opted for gradual iterations of criteria and categories rather than sweeping changes. Ironically, some changes rejected for the DSM-5 (for example, the adoption of a dimensional approach to personality disorder diagnosis) were implemented in the ICD-11—despite the constraints that the ICD's global focus places on innovation.

Many thinkers have pointed to a Kuhnian crisis of confidence in the ICD and DSM systems, which calls to mind the possibility of revolutionary paradigm shifts (Kendler & First,

2010; Phillips, 2013; Poland & Tekin, 2017; Solomon, 2022). We take it as given that there is significant interest in altering, reforming, or improving the classifications. This may involve iteration and gradual improvement but could also usher in a new phase characterized by more substantial innovation. It is, however, difficult to predict the future pace of scientific advances, and expectations that the next paradigm shift is just around the corner have not always been fulfilled.

From the innovator perspective, the entrenchment of DSM-ICD constructs creates resistance to change. Arguably, incentives to maintain the current system on the part of particular clinical specialties and research groups, the practical need to avoid disruptions to clinical care, and the reification of categories promotes some entrenchment of ICD and DSM classification. Another possible factor at play in the entrenchment is that diagnostic concepts such as depression and schizophrenia are embedded in folk psychology. In some cases, folk psychological terms (such as depression) have displaced professional terms (such as melancholia), and in other cases newly introduced professional terms gained a foothold in folk psychology (such as PTSD and anorexia).

Over the years, the ICD-DSM diagnostic categories and folk psychology have co-evolved, which may be one reason why even some scientists and clinicians who are skeptical about ICD-DSM categories continue to refer to categories such as depression, schizophrenia, and PTSD in research talks and papers. Practically speaking—and independent of forward-thinking scientific and clinical considerations—the entrenchment in folk psychology of ICD and DSM categories makes them very convenient to use as shorthand when discussing clinical syndromes, even if one has concerns about their validity and clinical utility.

One way to see the quest for innovation is that it is an attempt to introduce a new language for psychopathology. At first, learning new languages requires translating old into new. If so, one way to introduce new languages for psychopathology is to use the ICD-DSM categories as bridges to the new concepts. An example of a bridge question would be: why is it better to talk about internalizing disorders than depression? Another would be: how does the psychosis spectrum differ from schizophrenia? In theory at least, rather than being barriers for those who seek innovation, ICD-DSM constructs could play a role in promoting it.

References

American Psychiatric Association. (1952). *Diagnostic and statistical manual of mental disorders (DSM-I)* (3 ed.). American Psychiatric Association.

American Psychiatric Association. (1980). *Diagnostic and statistical manual of mental disorders* (3 ed.). American Psychiatric Association.

American Psychiatric Association. (2022). *Diagnostic and statistical manual of mental disorders, fifth edition, text revision (DSM-5-TR)*. American Psychiatric Press.

APA DSM Team. (2021). *Guide to submitting proposals for changes to DSM-5*. American Psychiatric Association. https://www.psychiatry.org/File%20Library/Psychiatrists/Practice/DSM/DSM5-Proposal-Submissions-General-Guidance.pdf

Anstey, P. R. (2011). *John Locke and natural philosophy*. Oxford University Press.

Appelbaum, P. S. (2024). Integrity is built into the process of developing DSM-5-TR. *Psychiatric News*. https://doi.org/10.1176/appi.pn.2024.03.3.36

Appelbaum, P. S., Leibenluft, E., & Kendler, K. S. (2021). Iterative revision of the DSM: An interim report from the DSM-5 steering committee. *Psychiatric Services*, *72*(11), 1348–1349. https://doi.org/10.1176/appi.ps.202100013

Bridgman, P. W. (1927). *The logic of modern physics*. Macmillan.

Caplan, P. J. (1995). *They say you're crazy: How the world's most powerful psychiatrists decide who's normal*. Addison-Wesley.

Cooper, J. (1982). The last big one? *British Journal of Psychiatry*, *141*(5), 531–532. https://doi.org/10.1017/S0007125000113212

Decker, H. S. (2013). *The making of DSM-III®: A diagnostic manual's conquest of American psychiatry*. Oxford University Press.

Engstrom, E. J., & Kendler, K. S. (2015). Emil Kraepelin: Icon and reality. *American Journal of Psychiatry*, *172*, 1190–1196.

Feighner, J. P., Robins, E., Guze, S. B., Woodruff, R. A., Winokur, G., & Munoz, R. (1972). Diagnostic criteria for use in psychiatric research. *Archives of General Psychiatry*, *26*, 57–63.

First, M. B. (2009). Harmonisation of ICD-11 and DSM-V: Opportunities and challenges. *British Journal of Psychiatry*, *195*(5), 382–390. https://doi.org/10.1192/bjp.bp.108.060822

First, M. B. (2010). Clinical utility in the revision of the Diagnostic and Statistical Manual of Mental Disorders (DSM). *Professional Psychology: Research and Practice*, *41*(6), 465–473. https://doi.org/10.1037/a0021511

First, M. B., Gaebel, W., Maj, M., Stein, D. J., Kogan, C. S., Saunders, J. B., Poznyak, V. B., Gureje, O., Lewis-Fernández, R., Maercker, A., Brewin, C. R., Cloitre, M., Claudino, A., Pike, K. M., Baird, G., Skuse, D., Krueger, R. B., Briken, P., Burke, J. D., . . . Reed, G. M. (2021). An organization- and category-level comparison of diagnostic requirements for mental disorders in ICD-11 and DSM-5. *World Psychiatry*, *20*(1), 34–51. https://doi.org/10.1002/wps.20825

Fleck, L. (1935/1979). *Genesis and development of a scientific fact* (F. Bradley & T. J. Trenn, Trans.). University of Chicago Press.

Frances, A. (2011). DSM-5 against everyone else: Research types just don't understand the clinical world. *Psychiatric Times*. http://www.psychiatrictimes.com/blog/dsm-5/content/article/10168/1981447

Frances, A. J., Widiger, T. A., & Pincus, H. A. (1989). The development of DSM-IV. *Archives of General Psychiatry*, *46*, 373–375.

Friesen, P. (2021). *Standpoint theory and the psy sciences: Can marginalization and critical engagement lead to an epistemic advantage?* University of Quebec at Montreal Philosophy of Psychiatry Webinar. https://www.philosophyofpsychiatry.com/webinar

Fulford, K. W. M., & Sartorius, N. (2009). The secret history of ICD and the hidden future of DSM. In M. Broomse & L. Bortolotti (Eds.), *Psychiatry as cognitve neuroscinece* (pp. 29–47). Oxford University Press.

Ghaemi, N. (November 2023). *Why DSM is mostly false*. Substack post. Retrieved April 24 from https://ghaemi.substack.com/p/why-dsm-is-mostly-false

Grob, G. N. (1991). Origins of DSM-I: A study in appearance and reality. *American Journal of Psychiatry*, *148*(4), 421–431. https://doi.org/10.1176/ajp.148.4.421

Gruenberg, E. M. (1968). Forward. In A. P. Association (Ed.), *DSM-II diagnostic and statistical manual of mental disorders*. American Psychiatric Association.

Hacking, I. (1990). *The taming of chance*. Cambridge University Press.

Hasin, D. S., O'Brien, C. P., Auriacombe, M., Borges, G., Kathleen Bucholz, Budney, A., Compton, W. M., Crowley, T., Ling, W., Petry, N. M., Schuckit, M., & Grant, B. F. (2013). DSM-5 criteria for substance use disorders: Recommendations and rationale. *American Journal of Psychiatry*, *170*(8), 834–851. https://doi.org/10.1176/appi.ajp.2013.12060782

Heckers, S., & Kendler, K. S. (2020). The evolution of Kraepelin's nosological principles. *World Psychiatry*, *19*(3), 381–388. https://onlinelibrary.wiley.com/doi/abs/10.1002/wps.20774

Hempel, C. G. (1961). Introduction to problems of taxonomy. In J. Zubin (Ed.), *Field studies in the mental disorders* (pp. 3–22). Grune and Stratton.

Horwitz, A. V. (2021). *DSM: A history of psychiatry's bible*. Johns Hopkins University Press.

Houts, A. C. (2000). Fifty years of psychiatric nomenclature: Reflections on the 1943 War Department Technical Bulletin, Medical 203. *Journal of Clinical Psychology*, *56*(7), 935–967. https://doi.org/10.1002/1097-4679(200007)56:7<935::aid-jclp11>3.0.co;2-8

Hyman, S. E. (2010). The diagnosis of mental disorders: The problem of reification. *Annual Review of Clinical Psychology*, *6*, 155–179.

Kamens, S. R., Cosgrove, L., Peters, S. M., Jones, N., Flanagan, E., Longden, E., Schulz, S., Robbins, B. D., Olsen, S., Miller, R., & Lichtenberg, P. (2019). Standards and guidelines for the development of diagnostic nomenclatures and alternatives in mental health research and practice. *Journal of Humanistic Psychology*, 59(3), 401–427. https://doi.org/10.1177/0022167818763862

Keeley, J. W., Chung, L., & Kleva, C. (2023). Classification in traditional nosologies. In R. F. Krueger & P. H. Blaney (Eds.), *Oxford textbook of psychopathology* (pp. 3–32). Oxford University Press.

Kendell, R. E. (1991). Relationship between the DSM-IV and the ICD-10. *Journal of Abnormal Psychology*, *100*(3), 297–301. https://doi.org/10.1037//0021-843x.100.3.297

Kendler, K. S., & First, M. B. (2010). Alternative futures for the DSM revision process: Iteration v. paradigm shift. *The British Journal of Psychiatry*, *197*, 263–265.

Kramer, M. (1968). Introduction: The history of the efforts to agree on an international classification of mental disorders. In A. P. Association (Ed.), *DSM-II diagnostic and statistical manual of mental disorders*. American Psychiatric Association.

Krueger, R. F., Kotov, R., Watson, D., Forbes, M. K., Eaton, N. R., Ruggero, C. J., Simms, L. J., Widiger, T. A., Achenbach, T. M., Bach, B., Bagby, R. M., Bornovalova, M. A., Carpenter, W. T., Chmielewski, M., Cicero, D. C., Clark, L. A., Conway, C., DeClercq, B., DeYoung, C. G., . . . Zimmermann, J. (2018). Progress in achieving quantitative classification of psychopathology. *World Psychiatry*, *17*(3), 282–293. https://doi.org/10.1002/wps.20566

Kuhn, T. S. (1970). *The structure of scientific revolutions* (2nd ed.). University of Chicago Press.

Kuhn, T. S. (1977). *The essential tension*. University of Chicago Press.

Kuhn, T. S. (1979). Foreward (B. Fred & T. J. Trenn, Trans.). In *Genesis and development of a scientific fact* (pp. v–xi). University of Chicago Press.

Kupfer, D. J., First, M. B., & Regier, D. A. (2002). *A research agenda for DSM-V*. American Psychiatric Association.

Lenzer, J. (2008). Review launched after Harvard psychiatrist failed to disclose industry funding. *British Medical Journal*, *336*(7657), 1327. https://doi.org/10.1136/bmj.39609.364688.DB

Marx, O. M. (1970). Nineteenth-century medical psychology: Theoretical problems in the work of Griesinger, Meynert, and Wernicke. *Isis*, *61*(3), 355–370. http://www.jstor.org/stable/229687

Menninger, K., Mayman, M., & Pruyser, P. (1963). *The vital balance*. The Viking Press.

Millon, T. (1986). On the past and future of the DSM-III: Personal recollections and projections. In T. Millon & G. L. Klerman (Eds.), *Contemporary directions in psychopathology: Toward the DSM-IV* (pp. 29–70). Guilford Press.

Moriyama, I. M., Loy, R. M., & Robb-Smith, A. H. T. (2011). *History of the statistical classification of diseases and causes of death* (H. M. Rosenberg & D. L. Hoyert, Eds.). National Center for Health Statistics.

National Conference on Medical Nomenclature. (1942). *Standard Nomenclature of Disease* (E. P. Jordan, Ed.). American Medical Association.

Petry, N. M., Rehbein, F., Ko, C. H., & O'Brien, C. P. (2015). Internet gaming disorder in the DSM-5. *Current Psychiatry Reports*, *17*(9), 72. https://doi.org/10.1007/s11920-015-0610-0

Phillips, J. (2013). The conceptual status of DSM-5 diagnoses. In *Making the DSM-5: Concepts and controversies* (pp. 143–157). Springer Science + Business Media. https://doi.org/10.1007/978-1-4614-6504-1_10

Poland, J., & Tekin, Ş. (2017). *Extraordinary science and psychiatry: Responses to the crisis in mental health research*. MIT Press.

Raines, G. N. (1952). Forward. In American Psychiatric Association (Ed.), *Diagnostic and statistical manual of mental disorders* (pp. v–xi). American Psychiatric Association Mental Hospital Service.

Raines, G. N. (1953). The new nomenclature. *The American Journal of Psychiatry*, *109*, 549–549.

Reed, G. M., First, M. B., Billieux, J., Cloitre, M., Briken, P., Achab, S., Brewin, C. R., King, D. L., Kraus, S. W., & Bryant, R. A. (2022). Emerging experience with selected new categories in the ICD-11: Complex PTSD, prolonged grief disorder, gaming disorder, and compulsive sexual behaviour disorder. *World Psychiatry*, *21*(2), 189–213. https://doi.org/10.1002/wps.20960

Regier, D. A., Narrow, W. E., Kuhl, E. A., & Kupfer, D. J. (2009). The conceptual development of DSM-V. *American Journal of Psychiatry*, *166*, 645–650.

Shedler, J., Beck, A., Fonagy, P., Gabbard, G. O., Gunderson, J., Kernberg, O., Michels, R., & Westen, D. (2010). Personality disorders in DSM-5. *American Journal of Psychiatry*, *167*, 1026–1028.

Society for Humanistic Psychology. (2011). *Open letter to the DSM-5 task force and the American Psychiatric Association*. http://www.ipetitions.com/petition/dsm5/

Solomon, M. (2022). On validators for psychiatric categories. *Philosophy of Medicine*, *3*(1), 1–23.

Spitzer, R. L. (2001). Values and assumptions in the development of DSM-III and DSM-III-R: An insider's perspective and a belated response to Sadler, Hulgus, and Agich's "On values in recent American psychiatric classification." *Journal of Nervous & Mental Disease*, *189*(6), 351–359. https://doi.org/10.1097/00005053-200106000-00002

Spitzer, R. L., Endicott, J., & Robins, E. (1978). Research diagnostic criteria. *Archives of General Psychiatry*, *35*, 773–782.

Spitzer, R. L., & Wilson, P. T. (1968). A guide to the American Psychiatric Association's new diagnostic nomenclature. *American Journal of Psychiatry*, *124*(12), 1619–1629. https://doi.org/10.1176/ajp.124.12.1619

Stengel, E. (1959). The classification of mental disorders. *Bulletin of the World Health Organization*, *21*, 601–663.

Wakefield, J. C. (2011). Should uncomplicated bereavement-related depression be reclassified as a disorder in the DSM-5? *The Journal of Nervous and Mental Disease*, *199*(3), 203–208.

World Health Organization. (2021). History of the development of the ICD. https://cdn.who.int/media/docs/default-source/classification/icd/historyoficd.pdf

World Health Organization. (2022). *International classification of diseases (11th revision)*. https://icd.who.int/

Zachar, P. (2022, November, 9). *Scientific evidence is the engine of change, but forward progress may also depend on practical, clinical considerations*. Bi-annual Meeting of the Philosophy of Science Association, Pittsburgh, PA.

Zachar, P., First, M. B., & Kendler, K. S. (2022). Revising substance-related disorders in the DSM-5: A history. *Journal of Studies on Alcohol and Drugs*, *83*(1), 99–105.

Zachar, P., & Kendler, K. S. (2017). The philosophy of nosology. *Annual Review of Clinical Psychology*, *13*, 49–71. https://doi.org/10.1146/annurev-clinpsy-032816-045020

PART II

Dimensional Approaches to Psychopathology

Origins, Research Advances, and Clinical Applications

CHAPTER 6

The Hierarchical Taxonomy of Psychology (HiTOP)

Origin, Development, and Future Directions

TAM PHAM AND MIRIAM K. FORBES

Introduction

Nosology, the classification of diseases or disorders, represents the systematic effort to organize diverse and complex clinical phenomena into meaningful and standardized descriptions of illness. In the field of psychopathology, the evolution of psychiatric nosology reflects the changing paradigms in our understanding of mental disorders, from the primordial attempts to categorize disorders based on spiritualistic perspectives to a more standardized approach influenced by clinical observations and scientific understandings. The 20th century witnessed the publication of the International Classification of Diseases (ICD) and the *Diagnostic and Statistical Manual of Mental Disorders* (DSM), which have defined the constructs we study and treat for decades. Nevertheless, as the chapters in this volume will no doubt serve to remind us, this journey is not without controversies and challenges. The inherent complexity and diversity of mental health conditions present difficulties in creating discrete categories that fully capture individuals' experiences. Issues such as cultural variability and dynamic changes in mental health over time further complicate the task of constructing a reliable organization of psychopathology.

Given the shortcomings of traditional classification systems like the ICD and DSM, the field has recently witnessed the emergence of alternative approaches to classification, such as the Hierarchical Taxonomy of Psychopathology (HiTOP; Kotov et al., 2017). The goal of this chapter is to briefly review important features of a useful nosology, describe the origin and structure of HiTOP, and discuss its implications for clinical practice, research endeavors, and the broader understanding of mental health within the context of an ever-evolving scientific landscape. Additionally, we will address some of the major criticisms of the quantitative approach to classification represented by HiTOP and describe ongoing efforts to address them.

Important Functions of a Nosology

A useful nosology for psychopathology goes beyond a rudimentary checklist of symptoms and diagnostic criteria. It serves as a dynamic and evolving tool that is expected to accurately reflect the underlying internal structures of outward clinical observations and ideally be practically useful in both research and clinical settings. In essence, the value of a classification system should be evaluated through the dual lenses of diagnostic validity and clinical utility

(Forbes et al., 2023d). These two concepts, though highly intertwined, are distinct, and both are essential.

Diagnostic validity can be considered in two parts: structural validity and external validity (Forbes et al., 2023d; Krueger & Eaton, 2012). Structural validity refers to the extent to which the psychiatric phenotypes are reliably defined within a nosology. This includes evaluating whether the phenotypes or the symptom sets are internally coherent—that is, symptoms assigned together are likely to co-occur—and distinct from each other. External validity, on the other hand, describes the extent to which the phenotypes correspond meaningfully to other constructs external to the system, whether they are stable over time and across different populations, and whether they can predict treatment outcomes and responses. Robins and Guze (1970) provided one of the earliest formal rubrics to evaluate the external validity of psychiatric diagnoses, which, over the years, has expanded to include 11 criteria (Andrews et al., 2009; Forbes et al., 2023d) spanning three temporal groups: antecedent (e.g., risk factors), concurrent (e.g., cognitive or emotional correlates), and predictive (e.g., treatment response). A diagnostic nosology that is both internally coherent and externally valid ensures that the working definitions of the psychiatric phenotypes are useful benchmarks to facilitate our understanding of the underlying liability of the observed psychopathology.

The clinical utility of a nosology is evaluated based on its feasibility in clinical settings (e.g., ease of use, time efficiency) and its ability to provide accurate clinical descriptions, facilitate communication between stakeholders, and guide decision-making in treatment planning and clinical management (Reed, 2010). In theory, a nosology may still be clinically useful to some extent with limited evidence of validity. For instance, despite accumulating evidence of their poor validity, descriptive and criteria-based nosologies such as the DSM have facilitated reliable descriptions, offering a common language to standardize diagnosis and facilitate communication in research and clinical settings (e.g., Abramowitz et al., 2019; Barlow, 2021; Clark & Beck, 2011; Martell et al., 2021).

However, the extent to which a nosology can assist sound clinical decisions (i.e., clinical utility) depends heavily on the validity of its clinical descriptions. Even the developers of the DSM stressed the focus on improving validity in each subsequent iteration (First et al., 2004; Frances et al., 1990). The assumption is that the lingua franca would pave the way for reliable research that shapes further revisions of the nosologies and moves diagnoses closer to validity. While this hypothesis is certainly reasonable in principle, emerging evidence from behavioral, neuroscience, and genetics research has suggested that it is unlikely to be realized for the DSM.

Current Nosologies and Their Limitations

A few decades after the introduction of modern classification systems (e.g., the DSM-III), evidence of their substantial limitations accumulated (Chmielewski et al., 2015; Hyman, 2007; Kapur et al., 2012; Kupfer et al., 2008; Regier et al., 2013; Sanislow et al., 2010; Spitzer et al., 2012; Wakefield, 2016; Whooley, 2014). The traditional categorical systems have not led to the anticipated validation of diagnostic entities, consequently limiting the practical utility of the nosologies in clinical settings (Reed, 2010). Notably, the lack of diagnostic validity means that there are often major misalignments between the descriptive DSM-defined categories and the symptomatic experiences of patients (Newson et al., 2021). In terms of diagnosis, the misalignments contribute significantly to a high proportion of patients either not meeting the criteria for any DSM-defined disorder, hence receiving the "Other Specified" diagnosis (Machado et al., 2007; Rajakannan et al., 2016; Verheul & Widiger, 2004), or concurrently meeting criteria for multiple disorders (Copeland et al., 2013; Hirschfeld, 2001; Maj, 2005).

The challenge of matching psychiatric presentations to the DSM-defined diagnostic categories is further exacerbated by the continual introduction of new categories and subtypes as an attempt to account for the high heterogeneity in symptom profiles within the disorders (Allsopp et al., 2019; Watson, 2003). In terms of treatment planning, the diagnostic decision also has a limited influence on the decision to treat, since people can experience significant symptom burdens without meeting the criteria (Newson et al., 2021). The rise in the adoption of transdiagnostic treatment (Barlow et al., 2017; Dalgleish et al., 2020; Gros, 2019; Schaeuffele et al., 2021; Sloan et al., 2017) also suggests that specific categories have become less relevant for practitioners in making treatment decisions. In a recent survey with more than 700 psychologists, less than one-third reported using the DSM for treatment planning, but almost two-thirds used the system for administration purposes such as using diagnostic codes for billing (Raskin et al., 2022).

Alternative Approaches

Amid the growing "disquiet in nosology" (Hyman, 2007, 2010; Ruggero et al., 2019), alternative approaches that aim to reconceptualize psychopathology have emerged. Notably, the Hierarchical Taxonomy of Psychopathology (HiTOP; Kotov et al., 2017) and the National Institute of Mental Health (NIMH)'s Research Domain Criteria (RDoC; Insel et al., 2010) stand out as the two efforts that have sparked the most substantial scientific discourse. In contrast with traditional nosologies that heavily rely on expert consensus, both HiTOP and RDoC have shifted the balance to prioritize empirical evidence in the conceptualization of psychopathology. This fundamental switch in approach has garnered considerable interest in the field, partly, because this "bottom-up" approach closely aligns with the long-sought "paradigm shift" toward the diagnostic validity (Maser et al., 2009)—a shift that the DSM-5 has been critiqued for failing to deliver (Whooley, 2014). More importantly, they offer a scientific alternative to the unintended "epistemic prison" (Hyman, 2010) created by DSM that impedes the search for etiology and knowledge about mental disorders—particularly when research-funding decisions have long been centered around DSM diagnostic constructs that lack validity (Insel et al., 2010).

RDoC and HiTOP both abandon the discrete architecture of traditional taxonomies, recognizing the evidence accumulated over decades that mental health exists along continuous dimensions rather than in distinct categories (Haslam et al., 2012, 2020). However, these efforts employ different strategies to address the stagnant progress to psychiatric validity. RDoC focuses on elucidating etiology, organizing its framework around neurobiological dimensions to delineate the underlying mechanisms of dysfunctions relevant to psychopathology (e.g., valance systems, cognitions, arousal regulation; Insel et al., 2010). At present, RDoC primarily serves as a research framework for etiology with limited clinical applicability, as it does not include the majority of clinical signs and symptoms (Clark et al., 2017).

In contrast, HiTOP remains agnostic to neurobiological bases and etiology. It focuses on empirically organizing psychopathology based on co-variation among dimensions of psychiatric indicators, including signs, symptoms, and maladaptive behaviors. The major motivation of HiTOP is to reconceptualize a nosology that aligns better with the symptomatic experiences of patients, with the view that reliable description is a necessary foundation for work that seeks to identify causal mechanisms. While the HiTOP framework shares a descriptive focus with the DSM, they differ in their approach to establishing the validity of the psychiatric phenotypes—groupings of signs and symptoms (Forbes et al., 2023d). The development and revisions of the DSM and ICD have placed more focus on establishing the external validity of the psychiatric phenotypes (i.e., categorial diagnoses in DSM and ICD), neglecting the foundational structural validity. This lack of structural validity means that the phenotypes may not provide coherent and reliable targets for inquiry, leading to issues with low reliability and reproducibility in research. As a result, studies using these phenotypes may struggle to draw clear conclusions about the causes and mechanisms of mental illness. This lack of structural validity also complicates efforts to identify effective interventions tailored to narrower symptom profiles, which are often lumped together under the broad, heterogeneous phenotype (i.e., categorical diagnosis). For instance, recent evidence suggests that adults with major depressive disorder can be assigned into subgroups based on their resting-state functional connectivity, with each group responding better to different treatments (Dunlop et al., 2017). One subgroup showed a higher remission rate following cognitive behavioral therapy, while the other had better outcomes with antidepressant treatment. Notwithstanding these differences, individuals in these subgroups receive the same DSM-defined diagnosis and are expected to receive the same treatment recommendation in clinical settings. This highlights the critical need for more-precise, structurally valid phenotypes to improve both the understanding of psychopathology and the tailoring of interventions to individual patients.

We will now shift to discussing the structure of the HiTOP framework, the accumulating evidence supporting the validity and utility of the HiTOP model, the primary limitations and relevant efforts underway in the HiTOP consortium to address them, and how the HiTOP framework can be integrated into research and clinical practice.

HiTOP: Origin and Structure

The History of Quantitative Psychopathology

Kotov and colleagues introduced the first version of the HiTOP model in 2017, presenting it as an empirically based, quantitative framework for the nosology of psychopathology. Though the model is relatively recent, the philosophy underpinning its quantitative approach to understanding mental health within a dimensional space was preceded by nearly a century of work in the history of clinical science. Factor analysis has long been used in past works to elucidate the natural organization of psychopathology. Early contributions include Moore's (1930) seminal work that discovered eight psychiatric syndromes underlying psychotic signs and symptoms. Similarly, Tellegen (1985) quantitatively studied the structure of mood, and Andrews et al. (1990) and Clark & Watson (1991) identified a general distress dimension underlying specific syndromes of anxiety and depression. Another notable example of the quantitative approach is the development of the Achenbach System of Empirically Based Assessment (ASEBA; Achenbach, 1966; Achenbach & Dumenci, 2001; Copeland, this volume), which remains a prominent set of assessment tools in child psychopathology in particular. Achenbach and colleagues quantitatively derived dimensional syndromes underlying children's emotional and behavioral problems, instead of relying on DSM-defined disorders, due to the "limited knowledge available regarding the taxonomy of child mental health problems" (Achenbach, 1966).

Quantitative classification has also been applied with success to other psychological domains, including the classifications of cognitive abilities (e.g., Cattell–Horn–Carroll model; Carroll, 1993), personality traits (e.g., Big-Five factor structure; Goldberg, 1993), and affect (e.g., Positive Activation–Negative Activation; Watson & Tellegen, 1985). The resulting factor analysis-based models have not only provided valuable insights into understanding individual differences but also received wide acceptance in their respective fields as effective guidelines in research for diagnostic assessment and clinical applications (Jewsbury et al., 2017; Markon et al., 2005; McGrew, 2009; Rubin & Talarico, 2009). Drawing from the success of the existing frameworks that provided useful classifications of individual differences, the HiTOP framework aims to be a quantitatively derived nosology of psychopathology that can move the field closer to identifying the causal mechanisms that underpin psychopathology and thus toward treatments that are more effective for more people.

Core Features of HiTOP Framework

At present, substantial evidence highlights three potential features with particular utility for organizing the structure of psychopathology. First, psychopathology is more accurately conceptualized as continuous dimensions of maladaptive emotions, cognitions, and behaviors, rather than discrete categorial disorders (Haslam et al., 2012, 2020). That is, individual differences in experiences of psychopathological signs and symptoms are a matter of degree, not kind (i.e., present versus absent). Second, dimensions of psychopathology are correlated with each other (Krueger & Markon, 2006; Lahey et al., 2017). This feature is most evident in the common co-occurrence among mental health conditions (Maj, 2005). Third, the patterns of correlations among the dimensions can be organized into a hierarchical structure, wherein higher-order dimensions summarize the co-occurring patterns of lower-order dimensions (Hagerty, 2023; Lahey et al., 2017; Markon et al., 2005). This hierarchical structure resembles the classifications of individual differences in other domains, such as personality traits, cognitive abilities, and affect, as previously discussed (Costa & McCrae, 2011; McGrew, 2009).

Accordingly, the HiTOP model is based on empirically derived dimensional phenotypes, organized hierarchically from narrow indicators of psychopathology (i.e., maladaptive traits and symptom components) to broader and more general phenotypes, based on structural evidence of their patterns of co-occurrence and co-variation. It is important to highlight that even though traditional DSM-defined disorders (e.g., major depressive disorder, social anxiety disorder) are not part of the official HiTOP framework, they have often been used in past studies as basic units of analysis to identify higher-order HiTOP dimensions. This is expected, especially in the early stages of development, since the extant literature and data are characterized by disorder-level assessment. In the following, we review the supporting evidence for the HiTOP structure, including the results obtained from both disorder- and symptom-level analysis.

Validity Evidence for HiTOP Framework

Structural Validity

According to the existing structural evidence, indicators of psychopathology can be reliably aggregated into increasingly broad dimensional phenotypes at higher-order levels in the HiTOP hierarchy (Forbes et al., 2021b; Kotov et al., 2020, 2021; Krueger et al., 2021; Watson et al., 2022). These levels are currently labeled as subfactor, spectrum, and superspectrum. Figure 6.1 illustrates an adapted version of the HiTOP working model.

Superspectra. At the top of the hierarchy is a superspectrum commonly referred to as the general factor of psychopathology (or "p factor"), which captures the positive manifold among varied domains of psychopathology (Caspi et al., 2014; Kotov et al., 2021; Lahey et al., 2012) but rests on shaky methodological foundations (e.g., Watts et al., 2024). This single overarching factor can be carved into three nested superspectra of emotional dysfunction, psychosis, and externalizing (Forbes et al., 2017b, 2021b; Kotov et al., 2017, 2021; Michelini et al., 2019), although the emotional dysfunction and psychosis superspectra are not currently part of the

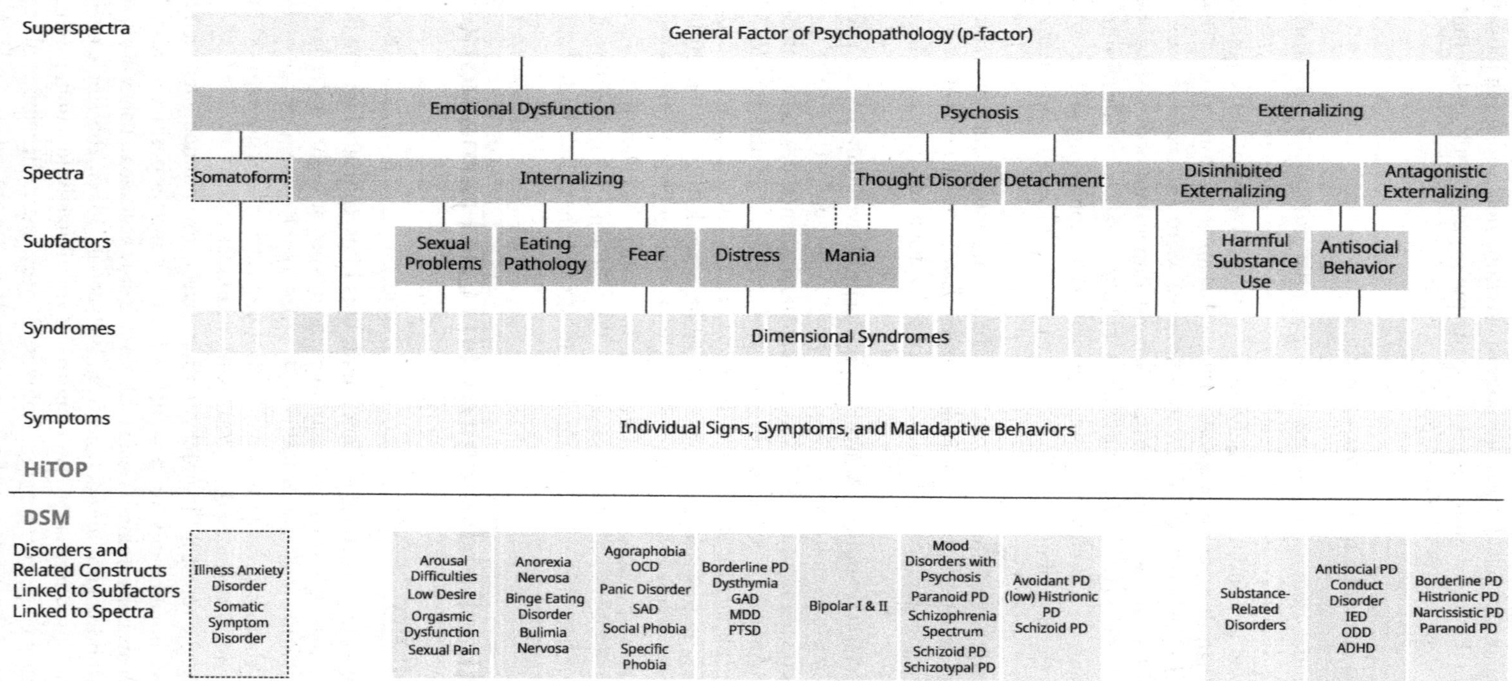

FIGURE 6.1 Adapted version of the current HiTOP model. Credit: The Official HiTOP Figure https://www.hitop-system.org/the-framework

Note. The emotional dysfunction and psychosis superspectra are not part of the current official model. DSM diagnoses are not included in the HiTOP model but are often used as units of measurement in disorder-level analysis.

official model. According to existing factor analytic evidence, emotional dysfunction emerges as the high-order factor capturing the empirical co-variation between the somatoform and internalizing spectra (Watson et al., 2022); externalizing captures the co-variation between the antagonistic externalizing and disinhibited externalizing spectra (Krueger et al., 2021); and psychosis captures the co-variation between the thought disorder and detachment spectra (Kotov et al., 2020).

Spectra. The dimensions at the spectrum level were among the first to emerge in the search for the structure of psychopathology and represent the most well-validated aspects of the framework (Kotov et al., 2017, 2021). Among these, the internalizing, antagonistic externalizing, disinhibited externalizing, thought disorder, and detachment spectra have been most consistently identified in the structural analyses of traditional Axis I and II disorders (Carragher et al., 2015; Cummings et al., 2014; Forbes et al., 2017a, 2017b; Forbush & Watson, 2013; Griffith et al., 2010; Krueger, 1999; Lahey et al., 2004, 2017; Røysamb et al., 2011; Widiger et al., 2019). Specifically, the internalizing spectrum typically emerges as the higher-order factor for emotionally focused presentations such as depressive, anxiety, trauma-based, and eating disorders. The disinhibited externalizing spectrum captures the impulse-control difficulties shared among conditions such as substance use, while the antagonistic externalizing spectrum captures the close connections among callous-unemotional presentations such as psychopathy and antisocial personality disorder (PD). Similarly, the thought disorder spectrum tends to emerge as the higher-order factor for cognitive-perceptual aberrations such as psychotic disorders or mania. The detachment spectrum is characterized by socioemotional withdrawal symptoms in avoidant, schizoid, or schizotypal PDs. When sufficient indicators for the (provisional) somatoform spectrum are included in analyses, it emerges as a distinct higher-order factor for bodily distress symptoms (Forbes et al., 2017b; Kotov et al., 2011; Markon, 2010).

Subfactors. At the subfactor level, structural analyses have also identified more narrowly defined dimensions nested within some of the spectra. The subfactors capture more specific patterns of co-variation—typically among observed indicators of psychopathology—and are therefore more homogenous than the higher-order spectra. Despite being less consistently identified than the higher-order spectra, several subfactors have been replicated across structural studies and are therefore included in the working HiTOP model. Within the internalizing spectrum, distress and fear subfactors were the earliest to emerge (Krueger, 1999); distress is defined by presentations related to pervasive negative emotionality such as depression, while fear is related to more acute, context-delimited forms of distress such as panic or specific phobia. Eating pathology and sexual problems are other subfactors that have emerged as distinct dimensions within the internalizing spectrum. They capture the commonalities shared among the relevant disorders defined in the DSM chapters (i.e., feeding and eating disorders, sexual dysfunctions) and among specific symptoms, such as binge eating for eating pathology or low sexual desire for sexual problems (Forbes et al., 2017a; Forbes & Schniering, 2013; Forbush et al., 2010, 2017; Forbush & Watson, 2013). Mania, subsuming presentations related to manic episodes such as euphoric activation or hyperactive cognition, is currently a provisional interstitial subfactor that falls under both the internalizing and thought disorder spectra (Kotov et al., 2011; Ruggero et al., 2014).

Within the two externalizing spectra, harmful substance use and antisocial behavior are the only two subfactors that have been included in the current HiTOP model; harmful substance use consists of indicators for alcohol and other substance use disorders (SUDs), while antisocial behavior describes a constellation of behaviors that harm or violate the rights of others such as aggression or rule-breaking behavior (De Wit-De Visser et al., 2023). While evidence suggests that harmful substance use is uniquely subsumed within the disinhibited externalizing spectrum, antisocial behavior appears to be associated with both externalizing spectra (Krueger et al., 2007; Krueger & Tackett, 2016; Mullins-Sweatt et al., 2022). Currently, the model does not formally include any specific subfactors under thought disorder and detachment spectra, except for mania, which, as discussed, is linked to both thought disorder and internalizing.

Even though DSM-defined disorders are commonly used as the basic units of analysis in structural studies, their inherent heterogeneity poses significant challenges for elucidating the more homogenous constructs within HiTOP lower-level dimensions. As evident from disorder-level structural analyses, symptom components within a disorder can be mapped onto different higher-order dimensions. For instance, schizophrenia includes negative symptoms and positive symptoms that are subsumed within two different higher-order spectra: detachment and thought disorder, respectively (Cicero et al., 2019; Tiego et al., 2023). Similarly, DSM personality disorders such as antisocial PD or borderline PD encompass symptom components related to both antagonism and disinhibition (Krueger et al., 2021). As DSM disorders are often too coarse-grained to effectively identify more fine-grained constructs, further empirical refinement of HiTOP's lower-order structure through factor analyses of homogenous symptom-level indicators is needed (Mullins-Sweatt et al., 2022).

Symptoms. Most supporting evidence for the HiTOP structure is derived from disorder-level analyses (Grisanzio et al., 2018; Kotov et al., 2020; Krueger et al., 2021; Watson et al., 2022). Notably, in a meta-analysis that synthesized disorder-level results across diverse samples and study designs, Ringwald et al. (2021) found a five-factor model that corresponds well to the HiTOP spectra. However, the somatoform spectrum could not be evaluated in this study due to the lack of research in the extant literature. Structural analyses of symptom-level data have also generally found the higher-order levels of the model to be robust (Dornbach-Bender et al., 2017; Forbes et al., 2021a; Krueger et al., 2007; McNulty & Overstreet, 2014; Sellbom, 2017; Waszczuk et al., 2017a; Wright et al., 2013).

A recent symptom-level analysis with comprehensive coverage of psychopathology (Forbes et al., 2023b) also showed substantial convergence with the HiTOP model, finding constructs that resembled all of the current HiTOP subfactors and spectra, albeit with some changes in structure (e.g., harmful substance use and eating pathology emerging as distinct spectra, rather than subfactors). Forbes et al. (2023b) also identified new subfactors under the externalizing, internalizing, thought disorder, and somatoform spectra (Cicero et al., 2019; Kotov et al., 2016; Stanton et al., 2021; Watts et al., 2023a), an additional branch of the model in neurodevelopmental and cognitive difficulties spectra, and some reorganization of the symptoms typically bound together within DSM diagnoses (e.g., somatic symptoms of depression and anxiety forming part of a somatoform spectrum)—all highlighting the promise of symptom-level over disorder-level analysis for elucidating detailed structural models of psychopathology. At this early stage, studies are exploring different structural models, employing different indicators of psychopathology, and expanding analyses to diverse populations—each of which can lead to new insights and indicate potential revisions to the model. To ensure that HiTOP remains a dynamic and up-to-date framework that evolves with the literature, the HiTOP Revisions Workgroup—discussed later in this chapter—was established to support the ongoing systematic review and incorporation of emerging findings.

External Validity

The external validity of the HiTOP spectra has been extensively examined in studies of genetic vulnerabilities, neurobiological abnormalities, environmental risk factors, cognitive and emotional processing abnormalities, illness course, and treatment response (Conway et al., 2019; DeYoung et al., 2024; Hopwood et al., 2020; Kotov et al., 2017, 2020, 2021; Krueger et al.,

2021; Latzman & DeYoung, 2020; Ruggero, Kotov et al., 2019; Waszczuk et al., 2020; Watson et al., 2022). Empirical studies and systematic reviews have primarily examined the correlations between external validators and the core HiTOP dimensions to assess the coherence and discriminability of associations within and between dimensions (i.e., examining consistency in validator profiles for constructs on the same HiTOP dimension versus different dimensions).

Overall, studies have identified shared patterns for groups of DSM-defined disorders, symptom dimensions, and traits that reflect the same HiTOP dimensions, tentatively supporting the dimensional coherence (e.g., Kotov et al., 2020; Krueger et al., 2021; Waszczuk et al., 2020; Watson et al., 2022). In studies that examined associations across multiple dimensions, distinct patterns have sometimes also been observed, tentatively supporting the validity of the distinctions between the dimensions. For instance, distinct genetic factors have been identified for psychotic disorders versus non-psychotic disorders (Pettersson et al., 2016), and for internalizing disorders versus externalizing disorders (Kendler et al., 2011). Treatment efficacy appears to be different for the two externalizing spectra (Comer et al., 2013), with symptoms more characteristic of antagonism (i.e., oppositionality and noncompliance) showing better response to psychosocial treatment than symptoms of disinhibition (i.e., inattention and hyperactivity); and stimulant medications have demonstrated specific effectiveness in the management of the latter symptoms (Greenhill et al., 2006).

More important, relative to the DSM structure, the dimensional framework in HiTOP appears to map more closely onto the underlying patterns of genetic, environmental, and neurobiological vulnerabilities and abnormalities. To date, while no genetic or environmental risk factors have been found to be specific to a DSM-defined disorder, several have been observed to be differentially associated with HiTOP spectra (Dick et al., 2005; Hoy et al., 2023; Kendler et al., 2011; Keyes et al., 2012; McLaughlin et al., 2020). Similarly, most pharmacological and psychological treatments have been found to be efficacious across multiple diagnoses, in patterns that align with HiTOP dimensions, suggesting that these dimensions could capture specific shared underlying processes that benefit from the same intervention. For instance, antipsychotics were found to be effective for positive psychosis symptoms in thought disorders (Buchanan et al., 2010; Fusar-Poli et al., 2017; Lehman et al., 2004), and selective serotonin reuptake inhibitors for internalizing conditions (Gosmann et al., 2021). Direct comparisons between the two frameworks have found that HiTOP dimensions typically outperform the DSM-defined categorical disorders in explaining various neural, social, psychological, and social functioning outcomes (Conway et al., 2021; Forbush et al., 2017, 2018; Kim et al., 2021; Martin et al., 2018; Morey et al., 2012; Reininghaus et al., 2019; Waszczuk, 2021).

Clinical Utility of HiTOP Framework

Existing research on the clinical utility of psychiatric classification systems typically examines reliability, prognostic value, and clinicians' perception of its usefulness in the practice (First et al., 2004; Mullins-Sweatt et al., 2016; Reed, 2010). To date, there is limited data to support the clinical utility of the full HiTOP framework beyond the preliminary findings of the field trials that are underway. However, there is some work looking at specific dimensions in the model that indicate its potential to improve the clinical utility of mental health practice. In the following, we review these results, noting their limitations and the need for further research.

Direct comparisons between dimensions in HiTOP versus DSM diagnoses have shown that transdiagnostic dimensions exhibit significantly higher diagnostic reliability, including both test-retest and inter-rater reliability (Markon et al., 2011). They also demonstrate greater prognostic power for both disorder-specific outcomes (e.g., impairments secondary to eating disorders such as mood and self-perception, Forbush et al., 2017, 2023; subsequent mental disorder diagnoses, Kim & Eaton, 2015; community, physical, neural, cognitive functionings, and symptom remission, Martin et al., 2021) and non-disorder outcomes (e.g., suicidaility, Eaton et al., 2013). However, these head-to-head comparisons are few and remain limited in their coverage of the constructs in the HiTOP framework. Further research is needed that covers a wider variety of constructs, contexts, and purposes.

In studies that compared the clinical perception of categorical and dimensional frameworks, clinicians generally rate the dimensional approach as more useful in terms of its ability to facilitate communication and treatment planning (Bornstein & Natoli, 2019; Lowe & Widiger, 2009; Morey et al., 2014; Samuel & Widiger, 2006, 2011). However, these studies have predominantly focused on comparing dimensional and categorical models of personality disorders and therefore provided limited support for the clinical utility of the HiTOP model specifically. To date, a study by Balling et al. (2023) represents the best direct comparison of clinicians' perceptions of the utility of DSM diagnoses versus HiTOP spectra and superspectra: Clinicians reported that HiTOP dimensions were as useful as, or even more useful than, the DSM diagnoses for describing, communicating, and managing psychopathology. This finding is both surprising and understandable. On one hand, one would expect clinicians who are more well-trained in the DSM framework than in HiTOP to find the DSM easier to use and to be more effective in guiding treatment formulation. On the other hand, the findings align with past reports of clinicians rating traditional systems as having poor utility for treatment selection and prognosis (First et al., 2018), instead relying on signs, symptoms, transdiagnostic processes or outcomes to guide treatment planning (Schaeuffele et al., 2021; Waszczuk et al., 2017b). Notably, limitations in the methodology of Balling et al. (2023) include the use of fictional vignettes and differing procedures to evaluate the utility of the HiTOP and DSM frameworks, limiting the generalization of the results to what we might see in practice. Therefore, even though this study provides important preliminary evidence to counter the concerns about clinicians not being able to interpret and use the HiTOP interface (Haeffel et al., 2022), more systematic head-to-head comparisons with the DSM are needed to evaluate the clinical utility of HiTOP in assessment and for guiding treatment.

We propose that future studies should take into account clinicians' familiarity with both DSM and HiTOP (Raskin et al., 2022), and provide necessary guidelines to standardize the application of the frameworks to assessments, case formulation, and treatment planning. For instance, given that HiTOP requires a comprehensive assessment across the broad spectra of psychopathology, DSM-based assessment should also be conducted with the same level of comprehensiveness, using standardized tools such as the Structured Clinical Interview for DSM (SCID). Importantly, the clinical utility of HiTOP needs to be assessed across a variety of domains, including diagnostic reliability, prognostic value, and clinical perception. Longitudinal studies would be particularly helpful in determining which approach ultimately facilitates more efficacious care for clients and leads to better treatment outcomes.

Limitations of the Evidence Supporting HiTOP

In addition to the specific limitations in the clinical utility literature, there are several overarching limitations to the evidence base that underpins the HiTOP framework, including that much of the current evidence relies on DSM-defined disorders, examines narrow groups of disorders in a piecemeal fashion, and uses homogeneous samples. In the following, we will elaborate on the primary limitations of the current body of evidence and discuss pertinent efforts that are planned for, or required to, address them.

Heavy Reliance on DSM-defined Disorders

A key limitation in the evidence for the HiTOP framework stems from the heavy reliance on studies of DSM-defined disorders, the limitations of which serve as the primary motivation for developing HiTOP. Hierarchical exclusion rules for diagnoses can artificially shape results from analyses of patterns of comorbidity (Conway & Brown, 2018), as can the overlapping symptoms among DSM diagnoses. In a descriptive study, Forbes (2023a) examined the proportions of symptom overlap within and between the HiTOP spectra and subfactors—that is, the percentage of symptom criteria repeated in two or more DSM-defined disorders within the same and across different dimensions, respectively. The study highlighted substantial symptom repetition within some HiTOP dimensions where disorders that comprise the same dimension have many diagnostic criteria in common. For instance, 53% and 100% of the symptoms within substance use and mania, respectively, were part of the diagnostic criteria for two or more diagnoses in each dimension. The symptom overlaps may artificially inflate patterns of co-variations among the DSM-defined disorders and potentially bias the structural results. One could argue that the higher-order HiTOP dimensions are merely artefacts of the shared phenomenology (Borsboom, 2002). This concern is, however, unlikely the case; the disorder co-variation underlying HiTOP dimensions appeared to be stronger than the correlations attributable solely to the shared phenomenology (Forbes, 2023a), suggesting that the HiTOP dimensions also reflect reliable co-variation beyond their symptom overlap. Nonetheless, structural analyses relying on DSM-defined disorders could still be biased by the shared phenomenology. Further research is warranted to elucidate the extent to which patterns of co-variation are inflated by symptom overlaps (Lahey et al., 2018), and how accounting for these similarities may alter the structure of the hierarchical model.

The heavy reliance on DSM-defined disorders also poses challenges when interpreting findings related to disorders that are mapped onto multiple dimensions. For instance, many DSM-defined psychotic disorders (e.g., schizophrenia, schizoaffective disorder, or schizophreniform disorder) subsumed within both thought disorder and detachment spectra (Kotov et al., 2020). Consequently, apparent vulnerabilities or abnormalities indicated by the associations between validators and these heterogeneous disorders cannot be disentangled or attributed specifically to a particular HiTOP dimension (e.g., the shared genetic risk for psychosis-related disorders cannot be attributed to thought disorder or detachment, due to the disorders cross-loading under both spectra). The patterns of cross-loadings throughout the model mean that disorder-level studies offer limited evidence of specificity—sometimes even at the coarse-grained level of superspectrum (e.g., borderline PD spans the externalizing and emotional dysfunction superspectra)—and prevent efforts to validate the detailed levels of the model.

To move away from relying on DSM-defined disorders as the proxies for lower-order syndrome dimensions in both research and clinical assessment, the HiTOP consortium has proposed a two-pronged approach. The first effort, led by the Clinical Translation Workgroup, focuses on promoting the use of HiTOP-consistent measures in the short term. Specifically, the Clinical Translation Workgroup has identified a non-exhaustive list of existing measures, at https://www.hitop-system.org/hitop-friendly-measures, that assess psychopathology dimensionally and hierarchically. However, to ensure good coverage across the model, users have to administer several of the measures together. To that end, the Clinical Translation Workgroup has also created a battery—the HiTOP Digital Assessment and Tracker (HiTOP-DAT)– from the subset of the existing measures; it is available at https://www.hitop-system.org/hitop-digital-assessment-and-tracker-hitop-dat (Jonas et al., 2021). The measures included in HiTOP-DAT assess the majority of HiTOP traits and symptoms in an average of 45 minutes. Importantly, they are freely available and have community normative data that support the evaluation of symptom severity relative to community norms. Further discussion on how these symptom-level measures can be utilized in clinical research can be found in the integration section later in this chapter. The second effort, led by the Measure Development Workgroup, focuses on developing and disseminating a purpose-built measure of the full HiTOP model (Simms et al., 2022; see https://www.hitop-system.org/hitop-sr-adaptations for a preliminary research-ready version of the measure). This comprehensive HiTOP measure will allow for more fine-grained analyses at the levels of symptoms and traits, which, in turn, could facilitate progress in elucidating the lower levels of the hierarchy and clarifying the composition of higher-order dimensions. Additionally, the scale validation phase helps to minimize the redundancy issue related to symptom overlaps and improve the discrimination between the scales of different dimensions.

Scope of Analysis

Constructing a collective understanding of the structure of psychopathology is hampered by the significant differences in studies' analysis scope and methodologies. The majority of empirical studies have focused on specific spectra but relied on different measures and operationalized psychopathology in different ways—using the presence/absence of disorders, the count of symptoms, or individual scores on symptom or trait scales/subscales. Studies that have spanned multiple spectra often rely on a limited set of disorders selected by the authors as representative of each dimension. Moreover, the overall structure that emerges in structural analyses can vary depending on the range of indicators included. For instance, an analysis can fail to identify a dimension if its indicators are underrepresented or it can generate a "bloated specific" factor—a unique dimension that is artifactually formed—if a group of specific and closely related indicators are over-represented (Watts et al., 2023b). To construct a reliable and robust structure of psychopathology, more analyses need to be done with broad and detailed measurement of psychopathological indicators, and without relying on DSM diagnoses as the unit of measurement.

Relatedly, the current HiTOP framework does not cover the full breadth of DSM (Kotov et al., 2021), which, in turn, does not offer a comprehensive representation of experiences of psychopathology (Dalgleish et al., 2020; Newson et al., 2021). This both impedes the aim of the HiTOP Consortium to comprehensively conceptualize psychopathology and hampers the practical usefulness of HiTOP at present. Recognizing this limitation, the HiTOP consortium has set one of the priorities as extending the breadth of the framework. Recent studies have begun to include features from DSM chapters that have yet to be integrated, such as the symptoms from the DSM neurodevelopmental disorders chapter (Forbes et al., 2023b; Michelini et al., 2019; Noordhof et al., 2015; Stanton et al., 2023). Similarly, more studies have focused on examining conditions that remain provisional in the model due to insufficient existing analyses, such as mania (e.g., Stanton et al., 2023). With more evidence, we can expect the HiTOP model to change, ideally with wider coverage, more fine-grained details at the lower levels, and clarification of the provisional aspects of the framework. To facilitate the empirical modification of the model, the Revisions Workgroup has developed and implemented standardized principles and procedures for revision based on the strength of the evidence for a proposed change (Forbes et al., 2023d). Of relevance here, higher scores are awarded to studies with more breadth and that use dimensional measures rather than categorical diagnoses—prioritizing evidence that moves away from DSM-defined disorders.

Problems of Homogenous Samples

Another limitation of the current evidence lies in the homogeneity of the studied samples, which limits the generalizability of the HiTOP model. The data that underpins the current HiTOP model primarily draws from white, Western, and adult samples, often referred to as WEIRD samples (Henrich et al., 2010). Indeed, this is an issue that pervades the field of psychological science. It is entirely conceivable that the current structure is different in data from more diverse samples—consisting of individuals of different races, cultures, genders, or age groups (Rodriguez-Seijas et al., 2023). Consequently, given the mostly homogenous samples in the existing evidence base, it is prudent to avoid assuming that the current HiTOP model is universally applicable to people across all contexts. Instead, it may be advisable to develop separate models tailored to different samples and statistically compare them to identify any discrepancies. If necessary, consideration should be given to constructing multiple parallel frameworks to accommodate significant disparities.

To address these gaps, the Developmental and Diversity, Equity, and Inclusion Workgroups were formed. Both groups set out to empirically examine the current framework with understudied populations, including those outside the typical age range of 18 to 65 years, as well as racial/ethnic, sexual, and gender minorities (Cicero & Ruggero, 2021; Eaton et al., 2021; He & Li, 2021; Tackett & Hallquist, 2022). Their goal is to determine whether psychopathology might be organized differently for different populations. For instance, contextual norms specific to a population could moderate the association between behaviors and trait dimensions at the narrower levels, changing the structure and composition of the dimensions on higher-order levels. For sexual and gender minorities, where substance use may be more normative than in the general population, substance use may be a less informative marker of externalizing dimensions like trait impulsivity or disinhibition (Rodriguez-Seijas et al., 2024). On the other hand, harmful substance use is likely to be uncommon among children, thus, substance use in this age group may be related to more prominent antisocial and rule-breaking behaviors. Accordingly, these work groups intend to collaborate with the Measurement Development Workgroup to consider variations needed in the creation, validation, and refinement of HiTOP measures, to ensure their suitability across diverse groups and take group-specific contexts into account.

In summary, it is important to acknowledge that HiTOP remains a work in progress and has several major limitations that need addressing for it to fulfil its full potential. Ultimately, HiTOP as a research-grounded nosology must be able to accurately and effectively inform clinical practice and enhance mental health care. In the following section, we will discuss how HiTOP can be integrated into clinical research and practice.

Integration of HiTOP into Clinical Research

HiTOP provides an alternative set of clinical phenotypes that hold promise for overcoming the limitations of traditional diagnostic categories and offer several advantages for advancing research into the causes and consequences of psychopathology. First, as dimensional phenotypes exhibit greater reliability and validity than categorical diagnoses (Markon et al., 2011), HiTOP constructs could provide more reliable targets that enhance the statistical power and reproducibility in clinical research (Forbes et al., 2023c; Tiego et al., 2022). Various subfields, such as psychiatric genetics (Derks et al., 2022) and psychiatric neuroimaging (Zald & Lahey, 2017), have emphasized the need for detailed and empirical characterization of psychopathological components—also referred to as detailed phenotyping (Tiego et al., 2022) or deep phenotyping (Watts et al., 2023c)—to facilitate more precise and replicable research findings.

Second, HiTOP defines psychiatric phenotypes at different levels of specificity, allowing researchers to examine the associations with outcome variables at a specific level of resolution (e.g., fine-grained symptom components or broad spectra) or across multiple levels of resolution simultaneously. Such versatility has become increasingly relevant in modern psychiatric research, as emerging results illustrate that etiological and outcome factors can operate at different levels of specificity. For instance, distinct genetic variants have been identified for the transdiagnostic fear subfactor (Otowa et al., 2016) and the narrow symptom component of anhedonia (Ward et al., 2019). Similarly, although adverse environments, in general, have non-specific associations with a broad variety of psychopathology (Caspi & Moffitt, 2018; Forbes et al., 2020), specific types of adversity have been linked to specific symptom components (Bentall et al., 2012).

Third, dimensional sampling is potentially less resource-intensive and captures more representative samples than case-control designs, because participants are not pre-screened and excluded based on arbitrary cut-off points or comorbidity. Instead, every individual's symptom presentation and severity are characterized across a comprehensive suite of dimensions. As such, insights gained from HiTOP-guided studies could facilitate the generalizability and translation of findings into more varied patient populations.

The Utility Workgroup has published several guidelines to apply the HiTOP framework to research to capitalize on its advantages. Findings from HiTOP-guided studies could, in turn, facilitate its refinement and pave the way for realizing its full potential as an empirically defined nosology (Conway et al., 2019, 2022). As mentioned earlier, there are a variety of dimensional measures available to directly derive the dimensions represented in HiTOP (Conway et al., 2022; Simms et al., 2022). Alternatively, studies can apply latent variable models to existing (ideally symptom-level) data to statistically derive HiTOP dimensions (Bornovalova et al., 2020; Forbes et al., 2021a). This approach to assessment allows researchers to examine the association of psychopathology at varying levels of granularity with a given outcome, and potentially identify a level of specificity that can meaningfully explain the variability among individuals.

Examining dimensional data that span multiple levels of hierarchy and breadth (i.e., include multiple higher-order dimensions) could also help to resolve the ongoing limitations of the HiTOP model. For instance, studies that examine symptom-level data could elucidate the structure at lower-order levels currently obscured by categorical data (Forbes et al., 2023b). Given that the dimensions that emerge in structural analyses are particularly dependent on the scope of the analysis (i.e., the disorders or the specific signs and symptoms included), findings from analyses that incorporate data across higher-order domains, including indicators currently being underrepresented or not included in existing literature, could expand the breadth of the model and validate the placement of provisional dimensions—namely, the mania subfactor and somatoform spectrum.

There are also scientific benefits to integrating the HiTOP framework into longitudinal studies, as the dimensional phenotypes have the potential to capture the natural progression of mental illness over time. According to the clinical staging model of psychiatry (McGorry et al., 2006; Mei et al., this volume), mental illness can evolve through stages of increasing symptom severity, functional impairment, illness duration, and treatment resistance. Importantly, the level of symptom specificity also varies across the stages; early clinical phenotypes are characterized by non-specific and transdiagnostic symptoms (e.g., sleep disturbances or mood fluctuations) that could evolve into more specific and pronounced syndromes (e.g., anhedonia, delusions, or specific phobia) at later stages. The HiTOP structure provides an optimal framework for conceptualizing dimensional phenotypes at varying levels of symptom severity and specificity. Accordingly, longitudinal studies guided by HiTOP can help define psychopathology along the illness courses and identify important risk and protective factors that could reliably predict an individual's progression. Incorporating transdiagnostic dimensions in this line of research also allows for more accurate and early identification of at-risk populations, which, in turn, could facilitate the development and dissemination of preventative interventions.

Longitudinal studies that span developmental stages would also fill the gaps in the current framework that has mainly focused on between-individual variability with cross-sectional data from adults. Longitudinal studies, including ambulatory assessment, could examine within-individual patterns of variation (e.g., Wright et al., 2015; Zimmermann et al., 2019) and clarify the extent to which the HiTOP phenotypes are developmentally coherent (i.e., can be reliably identified across the lifespan; e.g., Tackett & Hallquist, 2022). Currently, evidence suggests that broad dimensions of internalizing, externalizing, and thought problems are replicated across different age groups (e.g., Achenbach, 2020; Eaton et al., 2011, 2015; Krueger, 1999). However, the narrower dimensions show less consistency; studies found that specific dimensions such as fear or distress can be reliably identified from early childhood while others only emerge from the broader dimensions at later stages of development (Forbes et al., 2016). Further longitudinal research is needed to determine the developmental continuity and changes in clinical phenotypes and subsequently inform future revisions for the model to become more developmentally appropriate.

Integration of HiTOP into Clinical Practice

In clinical practice, integrating HiTOP principles means encouraging clinicians to assess clients' presenting problems dimensionally at various levels of specificity and proceeding with case formulation and treatment planning based on the elevated domains in clients' symptom profiles (Hopwood et al., 2020; Ruggero, Kotov et al., 2019). While a HiTOP-based clinical interview is under development, clinicians can add existing HiTOP-friendly measures to their current assessment protocols, such as the HiTOP-DAT, which automatically generates a report upon completion and can be used for measurement-based care, tracking symptom change over time. Other existing measures have also been mapped onto specific HiTOP dimensions (Wendt et al., 2023).

With regard to treatment selection, although existing evidence for treatment specific to the HiTOP approach remains sparse (Cicero et al., 2024; Haeffel et al., 2022), research has demonstrated effectiveness for many of the existing transdiagnostic treatments, and some of the transdiagnostic treatment targets can be readily mapped to the existing dimensions in HiTOP (Dalgleish et al., 2020; Gros, 2019; Gutner & Presseau, 2019; Schaeuffele et al., 2021, 2024; Sloan et al., 2017). Additionally, since clinicians often already make treatment decisions based on transdiagnostic symptom profiles rather than diagnostic disorders (First et al., 2018; Jensen-Doss & Hawley, 2011; Waszczuk et al., 2017b), adopting a transdiagnostic dimensional approach to treatment planning would not be likely to require a significant shift in their decision-making processes. In fact, the HiTOP approach could provide a more standardized framework to guide the process of matching treatment to symptom profiles, instead of clinicians having to rely on clinical judgment and subjective expertise (Hagerty, 2023).

The Clinical Translation Workgroup has published several guidelines to apply the HiTOP framework to diagnostic assessments, case formulation, and treatment planning (Hagerty, 2023; Hopwood, 2018; Hopwood et al., 2020; Mullins-Sweatt et al., 2020; Ruggero et al., 2019). Notably, the hierarchical organization of the HiTOP framework allows for a stepwise approach to assessment and treatment, which could promote clinical efficiency and flexibility. In brief intervention and acute-care settings, assessment and treatment can primarily focus on higher-order phenotypes, targeting the transdiagnostic vulnerabilities (Barlow et al., 2017) and pathological processes (e.g., Barlow et al., 2020; Boelen, 2010; Boelen & van den Bout, 2010; Campbell-Sills & Barlow, 2007; Sloan et al., 2017; Tull et al., 2004; Turk et al., 2005). In theory, broad treatments targeting shared processes that underlie comorbid problems should lead to the most gains within a limited amount of time. For instance, if an initial screening revealed that the patient presented with elevated scores on internalizing spectrum, the clinician has the flexibility to focus on treating the higher-order phenotypes, using antidepressants or the Unified Protocol for Emotional Disorder (Barlow et al., 2020). If resources permit, further assessment for narrower forms of psychopathology can be performed. For instance, if a follow-up assessment using the Inventory of Depression and Anxiety Symptoms (IDAS-II; Watson et al., 2012) revealed that the patient's elevated score on internalizing was mainly driven by elevated scores on the lower-order dimensions of dysphoria, insomnia, and panic. The clinician has the flexibility to formulate a more in-depth case formulation to understand the processes that cause and maintain the presenting problems and choose to deliver more specific treatment such as sleep hygiene or hypnotic drugs for insomnia.

For this hypothetical approach to come to fruition, and more generally for the HiTOP framework to be fully ready for clinical application, much research is still required. Research into transdiagnostic dimensional treatment has grown exponentially over the last few decades, a trend expected to continue given the emergence of transdiagnostic frameworks, such as RDoC and HiTOP. However, much research is still required for the HiTOP framework to be fully ready for clinical application. Conway et al. (2023) outlined 10 important research areas and relevant hypotheses aimed at enhancing our general understanding of psychopathology and clarifying the potential of HiTOP as a nosology to improve mental health care. Among them, an important question is whether the HiTOP dimensions can effectively guide clinical decisions and improve treatment outcomes. Addressing this question requires randomized controlled trials to compare treatment efficacy between HiTOP-guided assessment and treatment planning versus traditional diagnostic-based practices. Another practical consideration is the need for ranges or thresholds on the dimension scores to guide clinical decisions. Even though the dimensional structure is a more reliable and valid conceptualization of psychopathology, clinical settings often necessitate dichotomous decisions—to hospitalize or to discharge, to deliver active treatment or not, and what diagnostic code to use for billing (Kendler, 2018). Conway et al. (2023) suggested the use of statistical deviance (i.e., standard deviations above or below the means) to dichotomize the symptom severity in the short term (Ruggero et al., 2019). The long-term vision is to rely on outcome data to empirically determine thresholds for specific clinical decisions (e.g., ranges that are significantly related to the risk of suicide attempt that warrants admission decision).

To date, the majority of the transdiagnostic treatments have been primarily developed for or mapped onto the internalizing domain (Hopwood et al., 2020). However, there is a pressing need for further research to develop or identify interventions capable of effectively alleviating symptoms in other higher-order and lower-order phenotypes and to compare their efficacy with the traditional method of matching interventions to categorical diagnoses. Mullins-Sweatt et al. (2020) demonstrated how such research endeavors could be conducted, particularly focusing on the treatment of personality pathology. Specifically, the authors recommend a three-step approach to empirically evaluate how existing treatments can be mapped onto HiTOP dimensions, including (1) developing a comprehensive list of evidence-based interventions, (2) generating hypotheses about which technique can address specific phenotype based on the extant literature, and (3) empirically testing the hypotheses using naturalistic research or randomized controlled trials.

Conclusion

While traditional nosologies like the DSM have laid the groundwork for psychiatric classification, they fall short in several critical areas. HiTOP offers a promising alternative for a more reliable and valid organization of mental health disorders. This chapter has presented evidence supporting the potential of the HiTOP framework in providing more valid and reliable phenotypes for research, facilitating the identification of underlying mechanisms, and improving the precision of clinical interventions. However, HiTOP is not without its limitations. Despite its strengths, the model still requires further refinement and validation before it can be fully integrated into clinical practice. The HiTOP Consortium was established to support this ongoing development, and its members have made significant strides in addressing the critical challenges of creating an empirically based psychiatric nosology. There is good reason to be optimistic that HiTOP represents a pivotal step toward breaking free of the "epistemic prison" that has hindered the field, paving the way for a unified approach to research and clinical practice in mental health, and ultimately enhancing the effectiveness of care.

References

Abramowitz, J. S., Deacon, B. J., & Whiteside, S. P. (2019). *Exposure therapy for anxiety: Principles and practice*. Guilford Publications.

Achenbach, T. M. (1966). The classification of children's psychiatric symptoms: A factor-analytic study. *Psychological Monographs: General and Applied*, *80*(7), 1–37. https://doi.org/10.1037/h0093906

Achenbach, T. M. (2020). Bottom-up and top-down paradigms for psychopathology: A half-century odyssey. *Annual Review of Clinical Psychology*, *16*, 1–24. https://doi.org/10.1146/annurev-clinpsy-071119-115831

Achenbach, T. M., & Dumenci, L. (2001). Advances in empirically based assessment: Revised cross-informant syndromes and new DSM-oriented scales for the CBCL, YSR, and TRF: Comment on Lengua, Sadowski, Friedrich, and Fisher (2001). *Journal of Consulting and Clinical Psychology*, *69*(4), 699–702. PMID: 11550735.

Allsopp, K., Read, J., Corcoran, R., & Kinderman, P. (2019). Heterogeneity in psychiatric diagnostic classification. *Psychiatry Research*, *279*, 15–22. https://doi.org/10.1016/j.psychres.2019.07.005

Andrews, G., Goldberg, D. P., Krueger, R. F., Carpenter, W. T., Hyman, S. E., Sachdev, P., & Pine, D. S. (2009). Exploring the feasibility of a meta-structure for DSM-V and ICD-11: Could it improve utility and validity?: Paper 1 of 7 of the thematic section: "A proposal for a meta-structure for DSM-V and ICD-11." *Psychological Medicine*, *39*(12), 1993–2000. https://doi.org/10.1017/S0033291709990250

Andrews, G., Stewart, G., Allen, R., & Henderson, A. S. (1990). The genetics of six neurotic disorders: A twin study. *Journal of Affective Disorders*, *19*(1), 23–29. https://doi.org/10.1016/0165-0327(90)90005-S

Balling, C. E., South, S. C., Lynam, D. R., & Samuel, D. B. (2023). Clinician perception of the clinical utility of the Hierarchical Taxonomy of Psychopathology (HiTOP) system. *Clinical Psychological Science*, 21677026221138. https://doi.org/10.1177/21677026221138818

Barlow, D. H. (2021). *Clinical handbook of psychological disorders: A step-by-step treatment manual*. Guilford Publications.

Barlow, D. H., Farchione, T. J., Bullis, J. R., Gallagher, M. W., Murray-Latin, H., Sauer-Zavala, S., Bentley, K. H., Thompson-Hollands, J., Conklin, L. R., Boswell, J. F., Ametaj, A., Carl, J. R., Boettcher, H. T., & Cassiello-Robbins, C. (2017). The unified protocol for transdiagnostic treatment of emotional disorders compared with diagnosis-specific protocols for anxiety disorders. *JAMA Psychiatry*, *74*(9), 875–884. https://doi.org/10.1001/jamapsychiatry.2017.2164

Barlow, D. H., Harris, B. A., Eustis, E. H., & Farchione, T. J. (2020). The unified protocol for transdiagnostic treatment of emotional disorders. *World Psychiatry*, *19*(2), 245–246. https://doi.org/10.1002/wps.20748

Bentall, R. P., Wickham, S., Shevlin, M., & Varese, F. (2012). Do specific early-life adversities lead to specific symptoms of psychosis? A study from the 2007 The Adult Psychiatric Morbidity Survey. *Schizophrenia Bulletin*, *38*(4), 734–740. https://doi.org/10.1093/schbul/sbs049

Boelen, P. (2010). Intolerance of uncertainty and emotional distress following the death of a loved one. *Anxiety, Stress, and Coping*, *23*(4), 471–478. https://doi.org/10.1080/10615800903494135

Boelen, P. A., & van den Bout, J. (2010). Anxious and depressive avoidance and symptoms of prolonged grief, depression, and post-traumatic stress disorder. *Psychologica Belgica*, *50*(1–2), 49–67. https://doi.org/10.5334/pb-50-1-2-49

Bornovalova, M. A., Choate, A. M., Fatimah, H., Petersen, K. J., & Wiernik, B. M. (2020). Appropriate use of bifactor analysis in psychopathology research: Appreciating benefits and limitations. *Biological Psychiatry*, *88*(1), 18–27. https://doi.org/10.1016/j.biopsych.2020.01.013

Bornstein, R. F., & Natoli, A. P. (2019). Clinical utility of categorical and dimensional perspectives on personality pathology: A meta-analytic review. *Personality Disorders: Theory, Research, and Treatment*, *10*(6), 479–490. https://doi.org/10.1037/per0000365

Borsboom, D. (2002). The structure of the DSM. *Archives of General Psychiatry*, *59*(6), 569–570.

Buchanan, R. W., Kreyenbuhl, J., Kelly, D. L., Noel, J. M., Boggs, D. L., Fischer, B. A., Himelhoch, S., Fang, B., Peterson, E., Aquino, P. R., & Keller, W. (2010). The 2009 schizophrenia PORT psychopharmacological treatment recommendations and summary statements. *Schizophrenia Bulletin*, *36*(1), 71–93. https://doi.org/10.1093/schbul/sbp116

Campbell-Sills, L., & Barlow, D. H. (2007). Incorporating emotion regulation into conceptualizations and treatments of anxiety and mood disorders. In James J. Gross (Ed.), *Handbook of emotion regulation* (pp. 542–559). The Guilford Press.

Carragher, N., Krueger, R. F., Eaton, N. R., & Slade, T. (2015). Disorders without borders: Current and future directions in the meta-structure of mental disorders. *Social Psychiatry and Psychiatric Epidemiology*, *50*(3), 339–350. https://doi.org/10.1007/s00127-014-1004-z

Carroll, J. B. (1993). *Human cognitive abilities: A survey of factor-analytic studies* (Issue 1). Cambridge University Press.

Caspi, A., Houts, R. M., Belsky, D. W., Goldman-Mellor, S. J., Harrington, H., Israel, S., Meier, M. H., Ramrakha, S., Shalev, I., Poulton, R., & Moffitt, T. E. (2014). The p factor: One general psychopathology factor in the structure of psychiatric disorders? *Clinical Psychological Science: A Journal of the Association for Psychological Science*, *2*(2), 119–137. https://doi.org/10.1177/2167702613497473

Caspi, A., & Moffitt, T. E. (2018). All for one and one for all: Mental disorders in one dimension. *American Journal of Psychiatry*, *175*(9), 831–844. https://doi.org/10.1176/appi.ajp.2018.17121383

Chmielewski, M., Clark, L. A., Bagby, R. M., & Watson, D. (2015). Method matters: Understanding diagnostic reliability in DSM-IV and DSM-5. *Journal of Abnormal Psychology*, *124*(3), 764–769. https://doi.org/10.1037/abn0000069

Cicero, D. C., Jonas, K. G., Li, K., Perlman, G., & Kotov, R. (2019). Common taxonomy of traits and symptoms: Linking schizophrenia symptoms, schizotypy, and normal personality. *Schizophrenia Bulletin*, *45*(6), 1336–1348. https://doi.org/10.1093/schbul/sbz005

Cicero, D. C., Ruggero, C. J., Balling, C. E., Bottera, A. R., Cheli, S., Elkrief, L., Forbush, K. T., Hopwood, C. J., Jonas, K. G., Jutras-Aswad, D., Kotov, R., Levin-Aspenson, H. F., Mullins-Sweatt, S. N., Johnson-Munguia, S., Narrow, W. E., Negi, S., Patrick, C. J., Rodriguez-Seijas, C., Sheth, S., . . . Thomeczek, M. L. (2024). State of the science: The Hierarchical Taxonomy of Psychopathology (HiTOP). *Behavior Therapy*, *55*(6), 1114–1129. https://doi.org/10.1016/j.beth.2024.05.001

Cicero, D., & Ruggero, C. (2021). Commentary—Opening a can of worms: The importance of testing the measurement invariance of hierarchical models of psychopathology—a commentary on He and Li (2020). *Journal of Child Psychology and Psychiatry*, *62*(3), 299–302. https://doi.org/10.1111/jcpp.13353

Clark, D. A., & Beck, A. T. (2011). *Cognitive therapy of anxiety disorders: Science and practice.* Guilford Press.

Clark, L. A., Cuthbert, B., Lewis-Fernández, R., Narrow, W. E., & Reed, G. M. (2017). Three approaches to understanding and classifying mental disorder: ICD-11, DSM-5, and the National Institute of Mental Health's Research Domain Criteria (RDoC). *Psychological Science in the Public Interest, 18*(2), 72–145.

Clark, L. A., & Watson, D. (1991). Tripartite model of anxiety and depression: Psychometric evidence and taxonomic implications. *Journal of Abnormal Psychology, 100*(3), 316–336. https://doi.org/10.1037/0021-843X.100.3.316

Comer, J. S., Chow, C., Chan, P. T., Cooper-Vince, C., & Wilson, L. A. S. (2013). Psychosocial treatment efficacy for disruptive behavior problems in very young children: A meta-analytic examination. *Journal of the American Academy of Child and Adolescent Psychiatry, 52*(1), 26–36. https://doi.org/10.1016/j.jaac.2012.10.001

Conway, C. C., & Brown, T. A. (2018). Evaluating dimensional models of psychopathology in outpatients diagnosed with emotional disorders: A cautionary tale. *Depression and Anxiety, 35*(9), 898–902. https://doi.org/10.1002/da.22740

Conway, C. C., Forbes, M. K., Forbush, K. T., Fried, E. I., Hallquist, M. N., Kotov, R., Mullins-Sweatt, S. N., Shackman, A. J., Skodol, A. E., South, S. C., Sunderland, M., Waszczuk, M. A., Zald, D. H., Afzali, M. H., Bornovalova, M. A., Carragher, N., Docherty, A. R., Jonas, K. G., Krueger, R. F., . . . Eaton, N. R. (2019). A Hierarchical Taxonomy of Psychopathology can transform mental health research. *Perspectives on Psychological Science: A Journal of the Association for Psychological Science, 14*(3), 419–436. https://doi.org/10.1177/1745691618810696

Conway, C. C., Forbes, M. K., & South, S. C. (2022). A Hierarchical Taxonomy of Psychopathology (HiTOP) primer for mental health researchers. *Clinical Psychological Science, 10*(2), 236–258. https://doi.org/10.1177/21677026211017834

Conway, C. C., Kotov, R., Krueger, R. F., & Caspi, A. (2023). Translating the Hierarchical Taxonomy of Psychopathology (HiTOP) from potential to practice: Ten research questions. *American Psychologist, 78*(7), 873–885. https://doi.org/10.1037/amp0001046

Conway, C. C., Krueger, R. F., HiTOP Consortium Executive Board, Cicero, D. C., DeYoung, C. G., Eaton, N. R., Forbes, M. K., Hallquist, M. N., Kotov, R., Latzman, R. D., Ruggero, C. J., Simms, L. J., Waldman, I. D., Waszczuk, M. A., Watson, D., Widiger, T. A., & Wright, A. G. C. (2021). Rethinking the diagnosis of mental disorders: Data-driven psychological dimensions, not categories, as a framework for mental-health research, treatment, and training. *Current Directions in Psychological Science, 30*(2), 151–158. https://doi.org/10.1177/0963721421990353

Copeland, W. E., Angold, A., Costello, E. J., & Egger, H. (2013). Prevalence, comorbidity, and correlates of DSM-5 proposed disruptive mood dysregulation disorder. *American Journal of Psychiatry, 170*(2), 173–179.

Costa, P. T., & McCrae, R. R. (2011, February 10). *The five-factor model of personality and its relevance to personality disorders* (world) [Research-article]. Https://Doi.Org/10.1521/Pedi.1992.6.4.343; Guilford Publications Inc. https://doi.org/10.1521/pedi.1992.6.4.343

Cummings, C. M., Caporino, N. E., & Kendall, P. C. (2014). Comorbidity of anxiety and depression in children and adolescents: 20 years after. *Psychological Bulletin, 140*(3), 816–845. https://doi.org/10.1037/a0034733

Dalgleish, T., Black, M., Johnston, D., & Bevan, A. (2020). Transdiagnostic approaches to mental health problems: Current status and future directions. *Journal of Consulting and Clinical Psychology, 88*(3), 179–195. https://doi.org/10.1037/ccp0000482

Derks, E. M., Thorp, J. G., & Gerring, Z. F. (2022). Ten challenges for clinical translation in psychiatric genetics. *Nature Genetics, 54*(10), 1457–1465. https://doi.org/10.1038/s41588-022-01174-0

De Wit-De Visser, B., Rijckmans, M., Vermunt, J. K., & van Dam, A. (2023). Pathways to antisocial behavior: A framework to improve diagnostics and tailor therapeutic interventions. *Frontiers in Psychology, 14*. 993090. https://doi.org/10.3389/fpsyg.2023.993090

DeYoung, C. G., Blain, S. D., Latzman, R. D., Grazioplene, R., Haltigan, J. D., Kotov, R., Michelini, G., Venables, N. C., Docherty, A. R., Goghari, V. M., Kallen, A. M., Martin, E. A., Palumbo, I. M., Patrick, C., Perkins, E. R., Shackman, A. J., Snyder, M. E., & Tobin, K. E. (2024). The Hierarchical Taxonomy of Psychopathology (HiTOP) and the search for neurobiological substrates of mental illness: A systematic review and roadmap for future research. *Journal of Psychopathology and Clinical Science*, *133*(8), 697–715. https://doi.org/10.31234/osf.io/yatw7

Dick, D. M., Viken, R. J., Kaprio, J., Pulkkinen, L., & Rose, R. J. (2005). Understanding the covariation among childhood externalizing symptoms: Genetic and environmental influences on conduct disorder, attention deficit hyperactivity disorder, and oppositional defiant disorder symptoms. *Journal of Abnormal Child Psychology*, *33*(2), 219–229. https://doi.org/10.1007/s10802-005-1829-8

Dornbach-Bender, A., Ruggero, C. J., Waszczuk, M. A., Gamez, W., Watson, D., & Kotov, R. (2017). Mapping emotional disorders at the finest level: Convergent validity and joint structure based on alternative measures. *Comprehensive Psychiatry*, *79*, 31–39. https://doi.org/10.1016/j.comppsych.2017.06.011

Dunlop, B. W., Rajendra, J. K., Craighead, W. E., Kelley, M. E., McGrath, C. L., Choi, K. S., Kinkead, B., Nemeroff, C. B., & Mayberg, H. S. (2017). Functional connectivity of the subcallosal cingulate cortex identifies differential outcomes to treatment with cognitive behavior therapy or antidepressant medication for major depressive disorder. *The American Journal of Psychiatry*, *174*(6), 533–545. https://doi.org/10.1176/appi.ajp.2016.16050518

Eaton, N. R., Krueger, R. F., Keyes, K. M., Skodol, A. E., Markon, K. E., Grant, B. F., & Hasin, D. S. (2011). Borderline personality disorder co-morbidity: Relationship to the internalizing–externalizing structure of common mental disorders. *Psychological Medicine*, *41*(5), 1041–1050. https://doi.org/10.1017/S0033291710001662

Eaton, N. R., Krueger, R. F., Markon, K. E., Keyes, K. M., Skodol, A. E., Wall, M., Hasin, D. S., & Grant, B. F. (2013). The structure and predictive validity of the internalizing disorders. *Journal of Abnormal Psychology*, *122*(1), 86–92. https://doi.org/10.1037/a0029598

Eaton, N. R., Rodriguez-Seijas, C., Carragher, N., & Krueger, R. F. (2015). Transdiagnostic factors of psychopathology and substance use disorders: A review. *Social Psychiatry and Psychiatric Epidemiology*, *50*(2), 171–182. https://doi.org/10.1007/s00127-014-1001-2

Eaton, N. R., Rodriguez-Seijas, C., & Pachankis, J. E. (2021). Transdiagnostic approaches to sexual- and gender-minority mental health. *Current Directions in Psychological Science*, *30*(6), 510–518. https://doi.org/doi.org/10.1177/09637214211043918

First, M. B., Pincus, H. A., Levine, J. B., Williams, J. B. W., Ustun, B., & Peele, R. (2004). Clinical utility as a criterion for revising psychiatric diagnoses. *American Journal of Psychiatry*, *161*(6), 946–954. https://doi.org/10.1176/appi.ajp.161.6.946

First, M. B., Rebello, T. J., Keeley, J. W., Bhargava, R., Dai, Y., Kulygina, M., Matsumoto, C., Robles, R., Stona, A.-C., & Reed, G. M. (2018). Do mental health professionals use diagnostic classifications the way we think they do? A global survey. *World Psychiatry*, *17*(2), 187–195. https://doi.org/10.1002/wps.20525

Forbes, M. K. (2023a). Implications of the symptom-level overlap among DSM diagnoses for dimensions of psychopathology. *Journal of Emotion and Psychopathology*, *1*(1), 104–112. https://doi.org/10.55913/joep.v1i1.6

Forbes, M. K., Baillie, A. J., Batterham, P. J., Calear, A. L., Kotov, R., Krueger, R. F., Markon, K., Mewton, L., Pellicano, L., Roberts, M., Rodriguez-Seijas, C., Sunderland, M., Watson, D., Watts, A. L., Wright, A. G. C., & Clark, L. A. (2023b). *Reconstructing psychopathology: A data-driven reorganization of the symptoms in DSM-5*. PsyArXiv. https://doi.org/10.31234/osf.io/7um9a

Forbes, M. K., Baillie, A. J., Eaton, N. R., & Krueger, R. F. (2017a). A place for sexual dysfunctions in an empirical taxonomy of psychopathology. *Journal of Sex Research*, *54*(4–5), 465–485. https://doi.org/10.1080/00224499.2016.1269306

Forbes, M. K., Fried, E. I., & Vaidyanathan, U. (2023c). Studying fine-grained elements of psychopathology to advance mental health science. *Journal of Psychopathology and Clinical Science*, *132*(7), 793–796. https://doi.org/10.1037/abn0000872

Forbes, M. K., Greene, A. L., Levin-Aspenson, H. F., Watts, A. L., Hallquist, M., Lahey, B. B., Markon, K. E., Patrick, C. J., Tackett, J. L., Waldman, I. D., Wright, A. G. C., Caspi, A., Ivanova, M., Kotov, R., Samuel, D. B., Eaton, N. R., & Krueger, R. F. (2021a). Three recommendations based on a comparison of the reliability and validity of the predominant models used in research on the empirical structure of psychopathology. *Journal of Abnormal Psychology*, *130*(3), 297–317. https://doi.org/10.1037/abn0000533

Forbes, M. K., Kotov, R., Ruggero, C. J., Watson, D., Zimmerman, M., & Krueger, R. F. (2017b). Delineating the joint hierarchical structure of clinical and personality disorders in an outpatient psychiatric sample. *Comprehensive Psychiatry*, *79*, 19–30. https://doi.org/10.1016/j.comppsych.2017.04.006

Forbes, M. K., Magson, N. R., & Rapee, R. M. (2020). Evidence that different types of peer victimization have equivalent associations with transdiagnostic psychopathology in adolescence. *Journal of Youth and Adolescence*, *49*(3), 590–604. https://doi.org/10.1007/s10964-020-01202-4

Forbes, M. K., Ringwald, W. R., Allen, T., Cicero, D. C., Clark, L. A., DeYoung, C. G., Eaton, N. R., Naragon-Gainey, K., Kotov, R., Krueger, R., Latzman, R. D., Martin, E. A., Ruggero, C., Waldman, I., Brandes, C. M., Fried, E. I., Goghari, V., Hankin, B., Sperry, S. H., . . . Wright, A. G. C. (2023d). Principles and procedures for revising the Hierarchical Taxonomy of Psychopathology. *Journal of Psychopathology and Clinical Science*, *133*(1), 4. https://doi.org/10.31234/osf.io/xr48p

Forbes, M. K., & Schniering, C. A. (2013). Are sexual problems a form of internalizing psychopathology? A structural equation modeling analysis. *Archives of Sexual Behavior*, *42*(1), 23–34. https://doi.org/10.1007/s10508-012-9948-0

Forbes, M. K., Sunderland, M., Rapee, R. M., Batterham, P. J., Calear, A. L., Carragher, N., Ruggero, C., Zimmerman, M., Baillie, A. J., Lynch, S. J., Mewton, L., Slade, T., & Krueger, R. F. (2021b). A detailed Hierarchical Model of Psychopathology: From individual symptoms up to the general factor of psychopathology. *Clinical Psychological Science*, *9*(2), 139–168. https://doi.org/10.1177/2167702620954799

Forbes, M. K., Tackett, J. L., Markon, K. E., & Krueger, R. F. (2016). Beyond comorbidity: Toward a dimensional and hierarchical approach to understanding psychopathology across the life span. *Development and Psychopathology*, *28*(4pt1), 971–986. https://doi.org/10.1017/S0954579416000651

Forbush, K. T., Chen, P.-Y., Hagan, K. E., Chapa, D. A. N., Gould, S. R., Eaton, N. R., & Krueger, R. F. (2018). A new approach to eating-disorder classification: Using empirical methods to delineate diagnostic dimensions and inform care. *International Journal of Eating Disorders*, *51*(7), 710–721. https://doi.org/10.1002/eat.22891

Forbush, K. T., Chen, Y., Chen, P.-Y., Bohrer, B. K., Hagan, K. E., Chapa, D. A. N., Christensen Pacella, K. A., Perko, V., Richson, B. N., Johnson Munguia, S. N., Thomeczek, M. L., Nelson, S. V., Christian, K., Swanson, T. J., & Wildes, J. E. (2023). Integrating "lumpers" versus "splitters" perspectives: Toward a hierarchical dimensional taxonomy of eating disorders from clinician ratings. *Clinical Psychological Science*, *12*(4), 625–643. https://doi.org/10.1177/21677026231186803

Forbush, K. T., Hagan, K. E., Kite, B. A., Chapa, D. A. N., Bohrer, B. K., & Gould, S. R. (2017). Understanding eating disorders within internalizing psychopathology: A novel transdiagnostic, hierarchical-dimensional model. *Comprehensive Psychiatry*, *79*, 40–52. https://doi.org/10.1016/j.comppsych.2017.06.009

Forbush, K. T., South, S. C., Krueger, R. F., Iacono, W. G., Clark, L. A., Keel, P. K., Legrand, L. N., & Watson, D. (2010). Locating eating pathology within an empirical diagnostic taxonomy: Evidence from a community-based sample. *Journal of Abnormal Psychology*, *119*(2), 282–292. https://doi.org/10.1037/a0019189

Forbush, K. T., & Watson, D. (2013). The structure of common and uncommon mental disorders. *Psychological Medicine*, *43*(1), 97–108. https://doi.org/10.1017/S0033291712001092

Frances, A., Pincus, H., Widiger, T., Davis, W., & First, M. (1990). DSM-IV: Work in progress. *American Journal of Psychiatry*, *147*(11), 1439–1448. PubMed. https://doi.org/10.1176/ajp.147.11.1439

Fusar-Poli, P., McGorry, P. D., & Kane, J. M. (2017). Improving outcomes of first-episode psychosis: An overview. *World Psychiatry*, *16*(3), 251–265. https://doi.org/10.1002/wps.20446

Goldberg, L. R. (1993). The structure of phenotypic personality traits. *The American Psychologist*, *48*(1), 26–34. https://doi.org/10.1037//0003-066x.48.1.26

Gosmann, N. P., Costa, M. de A., Jaeger, M. de B., Motta, L. S., Frozi, J., Spanemberg, L., Manfro, G. G., Cuijpers, P., Pine, D. S., & Salum, G. A. (2021). Selective serotonin reuptake inhibitors, and serotonin and norepinephrine reuptake inhibitors for anxiety, obsessive-compulsive, and stress disorders: A 3-level network meta-analysis. *PLoS Medicine*, *18*(6), e1003664. https://doi.org/10.1371/journal.pmed.1003664

Greenhill, L., Kollins, S., Abikoff, H., McCracken, J., Riddle, M., Swanson, J., McGough, J., Wigal, S., Wigal, T., Vitiello, B., Skrobala, A., Posner, K., Ghuman, J., Cunningham, C., Davies, M., Chuang, S., & Cooper, T. (2006). Efficacy and safety of immediate-release methylphenidate treatment for preschoolers with ADHD. *Journal of the American Academy of Child and Adolescent Psychiatry*, *45*(11), 1284–1293. https://doi.org/10.1097/01.chi.0000235077.32661.61

Griffith, J. W., Zinbarg, R. E., Craske, M. G., Mineka, S., Rose, R. D., Waters, A. M., & Sutton, J. M. (2010). Neuroticism as a common dimension in the internalizing disorders. *Psychological Medicine*, *40*(7), 1125–1136. https://doi.org/10.1017/S0033291709991449

Grisanzio, K. A., Goldstein-Piekarski, A. N., Wang, M. Y., Rashed Ahmed, A. P., Samara, Z., & Williams, L. M. (2018). Transdiagnostic symptom clusters and associations with brain, behavior, and daily function in mood, anxiety, and trauma disorders. *JAMA Psychiatry*, *75*(2), 201–209. https://doi.org/10.1001/jamapsychiatry.2017.3951

Gros, D. F. (2019). Efficacy of transdiagnostic behavior therapy across the affective disorders. *American Journal of Psychotherapy*, *72*(3), 59–66. https://doi.org/10.1176/appi.psychotherapy.20190007

Gutner, C. A., & Presseau, C. (2019). Dealing with complexity and comorbidity: Opportunity for transdiagnostic treatment for PTSD. *Current Treatment Options in Psychiatry*, *6*(2), 119–131. https://doi.org/10.1007/s40501-019-00170-2

Haeffel, G. J., Jeronimus, B. F., Kaiser, B. N., Weaver, L. J., Soyster, P. D., Fisher, A. J., Vargas, I., Goodson, J. T., & Lu, W. (2022). Folk classification and factor rotations: Whales, sharks, and the problems with the Hierarchical Taxonomy of Psychopathology (HiTOP). *Clinical Psychological Science: A Journal of the Association for Psychological Science*, *10*(2), 259–278. https://doi.org/10.1177/21677026211002500

Hagerty, S. L. (2023). Toward precision characterization and treatment of psychopathology: A path forward and integrative framework of the Hierarchical Taxonomy of Psychopathology and the Research Domain Criteria. *Perspectives on Psychological Science*, *18*(1), 91–109. https://doi.org/10.1177/17456916221079597

Haslam, N., Holland, E., & Kuppens, P. (2012). Categories versus dimensions in personality and psychopathology: A quantitative review of taxometric research. *Psychological Medicine*, *42*(5), 903–920.

Haslam, N., McGrath, M. J., Viechtbauer, W., & Kuppens, P. (2020). Dimensions over categories: A meta-analysis of taxometric research. *Psychological Medicine*, *50*(9), 1418–1432.

He, Q., & Li, J. J. (2021). Factorial invariance in hierarchical factor models of mental disorders in African American and European American youths. *Journal of Child Psychology and Psychiatry*, *62*(3), 289–298. https://doi.org/10.1111/jcpp.13243

Henrich, J., Heine, S. J., & Norenzayan, A. (2010). The weirdest people in the world? *The Behavioral and Brain Sciences*, *33*(2–3), 61–83; discussion 83–135. https://doi.org/10.1017/S0140525X0999152X

Hirschfeld, R. M. A. (2001). The comorbidity of major depression and anxiety disorders: Recognition and management in primary care. *Primary Care Companion to the Journal of Clinical Psychiatry*, *3*(6), 244–254. https://doi.org/10.4088/pcc.v03n0609

Hopwood, C. J. (2018). A framework for treating DSM-5 alternative model for personality disorder features. *Personality and Mental Health*, *12*(2), 107–125. https://doi.org/10.1002/pmh.1414

Hopwood, C. J., Bagby, R. M., Gralnick, T., Ro, E., Ruggero, C., Mullins-Sweatt, S., Kotov, R., Bach, B., Cicero, D. C., Krueger, R. F., Patrick, C. J., Chmielewski, M., DeYoung, C. G., Docherty, A. R., Eaton, N. R., Forbush, K. T., Ivanova, M. Y., Latzman, R. D., Pincus, A. L., . . . Zimmermann, J. (2020). Integrating psychotherapy with the Hierarchical Taxonomy of Psychopathology (HiTOP). *Journal of Psychotherapy Integration*, *30*(4), 477–497. https://doi.org/10.1037/int0000156

Hoy, N., Lynch, S. J., Waszczuk, M. A., Reppermund, S., & Mewton, L. (2023). Transdiagnostic biomarkers of mental illness across the lifespan: A systematic review examining the genetic and neural correlates of latent transdiagnostic dimensions of psychopathology in the general population. *Neuroscience & Biobehavioral Reviews*, *155*, 105431. https://doi.org/10.1016/j.neubiorev.2023.105431

Hyman, S. E. (2007). Can neuroscience be integrated into the DSM-V? *Nature Reviews Neuroscience*, *8*(9), 725–732.

Hyman, S. E. (2010). The diagnosis of mental disorders: The problem of reification. *Annual Review of Clinical Psychology*, *6*(1), 155–179. https://doi.org/10.1146/annurev.clinpsy.3.022806.091532

Insel, T., Cuthbert, B., Garvey, M., Heinssen, R., Pine, D. S., Quinn, K., Sanislow, C., & Wang, P. (2010). Research domain criteria (RDoC): Toward a new classification framework for research on mental disorders. *American Journal of Psychiatry*, *167*(7), 748–751.

Jensen-Doss, A., & Hawley, K. M. (2011). Understanding clinicians' diagnostic practices: Attitudes toward the utility of diagnosis and standardized diagnostic tools. *Administration and Policy in Mental Health and Mental Health Services Research*, *38*(6), 476–485. https://doi.org/10.1007/s10488-011-0334-3

Jewsbury, P. A., Bowden, S. C., & Duff, K. (2017). The Cattell–Horn–Carroll model of cognition for clinical assessment. *Journal of Psychoeducational Assessment*, *35*(6), 547–567. https://doi.org/10.1177/0734282916651360

Jonas, K., Stanton, K., Simms, L., Mullins-Sweatt, S., Gillett, D., Dainer, E., Nelson, B., Cohn, J. R., Guillot, S. T., & Kotov, R. (2021). *HiTOP digital assessment and tracker (HiTOP-DAT) manual*. Open Science Framework. https://doi.org/10.17605/OSF.IO/8HNGD

Kapur, S., Phillips, A. G., & Insel, T. R. (2012). Why has it taken so long for biological psychiatry to develop clinical tests and what to do about it? *Molecular Psychiatry*, *17*(12), 1174–1179. https://doi.org/10.1038/mp.2012.105

Kendler, K. S. (2018). Classification of psychopathology: Conceptual and historical background. *World Psychiatry*, *17*(3), 241–242. https://doi.org/10.1002/wps.20549

Kendler, K. S., Aggen, S. H., Knudsen, G. P., Røysamb, E., Neale, M. C., & Reichborn-Kjennerud, T. (2011). The structure of genetic and environmental risk factors for syndromal and subsyndromal common DSM-IV Axis I and All Axis II disorders. *The American Journal of Psychiatry*, *168*(1), 29–39. https://doi.org/10.1176/appi.ajp.2010.10030340

Keyes, K. M., Eaton, N. R., Krueger, R. F., McLaughlin, K. A., Wall, M. M., Grant, B. F., & Hasin, D. S. (2012). Childhood maltreatment and the structure of common psychiatric disorders. *The British Journal of Psychiatry*, *200*(2), 107–115. https://doi.org/10.1192/bjp.bp.111.093062

Kim, H., & Eaton, N. R. (2015). The hierarchical structure of common mental disorders: Connecting multiple levels of comorbidity, bifactor models, and predictive validity. *Journal of Abnormal Psychology*, *124*(4), 1064–1078. https://doi.org/10.1037/abn0000113

Kim, H., Turiano, N. A., Forbes, M. K., Kotov, R., Krueger, R. F., & Eaton, N. R. (2021). Internalizing psychopathology and all-cause mortality: A comparison of transdiagnostic vs. diagnosis-based risk prediction. *World Psychiatry*, *20*(2), 276–282. https://doi.org/10.1002/wps.20859

Kotov, R., Foti, D., Li, K., Bromet, E. J., Hajcak, G., & Ruggero, C. J. (2016). Validating dimensions of psychosis symptomatology: Neural correlates and 20-year outcomes. *Journal of Abnormal Psychology*, *125*(8), 1103–1119. https://doi.org/10.1037/abn0000188

Kotov, R., Jonas, K. G., Carpenter, W. T., Dretsch, M. N., Eaton, N. R., Forbes, M. K., Forbush, K. T., Hobbs, K., Reininghaus, U., Slade, T., South, S. C., Sunderland, M., Waszczuk, M. A., Widiger, T. A., Wright, A. G. C., Zald, D. H., Krueger, R. F., & Watson, D. (2020). Validity and utility of Hierarchical Taxonomy of Psychopathology (HiTOP): I. Psychosis superspectrum. *World Psychiatry*, *19*(2), 151–172. https://doi.org/10.1002/wps.20730

Kotov, R., Krueger, R. F., Watson, D., Achenbach, T. M., Althoff, R. R., Bagby, R. M., Brown, T. A., Carpenter, W. T., Caspi, A., Clark, L. A., Eaton, N. R., Forbes, M. K., Forbush, K. T., Goldberg, D., Hasin, D., Hyman, S. E., Ivanova, M. Y., Lynam, D. R., Markon, K., . . . Zimmerman, M. (2017). The Hierarchical Taxonomy of Psychopathology (HiTOP): A dimensional alternative to traditional nosologies. *Journal of Abnormal Psychology*, *126*(4), 454–477. https://doi.org/10.1037/abn0000258

Kotov, R., Krueger, R. F., Watson, D., Cicero, D. C., Conway, C. C., DeYoung, C. G., Eaton, N. R., Forbes, M. K., Hallquist, M. N., Latzman, R. D., Mullins-Sweatt, S. N., Ruggero, C. J., Simms, L. J., Waldman, I. D., Waszczuk, M. A., & Wright, A. G. C. (2021). The Hierarchical Taxonomy of Psychopathology (HiTOP): A quantitative nosology based on consensus of evidence. *Annual Review of Clinical Psychology*, *17*(1), 83–108. https://doi.org/10.1146/annurev-clinpsy-081219-093304

Kotov, R., Ruggero, C. J., Krueger, R. F., Watson, D., Yuan, Q., & Zimmerman, M. (2011). New dimensions in the quantitative classification of mental illness. *Archives of General Psychiatry*, *68*(10), 1003–1011. https://doi.org/10.1001/archgenpsychiatry.2011.107

Krueger, R. F. (1999). The structure of common mental disorders. *Archives of General Psychiatry*, *56*(10), 921–926. https://doi.org/10.1001/archpsyc.56.10.921

Krueger, R. F., & Eaton, N. R. (2012). Structural validity and the classification of mental disorders. In K. S. Kendler & J. Parnas (Eds.), *Philosophical issues in psychiatry II: Nosology* (pp. 199–212). Oxford University Press. https://doi.org/10.1093/med/9780199642205.003.0029

Krueger, R. F., Hobbs, K. A., Conway, C. C., Dick, D. M., Dretsch, M. N., Eaton, N. R., Forbes, M. K., Forbush, K. T., Keyes, K. M., Latzman, R. D., Michelini, G., Patrick, C. J., Sellbom, M., Slade, T., South, S. C., Sunderland, M., Tackett, J., Waldman, I., Waszczuk, M. A., . . . Kotov, R. (2021). Validity and utility of Hierarchical Taxonomy of Psychopathology (HiTOP): II. Externalizing superspectrum. *World Psychiatry*, *20*(2), 171–193. https://doi.org/10.1002/wps.20844

Krueger, R. F., & Markon, K. E. (2006). Reinterpreting comorbidity: A model-based approach to understanding and classifying psychopathology. *Annual Review of Clinical Psychology*, 2, 111–133. https://doi.org/10.1146/annurev.clinpsy.2.022305.095213

Krueger, R. F., Markon, K. E., Patrick, C. J., Benning, S. D., & Kramer, M. D. (2007). Linking antisocial behavior, substance use, and personality: An integrative quantitative model of the adult externalizing spectrum. *Journal of Abnormal Psychology*, *116*(4), 645–666. https://doi.org/10.1037/0021-843X.116.4.645

Krueger, R. F., & Tackett, J. L. (2016). The externalizing spectrum of personality and psychopathology: An empirical and quantitative alternative to discrete disorder approaches. In T. P. Beauchaine & S. P. Hinshaw (Eds.), *The Oxford handbook of externalizing spectrum disorders* (pp. 79–89). Oxford University Press.

Kupfer, D. J., First, M. B., & Regier, D. A. (2008). *A research agenda for DSM V*. American Psychiatric Association. http://doi.org/10.1176/appi.books.9780890427644

Lahey, B. B., Applegate, B., Hakes, J. K., Zald, D. H., Hariri, A. R., & Rathouz, P. J. (2012). Is there a general factor of prevalent psychopathology during adulthood? *Journal of Abnormal Psychology*, *121*(4), 971–977. https://doi.org/10.1037/a0028355

Lahey, B. B., Applegate, B., Waldman, I. D., Loft, J. D., Hankin, B. L., & Rick, J. (2004). The structure of child and adolescent psychopathology: Generating new hypotheses. *Journal of Abnormal Psychology*, *113*(3), 358–385. https://doi.org/10.1037/0021-843X.113.3.358

Lahey, B. B., Krueger, R. F., Rathouz, P. J., Waldman, I. D., & Zald, D. H. (2017). A Hierarchical causal taxonomy of psychopathology across the life span. *Psychological Bulletin*, *143*(2), 142–186. https://doi.org/10.1037/bul0000069

Lahey, B. B., Zald, D. H., Perkins, S. F., Villalta-Gil, V., Werts, K. B., Van Hulle, C. A., Rathouz, P. J., Applegate, B., Class, Q. A., Poore, H. E., Watts, A. L., & Waldman, I. D. (2018). Measuring the hierarchical general factor model of psychopathology in young adults. *International Journal of Methods in Psychiatric Research*, *27*(1), e1593. https://doi.org/10.1002/mpr.1593

Latzman, R. D., & DeYoung, C. G. (2020). Using empirically-derived dimensional phenotypes to accelerate clinical neuroscience: The Hierarchical Taxonomy of Psychopathology (HiTOP) framework. *Neuropsychopharmacology*, *45*(7), 1083–1085. https://doi.org/10.1038/s41386-020-0639-6

Lehman, A. F., Lieberman, J. A., Dixon, L. B., McGlashan, T. H., Miller, A. L., Perkins, D. O., Kreyenbuhl, J., American Psychiatric Association, & Steering Committee on Practice Guidelines. (2004). Practice guideline for the treatment of patients with schizophrenia, second edition. *The American Journal of Psychiatry*, *161*(2 Suppl), 1–56.

Lowe, J. R., & Widiger, T. A. (2009). Clinicians' judgments of clinical utility: A comparison of the DSM-IV with dimensional models of general personality. *Journal of Personality Disorders*, *23*(3), 211–229. https://doi.org/10.1521/pedi.2009.23.3.211

Machado, P. P., Machado, B. C., Gonçalves, S., & Hoek, H. W. (2007). The prevalence of eating disorders not otherwise specified. *International Journal of Eating Disorders*, *40*(3), 212–217.

Maj, M. (2005). "Psychiatric comorbidity": An artefact of current diagnostic systems? *The British Journal of Psychiatry: The Journal of Mental Science*, *186*, 182–184. https://doi.org/10.1192/bjp.186.3.182

Markon, K. E. (2010). Modeling psychopathology structure: A symptom-level analysis of Axis I and II disorders. *Psychological Medicine*, *40*(2), 273–288. https://doi.org/10.1017/S0033291709990183

Markon, K. E., Chmielewski, M., & Miller, C. J. (2011). The reliability and validity of discrete and continuous measures of psychopathology: A quantitative review. *Psychological Bulletin*, *137*(5), 856–879. https://doi.org/10.1037/a0023678

Markon, K. E., Krueger, R. F., & Watson, D. (2005). Delineating the structure of normal and abnormal personality: An integrative hierarchical approach. *Journal of Personality and Social Psychology*, *88*(1), 139–157. https://doi.org/10.1037/0022-3514.88.1.139

Martell, C. R., Dimidjian, S., & Herman-Dunn, R. (2021). *Behavioral activation for depression: A clinician's guide*. Guilford Publications.

Martin, E. A., Jonas, K. G., Lian, W., Foti, D., Donaldson, K. R., Bromet, E. J., & Kotov, R. (2021). Predicting long-term outcomes in first-admission psychosis: Does the Hierarchical Taxonomy of Psychopathology aid DSM in prognostication? *Schizophrenia Bulletin*, *47*(5), 1331–1341. https://doi.org/10.1093/schbul/sbab043

Martin, J., Taylor, M. J., & Lichtenstein, P. (2018). Assessing the evidence for shared genetic risks across psychiatric disorders and traits. *Psychological Medicine*, *48*(11), 1759–1774. https://doi.org/10.1017/S0033291717003440

Maser, J. D., Norman, S. B., Zisook, S., Everall, I. P., Stein, M. B., Schettler, P. J., & Judd, L. L. (2009). Psychiatric nosology is ready for a paradigm shift in DSM-V. *Clinical Psychology: Science and Practice*, *16*(1), 24–40. https://doi.org/10.1111/j.1468-2850.2009.01140.x

McGorry, P. D., Hickie, I. B., Yung, A. R., Pantelis, C., & Jackson, H. J. (2006). Clinical staging of psychiatric disorders: A heuristic framework for choosing earlier, safer and more effective interventions. *The Australian and New Zealand Journal of Psychiatry*, *40*(8), 616–622. https://doi.org/10.1080/j.1440-1614.2006.01860.x

McGrew, K. S. (2009). CHC theory and the human cognitive abilities project: Standing on the shoulders of the giants of psychometric intelligence research. *Intelligence*, *37*(1), 1–10.

McLaughlin, K. A., Colich, N. L., Rodman, A. M., & Weissman, D. G. (2020). Mechanisms linking childhood trauma exposure and psychopathology: A transdiagnostic model of risk and resilience. *BMC Medicine*, *18*(1), 96. https://doi.org/10.1186/s12916-020-01561-6

McNulty, J. L., & Overstreet, S. R. (2014). Viewing the MMPI–2–RF structure through the personality psychopathology five (PSY–5) lens. *Journal of Personality Assessment*, *96*(2), 151–157. https://doi.org/10.1080/00223891.2013.840305

Michelini, G., Barch, D. M., Tian, Y., Watson, D., Klein, D. N., & Kotov, R. (2019). Delineating and validating higher-order dimensions of psychopathology in the Adolescent Brain Cognitive Development (ABCD) study. *Translational Psychiatry*, *9*(1), 261. https://doi.org/10.1038/s41398-019-0593-4

Moore, T. V. (1930). The empirical determination of certain syndromes underlying praecox and manic-depressive psychoses. *The American Journal of Psychiatry*, *9*, 719–738. https://doi.org/10.1176/ajp.86.4.719

Morey, L. C., Hopwood, C. J., Markowitz, J. C., Gunderson, J. G., Grilo, C. M., McGlashan, T. H., Shea, M. T., Yen, S., Sanislow, C. A., Ansell, E. B., & Skodol, A. E. (2012). Comparison of alternative models for personality disorders, II: 6-, 8-, and 10-year follow-up. *Psychological Medicine*, *42*(8), 1705–1713. https://doi.org/10.1017/S0033291711002601

Morey, L. C., Skodol, A. E., & Oldham, J. M. (2014). Clinician judgments of clinical utility: A comparison of DSM-IV-TR personality disorders and the alternative model for DSM-5 personality disorders. *Journal of Abnormal Psychology*, *123*(2), 398–405. https://doi.org/10.1037/a0036481

Mullins-Sweatt, S. N., Bornovalova, M. A., Carragher, N., Clark, L. A., Corona Espinosa, A., Jonas, K., Keyes, K. M., Lynam, D. R., Michelini, G., Miller, J. D., Min, J., Rodriguez-Seijas, C., Samuel, D. B., Tackett, J. L., & Watts, A. L. (2022). HiTOP assessment of externalizing antagonism and disinhibition. *Assessment*, *29*(1), 34–45. https://doi.org/10.1177/10731911211033900

Mullins-Sweatt, S. N., Hopwood, C. J., Chmielewski, M., Meyer, N. A., Min, J., Helle, A. C., & Walgren, M. D. (2020). Treatment of personality pathology through the lens of the hierarchical taxonomy of psychopathology: Developing a research agenda. *Personality and Mental Health, 14*(1), 123–141. https://doi.org/10.1002/pmh.1464

Mullins-Sweatt, S. N., Lengel, G. J., & DeShong, H. L. (2016). The importance of considering clinical utility in the construction of a diagnostic manual. *Annual Review of Clinical Psychology, 12*(1), 133–155. https://doi.org/10.1146/annurev-clinpsy-021815-092954

Newson, J. J., Pastukh, V., & Thiagarajan, T. C. (2021). Poor separation of clinical symptom profiles by DSM-5 disorder criteria. *Frontiers in Psychiatry, 12*. 775762. https://www.frontiersin.org/journals/psychiatry/articles/10.3389/fpsyt.2021.775762

Noordhof, A., Krueger, R. F., Ormel, J., Oldehinkel, A. J., & Hartman, C. A. (2015). Integrating autism-related symptoms into the dimensional internalizing and externalizing model of psychopathology. The TRAILS Study. *Journal of Abnormal Child Psychology, 43*(3), 577–587. https://doi.org/10.1007/s10802-014-9923-4

Otowa, T., Hek, K., Lee, M., Byrne, E. M., Mirza, S. S., Nivard, M. G., Bigdeli, T., Aggen, S. H., Adkins, D., Wolen, A., Fanous, A., Keller, M. C., Castelao, E., Kutalik, Z., Van der Auwera, S., Homuth, G., Nauck, M., Teumer, A., Milaneschi, Y., . . . Hettema, J. M. (2016). Meta-analysis of genome-wide association studies of anxiety disorders. *Molecular Psychiatry, 21*(10), 1391–1399. https://doi.org/10.1038/mp.2015.197

Pettersson, E., Larsson, H., & Lichtenstein, P. (2016). Common psychiatric disorders share the same genetic origin: A multivariate sibling study of the Swedish population. *Molecular Psychiatry, 21*(5), 717–721. https://doi.org/10.1038/mp.2015.116

Rajakannan, T., Safer, D. J., Burcu, M., & Zito, J. M. (2016). National trends in psychiatric not otherwise specified (NOS) diagnosis and medication use among adults in outpatient treatment. *Psychiatric Services, 67*(3), 289–295. https://doi.org/10.1176/appi.ps.201500045

Raskin, J. D., Maynard, D., & Gayle, M. C. (2022). Psychologist attitudes toward DSM-5 and its alternatives. *Professional Psychology: Research and Practice, 53*(6), 553–563. https://doi.org/10.1037/pro0000480

Reed, G. M. (2010). Toward ICD-11: Improving the clinical utility of WHO's International Classification of mental disorders. *Professional Psychology: Research and Practice, 41*(6), 457–464. https://doi.org/10.1037/a0021701

Regier, D. A., Narrow, W. E., Clarke, D. E., Kraemer, H. C., Kuramoto, S. J., Kuhl, E. A., & Kupfer, D. J. (2013). DSM-5 field trials in the United States and Canada, part II: Test-retest reliability of selected categorical diagnoses. *American Journal of Psychiatry, 170*(1), 59–70. https://doi.org/10.1176/appi.ajp.2012.12070999

Reininghaus, U., Böhnke, J. R., Chavez-Baldini, U., Gibbons, R., Ivleva, E., Clementz, B. A., Pearlson, G. D., Keshavan, M. S., Sweeney, J. A., & Tamminga, C. A. (2019). Transdiagnostic dimensions of psychosis in the Bipolar-Schizophrenia Network on Intermediate Phenotypes (B-SNIP). *World Psychiatry, 18*(1), 67–76. https://doi.org/10.1002/wps.20607

Ringwald, W. R., Forbes, M. K., & Wright, A. G. C. (2021). Meta-analysis of structural evidence for the Hierarchical Taxonomy of Psychopathology (HiTOP) model. *Psychological Medicine, 53*(2), 533–546. https://doi.org/10.1017/S0033291721001902

Robins, E., & Guze, S. B. (1970). Establishment of diagnostic validity in psychiatric illness: Its application to schizophrenia. *American Journal of Psychiatry, 126*(7), 983–987.

Rodriguez-Seijas, C., Li, J. J., Balling, C., Brandes, C., Bernat, E., Boness, C. L., Forbes, M. K., Forbush, K. T., Joyner, K. J., Krueger, R. F., Levin-Aspenson, H. F., Michelini, G., Ro, E., Rutter, L., Stanton, K., Tackett, J. L., Waszczuk, M., & Eaton, N. R. (2023). Diversity and the Hierarchical Taxonomy of Psychopathology (HiTOP). *Nature Reviews Psychology, 2*(8), 483–495. https://doi.org/10.1038/s44159-023-00200-0

Rodriguez-Seijas, C., Rogers, B. G., Harkness, A., Safren, S. A., & Pachankis, J. E. (2024). ParTy 'n' Play: Associations between sex-related substance use and the disinhibited externalizing spectrum among gay and bisexual men. *Clinical Psychological Science, 12*(1), 83–97. https://doi.org/10.1177/21677026231158062

Røysamb, E., Tambs, K., Ørstavik, R. E., Torgersen, S., Kendler, K. S., Neale, M. C., Aggen, S. H., & Reichborn-Kjennerud, T. (2011). The joint structure of DSM–IV Axis I and Axis II disorders. *Journal of Abnormal Psychology, 120*(1), 198–209. https://doi.org/10.1037/a0021660

Rubin, D. C., & Talarico, J. M. (2009). A comparison of dimensional models of emotion: Evidence from emotions, prototypical events, autobiographical memories, and words. *Memory (Hove, England)*, *17*(8), 802–808. https://doi.org/10.1080/09658210903130764

Ruggero, C. J., Callahan, J. L., Dornbach-Bender, A., Tackett, J. L., & Kotov, R. (2019). Disquiet in nosology: A primer on an emerging, empirically based approach to classifying mental illness and implications for training. *The Behavior Therapist*, *6*(42), 208–211.

Ruggero, C. J., Kotov, R., Hopwood, C. J., First, M., Clark, L. A., Skodol, A. E., Mullins-Sweatt, S. N., Patrick, C. J., Bach, B., Cicero, D. C., Docherty, A., Simms, L. J., Bagby, R. M., Krueger, R. F., Callahan, J. L., Chmielewski, M., Conway, C. C., De Clercq, B., Dornbach-Bender, A., . . . Zimmermann, J. (2019). Integrating the Hierarchical Taxonomy of Psychopathology (HiTOP) into clinical practice. *Journal of Consulting and Clinical Psychology*, *87*(12), 1069–1084. https://doi.org/10.1037/ccp0000452

Ruggero, C. J., Kotov, R., Watson, D., Kilmer, J. N., Perlman, G., & Liu, K. (2014). Beyond a single index of mania symptoms: Structure and validity of subdimensions. *Journal of Affective Disorders*, *161*, 8–15. https://doi.org/10.1016/j.jad.2014.02.044

Samuel, D. B., & Widiger, T. A. (2006). Clinicians' judgments of clinical utility: A comparison of the DSM-IV and five-factor models. *Journal of Abnormal Psychology*, *115*(2), 298–308. https://doi.org/10.1037/0021-843X.115.2.298

Samuel, D. B., & Widiger, T. A. (2011). Clinicians' use of personality disorder models within a particular treatment setting: A longitudinal comparison of temporal consistency and clinical utility. *Personality and Mental Health*, *5*(1), 10.1002/pmh.152. https://doi.org/10.1002/pmh.152

Sanislow, C. A., Pine, D. S., Quinn, K. J., Kozak, M. J., Garvey, M. A., Heinssen, R. K., Wang, P. S.-E., & Cuthbert, B. N. (2010). Developing constructs for psychopathology research: Research domain criteria. *Journal of Abnormal Psychology*, *119*(4), 631.

Schaeuffele, C., Meine, L. E., Schulz, A., Weber, M. C., Moser, A., Paersch, C., Recher, D., Boettcher, J., Renneberg, B., Flückiger, C., & Kleim, B. (2024). A systematic review and meta-analysis of transdiagnostic cognitive behavioural therapies for emotional disorders. *Nature Human Behaviour*, *8*(3), 493–509. https://doi.org/10.1038/s41562-023-01787-3

Schaeuffele, C., Schulz, A., Knaevelsrud, C., Renneberg, B., & Boettcher, J. (2021). CBT at the crossroads: The rise of transdiagnostic treatments. *International Journal of Cognitive Therapy*, *14*(1), 86–113. https://doi.org/10.1007/s41811-020-00095-2

Sellbom, M. (2017). Mapping the MMPI–2–RF specific problems scales onto extant psychopathology structures. *Journal of Personality Assessment*, *99*(4), 341–350. https://doi.org/10.1080/00223891.2016.1206909

Simms, L. J., Wright, A. G. C., Cicero, D., Kotov, R., Mullins-Sweatt, S. N., Sellbom, M., Watson, D., Widiger, T. A., & Zimmermann, J. (2022). Development of measures for the Hierarchical Taxonomy of Psychopathology (HiTOP): A collaborative scale development project. *Assessment*, *29*(1), 3–16. https://doi.org/10.1177/10731911211015309

Sloan, E., Hall, K., Moulding, R., Bryce, S., Mildred, H., & Staiger, P. K. (2017). Emotion regulation as a transdiagnostic treatment construct across anxiety, depression, substance, eating and borderline personality disorders: A systematic review. *Clinical Psychology Review*, *57*, 141–163. https://doi.org/10.1016/j.cpr.2017.09.002

Spitzer, R. L., Williams, J. B. W., & Endicott, J. (2012). Standards for DSM-5 reliability. *American Journal of Psychiatry*, *169*(5), 537–537. https://doi.org/10.1176/appi.ajp.2012.12010083

Stanton, K., DeLucia, E. A., Brown, M. F. D., & McDonnell, C. G. (2021). Advancing understanding of the classification of broad autism phenotype and attention-deficit/hyperactivity disorder symptom dimensions within the Hierarchical Taxonomy of Psychopathology. *Personality and Mental Health*, *15*(2), 113–123. https://doi.org/10.1002/pmh.1498

Stanton, K., Khoo, S., McDonnell, C. G., Andino, M. V., Sturgeon, T., & Aasen, L. (2023). An initial investigation of the joint classification of hypomania- and neurodevelopmental disorder-relevant dimensions within the hierarchical taxonomy of psychopathology. *Assessment*, *30*(2), 414–432. https://doi.org/10.1177/10731911211055670

Tackett, J. L., & Hallquist, M. (2022). The need to grow: Developmental considerations and challenges for modern psychiatric taxonomies. *Journal of Psychopathology and Clinical Science*, *131*(6), 660–663. https://doi.org/10.1037/abn0000751

Tellegen, A. (1985). Structures of mood and personality and their relevance to assessing anxiety, with an emphasis on self-report. In A. H. Turna & J. D. Maser (Eds.), *Anxiety and the anxiety disorders* (pp. 681–706). Routledge.

Tiego, J., Martin, E. A., DeYoung, C. G., Hagan, K. E., Cooper, S. E., Pasion, R., Satchell, L., Shackman, A. J., Bellgrove, M., & Fornito, A. (2022). *Precision behavioral phenotyping as a strategy for uncovering the biological correlates of psychopathology*. OSF Preprints. https://doi.org/10.31219/osf.io/geh6q

Tiego, J., Thompson, K., Arnatkeviciute, A., Hawi, Z., Finlay, A., Sabaroedin, K., Johnson, B., Bellgrove, M. A., & Fornito, A. (2023). Dissecting schizotypy and its association with cognition and polygenic risk for schizophrenia in a nonclinical sample. *Schizophrenia Bulletin*, *49*(5), 1217–1228. https://doi.org/10.1093/schbul/sbac016

Tull, M. T., Gratz, K. L., Salters, K., & Roemer, L. (2004). The role of experiential avoidance in posttraumatic stress symptoms and symptoms of depression, anxiety, and somatization. *The Journal of Nervous and Mental Disease*, *192*(11), 754–761. https://doi.org/10.1097/01.nmd.0000144694.30121.89

Turk, C. L., Heimberg, R. G., Luterek, J. A., Mennin, D. S., & Fresco, D. M. (2005). Emotion dysregulation in generalized anxiety disorder: A comparison with social anxiety disorder. *Cognitive Therapy and Research*, *29*(1), 89–106. https://doi.org/10.1007/s10608-005-1651-1

Verheul, R., & Widiger, T. A. (2004). A meta-analysis of the prevalence and usage of the personality disorder not otherwise specified (PDNOS) diagnosis. *Journal of Personality Disorders*, *18*(4), 309–319.

Wakefield, J. C. (2016). Diagnostic issues and controversies in DSM-5: Return of the false positives problem. *Annual Review of Clinical Psychology*, *12*, 105–132. https://doi.org/10.1146/annurev-clinpsy-032814-112800

Ward, J., Lyall, L. M., Bethlehem, R. A. I., Ferguson, A., Strawbridge, R. J., Lyall, D. M., Cullen, B., Graham, N., Johnston, K. J. A., Bailey, M. E. S., Murray, G. K., & Smith, D. J. (2019). Novel genome-wide associations for anhedonia, genetic correlation with psychiatric disorders, and polygenic association with brain structure. *Translational Psychiatry*, *9*(1), 327. https://doi.org/10.1038/s41398-019-0635-y

Waszczuk, M. A. (2021). The utility of hierarchical models of psychopathology in genetics and biomarker research. *World Psychiatry*, *20*(1), 65–66. https://doi.org/10.1002/wps.20811

Waszczuk, M. A., Eaton, N. R., Krueger, R. F., Shackman, A. J., Waldman, I. D., Zald, D. H., Lahey, B. B., Patrick, C. J., Conway, C. C., Ormel, J., Hyman, S. E., Fried, E. I., Forbes, M. K., Docherty, A. R., Althoff, R. R., Bach, B., Chmielewski, M., DeYoung, C. G., Forbush, K. T., . . . Kotov, R. (2020). Redefining phenotypes to advance psychiatric genetics: Implications from hierarchical taxonomy of psychopathology. *Journal of Abnormal Psychology*, *129*(2), 143–161. https://doi.org/10.1037/abn0000486

Waszczuk, M. A., Kotov, R., Ruggero, C., Gamez, W., & Watson, D. (2017a). Hierarchical structure of emotional disorders: From individual symptoms to the spectrum. *Journal of Abnormal Psychology*, *126*(5), 613–634. https://doi.org/10.1037/abn0000264

Waszczuk, M. A., Zimmerman, M., Ruggero, C., Li, K., MacNamara, A., Weinberg, A., Hajcak, G., Watson, D., & Kotov, R. (2017b). What do clinicians treat: Diagnoses or symptoms? The incremental validity of a symptom-based, dimensional characterization of emotional disorders in predicting medication prescription patterns. *Comprehensive Psychiatry*, *79*, 80–88. https://doi.org/10.1016/j.comppsych.2017.04.004

Watson, D. (2003). Subtypes, specifiers, epicycles, and eccentrics: Toward a more parsimonious taxonomy of psychopathology. *Clinical Psychology: Science and Practice*, *10*(2), 233–238. https://doi.org/10.1093/clipsy.bpg013

Watson, D., Levin-Aspenson, H. F., Waszczuk, M. A., Conway, C. C., Dalgleish, T., Dretsch, M. N., Eaton, N. R., Forbes, M. K., Forbush, K. T., Hobbs, K. A., Michelini, G., Nelson, B. D., Sellbom, M., Slade, T., South, S. C., Sunderland, M., Waldman, I., Witthöft, M., Wright, A. G. C., . . . Workgroup, H. U. (2022). Validity and utility of Hierarchical Taxonomy of Psychopathology (HiTOP): III. Emotional dysfunction superspectrum. *World Psychiatry*, *21*(1), 26–54. https://doi.org/10.1002/wps.20943

Watson, D., O'Hara, M. W., Naragon-Gainey, K., Koffel, E., Chmielewski, M., Kotov, R., Stasik, S. M., & Ruggero, C. J. (2012). Development and validation of new anxiety and bipolar symptom scales for an expanded version of the IDAS (the IDAS-II). *Assessment*, *19*(4), 399–420. https://doi.org/10.1177/1073191112449857

Watson, D., & Tellegen, A. (1985). Toward a consensual structure of mood. *Psychological Bulletin*, *98*(2), 219–235. https://doi.org/10.1037//0033-2909.98.2.219

Watts, A. L., Greene, A. L., Bonifay, W., & Fried, E. I. (2024). A critical evaluation of the p-factor literature. *Nature Reviews Psychology*, *3*(2), 108–122. https://doi.org/10.1038/s44159-023-00260-2

Watts, A. L., Greene, A. L., Ringwald, W., Forbes, M. K., Brandes, C. M., Levin-Aspenson, H. F., & Delawalla, C. (2023). Factor analysis in personality disorders research: Modern issues and illustrations of practical recommendations. *Personality Disorders*, *14*(1), 105–117. https://doi.org/10.1037/per0000581

Watts, A. L., Latzman, R. D., Boness, C. L., Kotov, R., Keyser-Marcus, L., DeYoung, C. G., Krueger, R. F., Zald, D. H., Moeller, F. G., & Ramey, T. (2023). New approaches to deep phenotyping in addictions. *Psychology of Addictive Behaviors: Journal of the Society of Psychologists in Addictive Behaviors*, *37*(3), 361–375. https://doi.org/10.1037/adb0000878

Watts, A. L., Watson, D., Heath, A. C., & Sher, K. J. (2023). Alcohol use disorder criteria exhibit different comorbidity patterns. *Addiction (Abingdon, England)*, *118*(8), 1457–1468. https://doi.org/10.1111/add.16121

Wendt, L. P., Jankowsky, K., Schroeders, U., London Personality and Mood Disorder Research Consortium, Nolte, T., Fonagy, P., Montague, P. R., Zimmermann, J., & Olaru, G. (2023). Mapping established psychopathology scales onto the Hierarchical Taxonomy of Psychopathology (HiTOP). *Personality and Mental Health*, *17*(2), 117–134. https://doi.org/10.1002/pmh.1566

Whooley, O. (2014). Nosological reflections: The failure of DSM-5, the emergence of RDoC, and the decontextualization of mental distress. *Society and Mental Health*, *4*(2), 92–110. https://doi.org/10.1177/2156869313519114

Widiger, T. A., Sellbom, M., Chmielewski, M., Clark, L. A., DeYoung, C. G., Kotov, R., Krueger, R. F., Lynam, D. R., Miller, J. D., Mullins-Sweatt, S., Samuel, D. B., South, S. C., Tackett, J. L., Thomas, K. M., Watson, D., & Wright, A. G. C. (2019). Personality in a hierarchical model of psychopathology. *Clinical Psychological Science*, *7*(1), 77–92. https://doi.org/10.1177/2167702618797105

Wright, A. G. C., Beltz, A. M., Gates, K. M., Molenaar, P. C. M., & Simms, L. J. (2015). Examining the dynamic structure of daily internalizing and externalizing behavior at multiple levels of analysis. *Frontiers in Psychology*, *6*, 1914. https://www.frontiersin.org/journals/psychology/articles/10.3389/fpsyg.2015.01914

Wright, A. G. C., Krueger, R. F., Hobbs, M. J., Markon, K. E., Eaton, N. R., & Slade, T. (2013). The structure of psychopathology: Toward an expanded quantitative empirical model. *Journal of Abnormal Psychology*, *122*(1), 281–294. https://doi.org/10.1037/a0030133

Zald, D. H., & Lahey, B. B. (2017). Implications of the hierarchical structure of psychopathology for psychiatric neuroimaging. *Biological Psychiatry: Cognitive Neuroscience and Neuroimaging*, *2*(4), 310–317. https://doi.org/10.1016/j.bpsc.2017.02.003

Zimmermann, J., Woods, W. C., Ritter, S., Happel, M., Masuhr, O., Jaeger, U., Spitzer, C., & Wright, A. G. C. (2019). Integrating structure and dynamics in personality assessment: First steps toward the development and validation of a personality dynamics diary. *Psychological Assessment*, *31*(4), 516–531. https://doi.org/10.1037/pas0000625

CHAPTER 7

Dimensionality in the Research Domain Criteria

Research Advances and Clinical Applications

CHARLES A. SANISLOW, REBECCA A. BERMAN, JENNIFER PACHECO, AND BRUCE N. CUTHBERT

Introduction

THE leadership of the National Institute of Mental Health (NIMH) put forth a goal in the NIMH 2008 Strategic Plan to "Develop, for research purposes, new ways of classifying mental disorders based on *dimensions of observable behavior and neurobiological measures*" (emphasis added, NIMH, 2008, p. 9). To facilitate progress on this goal, an internal working group was established at the NIMH, and efforts by this group orchestrated the development of the Research Domain Criteria (RDoC). The structure, goals, and process of development of the RDoC approach were detailed shortly thereafter (see Insel et al., 2010; Cuthbert & Insel, 2010a & b; Sanislow et al., 2010). Virtually every RDoC paper from the NIMH RDoC working group has been clear about the importance of a dimensional approach from the beginning[1] (Cuthbert & Insel, 2013; Cuthbert & Kozak, 2013; Insel & Cuthbert, 2009; Kozak & Cuthbert, 2016; Morris & Cuthbert, 2012; Sanislow et al., 2010), consistent with dimensional aspects across multiple measurement types that were set forth in prior decades (e.g., Cuthbert, 2005; Vaidyanathan et al., 2009). Pillar 2 of the "Seven Pillars of RDoC" explicitly detailed the importance of dimensions in RDoC (Cuthbert & Insel, 2013), and this bedrock principle was reiterated more recently by Morris and colleagues (2022): "The dimensional approach: assume dimensionality—among disorders and between illness and health—unless data show otherwise" (Morris et al., 2022, p. 4).

In this chapter, we first describe the scientific challenges that led to the proposal of RDoC, followed by a description of the RDoC framework and the ways that it has evolved since it was introduced. This introduction leads to a consideration of the dimensional principles of the RDoC model, where RDoC is compared to other approaches that are dimensionally based. Neural and psychological development is a key aspect of RDoC, and one that has garnered increasing attention, so we next devote attention to this, particularly because of the fundamental relevance of dimensional properties to human development. Then we turn to recent

[1] Some of the early reporting on RDoC (e.g., Insel et al., 2010) foregrounded biological elements in initial funding opportunities (e.g., emphasizing a link to a known neural circuit). This foregrounding may have overshadowed other important principles of RDoC, chief among them that the RDoC approach was dimensional; this problematic emphasis was squarely addressed in later publications (see Cuthbert & Insel, 2013; Cuthbert & Kozak, 2013; Kozak & Cuthbert, 2016).

clinical advances that have been well aligned with the RDoC framework. In concluding, we address some considerations for future directions.

Why RDoC? Historical Matters to the DSM-III and Beyond

The call for RDoC came in the midst of accelerating progress in scientific knowledge for genetics, neuroscience, behavioral science, and other areas. However, extensive new findings only served to highlight the plateau in mental health research as guided by the DSM. To break the mold of clinical research design using experimental groups defined by a DSM diagnosis, a new direction was needed. A summary of why the Research Domain Criteria project was initiated is useful to understand how dimensions fit into the overall concept and relate to other aspects. There are a number of principles involved, as well as a continuous evolution of the program and its many nuances. Accordingly, the account here is relatively brief, and the interested reader is recommended to consult other articles that contain a more extensive description (e.g., Cuthbert et al., 2023; Morris et al., 2022; Sanislow et al., 2010).

The goals of any medical specialty have been to relate symptoms to research findings that identify normal anatomy and/or physiology; determine the mechanisms that lead to the pathology of the symptoms; and find treatments that mitigate, cure, or prevent the illness. Nineteenth-century medicine saw gradual advances by working with diagnostic categories based on clinical description, particularly in the areas of infectious disease and overt medical conditions. For instance, the age-old condition of dropsy (more commonly known as edema) involved multiple causal physiological pathways that were unearthed by scientific advances in the mid-19th century. Progress in innumerable aspects of modern medical science has reduced morbidity and mortality for many (although far from all) illnesses for over a century.

It was only natural for psychiatry to follow this diagnostic model of delineating symptoms and then seeking new scientific advances that could illuminate the pathology (Cuthbert et al., 2023). But except for some unique cases (e.g., psychiatric symptoms stemming from syphilis), this approach to mental disorders did not lead to progress in the late 19th century. Scientists explored the anatomy of specific lesions or of disrupted brain connections but lacked the technologies to reach conclusive data (Stoyanov, Correia, & Cuthbert, 2019). Despite this shortcoming, Kraepelin and others codified a symptom-based categorical model of diseases such as dementia praecox (subsequently termed schizophrenia by Bleuler) and manic-depressive illness (later termed bipolar disorder).

The vacuum of progress resulted in psychoanalytic theories of mental illness taking root to become the dominant mode of psychiatry. Due at least in part to the idiosyncrasies of various schools of psychoanalytic thought as well as varying diagnostic criteria across the United States and Europe, diagnosis in psychiatry suffered from a lack of inter-clinician reliability relative to other medical specialties. By the 1960s, psychiatry in the United States needed a reliable system of diagnosis for research, insurance, and psychiatrists. Two marked initiatives in succession, one in the 1970s and the next in 1980, moved psychiatry into the modern era.

First, the Research Diagnostic Criteria (RDC), not to be confused with the Research Domain Criteria (RDoC), was developed by a cohort of psychiatrists at Washington University in the late 1970s, based extensively on the so-called Feighner Criteria published in 1972 (Feigner et al., 1972). The RDC aimed to advance the reliability of psychiatric research, with the premise that doing so would enhance the validity of psychiatric diagnosis (Spitzer, Endicott, & Robins, 1975, 1978). The RDC established a number of symptom-based disorders and introduced the polythetic criteria for making a diagnosis. This meant that disorder categories were determined by one or more symptom sets, and each set was assigned a number of symptoms; only a given number of varying symptoms were required to confer a diagnosis, for example, five or more symptoms from a total of eight were required for major depressive disorder.

The RDC offered a ready-made solution to construct expeditiously a clinical manual with mental disorder categories, as recommended in the first RDC publication (Spitzer et al., 1975). The American Psychiatric Association (APA) was quick to adopt these ideas for a new version of its *Diagnostic and Statistical Manual* (DSM), indicated by the statement in the 1978 RDC publication that " . . . many of the categories and criteria in the RDC are being considered for inclusion in the DSM-III" (Spitzer et al., 1978, p. 774). The second initiative was accordingly the publication of the DSM-III by the APA in 1980 only two years later, prompting a rapid acceleration of research and clinical work.

Innumerable papers and books have documented the progress in research and clinical utility that has been made over the nearly 45 years since DSM-III appeared. That progress is acknowledged. At the same time, however, it has also been noted that the burden of suffering of those with mental disorders has not been reduced in that time; if anything, morbidity and mortality have increased (Insel & Gogtay, 2014). The organized and semi-qualitatively diagnostic criteria of the DSM-III could have led to studies that caught up to other areas of medicine, as noted above: relating symptoms to research findings that identify normal anatomy and/or physiology (and behavior in the case of psychopathology); determining the mechanisms that lead to the pathology of the symptoms; and finding treatments that mitigate, cure, or prevent the illness. Unfortunately, this plan was not possible for mental illness. The urgent need to generate diagnostic entities for psychiatric disorders occurred in the mid-20th century, a time when there remained a near-total absence of scientific knowledge for discovering such aspects as genetics, anatomy, and neural systems as well as the behaviors that they implement. Instead, the disorders listed in the DSM-III of 1980 were defined almost entirely by signs and symptoms that were binary, well/ill categories that neglected dimensional aspects.

The disorders as listed in the new manual had evident value and moved the field into the modern age in many ways. However, the opportunity to make continual improvements as science increased its knowledge of basic functions, and then to apply them within and across various diagnoses, was lost not long after the DSM-III's beginning. The disorders became rapidly reified—that is, treated as a concrete entity (notwithstanding contrary comments in the preface of the DSM-III)—and treated as natural kinds rather than broad, heterogeneous syndromes with overlaps that had to be parsed (Hyman, 2010).

As research with the new system progressed, the idea that diagnostic classes were each distinct from the others, and from normal, proved to be false. As discussed over a decade ago, experienced researchers noted the "lack of a biological 'gold standard' definition of psychiatric illnesses"; instead, ". . . the field should focus on identifying biologically homogeneous subtypes that cut across phenotypic diagnosis" (Kapur, Phillips, & Insel, 2012, p. 1). The reification of disorder classes meant that studies would persist with categorical, symptom-based diagnostic practices; this prevented research grounded on innovative neurobiological and behavioral experimental designs (outside DSM diagnostic classes) that could move toward a valid understanding of disorders (Hyman, 2010).

The decades of persistent research efforts also made clear that defining psychiatric diagnoses categorically was an Achilles heel, and revealed that the nature of mental disorders should be more fully represented dimensionally (see Heckers, 2008; Heckers et al., 2022 Kupfer, First, & Regier, 2002). As former NIMH Director Steven Hyman noted, ". . . the essential features of psychiatric disorders are best captured dimensionally rather than in terms of distinct categories" (Hyman, 2021, p. 12).

Overall, it became clear from multiple perspectives that the axiom that validity would follow from reliability, as had been postulated by Robins and Guze (1970), was not going to work out. Those shortcomings were most pronounced in laboratory and genetic studies, and evident as the burgeoning knowledge in cognitive neuroscience did not advance psychopathology research.

This situation was what prompted one section of the 2008 NIMH Strategic Plan, whose theme headline was to "Develop, for research purposes, new ways of classifying mental disorders based on dimensions of observable behavior and neurobiological measures" (NIMH, 2008, p. 9). Fundamentally, this was an initiative to implement the long-lost ideal of relating specific symptoms to rapidly growing neurobehavioral research areas that can identify normal mechanisms and their dimensions of dysregulation. Further, the growth of science enables investigators to examine not simply one measure or data type with a particular symptom, but to acquire many data types that encourage integrative analyses that can provide an understanding of how various systems inter-relate. This effort is made even more complex by the fact that a given specific symptom may result due to various factors (equifinality), while a single factor may result in different symptoms (multifinality) (Cicchetti & Rogosch, 1996). However, this is the challenge if precision mental health is to progress.

A steering committee of NIMH staff convened in short order to discuss and implement the elements of the new strategy, organizing the process in early 2009 with the name of Research Doman Criteria (RDoC). To begin grounding psychopathology in scientific data, the first step for RDoC was to convene a series of workshops to define evidence-based biobehavioral constructs of healthy functional behaviors that were related to particular clinical problems when disrupted. The workshops each represented particular broad domains of functioning, which included negative valence, positive valence, cognition, social systems, and arousal/regulatory systems, with a subsequently added domain of motor systems. Participants in various fields from both clinical and/or basic areas, with expertise in studying humans and/or nonhuman animals, were invited to the workshops. They were asked to evaluate a list of potential constructs initially contributed by requested suggestions from the field and then debated by the steering committee to yield the draft set for consideration. The experts defined several related constructs for each domain that were considered as validated in the context of the RDoC project; each construct followed a definition that linked concomitant brain and behavior data (as per the Strategic Plan, ". . . dimensions of observable behavior and neurobiological measures" NIMH, 2008, p. 9).

The Strategic Plan also noted the need to extend the data types required for a sufficiently broad understanding of psychopathology: "This effort will require integration of genetic, neuroscience, imaging, behavioral, and clinical studies" (NIMH, 2008, p. 10). To inform investigators as to how this idea could be incorporated in a study design, the workshop participants were also asked to come up with a list of elements for each construct that were appropriate for several data types: genes, molecules, cells, circuits, physiology, behavior, and self-reports. The types were termed "Units of Analysis" to emphasize an integrative approach rather than the common, reductionistic "levels of analysis" phrase. The intent was twofold: first, to provide a ready-to-go list of measures for investigators who might study a validated construct; and second, to suggest the new kinds of measures that could be developed for investigators seeking to define a new construct (one of the major goals of the project). The result was a matrix of measures, with the constructs (nested within domains) in the rows and the various data types in the columns. The RDoC matrix was thus intended to be a heuristic, a scaffold upon which to organize dimensions for research design.

The matrix was only one part of the overall objective to provide a new and flexible path for research on psychopathology. Some researchers misunderstood the matrix, fearing that if it did not contain their particular construct of interest they could not conduct RDoC research (as though it were similar to the fixed number of DSM disorders). However, the goal was to provide examples of how the new research program could be conducted. It was stipulated—though not widely understood—that the initial steps of the project were only a start, and that the coming decades would grow and expand exponentially in multiple ways as researchers studied the complexity of brain and behavior and their dimensions of normal-to-abnormal functioning. Accounting for these increasing complexities requires multidimensional models that go beyond bivariate relations that may be implied by limiting aspects of the matrix structure (e.g., Bilder, Howe, & Sabb, 2013).

Parallel Development of Psychopathology Dimensions

Parallel to the development and the eventual birth of the new DSM in 1980, substantial progress was being made on the developmental psychopathology front as well as alternative approaches to the DSM. The developmental psychologist Thomas Achenbach (1966) codified the internalizing/externalizing distinction to capture two broad dimensions of childhood psychopathology: internalizing (anxiety or depression) and externalizing (oppositional or conduct problems). By the 1980s, the field of developmental psychopathology had become firmly ensconced in experimental methods, and embraced the tenet that ignoring dimensions in any nosology or taxonomy would neglect critically important variance for clinical research aimed at etiology (Chicchetti & Rizley, 1981; for a comprehensive retrospective on relation of developmental dimensions and RDoC, see Conradt, Crowell, & Cicchetti, 2021).

Later, Krueger's (1999) "The Structure of Common Mental Disorders" landmark paper identified a more elaborate factor structure that echoed Achenbach (1966), that more broadly applied the internalizing/externalizing factor structure to adult disorders by using DSM criteria. It also compellingly addressed the comorbidities and continuities of the categorically defined mental disorders by offering a statistically valid reorganization of the diagnostic criteria sets couched in hierarchical dimensions. Krueger's work marked a shift and further opened the door to dimensionalizing DSM mental disorders that had been unlocked earlier by other researchers (e.g., Clark & Watson, 1991). Over the years, researchers—mostly psychologists—labored to clarify dimensions of personality traits and temperament and then more broadly incorporated them into dimensions of psychopathology (Clark, 2005; Watson, 2005). In a thoughtful assessment of the state of the field, Clark and colleagues (2017) compared and contrasted leading diagnostic approaches that aimed to integrate categories and dimensions, and detailed the varied contributions made by the respective diagnostic systems that were examined. The spirit of this effort offered ideas on how the competing approaches could be leveraged with one another for better progress.

That progress notwithstanding, the categorical approach remained privileged in the DSM despite interest and efforts to incorporate dimensions. As another perspective, from that of clinical psychiatry and personality disorders, a notable effort to integrate dimensions into the DSM-5 demonstrated the challenges of such an effort. Dimensionalizing the personality disorders was suggested as a "test-case" for a dimensional model, which, if successful, would provide a sort of proof-of-concept for the clinical diagnoses more generally (First et al., 2002). However, the subsequent model, the Alternative Model for Personality Disorders (AMPD), was not fully adopted and instead relegated to its own section in the DSM-5, while the unchanged personality disorder model was retained in the personality disorder chapter. This was due in part to lack of consensus on the specifics of the dimensional model among the DSM-5 Personality Disorder Workgroup (see Zachar, Krueger, & Kendler, 2016). Interestingly, the fact that it had its own unique section—and was not placed in the traditional outside-the-mainstream category "disorders needing further study"—opened the door for it to be used clinically (Skodol et al., 2015). Moreover, the personality model in the eleventh edition of the

International Classification of Diseases is similar to the AMPD in most respects (ICD-11; WHO, 2024). Still, the process and outcome made clear certain challenges and barriers of integrating dimensions in the DSM.

Owing largely to efforts of clinical psychologists working at the intersection of psychopathological disorders and personality traits, the effort in this group to transition to dimensional diagnostic systems of mental disorders is now common, so much so that the issues at hand are "to do so cautiously and thoughtfully, rather than not to do so at all" (Hopwood et al., 2023, p. 1). Based on ample empirical evidence, a growing number of the scientific community supports the dimensional nature of mental disorders and of psychopathological mechanisms, for example, "... symptoms and impairments that constitute the building blocks of psychiatric disorders have been found to be continuously distributed in populations in terms of symptom number and severity with no evidence of discontinuities between affected and unaffected individuals" (Hyman, 2021, p. 12; see also Achenbach 2020; Barch et al., 2013; Groen-Blokhuis et al., 2014; Martin et al., 2014, 2015); importantly, the aforementioned building blocks include cognitive, behavioral, and neurobiological mechanisms.

On another front, armed with new research tools in the 1990s and 2000s, clinical scientists incorporated cognitive neuroscience to the study of psychopathology. Working in this framework, researchers naturally began to turn their attention to dimensions based on intermediate phenotypes, motivated to find valid biomarkers (e.g., Insel & Cuthbert, 2009; Meyer-Lindenberg & Weinberger, 2006). Modeled on the endophenotype concept from the field of genetics (see Gottesman & Gould, 2003), the idea of an intermediate phenotype is to identify features of psychopathology that are more proximal to psychological processes (e.g., working memory) or biological mechanisms (e.g., dopaminergic reward circuits) than were the standard clinically observed features that comprised clinical syndromes. The intermediate phenotype concept became a cornerstone of the RDoC approach and has become increasingly embraced by clinical scientists more generally (see Cannon & Keller, 2006; Miller & Rockstroh, 2013). Examples of intermediate phenotypes include attenuated striatal activity as an intermediate phenotype in symptoms of schizophrenia (Grimm et al, 2014), dimensional relations of striatal activity and reward processing (Krystal et al., 2020), or linear relationships between neurocognitive (circuit) deficits and genetic risk (familial distance from proband) (see Cannon et al., 2000).

In sum, although there was a recognition of the potential benefits of dimensional conceptualizations in psychiatry, psychology, and neuroscience, these fronts remained somewhat siloed, limiting cross-talk and impeding implementation of findings from integrative neuroscience to systematically clarify psychological mechanisms and clinically relevant behavior. In scientific peer review, the status quo for research funding remained harnessed to clinical syndromes of the DSM, impeding implementation of experimental psychopathology based on traditional experimental approaches (e.g., Lang, 1969; Maher, 1970). Such experimental approaches, in combination with the accumulating knowledge from integrative neuroscience, offered potential to advance the identification of treatment targets—behavioral and biological—which would subsequently lead to more effective treatments as well as open new doors for prevention. While the DSM served clinical purposes well, it was a rate-limiting step in research design. The RDoC initiative provides the flexibility of an integrative, dimensional approach to mental health research.

Dimensional Qualities of RDoC

What is a dimensional approach in the RDoC framework? One critical characteristic is that the dimension spans the full range of function, including normality. In other words, the

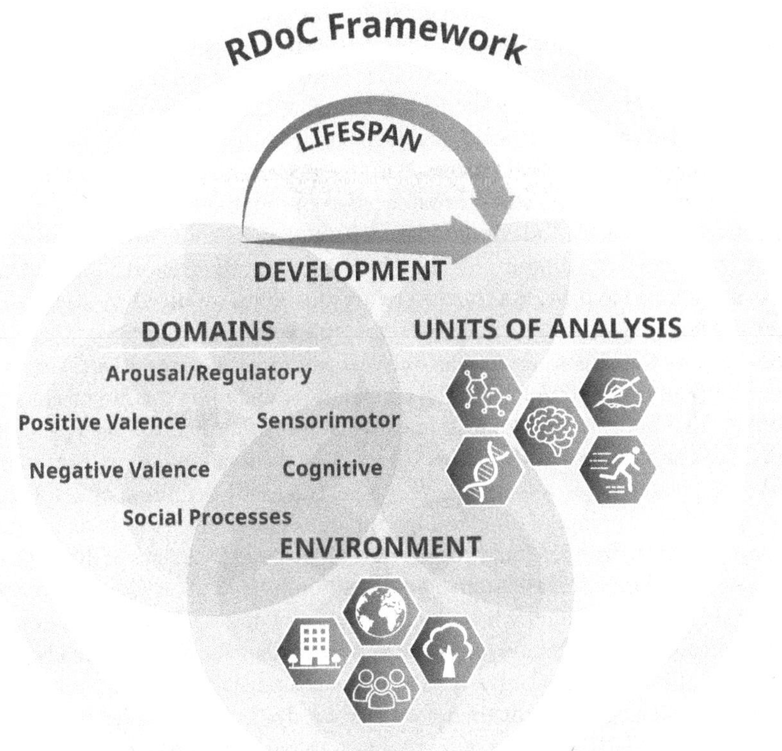

FIGURE 7.1 Research Domain Criteria Framework created by the RDoC group and reprinted with permission from NIH

"dimension" is not limited to only the span of the pathological range; the latter would be the case when, for example, dimensionalizing a DSM diagnosis set by summing the criteria as is currently the practice with the DSM Substance Use Disorders (SUDs). The complete range—including the span of normal function—allows the introduction of considerations that are potentially related to early stages of psychopathology. An early motivating force of the RDoC initiative was that many psychopathologies were defined in the "end-stage" of the disorder. Chronic mental illness, whether it was in the psychoses, the affective spectrum, severe personality pathology, or in the anxiety or trauma-related spectrum, was wrought with more comorbid conditions, often complicated by substance abuse and dependence. A section of the 2008 NIMH Strategic Plan outlined the need to focus on the onset or progression of symptoms and/or mechanisms, such that so-called pre-clinical states could actually make better diagnostic targets than the end-stage syndromes (NIMH, 2008).

This line of thinking was not new to RDoC or to the field of psychopathology research. Efforts at early intervention, for psychosis for example, began around 1990 (for a review of the early efforts of the modern approach, see Yung and McGorry, 1996). These studies heralded much progress, and clinically significant improvements in outcomes support the validity of these efforts, but progress was an uphill battle. In early efforts, adult disorders were retrofitted to the early stages, and this in combination with developmental principles such as equifinality and multifinality meant that outcomes could be overly narrow. In other words, the schizophrenia prodrome patient that did not "convert" to psychosis was not a "positive" case but was still clearly an individual who suffered clinical problems of a different outcome at the time of assessment (this problem will be considered in more detail in the developmental section). Early on, there also were controversies that held back progress, such as the idea of medicating adolescents with an antipsychotic medication before determining if schizophrenia was imminent. Only with the introduction of knowledge and methods from cognitive psychology and cognitive neuroscience, linked with human development, could better disorder treatment targets be identified (see Cannon, 2015 for a review). From these efforts, the Clinical Staging Model was developed to provide a framework for subclinical (or pre-clinical) states of mental disorder, (McGorry et al., 2006; see also Mei et al., this volume).

By not limiting the dimension to span only the pathological range, RDoC also emphasizes the importance of accounting for the full distribution, including the dimensions of normal functioning. That is, the idea is not to define the nature of this distribution a priori, but to examine the full range of functioning across the kinds of observation (i.e., units of analysis) provided as exemplars in the RDoC matrix. This is central to the definition of RDoC constructs, that they span the "full range of functioning from normal to abnormal." There are cases where mild forms of clinical disorder could progress into more severe versions of the same disorders. However, use of a different label interjects a discontinuity that otherwise should not be there (Kessler et al., 2003; see rejoinder by Regier, Narrow, & Rae, 2004). In some cases, there may be a developmental discontinuity; for instance, anhedonia in adolescence can be a precursor to adult schizophrenia. In other cases, adult disorders along potential continuums are instead conceptualized as categorically distinct, for instance, dysthymic disorder and major depressive disorder in DSM-IV. This line of reasoning resulted in the oxymoronic example of the concept of "double depression," that is, having two different "kinds" (dysthymia, major depression) of depression at once (Keller, Hirschfeld, & Hanks, 1997). In any event, dysthymia was replaced in DSM-5 by persistent depressive disorder, which included elements of dysthymia and chronic major depression.

A second consideration of the RDoC dimensional approach, in addition to spanning normal function, is the question of "where is the [ab]normal?" (see Galderisi et al., 2024). There are two parts in the answer to this question. First, we have to determine how to derive the cut point for where the line into illness is crossed (see Figure 1 in Kirkbride et al., 2024, p. 69); this is determined currently in the DSM by the number of symptoms from the polythetic set for a particular disorder, but might shift in the future to one or more quantitative measures that could employ multiple cut points (e.g., mild, moderate, severity pathology as well as risk levels that could promote prevention interventions). Cut points can also be modified as new data come in, something that is routinely done in most areas of medicine (and including the DSM in some cases) (Hyman, 2021). Second, we have to determine whether the dimensions are unipolar or bipolar. In terms of the question of polarity, for RDoC dimensions where a function is envisioned as normally distributed, is one tail of the distribution a superior function, while the other tail is considered pathology (akin to the way IQ is envisioned)? Or, is the peak of the normal distribution the ideal? These are empirical questions, and we would expect there could be cases of each, and we note that there are other approaches on underlying dimensions from dysfunction (see DeYoung & Krueger, 2023, for example).

We will detail in a later section the clinical relevance of one such example, where one tail of the distribution of the fear response is enhanced and associated with a single event exposure, while the other tail is where the fear response is blunted and associated with exposure to multiple traumatic events; those without traumatic exposure fall in the middle. This example illustrates bipolarity, where risk for psychopathology is found in the extremities of either tail of a single dimension. In contrast, a psychopathological mechanism or construct may be of clinical significance on only one tail of a dimension, either a high or low score on the featured dimension. Contrasted with bipolarity, this is what personality trait researchers identify as unipolarity (see Williams & Simms, 2018).

Finally, for purposes of clarity, we note distinctions of the nature of dimensions that are important to consider in the context of RDoC. In the RDoC framework, dimensions may be applied to different kinds of observations (i.e., units of analysis). In contrast to classic psychometric considerations of dimensions, which are typically limited to symptom scales or traits, RDoC dimensions can be multidimensional and reflect the strength of a neural circuit, or the performance on a behavioral task, or, as with the more traditional framing, self-reported (including clinically observed) symptom-based dimensions. Importantly for behavioral and neural dimensions in RDoC, the variants of the traditional psychometric properties need to be considered, for example, specificity and sensitivity (see Hajcak et al., 2017; Knodt et al., 2023; Weinberg & Hajcak, 2011).

Relation of RDoC to Other Dimensional Models

RDoC and DSM Dimensions

Diagnostic constructs such as those in the DSM or ICD, while imperfect, are based on kinds of evidence that range from clinical observation and consensus to having various levels of empirical support. It has been argued that DSM categories can be easily treated (converted) to dimensions, so that arguments over categories is a moot point (Kraemer, 2015; see also Kraemer, Noda, & O'Hara, 2004). Indeed, there are a range of approaches that have been used to treat DSM categories as dimensions for research purposes. One approach is to simply use a summation of criteria, though that approach is limited, because they only capture variance in the clinical range of the dimension and exclude the full range into normal function. Statistically, variance is further restricted by criterion representation of symptoms that are "present or absent," and so each item only represents clinically significant pathology (or present but of uncertain clinical significance in the typical "0," "1," or "2" ratings used in structured or semi-structured diagnostic interviews). The reliability of each judgment adds another source of error variance. There are other complications, too. Individual DSM criteria themselves are fallible—that is, no single criterion is predictive or necessary for a disorder to be present; criteria are also unequally weighted to the diagnostic prototype—that is, some criteria tend to be more correlated with the diagnosis than others. While maximum likelihood assumptions for methods such as structural equation modeling are robust to item level data, there are limitations when there is reason to expect that ordinal variables are not equidistant, or if putative distributions of categories are skewed, requiring special procedures (see Rhemtulla, Brosseau-Liard, & Savalei, 2012). There are other statistical work-arounds; for example, parceling diagnostic criteria in structural modeling is more likely to yield continuous variables with a normal distribution (e.g., Sanislow et al., 2009; see Little et al., 2002).

Several DSM diagnoses have now explicitly incorporated a dimensional frame, and while the dimensional aspects of these diagnoses are relevant to RDoC, certain cautionary notes are in order. Among these diagnoses are autism spectrum disorder (ASD), substance use disorders (SUD), and the dimensions within the AMPD. For ASD, the introduced three-point rating scale is largely constrained to severity and levels of support required, and supplements are a set of polythetic criteria that include items from the categorical autism (and previous DSM-IV Asperger's) diagnoses; from a dimensional RDoC standpoint, this system is unlikely to yield better phenotypes corresponding to mechanisms than the stand-alone diagnosis itself (or elements of the stand-alone diagnosis). Additionally, ASD remains categorically distinct because a boundary is implied from other forms of mental disorder.

For SUDs, a single set of dimensionally framed criteria are categorically applied to various kinds of substances. The dimensions consist of impairment ratings: mild (two to three criteria), moderate (four to five criteria), or severe (six or more criteria). This impairment rating has replaced the distinction between abuse and dependence in prior DSM editions. The polythetic criteria in the impairment scale, however, introduce a flaw, in that each criterion may contribute differently (in severity or by mechanism). Dependent variables for studying SUDs with an RDoC approach might include measures that are behavioral (e.g., number of drinks per day, similar to the "packs per day" used for cigarettes in general medicine), physiological (e.g., metabolites of alcohol breakdown), or structural (e.g., chronic changes in volume of frontal lobes).

Transdiagnosis and Intermediate Phenotypes

Dimensional approaches are also evident in the development of transdiagnostic constructs and intermediate phenotypes in specific areas of psychopathology. One such effort is David Barlow's "Unified Protocol for Transdiagnostic Treatment of Emotional Disorders" (UP) (see Barlow, Allen, & Choate, 2016; Barlow et al., 2017), which uses a "take all comers" approach to study emotional disorders and then systematically seeks to identify treatments for common transdiagnostic constructs. The UP emerged from studies begun in the 1990s that encouraged the study of higher-order dimensional traits common to depression and anxiety (Brown, Chorpita, & Barlow, 1998). This work reflects a dimensional and biobehaviorally minded approach, akin to RDoC, and the UP has evolved to offer a pragmatic treatment interventions for emotional disorders, targeting specific transdiagnostic functions such as cognitive flexibility and awareness of physical sensation (e.g., Ito et al., 2023). These interventions have proven efficacious in multiple settings (Barlow et al., 2020) and point to the benefit of looking across diagnostic boundaries to find functional constructs with clinical import.

Rumination is another example of a robust transdiagnostic construct that has emerged from the careful examination of dimensional functions. Rumination came into consideration in psychology and psychopathology following its introduction as part of the Response Style Theory of Nolen-Hoeksema (Nolen-Hoeksema, 1991). Ongoing research suggests that rumination may reflect genetic risk and serve as an intermediate phenotype for depression and anxiety disorders, representing a potential intermediate phenotype and an opportunity for determining mechanism and developing interventions (Chen & Li, 2013; Eszlari et al., 2019; Ruscio et al., 2015). As a construct, rumination exemplifies a transdiagnostic function that exists along a continuum, making it possible to characterize its normative range and identify maladaptive manifestations that cut across diagnostic categories (e.g., Luca, 2019; McLaughlin & Nolen-Hoeksema, 2011; Shaw et al., 2021). Rumination has also been incorporated into clinical staging models (e.g., Grierson, Hickie, Naismith, & Scott, 2016).

Structural (Hierarchical) Models

An increasing number of structural models, with intrinsic dimensional aspects due to hierarchical approaches, have appeared with constantly improving analytical computations (Lahey et al., 2021). Perhaps the most well known of the structural models is the Hierarchical Taxonomy of Psychopathology (HiTOP; Kotov et al., 2017), which hierarchically classifies psychopathological dimensions and is addressed directly by Pham and Forbes (this volume).

Both HiTOP and RDoC originated in response to limitations of the DSM classification scheme, and they have several core principles in common; the frameworks nevertheless have distinctive features and accompanying opportunities to contribute to mental health research. Accordingly, a brief joint description may illuminate how structural models can function and interact.

While the development of the HiTOP classification system was rooted in self- or collateral reported (or clinician rated) symptoms, efforts have expanded to incorporate genomics and neurobiology (see DeYoung et al., 2024). The RDoC framework emphasis on the use of multiple measures of psychopathology, including the integration of biological dimensions, can be traced to pre-RDoC proposals for a psychoneurometric approach to mental disorders. Specifically, work by Vaidyanathan and colleagues (Vaidyanathan et al., 2009) proposed a model to integrate the fear systems from experimental psychophysiology and the classification scheme similar to the HiTOP program announced several years later (Kotov et al., 2017). The psychoneurometric model focused on internalizing symptoms and bridged these symptoms to neurobiological processes, with example associations between physiological measures and psychopathological domains (Vaidyanathan et al., 2009; 2012). While this specific integration has not been formally realized, the psychoneurometric model illustrates one viable pathway to bring together complementary current aspects of HiTOP and RDoC dimensions (see also Michelini et al., 2021). These proposals, so long as they avoid reifying the notion of fixed or prescriptive constructs, hold promise for connecting these related frameworks, which agree on the fundamental dimensionality of constructs related to mental health.

In summary, there now exist a number of influential frameworks and proposals, in addition to RDoC, that acknowledge the importance of dimensionality in understanding mental disorders. While each instantiation brings different strengths and limitations to the study of psychopathology, they represent the overall shift toward incorporating dimensional aspects, and offer potential complementarities to advance both research and practice. We now turn to another key perspective that emphasizes the importance of dimensionality in the RDoC framework—namely, the role of development.

RDoC and Developmental Psychopathology Dimensions

The fluid nature of development, and the attention to potential precursors of overt disease and distress, meant that the field of developmental psychopathology was in many ways well aligned with key principles of RDoC prior to its launch (for examples, see Casey et al., 2014; Pacheco et al., 2022; Pine & Fox, 2015). In fact, this dimensional approach was already recognized by developmental psychopathologists in the 1980s, when Cicchetti and Rizley (1981) wrote about the study of child maltreatment: "any classification or nosology represents a rather futile effort to divide what is in reality a continuum into discrete categories . . . failure to attend to this major source of heterogeneity runs the very real risk of ignoring a source of variation that is crucial to an appreciation of the differing etiologies, sequelae, intergenerational transmission patterns, and treatment responses of different types of maltreatment" (Cicchetti & Rizley, 1981, p. 2, quoted in Conradt, Crowell, & Chicchetti, 2021, p. 1522). The principle of dimensionality was also familiar to the developmental field, because certain diagnostic categories were reserved for adults and simply unavailable for children and adolescents. As a result, many developmental researchers were accustomed to recruiting subjects not on the basis of a categorical diagnostic criterion but by using measures that captured relevant dimensions of function or the presence of increased risk (Achenbach, 1966; Casey et al., 2014; Mittal & Wakschlag, 2017).

In recent years, the importance of development across the lifespan has been explicitly highlighted as a key component to the RDoC framework (Garvey et al., 2016; NIMH, 2019; Pacheco et al., 2022) along with the intertwined role of environmental factors (Morris et al., 2022; Sanislow et al., 2022;). Successful implementation of RDoC research depends on accounting for the critical significance of development across the lifespan, not only for understanding mental disorders that manifest in childhood such as ASD and ADHD, but also for determining the precedents of disorders that have an onset in adolescence and adulthood. While "development" often refers to the rapid and conspicuous changes that mark infancy, childhood, and adolescence, leading into a more stable phase of adulthood, it is nonetheless important to acknowledge that there are developmental changes throughout the lifespan, where dimensional approaches continue to offer a valuable lens.

RDoC Developmental Themes

Why is the dimensional approach within RDoC well suited as a framework for developmental research? Four inter-related themes highlight the value of dimensionality in understanding developmental psychopathology and promoting mental well-being: (1) variability and individual trajectories, (2) normative behavior, (3) early detection and prevention, and (4) critical periods.

Variability and Individual Trajectories

Developmental research in general is exquisitely attuned to trajectories and individual variability. There is inherent appreciation, for example, that infants and children achieve key milestones according to unique trajectories. The field of developmental psychopathology has been shaped strongly by the concepts of equifinality and multifinality, as discussed in this chapter's introduction. As one example, the study of neurodevelopmental genetics has shown that multiple outcomes can emerge from homogeneous polygenetic pathways (Hyman, 2021; St. Pourcain et al., 2018). Other examples come from the work of Karalunas, Nigg, and colleagues, who have studied the trajectories of children diagnosed with ADHD (Karalunas et al., 2014; Nigg et al., 2004). This body of research has shown that a common ADHD diagnosis in childhood can take distinct trajectories into adulthood, with symptoms remitting in some individuals but not others. As described in more detail in the next section on clinical applications, the research has identified key dimensions of children's temperament and cognitive performance that help to predict ADHD severity in adulthood. Examples from genetic vulnerability in other forms of psychopathology include ASD and schizophrenia, which share a common phenotypic impairment in social communication, and common genetic vulnerabilities, but different temporal expressions (St. Pourcain et al., 2018). These observations emphasize that many factors contribute to final outcomes and support a dimensional view of the components that can affect an individual's trajectory (see also Pine & Fox, 2015; Seidlitz et al., 2020). In this view, multiple dimensions could converge in such a manner that a developmental tipping point is marked, introducing a shift into overt clinical psychopathology.

Normative Behavior

A second theme in developmental research, closely related to individual trajectories, is the importance of understanding normative behavior. The continuum of normal-to-abnormal function, which is central to the RDoC dimensional approach, comes into stark relief in the context of development. The same behaviors can be developmentally appropriate at one age but inappropriate or maladaptive at other ages (e.g., Wakschlag et al., 2014). This dynamic nature of development makes it essential to characterize normative behavior at all stages, to understand deviations that may be cause for concern (risk factor) or call for treatment intervention. This is another way in which developmental approaches are inherently dimensional—one needs to understand the range of behaviors that are functional for a given age range, and similarly chart normative neurodevelopmental trajectories (Bethlehem et al., 2022). The work of an international consortium of researchers (Uhlhaas et al., 2023) provides a good example, proposing a focus on youth mental health. They make a compelling case for accumulating normative data, with parallels to the role of growth charts in primary care. By tracking normative trends in the population—establishing ranges that in turn can be linked to functional outcomes—opportunities emerge for the early identification of trajectories that may result in health or risk for disease/disorder.

Longitudinal studies are of special value in mapping the range of normal-to-abnormal development, as they go beyond cross-sectional comparisons and allow finer-grained within-subject measurement of changes across time. On a large population scale, the NIH-led ABCD study characterizes a cohort of ~12,000 youth using multimodal measures from childhood (eight years of age) through adolescence and into early adulthood (Karcher & Barch, 2021 Volkow et al., 2018). ABCD exemplifies the benefit of dense longitudinal studies that span multiple geographical sites and—in keeping with RDoC principles—employ a variety of dimensional measures (cognition, sleep, environment) and methods (self-report, imaging, genetics). Recent studies have demonstrated the value of these large-scale data in advancing understanding for a range of topics, including functional connectomics (Busch et al., 2024), associations between network topographies and cognition (Keller et al., 2023), and interactions across environment, brain, and behavior (Zhi et al., 2024).

Early Detection and Intervention

A third critical facet of the dimensional approach in RDoC is its capacity to support early detection and intervention. Clinical syndromes, by the time they are diagnostically labeled, are often end-stage and do not offer ideal targets for intervention. In this way, categorical models preclude early interventions, whereas dimensional models can capture signals that allow for early detection and intervention before the manifestation of overt disorder. Within the context of development, however, functional impairments in childhood or adolescence may not simply be a "milder" form of adult psychopathology. As described above, the dynamic nature of different developmental stages must be accounted for when considering prevention and interventions; children are not just "mini-adults," and it is essential to characterize the temporal unfolding of symptomatology within the context of developmental stages. Pine and Fox (2015), for example, show that major domains of psychopathology (neurodevelopmental, psychotic, and emotional disorders) follow unique patterns. This kind of dimensional approach, with sensitivity to dynamics of development, lays essential groundwork for intervention.

The Clinical Staging Model of McGorry and colleagues (2006) similarly advocates for a dimensional approach, offering a clinical context for neurodevelopment. This model, which has its roots in the staging models of other areas of clinical medicine such as cancer, operationalizes the study of risk, onset, and progression of disorders, focusing on opportunities for intervention at the earliest possible stage (McGorry & Mei, 2018). The Clinical Staging Model has been implemented in youth mental health (Shah et al., 2022) and incorporated into recent studies that demonstrate its promise in identifying individuals at risk of developing severe symptomatology (Destrée et al., 2024). Although this model is described more fully in this volume (Mei et al., this volume), its significance warrants special consideration in the context of development and the RDoC framework. Specifically, it shares key principles of using objective measures to assess dimensions across diagnostic boundaries, and its longitudinal focus makes it a natural fit for understanding and intervening in the course of developmental change. As with RDoC, the staging model accounts that formative psychopathology is not necessarily a milder version of the "end-stage" diagnosis.

There are pragmatic challenges to the identification of early (developmental) forms of psychopathology that would provide prevention or treatment targets of early intervention. As Kessler and colleagues point out (Kessler, Merikangas, Berglund et al., 2003), health systems are typically built around the concept of disorders. Fundamental components of care, such as reimbursement and opportunity for specialty services, often depend on thresholds and a binary categorical diagnosis. Nevertheless, there have been promising signs from field testing of dimensional measures in the patient and clinician experience (Narrow et al., 2011), and dimensional principles have also been incorporated in the most recent manual for mental, behavioral, and neurodevelopmental disorders in the ICD-11. These dimensional implementations may be even more feasible in the developmental setting, given that many developmental researchers, clinicians, and educators are attuned to the aforementioned themes of individual trajectories and normative function. In schools, for example, interventional efforts often occur within ongoing monitoring of progress and an understanding of function in the appropriate context. Dimensional approaches may also be especially useful in light of the critical periods available in development, as described next.

Critical Periods

The fourth and final highlighted theme for dimensional developmental approaches is that of critical periods, or "sensitive periods." It is well established that there are distinct developmental phases with heightened plasticity and sensitivity to environmental exposures and experience. This plasticity has been long recognized as a property during infancy and early childhood development, and researchers have more recently demonstrated that adolescence is another key phase of sensitivity (Larsen & Luna, 2018; Nardou et al., 2019; Pattwell et al., 2012). Critical periods bring heightened risk, but also represent windows of opportunity for intervention. Adolescence, for example, is known as a period of significant change associated with increased risk for (and onset of) overt mental disorders (McLaughlin et al., 2022; Pine & Fox, 2015). Recent studies also demonstrate that targeted treatment during adolescence may mitigate the effects of early childhood deprivation (Colich et al., 2021; Gunnar et al., 2019). The dimensional approach, by acknowledging the range of potential function through these windows of plasticity, makes it possible to investigate targets of risk and harness potential interventions. As McLaughlin and Gabard-Durnam (2022) describe, it is possible to examine the developmental trajectory of specific RDoC domains, using multiple methodologies to determine whether plasticity is experience-expectant or experience-dependent, and tailoring interventions accordingly.

Integration of Themes: Dimensionality in Practice

Bringing these themes into practical context, a recent review by Astle and colleagues (Astle et al., 2022) puts forward a data-driven transdiagnostic approach to neurodevelopmental disorders. Their approach embodies several RDoC principles, including an integrative focus on dimensionality. They describe the merits of "functional recruitment" —relaxing strict categorical criteria and identifying study participants on the basis of relevant functional characteristics. For example, education research by Holmes and colleagues (Holmes et al., 2019, 2021) selected participants based on practitioner reports of difficulty with attention, learning, and memory. By recruiting a diverse population sample based on these functional domains, they were able to capture subthreshold impairments and identify new data-driven subgroups with distinct profiles, paving the way for more targeted interventions. The neurodevelopmental approach of Astle et al. also emphasizes the utility of functionally meaningful and dimensional measures, such as pragmatic challenges with language or social communication, that cut across diagnostic boundaries (e.g., Bishop & Norbury, 2002, Hawkins et al., 2016, Mareva et al., 2019). Lastly, they point out that models are valuable for charting changes across development, not only for individual dimensions but, critically, also for the relationship between dimensions (e.g., Kievit et al., 2019).

Recent research by Mahony and colleagues (2023) offers one such example of characterizing dimensional interactions in development. The study examined the relationship between dimensional measures of broad psychopathology and IQ, a common dimensional measure of cognitive function. In a general-population cohort of >2,500 youth aged 6 to 17, they observed that IQ was not uniformly associated with psychopathological measures. Instead, IQ was most strongly correlated with attentional and social impairments, and was associated with stronger coupling of specific problems, such as internalizing and repetitive behaviors. These findings have implications for interpreting standard clinical measures during development; more broadly, they show the benefit of delineating the relationships between dimensional domains.

As Astle et al. (2022) acknowledge, however, there are limitations to the dimensional approach to development, and we highlight two of these here. First, while a dimensional framework can identify data-driven subgroups and suggest mechanistic targets, more narrowly defined designs with set thresholds for developmental milestones may be better suited for establishing mechanism. In such cases, the dimensional approach is complemented by alternate methodologies that serve the question or problem at hand. Second, meaningful understanding of dimensions depends on choosing high-quality, valid measures and taking into account the population studied. Without judicious consideration of the selected measures and the sample population, dimensional models can be misleading at best and harmful at worst. For example, developmental "norms" determined in one cohort may not be generalizable to other cohorts, age groups, or social or cultural contexts. Careful attention to subpopulations and to the role of environment, including social determinants of health, will be essential to successful implementation of valid dimensional models in neurodevelopment. The concept of the *exposome* encompasses the many and various exposures that are encountered by individuals across the lifespan and is clearly intertwined with charting development. Studies have begun to examine how the exposome influences mental health, and continued use of the dimensional framework will be instrumental in advancing this critical line of research (Barzilay et al., 2022; Cardenas-Iniguez et al., 2024; Busch et al., 2025; Keller et al., 2024).

Clinical Applications and Treatment

From the outset, the NIMH RDoC work group has maintained that the framework is not a replacement for a clinical diagnostic manual. Moreover, history has shown that the goals of Research Diagnostic Criteria (RDC) from the 1970s and those of clinical diagnosis are not the same, and treating them as such does not work well. For RDoC, the goal has been to scaffold clinical research in ways that would elucidate valid behavioral and biological mechanisms relevant to manifest psychopathology, and to move toward ways of identifying multidimensional phenotypes with clinical relevance. Early discussion among the NIMH RDoC internal working group members about rough estimates for when RDoC might begin to have some clinical impact ranged from 20 to 30 years from when the project began. Broadly speaking, among the central aims of RDoC was to capitalize on connecting advances from integrative neural and behavioral science to better understand and treat human suffering. In that way, RDoC was conceptualized as an organizational toolbox, serving as a bridge to connect findings from basic research—where dimensions are often woven into the scientific landscape—to services and intervention research. There is a priority going forward to use RDoC principles and measures in services and intervention research and encourage clinical utility with RDoC-based research. Now in the midst of the second decade of its development, translational findings using the RDoC framework have begun to provide seeds for clinical trials research, and dimensional approaches have been central to this progress.

One of the early ideas for RDoC informed research was a "take all comers" strategy for participant recruitment, for instance, any and all patients seeking treatment at an anxiety disorders clinic. This is a useful strategy to overcome the artificially restricted variability inherent in researching clinical diagnoses that are over-specified. As an example, study participants might include patients at a specialty clinic for anxiety disorders regardless of which type of DSM anxiety disorder diagnosis might be assigned to each patient and include the possible presence of more than one diagnosis as well. Studies may also include diagnostic co-occurrence that has either simultaneous or longitudinal comorbidity. With simultaneous comorbidity, particularly where there is criterion overlap, a transdiagnostic dimension may be of interest. This approach has been developed prior to RDoC (Barlow, Allen, & Choate, 2016) and has been deployed in clinical trials with good results (e.g., Barlow, Farchione, Bullis et al., 2017). With longitudinal comorbidity, the developmental progression or course of a psychopathology dimension may be of interest—for example, reduction in heightened hypothalamic-pituitary-adrenal activity as the clinical presentation changes from anxiety symptoms to depression symptoms. Another strategy has been to study participants within a particular clinical diagnosis to address diagnostic heterogeneity or under-specification. As we have emphasized, independent variables are the dimensions that cross-cut the different disorders or span the heterogeneity of a single disorder (depending on the sample), and not the DSM diagnoses themselves. Thus, these example strategies illustrate how the RDoC dimensional approach can work in concert with the DSM, and that RDoC-themed research does not require the exclusion of DSM or ICD clinical diagnoses.

Fear Dimensions

Across the disorder categories for trauma and anxiety, recent research has demonstrated dimensional variations in fear reactivity across patient participants (Lang et al., 2018; McTeague & Lang, 2012; see also D'Andrea et al., 2013; Hopper et al., 2007; Sambuco et al., 2020). Instead of studying these disorders separately, an RDoC dimensional approach involves pooling study participants with anxiety and/or trauma-related disorders, and using dimensions—such as those common to fear systems—to characterize phenotypes that are rudiments of behavioral functioning. In an illustrative example of this research, investigators measured startle reactivity and found a continuum that helped to reclassify participants: high startle responses were characteristic of individuals who experienced a specific, single incident PTSD and specific phobia (highly specified), while low startle responses were associated with multiple incident PTSD and generalized anxiety disorder Lang et al. (2016). Of interest, arranging the range of anxiety disorder diagnoses (including PTSD) from most specified to least specified revealed a linear dimension of fear potentiation (Lang et al., 2016).

Another example of this approach in fear systems is a study of amygdala reactivity by Sambuco and colleagues (Sambuco et al., 2020). In this study, patient-participant groups were binned using the level of amygdala fMRI activation in response to viewing emotionally arousing relative to neutral scenes. This dimensional amygdala activation was then compared on a dimensional (factor) trauma score. Researchers found that participants showing the least responsiveness in amygdala activation (difference score based on scene type) reported the highest level of trauma. In these example studies, the independent and dependent variables were reversed compared to the traditional research designs. In the first example, the "dimension" from least specific to most specific (and orderly progression in between) was revealed post hoc; in the second, two dimensions were studied without regard to diagnosis. In both examples, by investigating the continuum of function, the research enables a re-ordering of patient-participants, potentially improving the understanding of mechanism and enabling more tailored interventions for the resultant groups.

Reward Dimensions

A prime reward-related example is the work of anhedonia, a core symptom of various psychiatric disorders including depression and schizophrenia. RDoC has facilitated the dissection of motivational systems and reward processing, particularly in distinguishing between "wanting" and "liking" aspects of reward (Berridge, Robinson, & Aldridge, 2009). Here, research has shown that liking a reward and wanting a reward are two distinct entities and are dissociable both psychologically and neurobiologically. In this case, liking refers to a more hedonic impact of the reward, and wanting refers to incentive salience. By understanding these distinct dimensions, and how they work together, researchers and clinicians can develop more targeted interventions for individuals experiencing reward-related disturbances, such as anhedonia. For instance, in clinical trials focused on addressing anhedonia, RDoC principles have guided the design and evaluation of interventions. Krystal et al. (2020) provided an example of a clinical trial that incorporated RDoC principles in investigating a treatment for anhedonia. The findings of Krystal et al. (2020) have now been expanded upon in several clinical trials, with promising results for the treatment of anhedonia and mood disorders. By aligning treatment strategies with specific dimensions of reward processing identified through RDoC, researchers aim to enhance treatment efficacy and tailor interventions to individual needs.

Psychosis Dimensions

An exemplar study that showcases the utility of a dimensional approach within the psychotic spectrum is the Bipolar-Schizophrenia Network for Intermediate Phenotypes (B-SNIP). This study, as outlined by Clementz et al. (2016), derived three biotypes from pooled participants with schizophrenia, schizoaffective disorder, and bipolar disorder with psychosis. The investigators characterized each participant using multiple measures, including behavioral tasks, structural and functional MRI, genetics, and EEG/ERP. From a principal components analysis, participants were identified along two dimensions: one involved behavioral task data, and the other comprised EEG/ERP measures. The two dimensions correlated at near zero, suggesting that they carried distinct information for characterizing participants; further, the behavioral tasks were linear from poor to good, while the EEG/ERP dimension was normal at the average and abnormal at the two tails of the distribution. These novel data demonstrated the importance of multiple dimensions for pinpointing different types of dimensions and indicating potential new mechanisms. Further, a cluster analysis from the two dimensions defined three distinct biotypes (clusters) that cut across diagnostic categories. These psychosis biotypes have since been replicated and validated in a second independent sample, demonstrating the robustness of the composite characterization (Clementz et al., 2022, and allowing the development of neurobehaviorally based hypotheses about optimal treatments. Building on these results and moving toward clinical applicability, the B-SNIP research consortium is developing tools to simplify the biotype differentiation process (Clementz et al., 2023). Clinical trials are now underway to test whether biotype classification can help predict responses to clozapine treatment on the basis of the bimodal EEG distribution (ClinicalTrials.gov ID NCT04580134). This body of work illustrates the translation of a dimensional approach and RDoC principles into real-world interventions for psychosis.

Cognitive Dimensions in a Neurodevelopmental Context

Another application of RDoC is to explore dimensions within the life-span development trajectory, which is highly heterogeneous. The work on longitudinal trajectories of ADHD offers a useful example. Karalunas, Nigg, and colleagues (detailed earlier in the development section) have shown distinct trajectories of subgroups of ADHD children based on dimensions of both temperament and cognitive profiles. Within the temperament subgroups, a group labeled as the "irritable" subgroup (which has higher ADHD symptoms, higher scores on anger scales, and lower scores on "soothability") is associated with a more challenging trajectory—including sustained ADHD symptoms into adulthood as well as a higher likelihood for future mental health-related diagnoses or problems functioning (Karalunas et al., 2014, 2019). With the cognitive subgroups, working memory was identified as a key indicator of disorder trajectory. If a childhood working memory deficit does not return to age-appropriate functioning by adolescence, this is indicative of a higher likelihood of sustained ADHD symptoms into adulthood. In contrast, the return of working memory to age-appropriate norms in adolescence is indicative of potential remittance of ADHD symptoms in adulthood. See Nigg (2022) for detailed review of these and related findings, and more elaboration of the complex role of working memory in ADHD and intervention strategies (Karalunas et al., 2017).

Deploying RDoC Dimensions Clinically: An Example

Building on dimensional findings of clinical relevance, such as those described above, RDoC is moving in the direction of larger-scale tests of clinical utility. A newly launched program exemplifies this direction, with the goal of harnessing dimensional behavioral measures and computational tools to improve precision mental health for all. Consistent with the RDoC framework, the NIMH recently called for studies that will generate clinical phenotypes to optimize evaluation at the level of the individual and inform clinical decision-making. The Individually Measured Phenotypes to Advance Computational Translation in Mental Health (IMPACT-MH; see NIMH, 2024) program aims to enable transdiagnostic, data-driven precision assessments in psychiatry. It will support studies that follow large cohorts of participants using behavioral measures and computational methods to refine clinical assessments, improve prognosis, and optimize treatment in persons with mental disorders.

These studies will integrate dimensional behavioral data with data from the clinical record, which can include conventional diagnostic information. One of the central goals is to ask, can low-cost, scalable behavioral measures be integrated with clinical records data to improve patient classification and prediction of individual trajectories? This research effort is emblematic of the dimensional principles espoused by RDoC and other dimensional frameworks, with a focus on characterizing functional domains along a continuum. The projects supported by the IMPACT-MH program are examining key functional dimensions, including cognition, reward processing, psychosis symptomatology, and sleep. Novel clinical phenotypes derived from individual participant-level measurements in these domains—novel in the sense that they are not derivative of DSM disorders per se—will foster more informative classification schemes, which will in turn be used to improve clinical practices and lead to the identification of specific pathology-related mechanisms.

Conclusions

We have shown that RDoC has helped to change the discourse of psychopathology research as evidenced by published research findings, NIMH extramural funded projects, and adoption/integration of RDoC principles in clinical research based in Europe and other areas of the world. Findings from RDoC-themed research now provide a basis for novel targets in clinical research. Indeed, this is an exciting time in psychopathology research, ripe for transition. As we have described, RDoC has its own unique approaches. Its central aspect is an emphasis on the full dimension of functioning. This includes both studies of normal behavioral constructs and the brain systems that implement them, and the gradual dysfunction that can eventually become overt problems extending in severity. The RDoC perspective includes both cross-section dimensions that represent a population distribution, and longitudinal dimensions that can occur during development when functional levels change within individuals. Further, the multiple data types involved in behavior and self-reports (e.g., from various brain networks and local circuits) are often only moderately correlated, requiring sophisticated analyses in order to understand the complex interactions in multiple systems.

RDoC research has continued to progress. Clinical applications from an RDoC perspective have been useful in such areas as fear, reward, and psychosis; further, clinical trials have been conducted in mood/anxiety disorders and psychotic samples. A quantum leap has recently been initiated, using multimodal measures and behavioral tasks in large cohorts of different types of participants, in order to employ machine learning algorithms that will seek to identify precision transdiagnostic phenotypes. Equally promising is the emphasis on child/adolescent trajectories, combining multiple measures in youth with exposome data in order to delineate overt functional problems for which prevention interventions can be developed before manifest symptoms are apparent.

All of the RDoC-based research projects routinely include dimensional data in order to understand the nature of psychopathology, and how to prevent or mitigate it. In addition, the importance of quantitative dimensions is recognized increasingly in the future as a way to consider cut points for multiple subcategories (re: severity or similar bins) on continuous data, as well as to change such points when epidemiological data indicate revision (as, e.g., blood pressure data). As summarized succinctly in a recent consummate essay, "Clinical description, laboratory studies, and family (now genetic) studies do not converge at all on distinct categories. Rather, modern studies are consistent with psychiatric disorders as heterogeneous quantitative deviations from health (Hyman, 2021, p. 6)."

What the future holds depends on shifts in the extant research frame. As described in this chapter and demonstrated throughout this volume, the field has set the stage for dimensional approaches to research, diagnose, and treat/prevent psychopathology. RDoC is only one line of this effort. Among the approaches detailed in this volume are the contemporary efforts of the HiTOP that applies empirical methods to organize clinical symptoms into coherent dimensions (see Pham & Forbes, this volume, and Kotov, Krueger, & Watson, 2018); Network Analysis, an approach that delineates dimensions of interrelating symptoms and foregrounds those dimensions as causal (see Rodebaugh et al., this volume, and Borsboom & Cramer, 2013); and the Clinical Staging model, designed to expand the range of targets of intervention to include earlier stages in disease development that may be missed in pure categorical models (see Mei et al., this volume, and McGorry et al., 2006). Of these collective efforts, RDoC offers an approach to research that can both benefit from and leverage the range of efforts to enhance progress in a parallel yet interacting fashion (as suggested by Clark et al., 2017). While all of the different approaches share a broad, final aim (i.e., improve diagnosis and in turn treatment of mental disorders), it is important to recognize that all approaches do not have the same immediate goals to reach that aim. It may be hoped that the coming decades will record significant advances in the ways that dimensional approaches advance the understanding of psychopathology—fostered by collaborations among the various projects that provide distinct but compatible perspectives.

References

Achenbach, T. M. (1966). The classification of children's psychiatric symptoms: A factor-analytic study. *Psychological Monographs*, 80, 1–37. http://dx.doi.org/10.1037/h0093906

Achenbach, T. M. (2020). Paradigms for psychopathology: A half-century odyssey. *Annual Review of Clinical Psychology*, *16*, 1–24. https://doi.org/10.1146/annurev-clinpsy-071119–115831

Astle, D. E., Holmes, J., Kievit, R., & Gathercole, S. E. (2022). Annual research review: The transdiagnostic revolution in neurodevelopmental disorders. *Journal of Child Psychology and Psychiatry, and Allied Disciplines*, 63(4), 397–417. https://doi.org/10.1111/jcpp.13481

Barch, D. M., Bustillo, J., Gaebel, W., Gur, R., Heckers, S., Malaspina, D., Owen, M. J., Schultz, S., Tandon, R., Tsuang, M., Van Os, J., & Carpenter, W. (2013). Logic and justification for dimensional assessment of symptoms and related clinical phenomena in psychosis: Relevance to DSM-5. *Schizophrenia Research*, *150*, 15–20. https://doi.org/10.1016/j.schres.2013.04.027.

Barlow, D. H., Allen, L. B., Choate, M. L. (2016). Toward a unified treatment for emotional disorders—Republished article. *Behavior Therapy*, *47*(6):838–853. https://doi.org/10.1016/j.beth.2016.11.005

Barlow, D. H., Farchione, T. J., Bullis, J. R., Gallagher, M. W., Murray-Latin, H., Sauer-Zavala, S., Bentley, K. H., Thompson-Hollands, J., Conklin, L. R., Boswell, J. F., Ametaj, A., Jenna R. Carl, J. R., Boettcher, H. T., & Cassiello-Robbins, C. (2017). The unified protocol for transdiagnostic treatment of emotional disorders compared with diagnosis-specific protocols for anxiety disorders: A randomized clinical trial. *JAMA Psychiatry*, *74*(9), 875–884. https://doi.org/10.1001/jamapsychiatry.2017.2164

Barlow, D. H., Harris, B. A., Eustis, E. H., & Farchione, T. J. (2020). The unified protocol for transdiagnostic treatment of emotional disorders. *World Psychiatry: Official Journal of the World Psychiatric Association*, 19(2), 245–246. https://doi.org/10.1002/wps.20748

Barzilay, R. Pries, L. K., Moore, T. M., Gur, R. E., van Os, J., Rutten, B.P. F., & Guloksuz, S. (2022). Exposome and trans-syndromal developmental trajectories toward psychosis. *Biological Psychiatry Global Open Science*, *2*(3), 197–205. https://doi.org/10.1016/j.bpsgos.2022.05.001

Berridge, K. C., Robinson, T. E., & Aldridge J. W. (2009). Dissecting components of reward: 'Liking', 'wanting', and learning. *Current Opinion in Pharmacology*, *9*(1), 65–73. https://doi.org/10.1016/j.coph.2008.12.014

Bethlehem, R. A. I., Seidlitz, J., White, S. R., Vogel, J. W., Anderson, K. M., Adamson, C., Adler, S., Alexopoulos, G. S., Anagnostou, E., Areces-Gonzalez, A., Astle, D. E., Auyeung, B., Ayub, M., Bae, J., Ball, G., Baron-Cohen, S., Beare, R., Bedford, S. A., Benegal, V., . . . Alexander-Bloch, A. F. (2022). Brain charts for the human lifespan. *Nature*, *604*(7906), 525–533. https://doi.org/10.1038/s41586-022-04554-y

Bilder, R. M., Howe, A. G., & Sabb, F. w. (2013). Multilevel models from biology to psychology: Mission impossible? *Journal of Abnormal Psychology*, *122*(3), 917–927. https://doi.org/10.1037/a0032263

Bishop, D., & Norbury, C. (2002). Exploring the borderlands of autistic disorder and specific language impairment: A study using standardised diagnostic instruments. *Journal of Child Psychology and Psychiatry, and Allied Disciplines*, 43(7), 917–929. https://doi.org/10.1111/1469-7610.00114

Borsboom, D. & Cramer, A. O. (2013). Network analysis: an integrative approach to the structure of psychopathology. *Annual Review of Clinical Psychology*, *9*, 91–121.

Brown, T. A., Chorpita, B. F., & Barlow, D. H. (1998). Structural relationships among dimensions of the DSM-IV anxiety and mood disorders and dimensions of negative affect, positive affect, and

autonomic arousal. *Journal of Abnormal Psychology, 107*(2), 179–192. https://doi.org/10.1037//0021-843x.107.2.179
Busch, E., Conley, M. & Baskin-Sommers, A. (2025). Manifold learning uncovers nonlinear interactions between the adolescent brain and environment that predict emotional and behavioral problems. *Biological Psychiatry: Cognitive Neuroscience and Neuroimaging, 10*, 463–474. https://doi.org/10.1016/j.bpsc.2024.07.001
Busch, E. L., Rapuano, K. M., Anderson, K. M., Rosenberg, M. D., Watts, R., Casey, B. J., Haxby, J. V., & Feilong, M. (2024). Dissociation of reliability, heritability, and predictivity in coarse- and fine-scale functional connectomes during development. *The Journal of Neuroscience: The Official Journal of the Society for Neuroscience, 44*(6), 1–16. https://doi.org/10.1523/JNEUROSCI.0735-23.2023
Cannon, T. D. (2015). How schizophrenia develops: Cognitive and brain mechanisms underlying onset of psychosis. *Trends in Cognitive Science, 19*(12), 744–756. https://doi.org/10.1016/j.tics.2015.09.009. Epub 2015 Oct 19. PMID: 26493362; PMCID: PMC4673025.
Cannon, T. D., Huttunen, M. O., Lonnqvist, J., Tuulio-Henriksson, A., Pirkola, T., Glahn, D., Finkelstein, J., Hietanen, M., Kaprio, J., & Koskenvuo M. (2000). The inheritance of neuropsychological dysfunction in twins discordant for schizophrenia. *American Journal of Human Genetics, 67*(2), 369–82. https://doi.org/10.1086/303006.
Cannon, T. D., Keller, M. C. (2006). Endophenotypes in the genetic analyses of mental disorders. *Annual Review of Clinical Psychology, 2*, 267–290.
Cardenas-Iniguez, C., Schachner, J. N., Ip, K. I., Schertz, K. E., Gonzalez, M. R., Abad, S., & Herting, M. M. (2024). Building towards an adolescent neural urbanome: Expanding environmental measures using linked external data (LED) in the ABCD study. *Developmental Cognitive Neuroscience, 65*, 101338. https://doi.org/10.1016/j.dcn.2023.101338
Casey, B. J., Oliveri, M. E., Insel, T. (2014). A neurodevelopmental perspective on the Research Domain Criteria (RDoC) framework. *Biological Psychiatry, 76*(5), 350–353.
Chen J, Li X. (2013). Genetic and environmental influences on adolescent rumination and its association with depressive symptoms. *Journal of Abnormal Child Psychology, 41*(8):1289–98. https://doi.org/10.1007/s10802-013-9757-5.
Cicchetti, D., & Rizley, R. (1981). Developmental perspectives on the etiology, intergenerational transmission, and sequelae of child maltreatment. *New Directions for Child and Adolescent Development, 1981*(11), 31–55. https://experts.umn.edu/en/publications/developmental-perspectives-on-the-etiology-intergenerational-tran-2
Cicchetti, D., & Rogosch, F. A. (1996). Equifinality and multifinality in developmental psychopathology. *Development and Psychopathology, 8*(4), 597–600. https://doi.org/10.1017/S0954579400007318
Clark, L. A. (2005). Temperament as a unifying basis for personality and psychopathology. *Journal of Abnormal Psychology, 114*(4), 505–521. https://doi.org/10.1037/0021-843X.114.4.505
Clark, L. A., Cuthbert, B. N., Lewis-Fernández, R., Narrow, W. E., & Reed, G. M. (2017). Three approaches to understanding and classifying mental disorder: ICD-11, DSM-5, and the national institute of mental health's Research Domain Criteria (RDoC). *Psychological Science in the Public Interest, 18*(2), 72–145. https://doi.org/10.1177/1529100617727266
Clark, L. A., & Watson, D. (1991). Tripartite model of anxiety and depression: Psychometric evidence and taxonomic implications. *Journal of Abnormal Psychology, 100*, 316–336. dx.doi.org/10.1037/0021843X.100.3.316
Clementz, B. A., Chattopadhyay, I., Trotti, R. L., Parker, D. A., Gershon, E. S., Hill, S. K., Ivleva, E. I., Keedy, S. K., Keshavan, M. S., McDowell, J. E., Pearlson, G. D., Tamminga, C. A., & Gibbons, R. D. (2023). Clinical characterization and differentiation of B-SNIP psychosis biotypes: Algorithmic diagnostics for efficient prescription of treatments (ADEPT)-1. *Schizophrenia Research, 260*, 143–151. https://doi.org/10.1016/j.schres.2023.08.006
Clementz, B. A., Parker, D. A., Trotti, R. L., McDowell, J. E., Keedy, S. K., Keshavan, M. S., Pearlson, G. D., Gershon, E. S., Ivleva, E. I., Huang, L.-Y., Hill, S. K., Sweeney, J. A., Thomas, O., Hudgens-Haney, M., Gibbons, R. D., & Tamminga, C. A. (2022). Psychosis biotypes: Replication and validation from the b-snip consortium. *Schizophrenia Bulletin, 48*(1), 56–68. https://doi.org/10.1093/schbul/sbab090

Clementz, B. A., Sweeney, J. A., Hamm, J. P., Ivleva, E. I., Ethridge, L. E., Pearlson, G. D., Keshavan, M. S., Tamminga, C. A. (2016). Identification of distinct psychosis biotypes using brain-based biomarkers. *American Journal of Psychiatry, 173*(4), 373–384. https://doi.org/10.1093/schbul/sbab090. Erratum in: *American Journal of Psychiatry*. 2016 Feb 1;173(2):198. https://doi.org/10.1176/appi.ajp.2015.1732correction1.

Colich, N. L., Sheridan, M. A., Humphreys, K. L., Wade, M., Tibu, F., Nelson, C. A., Zeanah, C. H., Fox, N. A., & McLaughlin, K. A. (2021). Heightened sensitivity to the caregiving environment during adolescence: Implications for recovery following early-life adversity. *Journal of Child Psychology and Psychiatry, and Allied Disciplines, 62*(8), 937–948. https://doi.org/10.1111/jcpp.13347

Conradt, E., Crowell, S. E., & Cicchetti, D. (2021). Using development and psychopathology principles to inform the Research Domain Criteria (RDoC) framework. *Developmental Psychopathology, 33*(5), 1521–1525. https://doi.org/10.1017/s0954579421000985

Cuthbert, B. N. (2005). Dimensional models of psychopathology: Research agenda and clinical utility. *Journal of Abnormal Psychology, 114*(4), 565–569. https://doi.org/10.1037/0021-843X.114.4.565

Cuthbert, B. N., & Insel, T. R. (2010a). Toward new approaches to psychotic disorders: The NIMH Research Domain Criteria project. *Schizophrenia Bulletin, 36*(6): 1061–1062. PMCID: PMC2963043

Cuthbert. B. N., & Insel, T. R. (2010b). The data of diagnosis: New approaches to psychiatric classification. *Psychiatry, 73*(4): 311–314. PMID: 21198381

Cuthbert, B. N., & Insel, T. R. (2013). Toward the future of psychiatric diagnosis: The seven pillars of RDoC. *BMC Medicine, 11*, 126. http://dx.doi.org/10.1186/1741-7015-11-126

Cuthbert, B. N., & Kozak, M. J. (2013). Constructing constructs for psychopathology: The NIMH research domain criteria. *Journal of Abnormal Psychology, 122*(3), 928–937. https://doi.org/10.1037/a0034028

Cuthbert, B. N., Miller, G. A., Sanislow, C. A., & Vaidyanathan, U. (2023). The Research Domain Criteria Project: Integrative translation for psychopathology. In R. Krueger and P. Blaney (Eds.), *Oxford textbook of psychopathology* (4th edition). Oxford University Press.

D'Andrea, W., Pole, N., DePierro, J., Freed, S., & Wallace, D. B. (2013). Heterogeneity of defensive responses after exposure to trauma: Blunted autonomic reactivity in response to startling sounds. *International Journal of Psychophysiology, 90*, 80–89. https://doi.org/10.1016/j.ijpsycho.2013.07.008

Destrée, L., McGorry, P., Chanen, A., Ratheesh, A., Davey, C., Polari, A., Amminger, P., Yuen, H. P., Hartmann, J., Dwyer, D., Spooner, R., & Nelson, B. (2024). Transdiagnostic risk identification: A validation study of the Clinical High At Risk Mental State (CHARMS) criteria. *Psychiatry Research*, 333, 115745. https://doi.org/10.1016/j.psychres.2024.115745

DeYoung, C. G., Blain, S. D., Latzman, R. D., Grazioplene, R. G., Haltigan, J. D., Kotov, R., Michelini, G., Venables, N. C., Docherty, A. R., Goghari, V. M., Kallen, A. M., Martin, E. A., Palumbo, I. M., Patrick, C. J., Perkins, E. R., Shackman, A. J., Snyder, M. E., & Tobin, K. E. (2024). The Hierarchical Taxonomy of Psychopathology and the search for neurobiological substrates of mental illness: A systematic review and roadmap for future research. *Journal of Psychopathology and Clinical Science, 133*(8), 697–715. https://doi.org/10.1037/abn0000903

DeYoung, C. G., & Krueger, R. F. (2023). A cybernetic perspective on the nature of psychopathology: Transcending conceptions of mental illness as statistical deviance and brain disease. *Journal of Psychopathology and Clinical Science, 132*(3), 228–237. https://doi.org/10.1037/abn0000541

Eszlari, N., Millinghoffer, A., Petschner, P., Gonda, X., Baksa, D., Pulay, A. J., Réthelyi, J. M., Breen, G., Deakin, J. F. W., Antal, P., Bagdy, G., & Juhasz, G. (2019). Genome-wide association analysis reveals KCTD12 and miR-383-binding genes in the background of rumination. *Translational Psychiatry*, 9(1):119. https://doi.org/10.1038/s41398-019-0454-1.

Feighner, J. P., Robins, E., Guze, S. B., Woodruff, R. A. Jr., Winokur, G., Munoz, R. (1972). Diagnostic criteria for use in psychiatric research. *Archive of General Psychiatry, 26*, 57–63.

First, M. B., Bell, C. C., Cuthbert, B., Krystal, J. H., Malison, R., Offord, D. R., Reiss, D., Shea, M. T., Widiger, T., & Wisner, K. L. (2002). Personality disorders and relational disorders: A research agenda for addressing crucial gaps in DSM. In D. J. Kupfer, M. B. First, & D. A. Regier (Eds.), *A research agenda for DSM—V* (pp. 123–199). American Psychiatric Association.

Galderisi, S. (2024). The need for a consensual definition of mental health. *World Psychiatry, 23*, 52–53.

Garvey, M., Avenevoli, S., & Anderson, K. (2016). The National Institute of Mental Health Research Domain Criteria and clinical research in child and adolescent psychiatry. *Journal of the American Academy of Child and Adolescent Psychiatry*, *55*(2): 93–98. https://doi.org/10.1016/j.jaac.2015.11.002

Gottesman, I. I., & Gould, T. D. (2003). The endophenotype concept in psychiatry: Etymology and strategic intentions. *American Journal of Psychiatry*, *160*, 636–645.

Grierson A., Hickie I., Naismith S., & Scott J. (2016). The role of rumination in illness trajectories in youth: Linking trans-diagnostic processes with clinical staging models. *Psychological Medicine*, *46*(12), 2467–2484.

Grimm, O., Heinz, A., Walter, H., Kirsch, P., Erk, S., Haddad, L., Plichta, M. M., Romanczuk-Seiferth, N, Pöhland, L., Mohnke, S., Mühleisen, T. W., Mattheisen, M.,Witt, S. H., Schäfer, A., Cichon, S., Nöthen, M., Rietschel, M., Tost, H., & Meyer-Lindenberg, A. (2014). Striatal response to reward anticipation: Evidence for a systems-level intermediate phenotype for schizophrenia. *JAMA Psychiatry*, *71*(5): 531–539. https://doi.org/10.1001/jamapsychiatry.2014.9

Groen-Blokhuis, M. M., Middeldorp, C. M., Kan, K. J., Abdellaoui, A., van Beijsterveldt, C. E. M., Ehli, E. A., Davies, G. E., Scheet, P. A., Xiao, X., Hudziak, J. J., Hottenga, J. J., Psychiatric Genomics Consortium ADHD Working Group, Neale, B. M., & Boomsma, D. I. (2014). Attention-deficit/hyperactivity disorder polygenic risk scores predict attention problems in a population-based sample of children. *Journal of the American Academy of Child and Adolescent Psychiatry*, *53*(10), 1123–1129.

Gunnar, M. R., DePasquale, C. E., Reid, B. M., Donzella, B., & Miller, B. S. (2019). Pubertal stress recalibration reverses the effects of early life stress in postinstitutionalized children. *Proceedings of the National Academy of Sciences of the United States of America*, *116*(48), 23984–23988. https://doi.org/10.1073/pnas.1909699116

Hajcak, G., Meyer, A., & Kotov, R. (2017). Psychometrics and the neuroscience of individual differences: Internal consistency limits between-subjects effects. *Journal of Abnormal Psychology*, *126*(6), 823–834. https://doi.org/10.1037/abn0000274

Hawkins, E., Gathercole, S., Astle, D., The Calm Team, & Holmes, J. (2016). Language problems and ADHD symptoms: How specific are the links? *Brain Sciences*, *6*(4), 50. https://doi.org/10.3390/brainsci6040050

Heckers, S. (2008). Making progress in schizophrenia research. *Schizophrenia Bulletin*, *34*(4), 591–594. https://doi.org/10.1093/schbul/sbn046

Heckers, S., Engstrom, E. J., & Kendler, K. S. (2022). "Manifestations of insanity": Kraepelin's final views on psychiatric nosology in their historical context. *Molecular Psychiatry*, *27*(1), 328–334. https://doi.org/10.1038/s41380-021-01232-9

Holmes, J., Bryant, A., CALM Team, & Gathercole, S. E. (2019). Protocol for a transdiagnostic study of children with problems of attention, learning and memory (CALM). *BMC Pediatrics*, *19*(1), 10. https://doi.org/10.1186/s12887-018-1385-3

Holmes, J., Guy, J., Kievit, R. A., Bryant, A., Mareva, S., CALM Team, & Gathercole, S. E. (2021). Cognitive dimensions of learning in children with problems in attention, learning, and memory. *Journal of Educational Psychology*, *113*(7), 1454–1480. https://doi.org/10.1037/edu0000644

Hopper, J. W., Frewen, P. A., van der Kolk, B. A., & Lanius, R. A. (2007). Neural correlates of re-experiencing, avoidance, and dissociation in PTSD: Symptom dimensions and emotion dysregulation in responses to script-driven trauma imagery. *Journal of Traumatic Stress*, *20*, 713–725. https://doi.org/10.1002/jts.20284

Hopwood, C. J., Morey, L. C., & Markon, K. E. (2023). What is a psychopathology dimension? *Clinical Psychology Review*, *106*, 1–10: 102356. https://doi.org/10.1016/j.cpr.2023.102356

Hyman, S. E. (2021). Psychiatric disorders: Grounded in human biology but not natural kinds. *Perspectives in Biology and Medicine*, *64*(1), 6–28. https://doi.org/10.1353/pbm.2021.0002

Hyman, S. H. (2010). The diagnosis of mental disorders: The problem of reification. *Annual Review of Clinical Psychology*, *6*, 12.1–12.25. https://doi.org/10.1146/annurev.clinpsy.3.022806.091532

Insel, T. R., & Cuthbert, B. N. (2009). Endophenotypes: Bridging genomic complexity and disorder heterogeneity. *Biological Psychiatry*, *66*(11), 988–989. https://doi.org/10.1016/j.biopsych.2009.10.008

Insel, T., Cuthbert, B., Garvey, M., Heinssen, R., Kozak, M., Pine, D. S., Quinn, K., Sanislow, C. A., & Wang, P. (2010). Research Domain Criteria (RDoC): Developing a valid diagnostic framework for research on mental disorders. *American Journal of Psychiatry*, *167*, 748–751. http://dx.doi.org/10.1176/appi.ajp.2010.09091379

Insel, T. R., Gogtay, N. (2014). National Institute of Mental Health clinical trials: New opportunities, new expectations. *JAMA Psychiatry*, *71*(7): 745–746. https://doi.org/10.1001/jamapsychiatry.2014.426

Ito, M., Horikoshi, M., Kato, N., Oe, Y., Fujisato, H., Yamaguchi, K., Nakajima, S., Miyamae, M., Toyota, A., Okumura, Y., & Takebayashi, Y. (2023). Efficacy of the unified protocol for transdiagnostic cognitive-behavioral treatment for depressive and anxiety disorders: A randomized controlled trial. *Psychological Medicine*, *53*(7), 3009–3020. https://doi.org/10.1017/S0033291721005067

Kapur, S., Phillips, A. G., & Insel, T. R. (2012). Why has it taken so long for biological psychiatry to develop clinical tests and what to do about it? *Molecular Psychiatry*, *12*, 1174–1179. https://doi.org/10.1038/mp.2012.105

Karalunas, S. L., Fair, D., Musser, E. D., Aykes, K., Iyer, S. P., Nigg, J. T. (2014). Subtyping attention-deficit/hyperactivity disorder using temperament dimensions: Toward biologically based nosologic criteria. *JAMA Psychiatry*, *71*(9), 1015–1024. https://doi.org/10.1001/jamapsychiatry.2014.763

Karalunas, S. L., Gustafsson, H. C., Dieckmann, N. F., Tipsord, J., Mitchell, S. H., & Nigg, J. T. (2017). Heterogeneity in development of aspects of working memory predicts longitudinal attention deficit hyperactivity disorder symptom change. *Journal of Abnormal Psychology*, *126*(6), 774–792. https://doi.org/10.1037/abn0000292

Karalunas, S. L., Gustafsson, H. C., Fair, D., Musser, E. D., & Nigg, J. T. (2019). Do we need an irritable subtype of ADHD? Replication and extension of a promising temperament profile approach to ADHD subtyping. *Psychological Assessment*, *31*(2), 236–247. https://doi.org/10.1037/pas0000664

Karcher, N. R., & Barch, D. M. (2021). The ABCD study: Understanding the development of risk for mental and physical health outcomes. *Neuropsychopharmacology*, *46*(1), 131–142. https://doi.org/10.1038/s41386-020-0736-6

Keller, A. S., Moore, T. M., Luo, A., Visoki, E., Gataviņš, M. M., Shetty, A., Cui, Z., Fan, Y., Feczko, E., Houghton, A., Li, H., Mackey, A. P., Miranda-Dominguez, O., Pines, A., Shinohara, R. T., Sun, K. Y., Fair, D. A., Satterthwaite, T. D., & Barzilay, R. (2024). A general exposome factor explains individual differences in functional brain network topography and cognition in youth. *Developmental Cognitive Neuroscience*, *66*, 101370. https://doi.org/10.1016/j.dcn.2024.101370

Keller, A. S., Pines, A. R., Shanmugan, S., Sydnor, V. J., Cui, Z., Bertolero, M. A., Barzilay, R., Alexander-Bloch, A. F., Byington, N., Chen, A., Conan, G. M., Davatzikos, C., Feczko, E., Hendrickson, T. J., Houghton, A., Larsen, B., Li, H., Miranda-Dominguez, O., Roalf, D. R. . . . & Satterthwaite, T. D. (2023). Personalized functional brain network topography is associated with individual differences in youth cognition. *Nature Communications*, *14*(1), 8411. https://www.nature.com/articles/s41467-023-44087-0

Keller, M., Hirschfeld, R., & Hanks, D. (1997). Double depression: A distinct subtype of unipolar depression *Journal of Affective Disorders*, *45*(1–2), 65–73.

Kessler, R. C., Merikangas, K. R., Berglund, P., Eaton, W. W., Koretz, D. S., Walters, M. S. (2003). Mild disorders should not be eliminated from the DSM-V. *Archive of General Psychiatry*, *60*, 1117–1122.

Kievit, R. A., Lindenberger, U., Goodyer, I. M., Jones, P. B., Fonagy, P., Bullmore, E. T., & Dolan, R. J. (2019). Mutualistic coupling between vocabulary and reasoning supports cognitive development during late adolescence and early adulthood. *Corrigendum. Psychological Science*, *30*(6), 955–959. https://doi.org/10.1177/0956797619843895

Kirkbride, J. B., Anglin, D. M., Colman, I., Dykxhoorn, J., Jones, P. B., Patalay, P., Pitman, A., Soneson, E., Steare, T., Wright, T., & Griffiths, S. L. (2024). The social determinants of mental health and disorder: Evidence, prevention and recommendations. *World Psychiatry*, *23*(1): 58–90. https://doi.org/10.1002/wps.21160

Knodt, A. R., Elliott, M. L., Whitman, E. T., Winn, A., Addae, A., Ireland, D., Poulton, R., Ramrakha, S., Caspi, A., Moffitt, T. E., & Hariri, A. R. (2023). Test–retest reliability and predictive utility of a macroscale principal functional connectivity gradient. *Human Brain Mapping*, *44*(18), 6399–6417.https://doi.org/10.1002/hbm.26517

Kotov, R., Krueger, R. F., & Watson, D. (2018). A paradigm shift in psychiatric classification: The Hierarchical Taxonomy of Psychopathology (HiTOP). *World Psychiatry*, *17*, 25–26.

Kozak, M. J., & Cuthbert, B. N. (2016). The NIMH Research Domain Criteria initiative: Background, issues, and pragmatics. *Psychophysiology*, *53*(3), 286–97. https://doi.org/10.1111/psyp.12518

Kraemer, H. C. (2015). Research Domain Criteria (RDoC) and the DSM—Two methodological approaches to mental health diagnosis. *JAMA: Psychiatry*, *72*(12), 1163–1164.

Kraemer, H. C., Noda, A., O'Hara, R. (2004). Categorical versus dimensional approaches to diagnosis: Methodological challenges. *Journal of Psychiatric Research*, *38*, 17–25. https://doi.org/10.1016/s0022-3956(03)00097-9

Krueger, R. F. (1999). The structure of common mental disorders. *Archives of General Psychiatry*, *56*(10), 921–926. https://doi.org/10.1001/archpsyc.56.10.921

Krystal, A. D., Pizzagalli, D. A., Smoski, M., Mathew, S. J., Nurnberger, J., Lisanby, S. H., Iosifescu, D., Murrough, J. W., Yang, H., Weiner, R. D., Calabrese, J. R., Sanacora, G., Hermes, G., Keefe, R. S. E., Song, A., Goodman, W., Szabo, S. T., Whitton, A. E., Gao, K., & Potter, W. Z. (2020). A randomized proof-of-mechanism trial applying the "fast-fail" approach to evaluating κ-opioid antagonism as a treatment for anhedonia. *Nature Medicine*, *26*(5), 760–768. https://doi.org/10.1038/s41591-020-0806-7

Kupfer, D. J., First, M. B., Regier, D. A. (2002). Introduction. In D. J. Kupfer, M. B. First, & D. A. Regier (Eds.), *A research agenda for DSM—V* (pp. xv–xxiii). American Psychiatric Association.

Lahey, B. B., Moore, T. M., Kaczkurkin, A. N., & Zald, D. H. (2021). Hierarchical models of psychopathology: Empirical support, implications, and remaining issues. *World Psychiatry*, *20*(1): 57–63. https://doi.org/10.1002/wps.20824.

Lang, P. J. (1969). The mechanics of desensitization and the laboratory study of human fear. In C.M. Franks (Ed.), *Behavior therapy: Appraisal and status* (pp. 160–191). McGraw-Hill.

Lang, P. J., Herring, D. R., Duncan, C., Richter, J., Sege, C. T., Weymar, M., Limberg, A., Hamm, A. O., & Bradley, M. M. (2018). The startle-evoked potential: Negative affect and severity of pathology in anxiety/mood disorders. *Biological Psychiatry*, 3(7), 626–634. https://doi.org/10.1016/j.bpsc.2017.07.006

Lang, P. J., McTeague, L. M., & Bradley, M. M. (2016). RDoC, DSM, and the reflex physiology of fear: A biodimensional analysis of the anxiety disorders spectrum. *Psychophysiology*, *53*(3), 336–347. https://doi.org/10.1111/psyp.12462

Larsen, B., & Luna, B. (2018). Adolescence as a neurobiological critical period for the development of higher-order cognition. *Neuroscience and Biobehavioral Reviews*, 94, 179–195. https://doi.org/10.1016/j.neubiorev.2018.09.005

Little, T. D., Cunningham, W. A., Shahar, G., & Widaman, K. F. (2002). To parcel or not to parcel: Exploring the question, weighing the merits. *Structural Equation Modeling*, 9, 151–173.

Luca, M. (2019). Maladaptive Rumination as a Transdiagnostic Mediator of Vulnerability and Outcome in Psychopathology. *Journal of Clinical Medicine Research*, 8(3). https://doi.org/10.3390/jcm8030314

Maher, B. (1970). Introduction to Psychopathology, McGraw Hill.

Mahony, B. W., Tu, D., Rau, S., Liu, S., Lalonde, F. M., Alexander-Bloch, A. F., Satterthwaite, T. D., Shinohara, R. T., Bassett, D. S., Milham, M. P., & Raznahan, A. (2023). IQ Modulates Coupling Between Diverse Dimensions of Psychopathology in Children and Adolescents. *Journal of the American Academy of Child and Adolescent Psychiatry*, 62(1), 59–73. https://doi.org/10.1016/j.jaac.2022.06.015

Mareva, S., CALM team, & Holmes, J. (2019). Transdiagnostic associations across communication, cognitive, and behavioural problems in a developmentally at-risk population: a network approach. *BMC Pediatrics*, 19(1), 452. https://doi.org/10.1186/s12887-019-1818-7

Martin, J. et al. (2014). "Genetic Risk for Attention-Deficit/Hyperactivity Disorder Contributes to Neurodevelopmental Traits in the General Population." *Biological Psychiatry* 76 (8), 664–761.

Martin, J. et al. (2015). "Neurocognitive Abilities in the General Population and Composite Genetic Risk Scores for Attention-Deficit Hyperactivity Disorder." *Journal of Child Psychology and Psychiatry*, *56*(6), 648–656.

McGorry, P. D., Hickie, I. B., Yung, A. R., Pantelis, C., & Jackson H.J. (2006). Clinical staging of psychiatric disorders: a heuristic framework for choosing earlier, safer and more effective interventions. *Australian & New Zealand. Journal of Psychiatry*, *40*(8), 616–622. doi: 10.1080/j.1440-1614.2006.01860.x

McGorry, P. D., & Mei, C. (2018). Early intervention in youth mental health: progress and future directions. *Evidence-Based Mental Health*, 21(4), 182–184. https://doi.org/10.1136/ebmental-2018-300060

McLaughlin, K. A., & Gabard-Durnam, L. (2022). Experience-driven plasticity and the emergence of psychopathology: A mechanistic framework integrating development and the environment into the Research Domain Criteria (RDoC) model. *Journal of Psychopathology and Clinical Science, 131*(6), 575–587. https://doi.org/10.1037/abn0000598.

McLaughlin, K. A., & Nolen-Hoeksema, S. (2011). Rumination as a transdiagnostic factor in depression and anxiety. *Behaviour Research and Therapy*, 49(3), 186–193. https://doi.org/10.1016/j.brat.2010.12.006

McTeague, L. M., & Lang, P. J. (2012). The anxiety spectrum and the reflex physiology of defense: From circumscribed fear to broad distress. *Depression and Anxiety*, 29, 264–281. doi: 10.1002/da.21891

Meyer-Lindenberg, A. & Weinberger, D. R. (2006) Intermediate Phenotypes and Genetic Mechanisms of Psychiatric Disorders. *Nature Reviews Neuroscience, 7*, 818–827. doi.org/10.1038/nrn1993

Michelini, G., Palumbo, I. M., DeYoung, C. G., Latzman, R. D., & Kotov, R. (2021). Linking RDoC and HiTOP: A new interface for advancing psychiatric nosology and neuroscience. *Clinical Psychology Review*, 86, 102025. https://doi.org/10.1016/j.cpr.2021.102025

Miller, G.A., & Rockstroh, B. (2013). Endophenotypes in psychopathology research: where do we stand? *Annual Review of Clinical Psychology*, 9, 177–213. doi:10.1146/annurev-clinpsy-050212-185540

Mittal, V. A, & Wakschlag, L. S. (2017). Research domain criteria (RDoC) grows up: Strengthening neurodevelopment investigation within the RDoC framework. *Journal of Affective Disorders, 216*, 30–35. doi: 10.1016/j.jad.2016.12.011

Morris S. E., & Cuthbert, B. N. (2012). Research Domain Criteria: Cognitive systems, neural circuits, and dimensions of behavior. *Dialogues in Clinical Neuroscience, 14*(1), 29–37. PMCID: PMC3341647

Morris, S. E., Sanislow, C. A., Pacheco, J., Vaidyanathan, U., Gordon, J. A., & Cuthbert, B. N. (2022). Revisiting the Seven Pillars of RDoC. *BMC Medicine, 22, Article number: 220*, 1 –11. doi.org/10.1186/s12916-022-02414-0

Nardou, R., Lewis, E. M., Rothhaas, R., Xu, R., Yang, A., Boyden, E., & Dölen, G. (2019). Oxytocin-dependent reopening of a social reward learning critical period with MDMA. *Nature, 569*(7754), 116–120. https://doi.org/10.1038/s41586-019-1075-9

Narrow, W. E., & Kuhl, E. A. (2011). Dimensional approaches to psychiatric diagnosis in DSM-5. *Journal of Mental Health Policy and Economics, 14*(4), 197–200.

National Institute of Mental Health (NIMH) (2008). The National Institute of Mental Health Strategic Plan. Bethesda, MD: Author. NIH Publication 08-6368 (PDF Version). Author. https://www.hsdl.org/?view&did=755067 (accessed March 4, 2024).

National Institute of Mental Health (NIMH). (2019). NIMH RDoC Initiative: Development and Environment in RDoC Workshop (2019). Research Domain Criteria (RDoC) initiative: Development and Environment in RDoC Workshop—Proceedings and thematic summary (PDF version). Bethesda, MD: Author. https://www.nimh.nih.gov/sites/default/files/documents/RDoC-Development-Environment-Workshop-Summary-508.pdf (accessed March 4, 2024).

National Institute of Mental Health (NIMH). (2024). The National Institute of Mental Health Individually Measured Phenotypes to Advance Computational Translation in Mental Health (IMPACT-MH). Bethesda, MD: Author. https://impact-mh.org (accessed March 4, 2024).

Nigg, J. T. (2022). Parsing ADHD with temperament traits. *Current Directions in Psychological Science*, 31(4), 324–332. https://doi.org/10.1177/09637214221098079

Nigg, J. T., Goldsmith, H. H., & Sachek, J. (2004). Temperament and attention deficit hyperactivity disorder: The development of a multiple pathway model. *Journal of Clinical Child and Adolescent Psychology*, 33(1), 42–53. https://doi.org/10.1207/S15374424JCCP3301_5

Nolen-Hoeksema, S. (1991). Responses to depression and their effects on the duration of depressive episodes. *Journal of Abnormal Psychology, 100*(4), 569–582. https://doi.org/10.1037//0021-843x.100.4.569

Pacheco, J., Garvey, M. A., Sarampote, C. S., Cohen, E. D., Murphy, E. R. & Friedman-Hill, S. R. (2022). Annual research review: The contributions of the RDoC research framework on understanding the neurodevelopmental origins, progression and treatment of mental illnesses. *Journal of Child Psychology and Psychiatry*, *63*(4), 360–376. https://doi.org/10.1111/jcpp.13543

Pattwell, S. S., Duhoux, S., Hartley, C. A., Johnson, D. C., Jing, D., Elliott, M. D., Ruberry, E. J., Powers, A., Mehta, N., Yang, R. R., Soliman, F., Glatt, C. E., Casey, B. J., Ninan, I., & Lee, F. S. (2012). Altered fear learning across development in both mouse and human. *Proceedings of the National Academy of Sciences of the United States of America*, *109*(40), 16318–16323. https://doi.org/10.1073/pnas.1206834109

Pine, D. S., & Fox, N. A. (2015). Childhood antecedents and risk for adult mental disorders. *Annual Review of Psychology*, *66*, 459–485. https://doi.org/10.1146/annurev-psych-010814-015038

Regier, D. A., Narrow, W. E., & Rae, D. S. (2004). For DSM-V, it's the "Disorder Threshold," stupid [letter]. *Archives of General Psychology*, *61*, 1052.

Rhemtulla, M., Brosseau-Liard, P. É., & Savalei, V. (2012). When can categorical variables be treated as continuous? A comparison of robust continuous and categorical SEM estimation methods under suboptimal conditions. *Psychological Methods*, *17*, 354–373.

Robins, E., & Guze, S. B. (1970). Establishment of diagnostic validity in psychiatric illness: Its application to schizophrenia. *The American Journal of Psychiatry*, *126*(7), 983–986. https://doi.org/10.1176/ajp.126.7.983

Ruscio, A. M., Gentes, E. L., Jones, J. D., Hallion, L. S., Coleman, E. S., & Swendsen, J. (2015). Rumination predicts heightened responding to stressful life events in major depressive disorder and generalized anxiety disorder. *Journal of Abnormal Psychology*, *124*(1), 17–26. https://doi.org/10.1037/abn0000025

Sambuco, N., Bradley, M., Herring, D., Hillbrandt, K., & Lang, P. J. (2020). Transdiagnostic trauma severity in anxiety and mood disorders: Functional brain activity during emotional scene processing. *Psychophysiology*, *57*(1), e13349. https://doi.org/10.1111/psyp.13349

Sanislow, C. A., Little, T. D., Ansell, E. B., Grilo, C. M., Daversa, M., Markowitz, J. C., Pinto, A., Shea, M. T., Yen, S., Skodol, A. E., Morey, L. C., Gunderson, J. G., Zanarini, M. C., & McGlashan, T. H. (2009). Ten-year stability and latent structure of the DSM-IV schizotypal, borderline, avoidant, and obsessive-compulsive personality disorders. *Journal of Abnormal Psychology*, *118*(3), 507–519.

Sanislow, C. A., Morris, S. E., Cuthbert, B. N., & Pacheco, J. (2022). Development and environment in the NIMH Research Domain Criteria. *Journal of Psychopathology and Clinical Science*, *131*, 653–659.

Sanislow, C. A., Pine, D. S., Quinn, K. J., Kozak, M. J., Garvey, M. A., Heinssen, R. K, Wang, P. S., & Cuthbert, B. N. (2010). Developing constructs for psychopathology research: Research Domain Criteria. *Journal of Abnormal Psychology*, *119*(4), 631–639.

Seidlitz, J., Nadig, A., Liu, S., Bethlehem, R. A. I., Vértes, P. E., Morgan, S. E., Váša, F., Romero-Garcia, R., Lalonde, F. M., Clasen, L. S., Blumenthal, J. D., Paquola, C., Bernhardt, B., Wagstyl, K., Polioudakis, D., de la Torre-Ubieta, L., Geschwind, D. H., Han, J. C., Lee, N. R., . . . Raznahan, A. (2020). Transcriptomic and cellular decoding of regional brain vulnerability to neurogenetic disorders. *Nature Communications*, *11*(1), 3358. https://www.nature.com/articles/s41467-020-17051-5

Shah, J. L., Jones, N., van Os, J., McGorry, P. D., & Gülöksüz, S. (2022). Early intervention service systems for youth mental health: Integrating pluripotentiality, clinical staging, and transdiagnostic lessons from early psychosis. *The Lancet. Psychiatry*, *9*(5), 413–422. https://doi.org/10.1016/S2215-0366(21)00467-3

Shaw, Z. A., Conway, C. C., & Starr, L. R. (2021). Distinguishing transdiagnostic versus disorder-specific pathways between ruminative brooding and internalizing psychopathology in adolescents: A latent variable modeling approach. *Research on Child and Adolescent Psychopathology*, *49*(10), 1319–1331. https://doi.org/10.1007/s10802-020-00714-8

Skodol, A. E., Morey, L. C., Bender, D. S., & Oldham, J. M. (2015). The alternative DSM-5 model for personality disorders: A clinical application. *American Journal of Psychiatry*, *172*(7): 606–613. https://doi.org/10.1176/appi.ajp.2015.14101220

Spitzer, R. L., Endicott, J., & Robins, E. (1975). Research Diagnostic Criteria for a selected group of functional Disorders. New York, New York Psychiatric Institute.

Spitzer, R. L., Endicott, J., Robins, E. (1978). Research Diagnostic Criteria: Rationale and reliability. *Archive of General Psychiatry*, *35*, 773–782.

St. Pourcain, B., Robinson, E. B., Anttila, V., Sullivan, B. B., Maller, J., Golding, J., Skuse, D., Ring, S., Evans, D. M., Zammit, S., Fisher, S. E., Neale, B. M., Anney, R. J. L., Ripke, S., Hollegaard, M. V., Werge, T., Ronald, A., Grove, J., Hougaard, D. M., . . . iPSYCH-SSI-Broad Autism Group (2018). ASD and schizophrenia show distinct developmental profiles in common genetic overlap with population-based social communication difficulties. *Molecular Psychiatry*, *23*(2), 263–270. https://doi.org/10.1038/mp.2016.198

Stoyanov, D., Telles-Correia, D., Cuthbert, B. N. (2019). The Research Domain Criteria (RDoC) and the historical roots of psychopathology: A viewpoint. *European Psychiatry*, *57*, 58–60. https://doi.org/10.1016/j.eurpsy.2018.11.007. Epub January 21, 2019.

Uhlhaas, P. J., Davey, C. G., Mehta, U. M., Shah, J., Torous, J., Allen, N., Avenevoli, S., Bella-Awusah, T., Chanen, A., Hai, Y., Chen, E., Correll, C. U., Q Do, K., Fisher, H., Frangou, S., Hickie, I., Keshavan, M. S., Konrad, K., Lee, F., . . . Wood, S. (2023). Towards a youth mental health paradigm: A perspective and roadmap. *Molecular Psychiatry*, *28*(8), 3171–3181. https://doi.org/10.1038/s41380-023-02202-z

Vaidyanathan, U., Nelson, L. D., & Patrick, C. J. (2012). Clarifying domains of internalizing psychopathology using neurophysiology. *Psychological Medicine*, *42*, 447–459. http://dx.doi.org/10.1017/S0033291711001528

Vaidyanathan, U., Patrick, C. J., & Cuthbert, B. N. (2009). Linking dimensional models of internalizing psychopathology to neurobiological systems: Affect-modulated startle as an indicator of fear and distress disorders and affiliated traits. *Psychological Bulletin*, *135*(6), 909–942. https://doi.org/10.1037/a0017222

Volkow, N. D., Koob, G. F., Croyle, R. T., Bianchi, D. W., Gordon, J. A., Koroshetz, W. J., Pérez-Stable, E. J., Riley, W. T., Bloch, M. H., Conway, K., Deeds, B. G., Dowling, G. J., Grant, S., Howlett, K. D., Matochik, J. A., Morgan, G. D., Murray, M. M., Noronha, A., Spong, C. Y., . . . Weiss, S. R. B. (2018). The conception of the ABCD study: From substance use to a broad NIH collaboration. *Developmental Cognitive Neuroscience*, *32*, 4–7. https://doi.org/10.1016/j.dcn.2017.10.002

Wakschlag, L. S., Briggs-Gowan, M. J., Choi, S. W., Nichols, S. R., Kestler, J., Burns, J. L., Carter, A. S., & Henry, D. (2014). Advancing a multidimensional, developmental spectrum approach to preschool disruptive behavior. *Journal of the American Academy of Child and Adolescent Psychiatry*, *53*(1), 82–96.e3. https://doi.org/10.1016/j.jaac.2013.10.011

Watson, D. (2005). Rethinking the mood and anxiety disorders: A quantitative hierarchical model for DSM-V. *Journal of Abnormal Psychology*, *114*, 522–536. https://doi.org/10.1037/0021-843X.114.4.522

Weinberg, A., & Hajcak, G. (2011). Longer term test–retest reliability of error-related brain activity. *Psychophysiology*, 48, 1420–1425. https://doi.org/10.1111/j.1469–8986.2011.01206.x

Williams, T. F., & Simms, L. J. (2018). Personality traits and maladaptivity: Unipolarity versus bipolarity. *Journal of Personality*, *86*(5), 888–901. https://doi.org/10.1111/jopy.12363

World Health Organization (WHO) (2024). New manual released to support diagnosis of mental, behavioural and neurodevelopmental disorders added in ICD-11. https://www.who.int/news/item/08-03-2024-new-manual-released-to-support-diagnosis-of-mental--behavioural-and-neurodevelopmental-disorders-added-in-icd11#:~:text=The%20ICD%2D11%20CDDR%20are,as%20nurses%2C%20occupational%20therapists%20and (accessed March 31, 2024).

Yung, A. R., & McGorry, P. D. (1996). The prodromal phase of first-episode psychosis: Past and current conceptualizations. *Schizophrenia Bulletin*, *22*(2), 353–370.

Zachar, P., Krueger, R. F., & Kendler, K. S. (2016). Personality disorder in DSM-5: An oral history. *Psychological Medicine*, *46*(1): 1–10. https://doi.org/10.1017/S0033291715001543

Zhi, D., Jiang, R., Pearlson, G., Fu, Z., Qi, S., Yan, W., Feng, A., Xu, M., Calhoun, V., & Sui, J. (2024). Triple interactions between the environment, brain, and behavior in children: An ABCD study. *Biological Psychiatry*, *95*(9), 828–838. https://doi.org/10.1016/j.biopsych.2023.12.019

CHAPTER 8

Network Theories of Psychopathology

THOMAS L. RODEBAUGH, JULIA LEVITAN, AND GABRIELLE R. MESSNER

Introduction

WHAT is central to depression? The answer depends on what the reader thinks depression is, as well as in what sense something could be central to it. Some might hold that depression is nothing but a fiction, agreed upon by our current society but with no central characteristics beyond what our society attributes to it. Others, perhaps adhering to a stringent version of a medical model, might affirm that what matters about depression is whether a person is depressed or not. Still others might view depression as one of several continuous dimensions on which people differ, or perhaps even a factor emerging from several such continuous dimensions, such as depressed mood and anhedonia.

Network theory offers a view on mental disorders that is distinct from those above. As first proposed by Borsboom (2008), network theory proposes a "causal systems perspective, which holds that disorders are causal networks consisting of symptoms and direct causal relations between them" (p. 1089). Network theory is often presented as opposing medical and latent-variable-based dimensional approaches. What is central to depression, from this point of view, is not just whether people are depressed or not. It is also not a set of underlying continuous dimensions explaining symptoms. Indeed, network theory suggests that what is central to depression may be quite complicated. It might be a specific symptom or set of symptoms, but it might also be no specific symptom. Instead, depression might have an empty center, and what is central to it might be all the relations between a set of symptoms.

In this chapter we argue that the proposed distinctions between network theory and other theories of psychopathology have some elements of truth, but these proposed distinctions have often been simplified or exaggerated. One key to understanding the network perspective and how it associates with other perspectives is to attend to what the typical practices are in the arena of network analysis, as well as whether such practices are distinct from those used in other frameworks. We view network theory's central thesis as the following: Multiple, ongoing causal processes lead to and maintain clinical problems, and understanding the complex causal networks that arise from these processes is necessary to making scientific and clinical progress. We review the literature that has accumulated around the concept of network theory. We find that much of this literature has ignored the central thesis of network theory and focused on using its associated methodologies, which include a set of statistical practices often referred to as network analyses. Network theory is not the only theory of psychopathology that has had this issue, but we expect progress to be more rapid when researchers attend to the central thesis of network theory. If the thesis is that clinical problems, like depression, involve complex causal processes, we need theories, data, and methods that can give insight into complex causal processes.

Origins of Network Theory

The formalization of a network theory perspective on psychopathology is most often attributed to Borsboom. Borsboom's (2008) theoretical article elegantly sets out multiple viewpoints on psychopathology and describes how these viewpoints comport with specific measurement models (e.g., the latent factor model for dimensional theories). The final model presented is a network model, which Borsboom refers to as a "causal systems perspective." Borsboom proposes that the relationships among symptoms reflect direct causal associations and argues that this perspective stands in opposition to conceptualizations of psychological disorders as categorical or continuous latent variables.

Although the application of this causal systems perspective to psychopathology was seen as novel, we (and others) see numerous conceptual precursors. Borsboom (2008) connects his proposed causal systems perspective to dynamical systems theory (Thelen & Smith, 1994), which conceptualizes developmental phenomena in terms of complex, nonlinear dynamic systems. Borsboom also references the causal modeling framework first proposed by Morton and Frith (1995), which is presented as a tool for visualizing the causal relations among biological, cognitive, and behavioral factors implicated in developmental disorders. McNally (2011, 2016) traces network theory back to Boyd's (1991) conceptualization of biological species as a cluster of properties that hang together and maintain homeostasis regardless of environmental fluctuations. Such conceptual models have undoubtedly influenced clinical psychologists who oppose essentialist accounts of psychopathology (i.e., which hold that features of a disorder arise from an underlying essence; Kendler et al., 2011). Although these ecological and developmental models provided a theoretical foundation for Borsboom's causal systems perspective, they stopped short of specifying methods to evaluate these causal relations empirically.

By contrast, van der Maas and colleagues (2006) present a way to empirically model the positive manifold of correlations among scores on cognitive tasks. That is, cognitive tasks tend to all correlate positively even when the tasks might otherwise be thought to be distinct (i.e., they display a positive manifold). We will return to the positive manifold repeatedly in this chapter, because psychological symptoms also typically display a positive manifold in cross-sectional data. Regarding cognitive tasks, van der Maas and colleagues argue that the positive manifold results from a system of reciprocal causation and interactions among different cognitive processes over the course of development, and provide a corresponding computational model. Like Borsboom (2008), the authors offer this model as an alternative to the prominent interpretation of the positive manifold as evidence of an underlying or latent variable (in the case of intelligence, this might be a general intelligence factor, *g*). However, the authors note that their simulations of the mutualism model and a latent factor model were statistically equivalent in several instances, a finding that recurs in the network literature.

Some years later, in their seminal paper, Cramer and colleagues (2012) posited a network theory of personality, proposing that personality dimensions are the result of a network of dependent factors, including behaviors, affect, and cognition. They distinguished this viewpoint from what they saw as the dominant theory that personality dimensions are latent constructs that inherently cause certain behaviors, affect, and cognition. It is not difficult for a reader interested in psychopathology to extend their arguments to that context. This paper sparked controversy and a series of responses. Some who disagreed with Cramer et al. (2012) argued for the precedence of the dominant theory (e.g., Guillaume–Hanes et al., 2012; Schimmack & Gere, 2012; Terracciano & McCrae, 2012). Others generally agreed with the premise put forth by Cramer and colleagues but noted potential problems or suggested areas of further research. For example, Costantini and Perugini (2012) pointed out that even network models of single items still involve aggregation, as do latent variable models. That is, even single item assessments (e.g., irritability) represent an aggregate of behavior, affect, and other factors. Accordingly, Constantini and Perugini called for a clearer description of the interplay between factor analysis and network analysis, which eventually came to fruition (see the section "Beyond Straw Men" below, among other sections). The authors also noted problems that can occur in visual inspection of network figures and uncritical acceptance of centrality indices, as both can be misleading (e.g., neither placement of nodes in a figure nor high centrality indices guarantee that a node is important).

Arguably the underlying themes that animate discussions of network theory versus other approaches are far older than suggested by the citations above. One frequently debated metaphor introduced by Cramer and colleagues (2012) is that a flock of birds is made of the set of relations among birds, not some unseen latent variable of flockness. That is, the flock is not really unitary, or perhaps we might call it only provisionally unitary: It could change at any moment, if a bird leaves the flock. The idea that what we often present as unitary may only be provisionally or fictionally unitary can be traced through both Western and Eastern philosophy (Giles, 1993). On the Western side we have David Hume declaring that the self is a fictional construct produced by the sensory impression that a set of parts are associated. On the Eastern side we have the Buddhist assertion that there is no central self, but only a group of components that we refer to, for convenience, as a self (again, see Giles, 1993 for an introduction to these concepts and comparison across cultures). It might appear fanciful to compare network theory to philosophical concepts from Hume or Buddhism, but we believe this comparison is more useful than it might first appear, and we will return to it.

Network Theory versus Other Approaches

When writing about network theory, researchers often assert that: (1) other approaches are categorical, network theory is not; (2) other approaches hypothesize single unitary latent causes, network theorists do not; (3) other approaches do not match clinician intuition, whereas network theory does. We believe these assertions lead to straw man arguments. That is, those researchers who have made these assertions argue for network theory by arguing against a simplistic (or straw man) version of other approaches, yet the proposed distinctions do not really separate network theory from other approaches as they are actually practiced, because the practice is not as simple as the straw man argument suggests. Again, we think focusing on practices is essential here, because we do not believe that any perspective can be understood apart from its associated practices. We should note here that some researchers and theorists who initially asserted these arguments have since been authors on papers that have modified or partially retracted them (Bringmann et al., 2022). Nevertheless, we find some of the reformulated arguments similarly straw-man-baiting, and many authors continue to recapitulate versions of these arguments. To avoid straw man arguments, we wish to be clear about what is typical about other approaches and network theory, which should lead us to an improved ability to assess the network theory literature.

First, contrary to the assertion that categorical approaches are concerned only with categories, proponents of such approaches routinely use continuous variables as well. Those using a categorical approach generally hold that categories are ultimately more important, useful, or descriptive of nature than continua. Meaningful levels of severity of a problem are typically acknowledged in the medical model, although the researchers doing the work may hold that the diagnosis is more important than the severity level. A person is only depressed if she has enough symptoms, but the number of symptoms she has may still have an impact. Indeed, the DSM has long included level of severity for multiple disorders (especially mood disorders) to be rated alongside the diagnoses themselves (American Psychiatric Association, 1987, 1994, 2013). Some authors have updated this argument and have asserted that network theory stands in contrast to biological models of psychopathology that assume symptoms are caused by biological processes (Bringmann et al., 2022). However, our point remains the same: In our experience it is rare to encounter researchers who hold that the only causes of mental disorders are biological, in the same way that it is rare to encounter researchers who assert, or even act as if, only categories are useful.

In addition, network theory, or at least network theory researchers, are not immune to the appeal of a categorical approach. Many network theory projects have involved researchers searching for "important" symptoms, which would seem to imply that some are not important. (The reader is invited to look in their preferred search engine for "psychopathology network analysis important symptoms" and review the results.) Given that the central thesis of network theory involves the direct relation among symptoms, it is far from obvious why a focus on a categorical distinction between important and less-important symptoms should emerge from this thesis. Network theorists also often study specific categorically defined populations, and the emphasis in early network literature on understanding comorbidity (e.g., Cramer et al., 2010) would have been an empty endeavor if categories were of no interest. The reader might protest that of course all researchers are obliged to work with both continua and categories, but we think it is important to emphasize that they really are not. If network theorists or medical model adherents really held that either categories or continua were not important, they would not be obliged to use both concepts. That they do use both concepts but with different emphases is exactly our point.

Similarly, contemporary dimensional approaches rarely hold that a given disorder is attributable to a single latent dimension, as often asserted by network theorists (for a review of this tendency and an alternate refutation, see Bringmann & Eronen, 2018). The Hierarchical Taxonomy of Psychopathology (HiTOP; see Pham et al., this volume) is one example. These approaches are far more likely to assert that mental disorders involve some combination of continuous latent dimensions. Thus, in these approaches it is not asserted that depression is caused by a single latent construct, but instead by more than one. Although this may seem to be a minor difference from what is typically asserted, given that some approaches taken by network theorists can involve a small number of causally connected symptoms (Wichers et al., 2020; Wichers & Groot, 2016), the clear distinction between the supposed latent approach and network approach only holds if we can say that one involves single causes and the other multiple causes. Notably, multiple network theory researchers appear to have accordingly deemphasized or dropped this argument (Bringmann et al., 2022), although, as noted above, the argument continues to be commonly repeated in the literature.

An important point here is that not all researchers use latent variables for the same reasons. For many latent variable theorists (whom we can perhaps refer to as "pragmatic"), latent variable models are primarily a solution to a measurement problem and not primarily causal models (Jonas & Markon, 2016). Whereas a network theorist might accuse the latent variable theorist of having a bad causal model, the pragmatic latent variable theorist might accuse a network theorist of bad measurement that can result in distortions in estimated relationships between variables (for a demonstration and a more technical treatment of the issues in the next paragraph, along with others of the same ilk, please see Hallquist et al., 2021).

A pragmatic latent variable theorist might point out to a network theorist that if we think symptoms cause other symptoms, this does not mean we think assessment items cause each other. For example, let's suppose that trouble sleeping causes irritability. What researchers have in their datasets are responses to items about trouble sleeping and irritability—and often a single item for each. On what grounds, the pragmatist wonders, can the network theorists assert that these single items are a good measure of the symptom itself? The pragmatist would prefer to use a latent variable model to handle the measurement challenge but would also point out that psychological symptoms cannot be observed directly. From this point of view there is no bottom to the search for the essential nature of either of these constructs at which we can stop invoking latent (that is, unobserved) variables. Unless one limits oneself to statements like, "saying you are having trouble sleeping causes saying you are irritable," then one is always invoking something beyond what is measured. Notably, trying to be objective does not eliminate this problem. How many nights of sleep measurement are enough to measure bad sleep? What kinds of sleep indices constitute bad sleep? How many judges are enough for determining level of irritability? If network theorists reject latent variables (and not all do), that does not solve this set of problems, it merely eliminates latent variables as the solution to them (cf. Costantini & Perugini, 2012; Schimmack & Gere, 2012).

Importantly, the problem may be more challenging than the preceding paragraph suggests. We see a more radical problem that the mere use of latent variables does not solve, but at least allows the potential to address more fully. Measurement models using latent variables offer the ability to handle sources of method variance or reporter bias that might otherwise contaminate symptom measures (Bauer et al., 2013; Rodebaugh et al., 2010). For example, it has been observed that people who are more likely to endorse standard negative affect items are also more likely to endorse socially undesirable affect items more generally (Pettersson & Turkheimer, 2013). Pettersson and Turkheimer demonstrated that people who endorse items such as "timid" also tend to endorse opposing but equally socially undesirable items such as "manic," although it seems implausible that timid people are really more likely to experience mania. This observation is not isolated and may vary across disorders. People with social anxiety disorder are more likely to report that they are worse on a variety of socially desirable dimensions (Moscovitch et al., 2009). People with the disorder are also more likely to report that their relationships in general are worse, a tendency that extends to ratings of specific friendships as well (Rodebaugh, 2009; Rodebaugh et al., 2014). Yet, their friends do not show such a clear tendency to rate the person with social anxiety disorder as a worse friend than someone without (Rodebaugh et al., 2014). If we want to know about processes within the friendships of people with the disorder, asking them about their friendships may not do the job. Similarly, if we want to know whether bad sleep leads to irritability, we do not want the estimated relationship to be biased by a tendency to complain generally or even to be excessively critical toward the self. It is not hard to find examples of such measurement minefields, but both network theorists and latent variable theorists routinely ignore them. Latent variable models can model such sources of bias relatively readily, but unfortunately they are rarely employed to do so.

A final proposition regarding network theory is that network theory matches clinician intuition better than other approaches. Sometimes the argument is presented in terms of network theory comporting with cognitive or cognitive-behavioral formulations of mental disorders (Bringmann et al., 2022), but the remaining points in this paragraph apply just as well to this version of the argument. We certainly agree that network theory does match an element of clinician intuition, in that clinicians generally prefer theories that include the diversity of experience they see in their clients (even those with identical disorders). However, other approaches also appeal to clinician intuition. Clinicians, including those with a cognitive-behavioral approach, spend most of their time discussing latent variables rather than observed facts. The idea that there are unobserved causes of mental disorders is inherent to the cognitive behavioral approach. Clinicians tell clients that automatic thoughts and underlying dysfunctional beliefs, which the client may be initially unaware of, cause their symptoms. More perniciously, all practitioners we know have struggled at times with assumptions we have made about clients based on their diagnoses or other characteristics; that is, we have categorized clients even when we know it is not helpful. We suspect that additional practitioners may unfortunately lump clients into categories without realizing they have done so, because this tendency is widespread among humans more generally: We like to put things, and people, into categories. Clinicians have all sorts of intuitions matching all sorts of theoretical approaches. That network theory aligns with some of these intuitions is not a firm ground to assess the quality of a theory.

Beyond Straw Men

The reader might infer based on this chapter so far that we believe network theory offers nothing additional beyond the other approaches noted above. On the contrary, if we remove the straw-man-baiting elements of the typically provided argument, we believe there are still some differences between network theory and the theories with which it is often compared. Network theory asserts that groups of causal processes lead to clinical problems, that some of these causal factors may include symptoms, and that ultimately understanding these complex causal networks is necessary to making scientific and clinical progress. From this point of view, putting people into categories is neither necessary nor sufficient for maximizing either scientific understanding or good clinical outcomes, whereas advocates of categorical systems would likely hold that it is necessary or sufficient in at least some cases. Further, from a network theory perspective, expectations are that underlying causal systems will be complex, not a few variables as implied by many other dimensional approaches. Notably, proponents of other dimensional approaches do not necessarily claim that causes are simple, but rather that a relatively small set of dimensions are the important ones. That is, such researchers typically examine a number of symptoms and propose that, relative to the number of symptoms, a smaller number of dimensions are important. Whether many mental disorders (as in HiTOP; see Pham et al., this volume) or a single mental disorder is analyzed (e.g., Mataix-Cols et al., 2005), those taking a dimensional approach assume that the important causes are likely to be fewer than the number of symptoms analyzed. In contrast, network theorists would generally expect that many causes are important and may not be reducible to any smaller set, although analyses of a small set of variables may sometimes help us understand the larger picture.

If we want to truly stop tempting straw man arguments, we should also address the question of network theory versus network analysis (see Sliptetz & Henry, this volume, for more on network analysis). Arguably, there was an early tendency to elide the distinction (e.g., Borsboom, 2008; Cramer et al., 2010). No doubt this was an efficient rhetorical device. Latent variable theories align particularly well with latent variable analyses, making the tendency to align network theory with existing network analytic methods useful for underlining differences. However, current evidence and theory highlight the lack of correspondence between network theory and any analytic framework (e.g., Bringmann & Eronen, 2018; Epskamp, Rhemtulla, et al., 2017). Again, this is not unique to network models: Latent and observed variable models are also not as distinct as one might think (Bentler & Molenaar, 2012). On a related note, an additional concept has emerged of network psychometrics (cf. Costantini et al., 2019). We define these as approaches designed to assess and improve the properties of measures for use in network analysis. Use of neither network analysis nor network psychometrics necessitates that one maintain a stance consistent with network theory.

A Review of Network Theory Literature

In the rest of this chapter, we will review the state of the evidence related to the network theory of psychopathology alongside practical and theoretical issues in pursuing it. We focus our review on work that has advanced our understanding of complex causal networks. For those readers who would prefer a more exhaustive survey, available reviews include an accounting of the publication patterns over 10 years of network perspective papers on psychopathology (Berta et al., 2022), as well as several narrative and systematic reviews (Borsboom et al., 2021; Contreras et al., 2019; Fried & Cramer, 2017; McNally, 2021; Monteleone & Cascino, 2021; Robinaugh et al., 2020),

A Cross-Section of the Literature

As already noted by systematic reviews (e.g., Robinaugh et al., 2020), the overwhelming preponderance of the literature purporting to focus on the network theory of psychopathology involves cross-sectional networks, typically fitted to self-report instrument items collected originally for other purposes. For example, Robinaugh and colleagues found 170 empirical studies that estimated a network structure of which 141 (83%) focused on cross-sectional data. We will not review evidence from these networks beyond making two points. First, there are good reasons to think they can assess some measure properties. That is, from a network psychometrics approach, such networks might allow the assessment of how well measurement functioned. Just as in latent variable models, we can use network analysis to uncover patterns of co-variance between items, and to the extent that we believe these items should co-vary, assessment of the strength of the co-variance allows inference about the quality of measurement, at least in terms of differentiating between people (e.g., the between level). On this latter point, one of the problems with cross-sectional data is that it tells us primarily about differences between people and how those differences relate to each other. However, sometimes this is precisely what we want to know about.

Yet, and second, in our view there is no reason to be optimistic that causal pathways can be recovered from such analyses. There are many reasons for this, perhaps best articulated in recent memory by Rohrer and colleagues (Rohrer, 2018; Rohrer et al., 2022). One way to approach the problem is to consider that any network analysis with cross-sectional data that includes more than two variables is implicitly a cross-sectional mediation analysis, which multiple authors have shown will result in biased pathways that can even switch sign relative to results returned from longitudinal data (Cole & Maxwell, 2003; Maxwell et al., 2011; Maxwell & Cole, 2007). Alternatively, one could focus on the framework of Pearl (2000), in which cross-sectional data is certainly used in some cases. However, Pearl also describes clearly how conditioning on a collider—a variable caused in part by at least two other variables in the analysis—will produce bias. For example, if both irritability and lack of sleep lead to depressed mood, including depressed mood as a predictor of either variable will lead to biased estimates. In cross-sectional data of psychological symptoms there is every reason to think that colliders will be frequent, and yet the data themselves offer us no clues about which variables might be colliders. In network analysis specifically, typical approaches to cross-sectional data condition all variables on one another, which seems sure to produce conditioning on a collider. For example, if it is true that both irritability and lack of sleep lead to depressed mood, a typical network analysis of depressive symptoms will have biased estimates, because all three variables will be conditioned on one another. In fact, to the extent that the proposition of complex causal structures among symptoms is correct, this will produce more colliders than if symptoms were not causing one another. The most complex causal network we could imagine for the three depressive symptoms we are thinking of is all of them causing one another over time. In that case, each variable would be a collider in the analysis of the other two, and thus paths from a cross-sectional network analysis will be biased in unpredictable ways. In short, although researchers have appeared optimistic that network analysis offers a special way to recover causal estimates not available from other methods, there is neither any evidence that they can do so nor any theoretical reason to think they should unless care is taken to deal appropriately with confounders and colliders (cf. Bringmann et al., 2022, who come to a similar conclusion via only partially overlapping arguments). Only theory and data that comport with that theory offer the possibility of meaningful causal inference. When theory predicts reciprocal, complex causal relationships among variables, longitudinal data or data from true experiments are useful: The problem of conditioning on a collider is not an issue if a cause is randomly assigned or multiple waves of data are included (cf. Rohrer et al. 2022).

The paragraph above will have new information for some readers, but most will be familiar with the idea that cross-sectional data are at least not ideal. It might appear paradoxical that so much of the network analysis literature rests on such data, but surely this has occurred because such studies are the easiest to do. Importantly, other literatures are just as vulnerable to this problem, including the latent variable literature. Using structural equation modeling does not banish these problems any more than using network analysis methods does.

A Central Issue

Moving beyond cross-sectional data, most studies that include longitudinal data focus on centrality indices. Centrality indices are easiest to understand if we keep social networks, one use of network analysis, in mind. In a social network, the person who is most connected to others will typically be depicted toward the center of a network figure. Indeed, although other placements of this person would be possible, none would be practical or informative, so this is what is typically done. This person is said to be central to the social network, and one might wonder, "how central are they?" Centrality indices attempt to quantify how central the person is, as well as how different people rank.

As reviewed cogently by Bringmann and colleagues (2019), centrality indices, which have been applied outside of social networks as well, represent an attempt to describe the role of an item in a network, and are often described as a way of determining the importance of the variable at hand. As also reviewed by Bringmann and colleagues, centrality indices had already been developed for other kinds of data and were thus readily available for researchers putting network analysis to use with symptom data. It seems to us that the emphasis on central symptoms puts the convenience cart before the theoretical horse: In many instances they are being used because they are available for use, rather than there being a strong theoretical basis for applying them to psychological symptoms. However, we are even more concerned that such indices may blind us to network theory's (initial) emphasis on the entirety of the network.

Bringmann and colleagues have pointed out that it is unclear whether we should think that centrality measures have anything to say about psychopathology (Bringmann et al., 2019), and we agree with this assessment. Bringmann and colleagues argue that certain assumptions are inherent to commonly used centrality indices, and these assumptions are incongruent with the theoretical understanding of how psychopathological symptoms connect to one another in a network. For example, Bringmann and colleagues note that one assumption of traditional centrality indices is that the network nodes are both distinct (i.e., do not overlap) and interchangeable. Such an assumption may hold for other types of networks. For example, in a social network in which each node represents an individual human being, each individual is typically understood as meaningfully distinct. Further, in many social networks each person is understood to be exchangeable for another in the analysis at hand. For example, for a person with 12 interpersonal relationships to be more central to the network than someone with 11 interpersonal relationships, we have to assume that these people are equivalent to each other in terms of what their relationships mean.

The assumptions of distinctness and equivalency can be questioned, even in social networks. For example, in some social networks not everyone is interchangeable: In a social network mapped onto a business, the hierarchy of positions within the company may mean that individuals should not be assumed to be equivalent. A high-level executive in the company may have fewer relationships, but these relationships may carry more weight and thus centrality indices may lead to false conclusions. A less obvious issue is that one can question that individual humans are really unitary in the sense assumed by centrality indices. As we discussed in the section regarding the origins of network theory, both Hume and Buddhists might assert instead that individuals are not really unitary, at least not in any absolute sense. As prefigured in Constantini and Perugini's early commentary (2012), the issue at hand is whether individual humans are a meaningful level of aggregation for the network. In some cases this may make sense; in others perhaps families, couples, or some other level of analysis is more appropriate.

We expect that most researchers would accept that considering individual humans as distinct and exchangeable would at least often make sense. In contrast, these assumptions seem very strange in psychopathological networks. Psychological symptoms often overlap such that judges are unlikely to agree on the appropriate level of aggregation. Are negative thoughts and negative affect distinct, because they are different aspects of experience (cognition versus emotion), or are they overlapping, because they are hypothesized to cause each other so quickly that only data at the level of seconds could distinguish them? Are items such as "sad" and "blue" distinct or not? Similarly, psychological symptoms often have different levels of importance such that most judges would agree that they are not interchangeable; as Bringmann and colleagues (2019) note, suicidal ideation is an exemplar here, because most judges would agree that it is inappropriate to consider this symptom of depression interchangeable with all others. Thus, the interpretability of centrality indices of psychopathological networks is limited by the violation of certain assumptions inherent to these indices.

There are other problematic assumptions of most centrality indices that Bringmann and colleagues (2019) review. For example, one is that the edges are always positive. Centrality indices were originally intended to represent some form of the shortest distance between nodes (shortest path lengths), with positive values counted as indications of closeness. However, in psychopathological networks, the sign of the value of an edge denotes the directionality of the relationship between nodes; a negative path doesn't make two nodes less related. For all of the issues raised by Bringmann and colleagues, one can imagine alternative metrics or methods that may be more appropriate. One example is the idea of expected influence (Robinaugh et al., 2016), which has the advantage of being a direct analogue to the familiar notions of regression coefficients and percentage of variance accounted for (regardless of the sign of the predictor). Researchers also have multiple tools at hand to test whether they should believe that nodes in the network are distinct; for example, Jones and colleagues describe a method assessing bridge centrality, which requires identification of communities of symptoms based on theory (Jones, Ma, et al., 2021). These tools and methods may help, but only if they answer to the needs of the specific analysis. Whether methods are old or new, their appropriate and successful use requires careful consideration of what we should expect from psychological networks. We expect more useful results from centrality metrics that are either created or applied with psychological data in mind, versus those merely imported from other fields.

However, we remain skeptical that centrality metrics are likely to provide much insight about psychopathology. Centrality metrics are summary statistics, yet network theory suggests that complex causal networks are what we need to understand. We have no doubt that summary statistics may be useful in specific situations, but we doubt they will well-characterize complex causal networks. For example, Robinaugh and colleagues (2019) demonstrate that a computational model of panic disorder, which includes only four psychological components, results in complex behavior that mimics panic symptoms over time (e.g., they simulate a panic attack under conditions of a biological challenge). In the network Robinaugh and colleagues present, which variable is central is immaterial: Each variable plays a role in the network such that changing the function of any individual variable will result in changes that cannot easily be inferred by examining the connections between nodes. Only knowledge of (and simulation of) the formal mathematical properties defining the relations between the nodes allows inference regarding the behavior of the network. We thus join Burger and colleagues (2020) in calling for formal computational models of psychopathological processes to move the field forward.

More specifically, as demonstrated by Robinaugh, Burger, and colleagues (Burger et al., 2020; Robinaugh et al., 2019), specifying a formal model allows us to simulate what might occur if we intervened on one or more of the variables modeled. Of course, this is exactly what many researchers are looking for when they seek central symptoms: They want to know which symptoms to intervene on. From a formal modeling perspective, it is obvious that the results of cross-sectional networks will generally not produce a viable model without additions. It is obvious, because most cross-sectional models, as observed by Robinaugh and colleagues (2020), display a positive manifold: Many symptoms correlate moderately positively with many other symptoms.

The positive manifold is so ubiquitous that it may seem strange to think that it implies that the resulting model is a poor basis for a formal model. Why would this be the case? A positive manifold, when interpreted naively, suggests the strong positive correlations indicate ongoing causal processes among the symptoms. In most cases, this simply cannot be accurate, because the model implied by such data would lead to ever-increasing levels of distress. When a person's irritability increases, so should their trouble sleeping, their depressed mood, and all the other positively correlated symptoms. We observe something quite different in the real world: People with disorders have times of increased and decreased distress, but most establish an equilibrium or homeostasis in the distressed state. When people have trouble sleeping, this does tend to increase their irritability, but also increases sleep-driven behavior such that trouble sleeping does not generally increase to its maximum for an extended period of time. Given these real-world observations, we can see that a model with a positive manifold must either (a) overstate the causal relationships between symptoms or (b) fail to include one or more casual processes that act to reduce the tendency of the system to lead to ever-increasing symptom levels. For example, the model proposed by Robinaugh and colleagues includes a negative feedback loop for avoidance, a negative relationship between escape and perceived threat, and an additional homeostatic mechanism. In cross-sectional data for panic disorder, we would expect both avoidance and perceived threat to be part of the positive manifold and have no notable negative relationships. We were unable to locate such an analysis regarding panic disorder that included perceived threat but did find two including anticipatory anxiety (which we take as a proxy for perceived threat) and avoidance: In both cases these symptoms indeed had only positive relationships with other symptoms (Cha et al., 2022; Kim et al., 2023), whereas the Robinaugh model specifies negative relationships. More generally, because the nodes that contribute the most to the positive manifold will have the highest centrality, and because the positive manifold is antithetical to a realistic (i.e., relatively steady-state) system, we have every reason to think that the results obtained from centrality of a cross-sectional network will not concord with results from formal modeling, even if the formal model were based on such a network to begin with. The necessary addition of negative feedback loops and homeostatic mechanisms will transform the relationships among the central variables and modify their role in the model.

Although cross-sectional networks may be one source of information to be used in constructing formal models, we have no confidence that relying on such models will be very useful unless supplemented by other sources of information. Burger and colleagues (2020) suggest idiographic models from longitudinal data and observation in combination with clinician observation to create formal models in a clinical context. Once such a model is constructed, simulating an intervention can lead to both tests of the model (in that its reaction should be consistent with known reactions to interventions) and possibilities for novel interventions. As Burger and colleagues note, however, use of such models in the realm of psychopathology continues to be rare. We hope the reader is persuaded to investigate this possibility further.

Reliability, Measurement, and Replication

Another major issue is whether network analysis produces reliable results. Researchers have proposed that typically used techniques do not produce reliable results (Forbes et al., 2017, 2021) and such critiques have been answered (Borsboom et al., 2017; Jones, Williams, et al., 2021), although not evidently to the satisfaction of the authors of the original critiques, who have continued to assert that networks as typically estimated are not reliable (Neal et al., 2022). Our read of this exchange is that the question of whether network results are reliable rests on the answer to the question, "Reliable for what?" For global network indices such as centrality indices, reliability may be about as good as one would typically expect for psychological data. For estimation of the values of specific pathways, the results may be less impressive.

We do not think this issue is primarily a problem of network theory or network analysis, but rather an issue of measurement. Indices that summarize across more data will generally be more reliable, just as two positively correlated items added together are more reliable than individual items. In a latent variable model in which individual items are used to estimate latent variables, we would thus put more faith in global fit indices and estimates of relationships between latent variables than we would in pathways from the latent variables to individual items. Similarly, if we were focusing on the pathways to individual items, we would put more faith in the replicability of the relative size of the pathways in comparison to each other rather than the precise numerical estimates. Indeed, Borsboom and colleagues (2017) point out that using the same methods as Forbes et al. (2017) do for network analysis can easily lead to the conclusion that latent variable models are not reliable, either. In turn, Forbes and colleagues (2017a) reply that in the case of network theory, the strength of various edges is often the stated primary research question.

The difference, from our point of view, is that in latent variable models, it is rare to define a latent variable by a single item, whereas in network analyses, nodes are often single items. We recommend caution in interpreting such results, whether the analysis is conducted under a network analysis framework, latent variable models, or something else. For example, Schuurman and Hamaker (2019) show that ignoring measurement error can produce spurious paths or cause true paths to be missed in a vector autoregression model, which is the typical model used for intensive longitudinal data, whether one prefers to use latent variables or a network structure. Thus, many (perhaps most) ecological momentary assessment (EMA) studies will have the same problem, because reliance on single items is typical. This methodological issue tells us something about evaluating early network theory results but does not tell us anything about network theory itself, or even its associated analytical techniques, other than the fact that it is not immune to the problems that have long bedeviled psychological research. Measurement is central to scientific progress (cf. Flake & Fried, 2020).

Thus, one way to grapple with the problem of reliability of networks is through enhancing reliability of measurement before fitting a network model. Another is to aggregate across multiple studies, as recently done by Isvoranu and colleagues (2021); the results of this investigation of post-traumatic stress disorder symptoms across studies suggests that results from any one study using typical methods should not be expected to yield definitive results. Again, part of this result must be due to the fact that no single scientific study should be expected to be definitive, but we think measurement issues compound this problem. Finally, some authors have investigated using Bayesian priors to inform network estimation when data are scarce (Burger et al., 2022; Terracciano & McCrae, 2012), which may also help to overcome shortcomings in measurement.

As this chapter progresses, we will focus increasingly on studies that examine groups and individuals over time. Accordingly, we should mention here that the issue of replicability is particularly pressing with such complex data. Bastiaansen and colleagues (2020) show convincingly that researcher choices regarding analysis can lead to very different conclusions regarding exactly the same data. Ensuring that research practices are replicable is more difficult when data and methods are complex, but this simply means it is all the more important to pursue these goals. We also suspect that researchers will need to go a step further and coordinate efforts to determine which methods are optimal for particular areas of study through careful examination of how different methods lead to different outcomes.

Network Analyses over Time

An astute reader might note that we have yet to recount any substantive findings from network analyses and wonder what kinds of network theory-related results we intend to review in more detail. Our first detailed look of the literature will focus on longitudinal data, with a heavy focus on idiographic and multi-level network analyses of symptoms over time. First, however, we will review the growing use of cross-lagged panel network (CLPN) models.

CLPN Models and the Challenge of Ergodicity

Our review of the literature found an increasing use of CLPN models. Most authors using this approach have cited Wysocki and colleagues' description of an approach in which many regressions are run to estimate prospective paths and the least absolute shrinkage and selection operator is used to reduce the risk of spurious paths (Wysocki et al., 2022, sometimes cited as Rhemtulla et al., 2022). In other words, whereas a more familiar cross-lagged panel model might focus on a few variables (e.g., hopelessness predicts depressive mood and itself over time), the CLPN approach allows the investigator to break apart a hopelessness scale into its items, and a depressive mood measure into its items. This approach leads to a potentially vast number of regressions being conducted, and the least absolute shrinkage and selection operator is used to reduce many of the obtained paths to zero and reduce the likelihood of false positive findings. This approach allows researchers to use now-familiar network methods with a longitudinal dataset with two or more waves. All of the papers on this topic appear, as best we can determine, to focus on datasets that were originally collected for other purposes (Bernstein et al., 2019; Funkhouser et al., 2021; Karalunas et al., 2021; Y. Li & Kwok, 2023; Savelieva et al., 2021; Zhang et al., 2024). Most of these authors focused on youth, although one focused on older adults (Savelieva et al., 2021). Most focused wholly or in part on depression or related issues, such as suicidality (Y. Li & Kwok, 2023), although one focused on attention deficit hyperactivity disorder (Karalunas et al., 2021).

Authors of the identified papers presented contemporaneous networks as well as lagged networks and generally appeared to give equal weight to both types of networks. Most also focused primarily on centrality indices in interpreting their results. In contrast, because the contemporaneous networks represent cross-sectional data, and due to the concerns we raise above, here we focus on the prospective networks. The overall impression from these papers is that authors found their results to primarily accord with previous findings in the same topic area. For example, authors of two studies concluded, in part, that their results supported the hopelessness theory of depression (Bernstein et al., 2019; Funkhouser et al., 2021). To the extent that the previous studies were in part founded on longitudinal data, such results should not be surprising: CLPN models are distinct from the more familiar cross-lagged panel models used in previous longitudinal research only in that they permit (but do not require) more variables and more paths. CLPN models should be expected to recover different paths only when (a) more variables are used in the analysis and (b) the smaller set of previously used variables did not adequately summarize the primary sources of variance in the data. The relative consistency between many CLPN results and established theory suggests that disaggregating scales or subscores into smaller units does not necessarily alter the interpretation of findings.

However, a secondary impression is that in many cases interpretation of the results are quite challenging. Take, for example, the analysis conducted by Savelieva and colleagues (2021). These authors report an analysis of 12 depression symptoms reported by 72,971 individuals, which means they, unusually, had the power and sample size needed to fully estimate a complex network. Given these data and especially because seven waves of data were modeled, the result is a series of densely connected networks in which visual interpretation of the models is essentially impossible: Every symptom appears to be prospectively related to every other symptom. If we were to ask these authors to not use centrality indices, they might have asked us, quite reasonably, what else they were supposed to do. One answer, as implied above, is formal computational modeling, which can provide an answer to the question of what the network would predict would occur if we intervened on a symptom (Burger et al., 2020).

All of the CLPN models have the appeal of arising from longitudinal data. This is arguably useful when attempting to infer causal pathways, in that the models the authors use account for previous measurement of the variables in the network in their prospective paths. However, our note above that CLPN models are in many ways equivalent to standard cross-panel models leads us to a problem. Lucas (2023) has shown that failure to account for random intercepts, or the fact that people have different baseline tendencies, can produce larger prospective effects than are observed when baseline tendencies are accounted for. In other words, a failure to separate between-person differences (e.g., in the intercepts or any other feature of the model) from within-person processes may lead to biased results. Preliminary work has suggested that CLPN is vulnerable to the same problem (Freichel et al., 2023). Thus, we can expect that these CLPN results will contain false positives compared to models that more properly separate within- from between-person variance.

The distinction between between- and within-person variance brings up a more essential problem with CLPN and, indeed, any method that focuses on a handful of timepoints. Such methods can certainly tell us, for example, whether a person who has higher suicidal ideation at Time 1 is likely to be a person who has higher depression than others at Time 2. In some cases, this may be exactly what we want to know. For example, we may want to predict which people should be contacted in the future for further screening. Counterintuitively, however, this result may tell us nothing about what is true over time for that specific person: Between-person analyses may not comment on within-person processes.

The potential for a lack of correspondence across between- and within-person processes may come as a surprise, because researchers often behave as if between-participant tests will yield results that apply to individuals over time. For example, the between-person finding of suicidal ideation leading to future depression is taken as an indication that if a person has high suicidal ideation today, they are more likely to be depressed at some point in the future. Although this may sometimes be true, both data and conceptual work reveal that such inferences run afoul of the ecological fallacy unless strict ergodicity holds, which seems unlikely for psychological processes (for more detail and a review of these issues, see Molenaar, 2004, 2007, 2013). In a brief and simplified form (and following the more detailed and technical observations by Molenaar, 2004), an ergodic process is one in which subsections of a process (here, people) are well represented by the features of the group. The reader could be forgiven for thinking that we have good reasons to think ergodicity might hold in psychological processes, but Molenaar (2004) shows clearly that ergodicity is easily violated and that we have every reason to think it is routinely violated in psychological processes in particular. We so routinely apply group-level results to individuals that it would be easy to conclude that we must have good reasons to assume ergodicity holds—and that it is the burden of researchers such as Molenaar to convince us that some processes are not ergodic. However, reviewing the arguments and evidence Molenaar presents leads to exactly the opposite conclusion. It is the burden of a researcher studying a group to demonstrate that group-level models represent individuals well. Failing to do so sees the researcher committing the ecological fallacy—assuming that between-person results are likely to apply to an individual. Our own initial efforts to investigate this issue have merely provided Molenaar and like-minded colleagues with further evidence that group-level models are not a good guide to individuals (Rodebaugh et al., 2023, 2024).

Accordingly, data that track processes within individuals is considerably more promising for understanding such processes. Bringmann and Eronen (2018) have gone so far as to assert that a focus on dynamic processes is a better way to articulate the difference between network theory and other approaches than the traditional arguments noted in section "Network Theory versus Other Approaches" (e.g., versus a contrast with categorical and latent variable models). In the rest of the chapter we will focus on network theory-related results that focus on models that at least potentially give us insight into processes in individuals.

Multi-level Vector Autoregression Models

Recent work has employed network analytic approaches to intensive longitudinal data to understand the dynamic relationships among symptoms. For example, as we will discuss in detail starting in the next paragraph, researchers have used multi-level vector autoregression (MLVAR) to estimate longitudinal networks of psychopathological symptoms. MLVAR models allow at least the possibility of examining the correspondence between a group-level model (which attempts to provide what is generally true of the group's paths) and individual models. Before reviewing substantive results, our review of the literature suggests a warning is in order.

MLVAR models are one of many vector autoregression approaches intended for intensive longitudinal data. For our current purposes, the reader who is not already familiar with vector autoregression can think of it as an approach that leads to a model in which we can use previous time points to predict either a person's state or a group's state at the current time point. Such an approach allows us to examine what predicts *when* a person's symptoms will be higher. With such models we are no longer focusing inadvertently on differences between people, but rather effects that play out in individuals over time.

Unsurprisingly, the more time points and more people are available for such analyses, the better our estimates can be expected to be. However, there seems to be some confusion in the literature as to how many of each is likely to lead to interpretable results. Part of the problem here is that, as noted by Bringmann and colleagues (2022), determining power for such models requires simulations: No single estimate of sample size is sufficient for determining whether power is adequate, because such models have a very large number of parameters, and power for each parameter depends on the overall set of interactions among variables. At the same time, we can draw some conclusions from several investigations of the performance of vector autoregression models (Lafit et al., 2021; Y. Li et al., 2022; Schultzberg & Muthén, 2018). Although these investigations examine a variety of different methods (e.g., multi-level vector autoregression using various methods of estimation, dynamic structural equation modeling, etc.), what is often underappreciated by researchers is that all of these approaches rely on the same basic model despite their different names: Vector autoregression is the foundation of the various methods used across these techniques (Piccirillo & Rodebaugh, 2019).

In each investigation the researchers set various levels of time points and sample size in their simulations, which tells us what level of each they consider too small to be worth investigating. Across these papers (Lafit et al., 2021; Y. Li et al., 2022; Schultzberg & Muthén, 2018) we observe an implicit anchor of approximately 100 or more people with 100 time points being a reasonable number. Li and colleagues specifically indicate that 60 time points or fewer was a small sample size in their view, whereas Lafit and colleagues start their simulations with 50. Schultzberg and Muthén, in contrast, start with as few as 10 of each, yet never find an indication that such a small sample size is remotely acceptable for the kinds of models likely in psychopathology research. For a model in which a single variable predicts itself, and that autoregression is modeled at the between-level with additional observed between-level variables, 10 time points might be sufficient if the sample size is 150 or higher. Yet, their results indicate that this does not always hold depending on the complexity of the overall model—and, again, this is a model in which a single variable is observed over time. If researchers want to know whether they have sufficient power for MLVAR, a simulation is highly recommended. If a simulation is not within the researchers' reach, they should be warned that when either number of time points or number of participants is below 50, they are on very shaky ground indeed. Accordingly, we will not review the substantive results of two reports we located in which time points were considerably below 50 without any power analysis provided to justify analyzing the data in question (Hoffart et al., 2019; Holzhauer et al., 2020). Unfortunately, there are simply no grounds to think that these analyses provide meaningful information.

Fortunately, other researchers have used more appropriate numbers of time points and participants in projects focusing on depression (de Vos et al., 2017; Marian et al., 2023) and post-traumatic stress disorder (PTSD; Greene et al., 2020; McGhie & McNally, 2023); although it must be noted that most skirted the lower edge of what the simulation studies above might lead us to expect to be a plausible lower bound, either in terms of participants or time points. All of these papers had a focus on in-strength and out-strength centrality indices (also known as just in-strength and out-strength). Here, in-strength centrality means the degree to which a symptom was predicted by the network of symptoms at the previous time point. In contrast, out-strength centrality refers to the degree to which a symptom predicted the network of symptoms at the next time point. None of these studies showed overlap in measures, samples, or methods that would allow ready comparison between their findings. For example, de Vos and colleagues (2017) estimated within-level temporal networks of positive and negative affect items in both adults with major depressive disorder (MDD) and healthy control (HC) adults. In the MDD network, the node with the highest in-strength centrality was tenseness, and the node with the highest out-strength centrality was cheerfulness. These findings contrasted with the findings of Marian and colleagues (2023), who also used MLVAR to estimate a temporal network of depression and anxiety symptoms within an undiagnosed sample of undergraduate students. They found that difficulty concentrating had the highest out-strength centrality, followed by worry, anhedonia, and sad mood. Restlessness showed the highest in-strength centrality, followed by worry and fatigue. Overall, despite the fact that both studies focused on MDD, there is little that unites them in method or findings.

Both McGhie and McNally (2023) and Greene and colleagues (2020) examined how PTSD networks predicted affect, although they focused on different forms of affect. Both used bridge centrality to estimate the dynamic associations between affect and PTSD symptoms. Bridge centrality (which is also referred to as bridge strength and bridge expected influence) is the degree to which a node is a plausibly strong path between sets of nodes. For example, in psychopathology networks, bridge centrality can be used to demonstrate the degree to which symptoms of one disorder are strongly associated with symptoms of a second, commonly comorbid disorder (e.g., how they "bridge" two groups of symptoms; Marian et al., 2023). Here, however, McGhie and McNally and Greene and colleagues utilized bridge centrality to investigate the temporal relationships between PTSD symptoms and momentary mood (i.e., affect). Specifically, they used bridge in-strength centrality to show how one mood node could be predicted by all PTSD nodes, and vice versa. They also used bridge in-strength centrality to show how one mood node could predict all PTSD nodes (and vice versa).

McGhie and McNally (2023) found that the PTSD symptoms of feeling distant from others and feeling on edge, separately, negatively predicted positive affect at the next time point (i.e., highest respective bridge out-strength centrality). Against their expectation, positive affect nodes did not have any meaningful bridge centrality indices. Greene and colleagues (2020) conducted a similar study but measured PTSD symptoms and negative affect. They found that sadness and fear each predicted PTSD symptoms at the next time point (highest respective bridge out-strength centrality); sadness, fear, and stress were also each found to be predicted by PTSD symptoms at the previous time point (highest respective bridge in-strength centrality). Regarding PTSD symptoms, arousal predicted negative affect at the next time point (highest bridge out-strength centrality); and helplessness and feeling overwhelmed were most predicted by negative affect at the previous time point (highest respective bridge in-strength centrality). Taken together, these studies support different PTSD symptoms having differential dynamic relationships with positive and negative affect. However, although the authors across these studies essentially used the same PTSD measure, they collapsed the symptoms into different nodes, in addition to focusing on different types of affect. The MLVAR literature overall clearly indicates that it will be difficult to compare studies that present network analyses of psychopathology unless consistent items and methods are used, which will require collaboration among researchers focusing on a specific topic.

Notably, some of these authors focused on how their group-level results applied to individuals and some did not. One of the appealing uses of MLVAR, as alluded to above (see "CLPN Models and the Challenge of Ergodicity"), is the option to examine variance in paths (e.g., do people differ significantly on a given path) and output estimated individual networks (Bringmann et al., 2013). In their study, deVos and colleagues (2017) visually inspected individual models and reported that they were clearly distinct from one another. McGhie and McNally (2023) also examined individual models and generally observed that group-level paths were rare in individual models, although they correctly noted that this might be due to power or true differences between individuals. Such findings comport with a more general finding, extending beyond research focused on networks per se, that when group-level models are examined in individuals, what is true for the group may apply to very few individuals (Rodebaugh et al., 2023, 2024).

Fully Idiographic Vector Autoregression

Another option for investigating the relationship between symptoms and other factors over time is to focus entirely on individuals. Such models also use vector autoregression, in this case without the multi-level component—instead of modeling individuals nested within a group, the studies we discuss here modeled individuals. Again, the focus is on what factors predict *when* individuals experience higher levels of symptoms: What other factors from previous time points predict distress at a given time. Such investigations have one overwhelming conclusion in common: Individuals, however homogeneous, show very different paths. For example, Fisher and colleagues (2017) examined both the nomothetic (i.e., group-level) and idiographic (i.e., person-specific) contemporaneous correlations and temporal dynamics between mood and anxiety symptoms in a sample of participants with generalized anxiety disorder, major depressive disorder, or both. These authors did provide overall group-level findings, but we will focus on idiographic findings here. For the idiographic results, the authors selected exemplar models based on centrality indices. For each, the nodes that showed the greatest centrality, in-strength, and out-strength were not only different across the idiographic models, but also different from the nomothetic results. That is, not only were individuals different from one another regarding which nodes were flagged as important, but the group-level results would not have given any indication of what nodes would be important for any individual. Additional idiographic models were supplied in a supplement and make it clear that results varied widely across idiographic models.

In another study, Piccirillo and Rodebaugh (2022) compared group-level and person-specific symptom networks for women with comorbid social anxiety disorder and major depressive disorder. These authors again used methods to draw together group-level findings, but here we will focus on their individual models. At the person-specific level, temporal VAR models were sparse and the most common directed paths were the autoregression of feeling sad, feeling accomplished, and avoiding social situations. That is, the most common paths for individuals were variables predicting themselves. Piccirillo and Rodebaugh (2022) selected the three participants who provided the most data to examine person-specific differences in the temporal VAR models. Their models varied considerably. For example, different variables (e.g., feeling lonely, feeling calm, and feeling anxious) exhibited the largest expected influence in each model. Additionally, one person-specific model included positive autoregressive effects for both depressed mood and social avoidance, whereas another included only the positive autoregressive effect for depressed mood, and the third did not include any significant temporal effects at all. Overall, there was considerable heterogeneity and little relation between the group- and individual-level models.

Multiple idiographic studies of psychopathology have been conducted with the express purpose of investigating whether such models would be useful clinically. For example, Frumkin and colleagues (2020) invited clients seeking therapy to generate predictions about the contemporaneous and directed relationships between their symptoms and compared these predictions to idiographic graphical VAR models. Predictions by clients appeared unrelated to the final models, often in part because clients expected far more paths than were seen in their models. One of the most striking aspects of the models from the point of view of psychopathology is how few paths were recovered, which we will discuss below (see "Idiography Part One"). This study otherwise focused primarily on clinical application of models rather than psychopathology per se. Similarly, Levinson and colleagues (2023) investigated whether idiographic networks could be used with clients with eating disorders to direct treatment. A few conclusions can be drawn that are related to psychopathology more specifically. First, these authors also found directed networks that were empty; contemporaneous networks were also sometimes quite sparse. Second, selecting items based on centrality indices led to a wide variety of symptoms being targeted, with no apparent relationships to which diagnoses a client had. Third, and in keeping with the initial observations in this section, the main impression was of a wide variety of networks despite the relative homogeneity of the clients regarding symptomatology.

Idiography Part One: The Horror of the Empty Networks

Many studies in which authors examine participants idiographically over time have found many networks without directed paths. Given such results, alongside our own experiences with idiographic networks (including those presented by Frumkin et al., 2020), we offer an observation and a warning in interpreting this literature: Empty prospective networks (i.e., those without statistically significant prospective paths) are common, to the extent that they should be expected. That is, both contemporaneous networks and the group-level estimates for directed paths will often show many significant pathways. Yet, examining the prospective networks of at least some individuals, even within a group that shows prospective paths, will often show few, if any, prospective pathways. One solution to this conundrum is to accept that many aspects of the relations among symptoms will be encoded in the contemporaneous networks (cf. Epskamp et al., 2018). Yet, many researchers would prefer to uncover prospective paths, under the assumption that these more clearly imply plausible causal pathways. From that perspective, it is unsettling to find that models often have very few such paths.

For example, Piccirillo and Rodebaugh (2022) examined women with social anxiety disorder and focused their discussion on the contemporaneous networks, noting that the temporal networks were sparse. Examining the temporal networks provided in supplement, we can see that few paths were found for any individuals. Of the potential prospective relationships among the twelve variables, only four prospective paths materialized once autoregressive relationships were ignored. This occurred despite the fact that the variables selected for the networks included both social anxiety disorder and depression symptoms, alongside factors thought to directly influence those symptoms (e.g., exercise, social avoidance). In another example, Levinson and colleagues (2023) found many directed paths for some clients but relatively few for most. Multi-level techniques that provide individual paths can also produce this kind of finding; McGhie and McNally (2023) reported that, in their MLVAR PTSD-only network, fewer than 29% of individual models had directed paths.

When thinking about these networks, researchers typically expect many significant paths, in part because they are used to longitudinal analyses with many significant paths. However, there are several reasons to expect that the typical idiographic network should not show similar findings to typical longitudinal analyses. First, many methods for idiographic modeling assume that the true number of pathways is small. As pointed out previously, if a method presumes sparseness, the fact that the resulting network is sparse may merely reflect the method used (Epskamp, Kruis, et al., 2017). Another method that does not assume sparseness might return a larger number of prospective paths, as found, for example, by Fisher and colleagues (2017), who reported a much higher number of prospective paths (primarily among symptoms of anxiety and depression) when using an automated search algorithm than did Piccirillo and Rodebaugh (2022) when using a more common method that assumes sparseness.

Second, typical longitudinal analyses on groups involve relatively few measures with a large number of items assessed across weeks or months. Idiographic networks typically focus on shorter time lags and not only more variables overall, but also assessments that have weaker measurement properties. All of these methodological differences should be expected to attenuate any effects found in idiographic networks versus between-participant longitudinal studies. More reliable measures should make it easier to detect effects, and effects across constructs have more time to occur if the time period is longer. On a related note, a recent guide to the number of time points and variables that can be used with idiographic analyses might suggest that many published studies are quite underpowered (Mansueto et al., 2023). Mansueto and colleagues (2023) found that unless the number of time points exceeded 100, it was advisable to reduce the number of variables modeled to six or fewer; many of the papers we reviewed either did not reliably have more than 100 time points per person, modeled well over six variables, or both.

Third, one of the key factors that make idiographic models appealing is that they avoid the ecological fallacy. As noted above (see "CLPN Models and the Challenge of Ergodicity"), there is no basis for the assumption that between-participant effects should generalize to within-person processes. Thus, expecting within-person analyses to yield results similar to those from between-participant longitudinal modeling commits that very fallacy. We have every reason to think within-participant results may be very different than those found between participants. Finally, it is important to note that our intuitions about how large prospective effects should be even in between-participant research may be distorted by methodological limitations of most extant studies. As noted above (see "CLPN Models and the Challenge of Ergodicity"), typical cross-lagged panel models used in the literature will tend to overestimate prospective effects (Lucas, 2023). Thus, the bigger problem may be that we have bad intuitions about how easy it is to predict one construct from another as a result of methodological limitations of previous work.

If empty prospective networks are both common and represent the facts of psychological processes, one implication is that the important causes in psychological processes simply do not unfold over the course of hours (i.e., the time frame typically used). Perhaps many run over the course of seconds, whereas others run over the course of months. If our analyzed time scale does not encompass these periods, whether because they are much longer or much shorter, we cannot expect to recover the effects we expect (as demonstrated, for example, by Haslbeck & Ryan, 2022). Put simply, we cannot simply pick a time course because it is convenient. We must choose time courses based on our theoretical or empirical understanding of how processes occur. Of course, if network theory is fundamentally incorrect about psychological disorders, and symptoms do not in any meaningful way cause one another, empty networks should also be typical.

Idiography Part Two: The Existential Terror of Disaggregation

If the appeal of idiographic networks is avoiding the ecological fallacy, the implied underlying existential terror for psychologists is the possibility that all people must be understood as individuals. To see why this is an existential threat and not a reassuring saying on a greeting card, consider how a psychologist should answer what their idiographic networks mean for dealing with a new individual. Unless their idiographic networks are very similar across participants, the psychologist would have to answer that the new participant must also be studied. And the next participant. And the next. We need some way to generalize lest our ability to gain knowledge creeps in such a petty pace from day to day that we fall into an abyss of endless study.

It is often unclear how to combine idiographic models into any statements or claims about groups. On one hand, several methods promise to aggregate individual analyses, but all do so under assumptions that may be frequently violated (Asparouhov et al., 2018; Beltz & Gates, 2017; Bringmann et al., 2013; Lane & Gates, 2017). In some cases, it is even questionable whether the resulting model can really be referred to as idiographic (i.e., because individual paths are only estimated relative to the group to begin with; Asparouhov et al., 2018; Bringmann et al., 2013). Efforts to compare different methods that aggregate across idiographic networks are rare (we have found none in our review, although we know of some ongoing efforts). Such examinations will be essential moving forward so that we can have a better idea under what circumstances these methods may yield useful information.

We can reassure ourselves somewhat that aggregating across individuals at least sometimes yields valid results. For example, the interventions we have derived from between-participant comparisons are not suspect, because the design equates across individuals. What participants have in common is their assignment on the variable we controlled ourselves, the independent variable. However, it is exactly these sorts of designs that researchers are now struggling to improve with idiographic models. Any results that we would hope to have an application on the population level must ultimately make the journey back to between-participant guidelines. For example, many have hoped that idiographic networks will improve treatments via individualizing those treatments. However, idiographic networks only individualize treatments through changing existing treatments (in form or emphasis), and changing a treatment does not guarantee it will be improved over what would have been done without the idiographic model. Some standard of comparison is needed, and this can only be done at the between-participants level. However, this is appropriate, because what treatment works for whom is a between-participants question. This does not mean, for example, that treatment can't be individualized, but it does mean that the means of individualizing it must be systematic and compared to an equally systematically provided non-individualized therapy.

Idiography Part Three: Adventures in Application

One way to resolve the difficulty of aggregation of individuals is to go ahead and analyze one individual at a time. Indeed, several authors have discussed the possibility of using idiographic networks for treatment purposes, with varying levels of optimism (Frumkin et al., 2020; Levinson et al., 2021; Rodebaugh et al., 2020; von Klipstein et al., 2020). Here we will confine our discussion to factors brought up by these discussions that also affect what we can expect these methods to reveal about psychopathology.

All current approaches that result in idiographic networks of more than two symptoms involve, at a minimum, a vector autoregressive method (Lütkepohl, 2005) and an algorithm or tuning parameter designed to handle the large number of parameters that can result (cf. Piccirillo et al., 2019; Piccirillo & Rodebaugh, 2019). In vector autoregression, the results of idiographic networks involve (1) stationary prospective effects that are (2) locked to the time scale of observations. We have discussed above the issue of analyses being locked to a single time scale (see "Idiography Part Two"), but stationarity (the quality of a model having all stationary effects) deserves separate discussion.

Stationarity is a formal assumption of vector autoregressive approaches and is often listed as a limitation of the method in discussions of idiographic models. However, we think the issue is more fundamental than is often appreciated. To illustrate what is meant by stationarity, we will take a simple model in which difficulty sleeping predicts irritability for a client. When we assume stationarity for this specific prediction, this means we are assuming that neither the mean nor variance of irritability is systematically changing over time. Further, we also assume that the paths predicting irritability (here, its past measurement and past difficulty sleeping) also do not change over the course of the assessments. If any of these parameters change systematically over the course of the assessment, the estimates of the model will be incorrect. Changes in the means of variables are not too difficult to handle; the variables can be detrended or time can be included if the modeling approach allows it. However, relationships between variables are more challenging. For example, say that the person being assessed encountered some psychoeducation about sleep halfway through the assessment period that alleviated their irritability about sleep. As a result, for this individual, sleep difficulty leads to higher irritability early in the assessment period, but this relationship diminishes. In this case vector autoregressive methods clearly give us the wrong result, in that it gives us a single parameter that is incorrect for at least most points during the assessment period.

There are two issues we want to point out about stationarity that affect our interpretation of psychopathological networks. The first is that the issue is implicit in any statistical analysis: It is not just an esoteric property of vector autoregression. Any statistical method that returns a single value for the relationship between two variables assumes stationarity implicitly. If we use a cross-sectional regression analysis in a thousand participants and claim that we now know that difficulty sleeping has a moderate relationship with irritability, either our statement has no meaning or we are assuming that stationarity holds. The majority of methods discussed in this book make such assumptions, and we generally do not know how reasonable such assumptions are. The second point is that there are methods of testing whether stationarity holds, although these are generally thought to require many time points (more than typically seen in the idiographic analysis literature) (Bringmann et al., 2015; Bringmann et al., 2017; Haslbeck et al., 2021; R. Li et al., 2017). Such methods have yet to be applied, to our knowledge, in such a way that a network of many symptoms could be examined simultaneously, although Nemesure and colleagues (2024, see next paragraph of this section) recently simulated such an analysis through many separate analyses that were then combined. However, the initial findings strongly suggest to us that stationarity may frequently be violated. If this is the case, it adds an additional level of complexity to an already complex set of problems.

When using idiographic data to inform treatment, frequent violations of stationarity would lead to different conclusions about idiographic networks based on when the person was assessed. Indeed, knowledge of this possibility may explain why researchers have largely focused on networks generated prior to treatment rather than during treatment (Frumkin et al., 2020; Levinson et al., 2021; von Klipstein et al., 2020): Such researchers are betting that stationarity is more likely before treatment than during it. However, there is no guarantee that these researchers are right. Indeed, initial depictions of violations of stationarity were obtained outside of treatment (Bringmann et al., 2015). Using techniques introduced by Bringmann and colleagues, Nemesure and colleagues (2024) recently provided evidence that, in a group of 105 individuals with MDD, most ($n = 89$) showed changes in their networks such that the most influential symptom in their network changed over the course of 90 days. We expect researchers focused on psychopathology, rather than treatment, to wrestle further with this issue in the future. If relationships among symptoms routinely change over time, our models will not only require data over time, but also theories about how processes change over time.

Idiography Part Four: Early Warning Signs

Network theory is consistent with principles of complex dynamical systems theory used to examine systems and change processes in fields ranging from ecology to psychopathology. It is unsurprising then that researchers interested in detecting and predicting critical symptom changes in psychopathology have drawn inspiration from the phenomenon of early warning signals (EWS; Scheffer et al., 2009), in which changes in variables or relationships between variables can presage important outcomes. From a dynamical systems perspective, individual symptom networks represent complex systems of interacting components, which may shift between various stable states (e.g., adaptive and maladaptive, desirable and undesirable, etc.). The assumption here is that symptoms generally move into a homeostatic state in which each symptom has a relatively stable role, until some shift happens in the system that moves the initial stable role to a new one as the system moves to a new homeostatic stable state. Notably, there are strong reasons to think that various physical systems behave in this way, but it is not yet clear that psychological symptoms do.

These shifts may be preceded by EWS of destabilization in the temporal dynamics of variables in the system, as reviewed recently by Tonge and colleagues (2024). For example, the system may show signs of a critical slowing down (CSD) prior to an impending shift from a desirable to undesirable state, wherein even small perturbations (e.g., a stressor) cause the system to return to the desirable state more slowly. As also reviewed by Tonge and colleagues, CSD is typically detected using statistical indices such as increased autocorrelations and variance within elements in the system (e.g., symptom states), and increased spatial correlation (i.e., the strength of connections among elements in the system). These indices are referred to collectively as EWS. As may be obvious from the description above, such phenomena simply cannot be detected without many measurements being obtained. In the case of psychological symptoms, EMA is typically required.

Researchers have emphasized the potential clinical utility of EWS for the detection, prediction, and prevention of episodes of psychopathology. The majority of studies have investigated the use of EWS to detect and predict recurrent depressive episodes (Tonge et al., 2024; Wichers et al., 2020; Wichers & Groot, 2016); whereas others have examined EWS in the context of bipolar disorder (Bos et al., 2022), transdiagnostic symptom changes (Schreuder et al., 2020; Wichers et al., 2019), and processes of change in psychotherapy (Helmich et al., 2023; Olthof et al., 2020). Several studies in the last decade have reported group-level associations between EWS and change in symptoms (Curtiss et al., 2023; Schreuder et al., 2020; van de Leemput et al., 2014). However, fewer studies to date have realized the purported clinical utility of EWS to temporally predict qualitative shifts in psychopathology at the individual level (Bos et al., 2022; Tonge et al., 2024; Wichers et al., 2020; Wichers & Groot, 2016). Two notable studies by Wichers and colleagues investigated CSD as an indicator of depressive relapse using fully idiographic methods. In one case study, the authors examined autocorrelations of positive and negative affect rated multiple times per day by a patient undergoing a gradual discontinuation from antidepressant medication (Wichers & Groot, 2016). The authors found that a statistically significant shift in depressive symptoms was preceded by CSD, as evidenced by rising autocorrelations and variance, as well as stronger associations among symptom states.

In a follow-up study, the authors reported similar findings for one individual who reported a sudden increase in depressive symptoms and found that the autocorrelation and variance of EMA ratings of feeling down increased before the symptom transition (Wichers et al., 2020). The authors also found that internode connectivity between the 10 momentary mental states rated during the EMA period increased prior to the symptom transition. Notably, the authors conducted post hoc analyses with EMA data from participants who did not report a steep increase in depressive symptoms and found only one false positive EWS (e.g., a rising autocorrelation that did not precede a significant symptom transition).

However, the authors of several recent studies have questioned the sensitivity and specificity of EWS. Bos and colleagues (2022) examined EWS as predictors of manic and depressive episodes at both the group and individual levels. At the group level, the authors found evidence of false negatives, which indicated that EWS were not always detected prior to a symptom transition (Bos et al., 2022). Tonge and colleagues (2024) similarly found that although EWS were sensitive predictors of depressive relapse for one participant, there were false positive EWS prior to fluctuations in depressive symptoms that did not meet criteria for depressive relapse.

Despite theoretical emphasis on complex dynamical systems, relatively few EWS studies leverage indices of network connectivity per se. Although Wichers et al. (2016) established internode network connectivity as one of three standard metrics of EWS, other studies that have included network connectivity as an EWS index did not find evidence that it predicted significant changes in depressive symptoms (Curtiss et al., 2023). Further, most studies in this body of literature only examine temporal autocorrelation and variance from either a single variable, or one variable at a time (i.e., without consideration of relationships among variables; Bos et al., 2022; Helmich et al., 2023; Schreuder et al., 2020). The authors make (or at least entertain) the assumption that changes in a single variable either reflect or cause change in an overall network, but they do not necessarily model such a network directly. Thus, as we imply above, thinking in terms of complex causal symptoms (and thus using network theory) does not require the use of network analysis per se; nor does it require the use of many variables.

Others have taken a different approach to the same problem. Instead of trying to detect EWS reflecting changes in a network, these authors have focused on attempting to detect an oncoming depressive episode based on changes in symptom levels. Smit and Snippe (2023) detected increases in the day average of a given symptom state (e.g., restlessness) using the exponentially weighted moving average, and these increases preceded the recurrence of depressive symptoms. This finding suggests that close examination of fluctuations in suspected prodromal symptoms may be as effective as autocorrelations and other EWS. Snippe and colleagues (2023) reported similar findings, although with worry and negative thoughts about the self proving to be sensitive indicators. The fact that mean levels of certain symptoms tend to rise ahead of depressive episodes could be taken as an indication of changes in a network of symptoms, but it is not strictly necessary to do so. Instead, it could be that the authors have simply identified the most sensitive leading indicators of a rise in depression as a unitary syndrome. Thus, EWS of this sort are less clearly aligned with a complex causal systems perspective.

Conclusion

We have argued that the network theory of psychopathology has, at its heart, the proposition that multiple, ongoing causal processes lead to and maintain clinical problems, and understanding the complex causal networks that arise from these processes is necessary to make scientific and clinical progress. The network theory of psychopathology is a relatively recent innovation that arose with claims that it is distinct from other perspectives, such as latent variable models and the medical model (Borsboom, 2008; Cramer et al., 2012). In application, however, network theory has much in common with these other perspectives: Researchers tend to use the data and tools that are easily available. Accordingly, since the network perspective was first proposed, the vast majority of applications have focused on cross-sectional data. Even if the reader holds out hope that each of these individual studies might contribute to understanding complex causal symptoms, it is hard to escape the conclusion that such efforts are over-represented in the literature.

We suspect a critical and thoroughgoing look at any perspective on psychopathology would have similar findings: Our data and methods are all too frequently insufficient for testing our theories. Fortunately, some researchers associated with network theory have made advances that bring us closer to testing propositions about complex causal networks. Based on their results and arguments, we are convinced that (1) no particular analytical method is required when testing propositions of network theory (i.e., network analysis is distinct from network theory); (2) off-the-shelf centrality indices may have their uses but should be examined carefully and might be better replaced by alternatives designed specifically for psychological data; and (3) a true reckoning with a complex causal symptoms perspective requires us to venture at the outer limits of such challenging frontiers as idiography, varying timescales, time-varying effects, and formal computational models.

Bringmann and Eronen (2018) suggest that rather than a contrast between a network perspective and other approaches such as the use of latent variables, it is more useful to contrast (1) static versus dynamic approaches and (2) symptom versus syndrome perspectives. We are not so sure about symptoms versus syndromes being a crucial dimension. On that point we return to the viewpoints of Hume and Buddhist philosophers, as well as Constantini and Perugini (2012). A typical network perspective is that syndromes are made of symptoms, such that we should study symptoms. Yet, we can continue to disaggregate symptoms, as well. Difficulty sleeping involves time to sleep onset, amount of waking, progression through stages of sleep, etc. We see both symptoms and syndromes as provisional aggregates that may be useful. We find it implausible, though, that one level will necessarily be more useful than another in all circumstances.

We agree, however, with Bringmann and Eronen (2018) on the crucial distinction between static and dynamic approaches, or perhaps more precisely we believe that dynamic approaches are the best bet for moving our understanding forward. Complex causal networks cannot be understood with models built on static simple data, regardless of how many symptoms are in the dataset. At least, that is our view on the topic, and thus our review is consistent with that reading. Others may see network theory differently and might prefer another recent review that provides more depth regarding findings from cross-sectional networks (Borsboom et al., 2021; Contreras et al., 2019; Fried & Cramer, 2017; McNally, 2021; Monteleone & Cascino, 2021; Robinaugh et al., 2020). What constitutes network theory, or any scientific perspective, is also provisional. Perhaps some readers who thought they would reject the network perspective have been surprised by this chapter. Perhaps they have had complaints about the network literature but are happy to endorse a complex causal symptoms perspective. If so, we urge such readers to take what parts are useful from the aggregate that people call the network perspective and join us in using dynamic data to better understand the complex causal processes essential to understanding psychopathology.

References

American Psychiatric Association. (1987). *Diagnostic and statistical manual of mental disorders: DSM-III-R* (3rd ed., revised). American Psychiatric Association.

American Psychiatric Association. (1994). *Diagnostic and statistical manual of mental disorders: DSM-IV* (4th ed.). American Psychiatric Association.

American Psychiatric Association. (2013). *Diagnostic and statistical manual of mental disorders: DSM-5* (5th ed.). American Psychiatric Association. http://www.PsychiatryOnline.org

Asparouhov, T., Hamaker, E. L., & Muthén, B. (2018). Dynamic structural equation models. *Structural Equation Modeling: A Multidisciplinary Journal, 25*(3), 359–388.

Bastiaansen, J. A., Kunkels, Y. K., Blaauw, F. J., Boker, S. M., Ceulemans, E., Chen, M., Chow, S. M., de Jonge, P., Emerencia, A. C., Epskamp, S., Fisher, A. J., Hamaker, E. L., Kuppens, P., Lutz, W., Meyer, M. J., Moulder, R., Oravecz, Z., Riese, H., Rubel, J., . . . Bringmann, L. F. (2020). Time to get personal? The impact of researchers choices on the selection of treatment targets using the experience sampling methodology. *Journal of Psychosomatic Research, 137*, 110211. https://doi.org/10.1016/j.jpsychores.2020.110211

Bauer, D. J., Howard, A. L., Baldasaro, R. E., Curran, P. J., Hussong, A. M., Chassin, L., & Zucker, R. A. (2013). A trifactor model for integrating ratings across multiple informants. *Psychological Methods, 18*(4), 475–493. https://doi.org/10.1037/a0032475

Beltz, A. M., & Gates, K. M. (2017). Network mapping with GIMME. *Multivariate Behavioral Research, 52*(6), 789–804. https://doi.org/10.1080/00273171.2017.1373014

Bentler, P. M., & Molenaar, P. C. M. (2012). The Houdini transformation: True, but illusory. *Multivariate Behavioral Research, 47*(3), 442–447. https://doi.org/10.1080/00273171.2012.673941

Bernstein, E. E., Kleiman, E. M., van Bork, R., Moriarity, D. P., Mac Giollabhui, N., McNally, R. J., Abramson, L. Y., & Alloy, L. B. (2019). Unique and predictive relationships between components of cognitive vulnerability and symptoms of depression. *Depression and Anxiety, 36*(10), 950–959. https://doi.org/10.1002/da.22935

Berta, A., Miguel Ángel, C., Clara, G.-S., & Rubén, H. (2022). A bibliometric analysis of 10 years of research on symptom networks in psychopathology and mental health. *Psychiatry Research, 308*, 114380. https://doi.org/10.1016/j.psychres.2021.114380

Borsboom, D. (2008). Psychometric perspectives on diagnostic systems. *Journal of Clinical Psychology, 64*(9), 1089–1108. https://doi.org/10.1002/jclp.20503

Borsboom, D., Deserno, M. K., Rhemtulla, M., Epskamp, S., Fried, E. I., McNally, R. J., Robinaugh, D. J., Perugini, M., Dalege, J., Costantini, G., Isvoranu, A.-M., Wysocki, A. C., van Borkulo, C. D., van Bork, R., & Waldorp, L. J. (2021). Network analysis of multivariate data in psychological science. *Nature Reviews Methods Primers, 1*(1), 1–18, Article 1. https://doi.org/10.1038/s43586-021-00055-w

Borsboom, D., Fried, E. I., Epskamp, S., Waldorp, L. J., van Borkulo, C. D., van der Maas, H. L. J., & Cramer, A. O. J. (2017). False alarm? A comprehensive reanalysis of "Evidence that psychopathology symptom networks have limited replicability" by Forbes, Wright, Markon, and Krueger (2017). *Journal of Abnormal Psychology, 126*(7), 989–999. https://doi.org/10.1037/abn0000306

Bos, F. M., Schreuder, M. J., George, S. V., Doornbos, B., Bruggeman, R., van der Krieke, L., Haarman, B. C. M., Wichers, M., & Snippe, E. (2022). Anticipating manic and depressive transitions in patients with bipolar disorder using early warning signals. *International Journal of Bipolar Disorders, 10*(1), 12. https://doi.org/10.1186/s40345-022-00258-4

Boyd, R. (1991). Realism, anti-foundationalism and the enthusiasm for natural kinds. *Philosophical Studies: An International Journal for Philosophy in the Analytic Tradition, 61*(1/2), 127–148.

Bringmann, L. F., Albers, C., Bockting, C., Borsboom, D., Ceulemans, E., Cramer, A., Epskamp, S., Eronen, M. I., Hamaker, E., Kuppens, P., Lutz, W., McNally, R. J., Molenaar, P., Tio, P., Voelkle, M. C., & Wichers, M. (2022). Psychopathological networks: Theory, methods and practice. *Behaviour Research and Therapy, 149*, 104011. https://doi.org/10.1016/j.brat.2021.104011

Bringmann, L. F., Elmer, T., Epskamp, S., Krause, R. W., Schoch, D., Wichers, M., Wigman, J. T. W., & Snippe, E. (2019). What do centrality measures measure in psychological networks? *Journal of Abnormal Psychology, 128*(8), 892–903. https://doi.org/10.1037/abn0000446

Bringmann, L. F., & Eronen, M. I. (2018). Don't blame the model: Reconsidering the network approach to psychopathology. *Psychological Review, 125*(4), 606–615. https://doi.org/10.1037/rev0000108

Bringmann, L. F., Hamaker, E. L., Vigo, D. E., Aubert, A., Borsboom, D., & Tuerlinckx, F. (2017). Changing dynamics: Time-varying autoregressive models using generalized additive modeling. *Psychological Methods, 22*(3), 409–425. https://doi.org/10.1037/met0000085

Bringmann, L. F., Vissers, N., Wichers, M., Geschwind, N., Kuppens, P., Peeters, F., Borsboom, D., & Tuerlinckx, F. (2013). A network approach to psychopathology: New insights into clinical longitudinal data. *PLoS One, 8*(4), e60188. https://doi.org/10.1371/journal.pone.0060188

Bringmann, L., Ferrer, E., Hamaker, E., Borsboom, D., & Tuerlinckx, F. (2015). Modeling nonstationary emotion dynamics in dyads using a semiparametric time-varying vector autoregressive model. *Multivariate Behavioral Research, 50*(6), 293–314. https://doi.org/10.1080/00273171.2015.1120182

Burger, J., Ralph-Nearman, C., & Levinson, C. A. (2022). Integrating clinician and patient case conceptualization with momentary assessment data to construct idiographic networks: Moving toward personalized treatment for eating disorders. *Behaviour Research and Therapy, 159*, 104221. https://doi.org/10.1016/j.brat.2022.104221

Burger, J., van der Veen, D. C., Robinaugh, D. J., Quax, R., Riese, H., Schoevers, R. A., & Epskamp, S. (2020). Bridging the gap between complexity science and clinical practice by formalizing idiographic theories: A computational model of functional analysis. *BMC Medicine, 18*(1), 99. https://doi.org/10.1186/s12916-020-01558-1

Cha, E. J., Hong, S., Park, D.-H., Ryu, S.-H., Ha, J. H., & Jeon, H. J. (2022). A network analysis of panic symptoms in relation to depression and anxiety sensitivity in patients with panic disorder. *Journal of Affective Disorders, 308*, 134–140. https://doi.org/10.1016/j.jad.2022.04.062

Cole, D. A., & Maxwell, S. E. (2003). Testing mediational models with longitudinal data: Questions and tips in the use of structural equation modeling. *Journal of Abnormal Psychology, 112*(4), 558–577. https://doi.org/10.1037/0021-843X.112.4.558

Contreras, A., Nieto, I., Valiente, C., Espinosa, R., & Vazquez, C. (2019). The study of psychopathology from the network analysis perspective: A systematic review. *Psychotherapy and Psychosomatics, 88*(2), 71–83. https://doi.org/10.1159/000497425

Costantini, G., & Perugini, M. (2012). The definition of components and the use of formal indexes are key steps for a successful application of network analysis in personality psychology. *European Journal of Personality, 26*(4), 434–435. https://doi.org/10.1002/per.1869

Costantini, G., Richetin, J., Preti, E., Casini, E., Epskamp, S., & Perugini, M. (2019). Stability and variability of personality networks. A tutorial on recent developments in network psychometrics. *Personality and Individual Differences, 136*, 68–78. https://doi.org/10.1016/j.paid.2017.06.011

Cramer, A. J., Waldorp, L. J., van der Maas, H. J., &. Borsboom, D. (2010). Comorbidity: A network perspective. *Behavioral and Brain Sciences, 33*, 137–150. https://doi.org/10.1017/S0140525X09991567

Cramer, A. O. J., Van der Sluis, S., Noordhof, A., Wichers, M., Geschwind, N., Aggen, S. H., Kendler, K. S., & Borsboom, D. (2012). Dimensions of normal personality as networks in search of equilibrium: You can't like parties if you don't like people. *European Journal of Personality, 26*(4), 414–431. https://doi.org/10.1002/per.1866

Cramer, A. O. J., Waldorp, L. J., Maas, H. L. J. van der, & Borsboom, D. (2010). Comorbidity: A network perspective. *Behavioral and Brain Sciences, 33*(2–3), 137–150. https://doi.org/10.1017/S0140525X09991567

Curtiss, J. E., Mischoulon, D., Fisher, L. B., Cusin, C., Fedor, S., Picard, R. W., & Pedrelli, P. (2023). Rising early warning signals in affect associated with future changes in depression: A dynamical systems approach. *Psychological Medicine, 53*(7), 3124–3132. https://doi.org/10.1017/S0033291721005183

de Vos, S., Wardenaar, K. J., Bos, E. H., Wit, E. C., Bouwmans, M. E. J., & Jonge, P. de. (2017). An investigation of emotion dynamics in major depressive disorder patients and healthy persons using sparse longitudinal networks. *PLOS ONE, 12*(6), e0178586. https://doi.org/10.1371/journal.pone.0178586

Epskamp, S., Kruis, J., & Marsman, M. (2017). Estimating psychopathological networks: Be careful what you wish for. *PLOS ONE, 12*(6), e0179891. https://doi.org/10.1371/journal.pone.0179891

Epskamp, S., Rhemtulla, M., & Borsboom, D. (2017). Generalized network psychometrics: Combining network and latent variable models. *Psychometrika, 82*(4), 904–927. https://doi.org/10.1007/s11336-017-9557-x

Epskamp, S., van Borkulo, C. D., van der Veen, D. C., Servaas, M. N., Isvoranu, A.-M., Riese, H., & Cramer, A. O. J. (2018). Personalized network modeling in psychopathology: The importance of contemporaneous and temporal connections. *Clinical Psychological Science, 6*(3), 416–427. https://doi.org/10.1177/2167702617744325

Fisher, A. J., Reeves, J. W., Lawyer, G., Medaglia, J. D., & Rubel, J. A. (2017). Exploring the idiographic dynamics of mood and anxiety via network analysis. *Journal of Abnormal Psychology, 126*(8), 1044–1056. https://doi.org/10.1037/abn0000311

Flake, J. K., & Fried, E. I. (2020). Measurement schmeasurement: Questionable measurement practices and how to avoid them. *Advances in Methods and Practices in Psychological Science, 3*(4), 456–465. https://doi.org/10.1177/2515245920952393

Forbes, M. K., Wright, A. G. C., Markon, K. E., & Krueger, R. F. (2017). Evidence that psychopathology symptom networks have limited replicability. *Journal of Abnormal Psychology, 126*(7), 969–988. https://doi.org/10.1037/abn0000276

Forbes, M. K., Wright, A. G. C., Markon, K. E., & Krueger, R. F. (2017a). Further evidence that psychopathology networks have limited replicability and utility: Response to Borsboom et al. (2017) and Steinley et al. (2017). *Journal of Abnormal Psychology, 126*(7), 1011–1016. https://doi.org/10.1037/abn0000313

Forbes, M. K., Wright, A. G. C., Markon, K. E., & Krueger, R. F. (2021). Quantifying the reliability and replicability of psychopathology network characteristics. *Multivariate Behavioral Research, 56*(2), 224–242. https://doi.org/10.1080/00273171.2019.1616526

Freichel, R., Veer, I., Wiers, R., McNally, R. J., & Epskamp, S. (2023). *Cross-lagged panel models for studying psychopathology: A comparative overview of structural equation and panel network approaches.* Open Science Foundation. https://doi.org/10.31234/osf.io/b94qt

Fried, E. I., & Cramer, A. O. J. (2017). Moving forward: Challenges and directions for psychopathological network theory and methodology. *Perspectives on Psychological Science, 12*(6), 999–1020. https://doi.org/10.1177/1745691617705892

Frumkin, M. R., Piccirillo, M. L., Beck, E. D., Grossman, J. T., & Rodebaugh, T. L. (2020). Feasibility and utility of idiographic models in the clinic: A pilot study. *Psychotherapy Research, 31*(4), 520–534. https://doi.org/10.1080/10503307.2020.1805133

Funkhouser, C. J., Chacko, A. A., Correa, K. A., Kaiser, A. J. E., & Shankman, S. A. (2021). Unique longitudinal relationships between symptoms of psychopathology in youth: A cross-lagged panel network analysis in the ABCD study. *Journal of Child Psychology and Psychiatry, 62*(2), 184–194. https://doi.org/10.1111/jcpp.13256

Giles, J. (1993). The no-self theory: Hume, Buddhism, and personal identity. *Philosophy East and West, 43*(2), 175–200. https://doi.org/10.2307/1399612

Greene, T., Gelkopf, M., Fried, E. I., Robinaugh, D. J., & Lapid Pickman, L. (2020). Dynamic network analysis of negative emotions and dsm-5 posttraumatic stress disorder symptom clusters during conflict. *Journal of Traumatic Stress, 33*(1), 72–83. https://doi.org/10.1002/jts.22433

Guillaume–Hanes, E., Morse, P., & Funder, D. (2012). Network models in the organization of personality. *European Journal of Personality, 26*(4), 439–440. https://doi.org/10.1002/per.1872

Hallquist, M. N., Wright, A. G. C., & Molenaar, P. C. M. (2021). Problems with centrality measures in psychopathology symptom networks: Why network psychometrics cannot escape psychometric theory. *Multivariate Behavioral Research, 56*(2), 199–223. https://doi.org/10.1080/00273171.2019.1640103

Haslbeck, J. M. B., Bringmann, L. F., & Waldorp, L. J. (2021). A tutorial on estimating time-varying vector autoregressive models. *Multivariate Behavioral Research, 56*(1), 120–149. https://doi.org/10.1080/00273171.2020.1743630

Haslbeck, J. M. B., & Ryan, O. (2022). Recovering within-person dynamics from psychological time series. *Multivariate Behavioral Research, 57*(5), 735–766. https://doi.org/10.1080/00273171.2021.1896353

Helmich, M. A., Smit, A. C., Bringmann, L. F., Schreuder, M. J., Oldehinkel, A. J., Wichers, M., & Snippe, E. (2023). Detecting impending symptom transitions using early-warning signals in individuals receiving treatment for depression. *Clinical Psychological Science, 11*(6), 994–1010.

Hoffart, A., Langkaas, T. F., Øktedalen, T., & Johnson, S. U. (2019). The temporal dynamics of symptoms during exposure therapies of PTSD: A network approach. *European Journal of Psychotraumatology, 10*(1), 1618134. https://doi.org/10.1080/20008198.2019.1618134

Holzhauer, C. G., Hildebrandt, T., Epstein, E., McCrady, B., Hallgren, K. A., & Cook, S. (2020). Mechanisms of change in female-specific and gender-neutral cognitive behavioral therapy for women with alcohol use disorder. *Journal of Consulting and Clinical Psychology, 88*(6), 541–553. https://doi.org/10.1037/ccp0000492

Isvoranu, A.-M., Epskamp, S., & Cheung, M. W.-L. (2021). Network models of posttraumatic stress disorder: A meta-analysis. *Journal of Abnormal Psychology, 130*(8), 841–861. https://doi.org/10.1037/abn0000704

Jonas, K. G., & Markon, K. E. (2016). A descriptivist approach to trait conceptualization and inference. *Psychological Review, 123*(1), 90–96. https://doi.org/10.1037/a0039542

Jones, P. J., Ma, R., & McNally, R. J. (2021). Bridge centrality: A network approach to understanding comorbidity. *Multivariate Behavioral Research, 56*(2), 353–367. https://doi.org/10.1080/00273171.2019.1614898

Jones, P. J., Williams, D. R., & McNally, R. J. (2021). Sampling variability is not nonreplication: A Bayesian reanalysis of Forbes, Wright, Markon, and Krueger. *Multivariate Behavioral Research, 56*(2), 249–255. https://doi.org/10.1080/00273171.2020.1797460

Karalunas, S. L., Antovich, D., Goh, P. K., Martel, M. M., Tipsord, J., Nousen, E. K., & Nigg, J. T. (2021). Longitudinal network model of the co-development of temperament, executive functioning, and psychopathology symptoms in youth with and without ADHD. *Development and Psychopathology, 33*(5), 1803–1820. https://doi.org/10.1017/S0954579421000900

Kendler, K. S., Zachar, P., & Craver, C. (2011). What kinds of things are psychiatric disorders? *Psychological Medicine, 41*(6), 1143–1150. https://doi.org/10.1017/S0033291710001844

Kim, H.-J., Lee, S.-H., & Pae, C. (2023). Gender differences in anxiety and depressive symptomatology determined by network analysis in panic disorder. *Journal of Affective Disorders*, *337*, 94–103. https://doi.org/10.1016/j.jad.2023.05.087

Lafit, G., Adolf, J. K., Dejonckheere, E., Myin-Germeys, I., Viechtbauer, W., & Ceulemans, E. (2021). Selection of the number of participants in intensive longitudinal studies: A user-friendly shiny app and tutorial for performing power analysis in multilevel regression models that account for temporal dependencies. *Advances in Methods and Practices in Psychological Science*, *4*(1), 1–24. https://doi.org/10.1177/2515245920978738

Lane, S. T., & Gates, K. M. (2017). Automated selection of robust individual-level structural equation models for time series data. *Structural Equation Modeling: A Multidisciplinary Journal*, *24*(5), 768–782. https://doi.org/10.1080/10705511.2017.1309978

Levinson, C. A., Hunt, R. A., Keshishian, A. C., Brown, M. L., Vanzhula, I., Christian, C., Brosof, L. C., & Williams, B. M. (2021). Using individual networks to identify treatment targets for eating disorder treatment: A proof-of-concept study and initial data. *Journal of Eating Disorders*, *9*(1), 147. https://doi.org/10.1186/s40337-021-00504-7

Levinson, C. A., Williams, B. M., Christian, C., Hunt, R. A., Keshishian, A. C., Brosof, L. C., Vanzhula, I. A., Davis, G. G., Brown, M. L., Bridges-Curry, Z., Sandoval-Araujo, L. E., & Ralph-Nearman, C. (2023). Personalizing eating disorder treatment using idiographic models: An open series trial. *Journal of Consulting and Clinical Psychology*, *91*(1), 14–28. https://doi.org/10.1037/ccp0000785

Li, R., Dziak, J. J., Tan, X., Huang, L., Wagner, A. T., & Yang, J. (2017). *TVEM (time-varying effect model) SAS macro users' guide (Version 3.1.1)*. The Methodology Center, Penn State. http://methodology.psu.edu.

Li, Y., & Kwok, S. Y. C. L. (2023). A longitudinal network analysis of the interactions of risk and protective factors for suicidal potential in early adolescents. *Journal of Youth and Adolescence*, *52*(2), 306–318. https://doi.org/10.1007/s10964-022-01698-y

Li, Y., Wood, J., Ji, L., Chow, S.-M., & Oravecz, Z. (2022). Fitting multilevel vector autoregressive models in stan, jags, and mplus. *Structural Equation Modeling: A Multidisciplinary Journal*, *29*(3), 452–475. https://doi.org/10.1080/10705511.2021.1911657

Lucas, R. E. (2023). Why the cross-lagged panel model is almost never the right choice. *Advances in Methods and Practices in Psychological Science*, *6*(1), 25152459231158378. https://doi.org/10.1177/25152459231158378

Lütkepohl, H. (2005). *New introduction to multiple time series analysis* (13961076). Springer. Publisher description http://www.loc.gov/catdir/enhancements/fy0663/2005927322-d.html Table of contents only http://www.loc.gov/catdir/enhancements/fy0824/2005927322-t.html

Mansueto, A. C., Wiers, R. W., Van Weert, J. C. M., Schouten, B. C., & Epskamp, S. (2023). Investigating the feasibility of idiographic network models. *Psychological Methods*, *28*(5), 1052–1068. https://doi.org/10.1037/met0000466

Marian, S., Costantini, G., Macsinga, I., & Sava, F. A. (2023). The dynamic interplay of anxious and depressive symptoms in a sample of undergraduate students. *Journal of Psychopathology and Behavioral Assessment*, *45*(1), 150–159. https://doi.org/10.1007/s10862-022-10014-8

Mataix-Cols, D., do Rosario-Campos, M. C., & Leckman, J. F. (2005). A multidimensional model of obsessive-compulsive disorder. *American Journal of Psychiatry*, *162*(2), 228–238. https://doi.org/10.1176/appi.ajp.162.2.228

Maxwell, S. E., & Cole, D. A. (2007). Bias in cross-sectional analyses of longitudinal mediation. *Psychological Methods*, *12*(1), 23–44. https://doi.org/10.1037/1082-989X.12.1.23

Maxwell, S. E., Cole, D. A., & Mitchell, M. A. (2011). Bias in cross-sectional analyses of longitudinal mediation: Partial and complete mediation under an autoregressive model. *Multivariate Behavioral Research*, *46*(5), 816–841. https://doi.org/10.1080/00273171.2011.606716

McGhie, S. F., & McNally, R. J. (2023). Posttraumatic stress disorder symptoms and positive affect: Individual and multilevel dynamic networks. *Psychological Trauma: Theory, Research, Practice, and Policy*, *17*(3), 593–602. https://doi.org/10.1037/tra0001605

McNally, R. J. (2011). *What is mental illness?* Harvard University Press. https://doi.org/10.4159/9780674059481

McNally, R. J. (2016). Can network analysis transform psychopathology? *Behaviour Research and Therapy*, *86*, 95–104. https://doi.org/10.1016/j.brat.2016.06.006

McNally, R. J. (2021). Network analysis of psychopathology: Controversies and challenges. *Annual Review of Clinical Psychology*, *17*(1), 31–53. https://doi.org/10.1146/annurev-clinpsy-081219-092850

Molenaar, P. C. M. (2004). A manifesto on psychology as idiographic science: Bringing the person back into scientific psychology, this time forever. *Measurement: Interdisciplinary Research and Perspectives*, 2(4), 201–218. https://doi.org/10.1207/s15366359mea0204_1

Molenaar, P. C. M. (2007). Psychological methodology will change profoundly due to the necessity to focus on intra-individual variation. *Integrative Psychological & Behavioral Science*, *41*(1), 35–40. https://doi.org/10.1007/s12124-007-9011-1

Molenaar, P. C. M. (2013). On the necessity to use person-specific data analysis approaches in psychology. *European Journal of Developmental Psychology*, *10*(1), 29–39. https://doi.org/10.1080/17405629.2012.747435

Monteleone, A. M., & Cascino, G. (2021). A systematic review of network analysis studies in eating disorders: Is time to broaden the core psychopathology to non specific symptoms. *European Eating Disorders Review*, 29(4), 531–547. https://doi.org/10.1002/erv.2834

Morton, J., & Frith, U. (1995). Causal modeling: A structural approach to developmental psychopathology. In *Developmental psychopathology, Vol. 1: Theory and methods* (pp. 357–390). John Wiley & Sons.

Moscovitch, D. A., Orr, E., Rowa, K., Reimer, S. G., & Antony, M. M. (2009). In the absence of rose-colored glasses: Ratings of self-attributes and their differential certainty and importance across multiple dimensions in social phobia. *Behaviour Research and Therapy*, *47*(1), 66–70. https://doi.org/10.1016/j.brat.2008.10.007

Neal, Z. P., Forbes, M. K., Neal, J. W., Brusco, M. J., Krueger, R., Markon, K., Steinley, D., Wasserman, S., & Wright, A. G. C. (2022). Critiques of network analysis of multivariate data in psychological science. *Nature Reviews Methods Primers*, 2(1), 66–70, Article 1. https://doi.org/10.1038/s43586-022-00177-9

Nemesure, M. D., Collins, A. C., Price, G. D., Griffin, T. Z., Pillai, A., Nepal, S., Heinz, M. V., Lekkas, D., Campbell, A. T., & Jacobson, N. C. (2024). Depressive symptoms as a heterogeneous and constantly evolving dynamical system: Idiographic depressive symptom networks of rapid symptom changes among persons with major depressive disorder. *Journal of Psychopathology and Clinical Science*, *133*(2), 155–166. https://doi.org/10.1037/abn0000884

Olthof, M., Hasselman, F., Strunk, G., Van Rooij, M., Aas, B., Helmich, M. A., Schiepek, G., & Lichtwarck-Aschoff, A. (2020). Critical fluctuations as an early-warning signal for sudden gains and losses in patients receiving psychotherapy for mood disorders. *Clinical Psychological Science*, *8*(1), 25–35. https://doi.org/10.1177/2167702619865969

Pearl, J. (2000). *Causality: Models, reasoning, and inference* (11768929). Cambridge University Press. Table of contents http://www.loc.gov/catdir/toc/cam024/99042108.html Publisher description http://www.loc.gov/catdir/description/cam0210/99042108.html Contributor biographical information http://www.loc.gov/catdir/enhancements/fy1001/99042108-b.html

Pettersson, E., & Turkheimer, E. (2013). Approach temperament, anger, and evaluation: Resolving a paradox. *Journal of Personality and Social Psychology*, *105*(2), 285–300. https://doi.org/10.1037/a0033046

Piccirillo, M. L., Beck, E. D., & Rodebaugh, T. L. (2019). A clinician's primer for idiographic research: Considerations and recommendations. *Behavior Therapy*, *50*(5), 938–951. https://doi.org/10.1016/j.beth.2019.02.002

Piccirillo, M. L., & Rodebaugh, T. L. (2019). Foundations of idiographic methods in psychology and applications for psychotherapy. *Clinical Psychological Review*. https://doi.org/10.1016/j.cpr.2019.01.002

Piccirillo, M. L., & Rodebaugh, T. L. (2022). Personalized networks of social anxiety disorder and depression and implications for treatment. *Journal of Affective Disorders*, *298*(Part A), 262–276. https://doi.org/10.1016/j.jad.2021.10.034

Robinaugh, D., Haslbeck, J., Waldorp, L., Kossakowski, J. J., Fried, E., Millner, A., McNally, R., Ryan, O., de Ron, J., van der Maas, H., van Nes, E., Scheffer, M., Kendler, K., & Borsboom, D. (2019). *Advancing the network theory of mental disorders: A computational model of panic disorder*. https://doi.org/10.31234/osf.io/km37w

Robinaugh, D. J., Hoekstra, R. H. A., Toner, E. R., & Borsboom, D. (2020). The network approach to psychopathology: A review of the literature 2008–2018 and an agenda for future research. *Psychological Medicine*, *50*(3), 353–366. https://doi.org/10.1017/S0033291719003404

Robinaugh, D. J., Millner, A. J., & McNally, R. J. (2016). Identifying highly influential nodes in the complicated grief network. *Journal of Abnormal Psychology*, *125*(6), 747–757. https://doi.org/10.1037/abn0000181

Rodebaugh, T. L. (2009). Social phobia and perceived friendship quality. *Journal of Anxiety Disorders*, *23*(7), 872–878. https://doi.org/10.1016/j.janxdis.2009.05.001

Rodebaugh, T. L., Frumkin, M. R., & Piccirillo, M. L. (2020). The long road from person-specific models to personalized mental health treatment. *BMC Medicine*, *18*(1), 365. https://doi.org/10.1186/s12916-020-01838-w

Rodebaugh, T. L., Gianoli, M. O., Turkheimer, E., & Oltmanns, T. F. (2010). The interpersonal problems of the socially avoidant: Self and peer shared variance. *Journal of Abnormal Psychology*, *119*(2), 331–340. https://doi.org/10.1037/a0019031

Rodebaugh, T. L., Grossman, J. T., Tonge, N. A., Shin, J., Frumkin, M. R., Rodriguez, C. R., Ortiz, E. G., & Piccirillo, M. L. (2024). Avoidance and fear day by day in social anxiety disorder. *Psychotherapy Research*, *35*(2), 282–295. https://doi.org/10.1080/10503307.2023.2297994

Rodebaugh, T. L., Lim, M. H., Fernandez, K. C., Langer, J. K., Weisman, J. S., Tonge, N., Levinson, C. A., & Shumaker, E. A. (2014). Self and friend's differing views of social anxiety disorder's effects on friendships. *Journal of Abnormal Psychology*, *123*(4), 715–724. https://doi.org/10.1037/abn0000015

Rodebaugh, T. L., Piccirillo, M. L., Frumkin, M. R., Kallogjeri, D., Gerull, K. M., & Piccirillo, J. F. (2023). Investigating individual variation using dynamic structural equation modeling: A tutorial with tinnitus. *Clinical Psychological Science*, *11*(3), 574–591. https://doi.org/10.1177/21677026221129279

Rohrer, J. M. (2018). Thinking clearly about correlations and causation: Graphical causal models for observational data. *Advances in Methods and Practices in Psychological Science*, *1*(1), 27–42. https://doi.org/10.1177/2515245917745629

Rohrer, J. M., Hünermund, P., Arslan, R. C., & Elson, M. (2022). That's a lot to process! Pitfalls of popular path models. *Advances in Methods and Practices in Psychological Science*, *5*(2), 25152459221095827. https://doi.org/10.1177/25152459221095827

Savelieva, K., Komulainen, K., Elovainio, M., & Jokela, M. (2021). Longitudinal associations between specific symptoms of depression: Network analysis in a prospective cohort study. *Journal of Affective Disorders*, *278*, 99–106. https://doi.org/10.1016/j.jad.2020.09.024

Scheffer, M., Bascompte, J., Brock, W. A., Brovkin, V., Carpenter, S. R., Dakos, V., Held, H., van Nes, E. H., Rietkerk, M., & Sugihara, G. (2009). Early-warning signals for critical transitions. *Nature*, *461*(7260), 53–59. https://doi.org/10.1038/nature08227

Schimmack, U., & Gere, J. (2012). The utility of network analysis for personality psychology. *European Journal of Personality*, *26*(4), 446–447. https://doi.org/10.1002/per.1876

Schreuder, M. J., Hartman, C. A., George, S. V., Menne-Lothmann, C., Decoster, J., van Winkel, R., Delespaul, P., De Hert, M., Derom, C., Thiery, E., Rutten, B. P. F., Jacobs, N., van Os, J., Wigman, J. T. W., & Wichers, M. (2020). Early warning signals in psychopathology: What do they tell? *BMC Medicine*, *18*(1), 269. https://doi.org/10.1186/s12916-020-01742-3

Schultzberg, M., & Muthén, B. (2018). Number of subjects and time points needed for multilevel time-series analysis: A simulation study of dynamic structural equation modeling. *Structural Equation Modeling*, *25*(4), 495–515. https://doi.org/10.1080/10705511.2017.1392862

Schuurman, N. K., & Hamaker, E. L. (2019). Measurement error and person-specific reliability in multilevel autoregressive modeling. *Psychological Methods*, *24*(1), 70–91. https://doi.org/10.1037/met0000188

Snippe, E., Smit, A. C., Kuppens, P., Burger, H., & Ceulemans, E. (2023). Recurrence of depression can be foreseen by monitoring mental states with statistical process control. *Journal of Psychopathology and Clinical Science*, *132*(2), 145–155. https://doi.org/10.1037/abn0000812

Terracciano, A., & McCrae, R. R. (2012). Why do (some) birds flock? Causality and the structure of characteristic adaptations. *European Journal of Personality*, *26*(4), 449–450. https://doi.org/10.1002/per.1878

Thelen, E., & Smith, L. B. (1994). *A dynamic systems approach to the development of cognition and action* (1st MIT pbk. ed.). MIT Press. https://catalog.lib.unc.edu/catalog/UNCb3998124

Tonge, N. A., Miller, J. P., Kharasch, E. D., Lenze, E. J., & Rodebaugh, T. L. (2024). An investigation of the potential clinical utility of critical slowing down as an early warning sign for recurrence of depression. *Journal of Behavior Therapy and Experimental Psychiatry*, *82*, 101922. https://doi.org/10.1016/j.jbtep.2023.101922

van de Leemput, I. A., Wichers, M., Cramer, A. O. J., Borsboom, D., Tuerlinckx, F., Kuppens, P., van Nes, E. H., Viechtbauer, W., Giltay, E. J., Aggen, S. H., Derom, C., Jacobs, N., Kendler, K. S., van der Maas, H. L. J., Neale, M. C., Peeters, F., Thiery, E., Zachar, P., & Scheffer, M. (2014). Critical slowing down as early warning for the onset and termination of depression. *PNAS Proceedings of the National Academy of Sciences of the United States of America*, *111*(1), 87–92. https://doi.org/10.1073/pnas.1312114110

van der Maas, H. L. J., Dolan, C. V., Grasman, R. P. P. P., Wicherts, J. M., Huizenga, H. M., & Raijmakers, M. E. J. (2006). A dynamical model of general intelligence: The positive manifold of intelligence by mutualism. *Psychological Review*, *113*(4), 842–861. https://doi.org/10.1037/0033-295X.113.4.842

von Klipstein, L., Riese, H., van der Veen, D. C., Servaas, M. N., & Schoevers, R. A. (2020). Using person-specific networks in psychotherapy: Challenges, limitations, and how we could use them anyway. *BMC Medicine*, *18*(1), 345. https://doi.org/10.1186/s12916-020-01818-0

Wichers, M., & Groot, P. C. (2016). Critical slowing down as a personalized early warning signal for depression. *Psychotherapy and Psychosomatics*, *85*(2), 114–116.

Wichers, M., Schreuder, M. J., Goekoop, R., & Groen, R. N. (2019). Can we predict the direction of sudden shifts in symptoms? Transdiagnostic implications from a complex systems perspective on psychopathology. *Psychological Medicine*, *49*(3), 380–387. https://doi.org/10.1017/S0033291718002064

Wichers, M., Smit, A. C., & Snippe, E. (2020). Early warning signals based on momentary affect dynamics can expose nearby transitions in depression: A confirmatory single-subject time-series study. *Journal for Person-Oriented Research*, *6*(1), 1–15, Article 1. https://doi.org/10.17505/jpor.2020.22042

Wysocki, A., Bork, R. van, Cramer, A., & Rhemtulla, M. (2022). *Cross-lagged network models*. Open Science Framework. https://doi.org/10.31234/osf.io/vjr8z

Zhang, C., Huang, J., & Xu, W. (2024). Longitudinal relationships between depressive symptoms and generalized anxiety symptoms in adolescents: A cross-lagged network analysis. *Journal of Youth and Adolescence*, *53*, 1918–1927. https://doi.org/10.1007/s10964-024-01961-4

CHAPTER 9

The Dimensionalization of Personality Pathology

The State of the Science

CARLA SHARP AND KIRAN BOONE

Introduction

THE advantages of dimensional approaches to psychopathology for the understanding, assessment, and treatment of mental disorders are well documented. Since the 1950s, there have been persistent calls for the dimensionalization of psychopathology (e.g. Frances, 1993; Holzberg & Wittenborn, 1953; Tyrer & Alexander, 1979; Wittenborn, Holzberg, & Simon, 1953). In this chapter, we provide an update on the state of the science with regard to the dimensionalization of psychopathology, specifically as it pertains to personality pathology. We begin with a brief discussion of the rationale for this dimensionalization. We then present two recent dimensional classification systems for personality disorder that emerged from the drive toward dimensionalization: the DSM-5-TR (2024) Alternative Model for Personality Disorder (AMPD) and the ICD-11 (WHO, 2022) diagnostic criteria for personality disorder. We focus our discussion on the distinct and dimensionally distributed single indicator of personality pathology that was introduced to address the problems of the categorical system—that is, Level of Personality Functioning (LPF). We lay out the argument for why a distinct, dimensionally distributed single indicator of personality pathology is necessary, centering our argument around its function in explaining the onset of personality disorder. In short, we argue that other indicators of personality disorder (such as traits) represent continuous, non-distinctive features of personality disorder, falling short of providing the kind of information necessary to optimize clinical utility in the diagnosis of personality disorder. In presenting our argument, an obvious tension is revealed: while personality pathology is best represented by a single underlying dimension of personality pathology, this dimension may be distinct from other dimensions of psychopathology, signaling a distinct class of psychopathology that potentially undermines a fully dimensionalized view of psychopathology. Therefore, in the final section of the chapter, we address the implications of our perspective for other dimensional models of psychopathology. We conclude with a section on future directions for research.

The Dimensionalization of Personality Pathology

Problems with the Categorical System for the Diagnosis of Personality Disorder

Section II of the DSM-5 (Diagnostic Criteria and Codes) currently contains 10 personality disorders that are diagnosed with polythetic criterion sets, including schizotypal, schizoid, paranoid, antisocial, borderline, narcissistic, histrionic, avoidant, dependent, and obsessive-compulsive personality disorders. Personality disorders, like most other disorders in the DSM, are viewed as discrete entities delimited from one another and from other psychiatric disorders. The limitations of a categorical approach to the diagnosis of personality disorder have been well documented over the last 50 years (Clark, 2007; Frances, 1993; Krueger & Eaton, 2010; Livesley, 1998; Oldham & Skodol, 2000; Skodol et al., 2011; Tyrer & Alexander, 1979; Widiger & Clark, 2000; Widiger & Trull, 2007). First, personality disorders, especially when assessed in rigorous research studies employing interview-based assessment tools, are highly comorbid with one another, such that a patient diagnosed with one personality disorder is likely to be diagnosed with at least two or three additional personality disorders (Eaton, South, & Krueger, 2015; Trull & Durrett, 2005). In clinical practice, this problem manifests in clinicians' struggles to fit an individual patient into any one specific category, resulting in either the underdiagnosis of personality disorder, or the use of Personality Disorder Not Otherwise Specified (PD-NOS-)—which turns out to be the most diagnosed personality disorder—(-e.g., Verheul, Bartak, & Widiger, 2007). Second, due to polythetic criteria sets, individuals who meet criteria for a personality disorder differ in marked ways from one another. In some cases, individuals meeting criteria for the same personality disorder may have only one feature in common. This is problematic for a diagnostic label, because it implies that individuals in the same diagnostic class may actually resemble one another in very limited ways. Third, diagnostic thresholds (e.g., the five out of nine requirement for borderline personality disorder) are arbitrary, calling into question whether individuals above and below clinical threshold really differ from one another in the clinically significant way the diagnosis implies. Fourth, high levels of heterogeneity and comorbidity and/or co-occurrence among personality disorders have resulted in failed attempts to identify 10 discrete disorders through factor analyses (Sheets & Craighead, 2007). Meta-analyses show that instead of 10 specific factors (e.g., a borderline personality factor) that each explain co-variation of a set of symptoms (e.g., the nine borderline criteria), significant cross-loading of personality disorder symptoms occur with no clear 10-factor structure emerging in the data (Sheets & Craighead, 2007).

Taken together, high levels of comorbidity, heterogeneity within disorder, and the associated failure to demonstrate 10 discrete categories in factor analyses call into question the existence of PD as discrete entities. Indeed, with such porous boundaries, it is also no surprise that progress has been slow to demonstrate any unique antecedents, correlates, or outcomes for personality disorder that are distinguishable from other disorders. While it is true that cognitive, emotional, and psychophysiological antecedents, correlates, and outcomes have been identified for borderline personality disorder, and to some extent for antisocial, schizotypal, and avoidant personality disorder, this is not the case for the other PDs. Moreover, even when antecedent risk factors (e.g., maltreatment, adversity), correlates (e.g., emotion dysregulation, mentalization difficulties), and outcomes (e.g., functional impairment, suicidal behavior) have been identified, they tend to be non-specific to personality disorder, and appear to be ubiquitous across PDs, failing to identify any unique validators for individual PDs.

Taken together, the issues summarized above naturally pose many practical challenges for the assessment, diagnosis, and treatment planning and implementation for personality disorder. Studies have shown that with the exception of antisocial personality disorder, weak interrater reliability and test-retest reliability pervades categorially defined PD assessment and diagnosis, unless clinicians are aided by the use of a semi-structured interview that provides specific questions for each diagnostic criterion (Widiger & Frances, 1987). If categories do not exist as described in the DSM, and if they cannot be reliably identified by front-line clinicians doing unstructured clinical interviews, how reasonable is it to develop and evaluate treatment manuals for each disorder as if they were discrete? Indeed, research shows that clinicians end up discarding the rigid use of individualized treatment manuals to more eclectically personalize treatment. While eclectic integration provides an immediate practical solution for front-line clinicians, it poses a challenge for evidence-based practice with millions of dollars spent on developing, evaluating, training, supervising, and implementing adherent treatment protocols that are not used as designed, because they fail to adequately fit the symptom presentation of real-life patients (e.g., Chorpita et al., 2011; Wampold & Imel, 2015).

The final problem with PD categories we would like to highlight is the stigma associated with them. Personality disorders are highly stigmatized (Sheehan, Nieweglowski, & Corrigan, 2016). Borderline personality disorder (BPD), in particular, is viewed as the most stigmatized of all the personality disorders, especially among healthcare providers (Bonnington & Rose, 2014). In addition, Sheehan et al.'s (2016) review concluded that general public knowledge of personality disorders is low and that personality disorders are not necessarily viewed as illness, but rather as misbehavior. The question then arises as to whether a more dimensionalized system can reduce stigmatization, and if so, how.

DSM-5 Alternative Model for Personality Disorder

Against the background of these challenges, the DSM-5 personality and personality disorder work group proposed to replace the 10 categorical PD diagnoses with a single indicator of PD, emphasizing that all individuals with personality pathology share a common core feature—that is, maladaptive self and interpersonal functioning. They named this common (shared) dimension the Level of Personality Functioning (LPF) and defined it as a unidimensional severity criterion common to all personality disorder manifestations (see Table 9.1 for an abbreviated LPF scale). LPF is viewed as a parsimonious solution to eliminate comorbidity, as well as the need for non-descript PD diagnoses such as PD-NOS, thereby facilitating PD diagnosis and treatment for individuals with an underdiagnosed and stigmatized condition. In addition, beyond clinical utility, from a structural point of view, the expectation was that an alternative representation of the true co-variation of PD symptoms would be described that more accurately corresponds to the way maladaptive traits associate with one another.

As shown in Table 9.1, the DSM-5 Level of Personality Functioning Scale (LPFS) describes identity and self-direction as the main defining features of self-functioning, and empathy and intimacy as the main defining features of interpersonal functioning. Identity, self-direction, empathy, and intimacy are rated by a clinician on a five-point Likert scale from zero to four. Personality functioning scored at a zero indicates healthy personality functioning (an integrated sense of self, strong reflective capacities, differentiated emotional life, self-directedness, the capacity to empathically reflect and integrate the perspective of others, and strong and mutually rewarding relationships). A rating of one indicates some challenges in the domains of self- and interpersonal functioning, which are not significant enough to be considered clinically meaningful. A rating of two begins to indicate a clinical level of personality functioning, including an incoherent sense of self, lack of self-directedness, marked impairment in

TABLE 9.1 Level of Personality Functioning Scale

Level of Impairment	Self		Interpersonal	
	Identity	Self-direction	Empathy	Intimacy
0 Little or No Impairment	Awareness of a unique self with role-appropriate boundaries; positive and accurate self-esteem; full range of emotions.	Sets reasonable goals; appropriate and fulfilling standards of behavior; can reflect on and make meaning of internal experience.	Understands others' experiences, motivations, and perspectives; aware of effect of actions on others.	Multiple satisfying, enduring, reciprocal relationships; strives for cooperation and mutual benefit.
1 Some impairment	Intact sense of self but less clear in times of distress; self-esteem diminished at times; restricted range of emotions and strong emotions may be distressing.	Excessively goal-directed, goal-inhibited, or conflicted; unrealistic or inappropriate standards of behavior; may overemphasize intellectual or emotional self-reflection.	Somewhat compromised understanding of others' experiences and motivations; resists different perspectives; inconsistent awareness of effect of actions on others.	Enduring relationships with some limitations on depth, satisfaction, and meaningful expression; cooperation may be limited by unrealistic standards.
2 Moderate impairment	Depends on others for identity definition; vulnerable, inflated, or deflated self-esteem; emotion regulation depends on external evaluation.	Goals are a means for gaining external approval; standards of behavior are inauthentic and unreasonably high or low; impaired self-reflection.	Excessively self-referential in considering others' experiences, motivations, and perspectives; unaware, unconcerned, or unrealistic about effect of actions on others.	Superficial connections; close relationships are based on meeting own needs; does not see relationships as reciprocal, cooperates for personal gain.
3 Severe impairment	Weak sense of self, poor or rigid boundaries, emptiness; fragile, un-nuanced self-esteem influenced by events; rapidly shifting emotions or chronic despair.	Difficulty setting or achieving goals; standards of behavior are unclear or contradictory, life is seen as meaningless or dangerous; significantly compromised self-reflection.	Poor understanding of others' experiences and motivations; threatened by different perspectives; confused or unaware of the effect of actions on others.	Few positive connections; close relationships are based on absolute need for others or expectations of abuse or abandonment; low mutuality, disrupted cooperation.
4 Extreme impairment	Virtually no sense of self, confused or no boundaries; weak self-image threatened by others; emotions are incongruent with context or internal experience.	Goals are unrealistic or incoherent, poor differentiation of thoughts from actions; no standards of behavior; profoundly impaired self-reflection.	Pronounced inability to understand others' experiences and motivations; no attention to different perspectives; social interactions can be confusing and disorienting.	Disinterest or expectation of harm in relationships; sees relationships in terms of comfort vs pain; social behavior is not reciprocal but seeks fulfillment of needs.

empathy, and problems in maintaining relationships. A rating of three indicates severe impairment in self- and interpersonal functioning. A rating of four indicates almost complete breakdown in self- and interpersonal functioning, including virtually absent experience of self as an autonomous agent, poor self/other boundaries, distorted self-image and appraisal, incongruence in inner experience of emotions, poor self-directedness and self-reflection, lack of internal standards to guide behavior, pronounced inability to consider the perspectives or feelings of others, disorienting and confusing interactions with others, and complete lack of reciprocity in relationships marked by disinterest or disorganization and conflict.

Once a clinician has assigned a rating on the dimension of LPF, they proceed to assess the "flavor," style, or manifestation of personality dysfunction by evaluating an individual's traits, which are hierarchically organized within five trait domains broadly mirroring the Big Five trait structure of basic personality, including negative affectivity (neuroticism), detachment (introversion), antagonism (low agreeableness), disinhibition (low conscientiousness), and psychoticism (openness) (Widiger & Simonsen, 2005). To rate traits, facets, and domains, the clinician may use the Personality Inventory for DSM-5 (PID-5) (Krueger, Derringer, Markon, Watson, & Skodol, 2012), which is freely available on the DSM web pages.

The proposed AMPD was accepted with great excitement among most of the research community; however, at the time, the American Psychiatric Association determined that critical elements of its empirical basis were still lacking. The AMPD was therefore relegated to Section III of the DSM-5 for further study while the original 10 categorical PDs were retained in the main section (Section II) of the DSM-5.

The ICD-11 Criteria for the Diagnosis of PD

In contrast, the World Health Organization fully embraced a dimensionalized approach to the diagnosis of PD when it published the ICD-11 in 2022 (Mulder, 2021; World Health Organization, 2019). The ICD-11 mirrors the AMPD with its entry criterion of maladaptive self- and interpersonal functioning as a single indicator of personality disturbance, and makes the specification of maladaptive trait manifestation optional. In other words, all that is needed for a diagnosis of PD in the ICD-11 is the evaluation of an individual's self- and interpersonal functioning. Describing the style in which personality disturbance manifests is an option for clinicians and not conditional to the diagnosis. Two other features of the ICD-11 system distinguish it from the AMPD. First, psychoticism is represented elsewhere in the ICD-11 and, instead, anankastia (compulsive) traits are included as a fifth trait domain. Finally, to facilitate a crosswalk with the traditional categorical system so that services can transition to the new system, a borderline specifier was retained. All other personality disorder categories were removed from the criteria set.

Summary: The Dimensionalization of Personality Pathology

Both the AMPD and ICD-11 represent dimensionalized approaches to psychopathology in two important ways. First, these models identify underlying dimensions (or spectra) that account for co-variance of multiple symptoms or disorders at the observed level. Thus, the LPF is a dimension that accounts for the co-variance of the symptoms of all personality disorders. Similarly, maladaptive trait domains represent five dimensions that account for the co-variance of subsets of personality disorder symptoms. Whether one dimension (LPF) or five dimensions (trait domains) or a combination of the two are necessary remains a hotly debated issue (Morey, 2019b, 2019c; Sleep, Lynam, Widiger, Crowe, & Miller, 2019; Widiger et al., 2019), which we will return to later in the chapter.

The second way in which these systems represent dimensionality is by allowing for severity ratings. An individual no longer has or does not have a personality disorder, but instead lies on a continuum of severity of personality pathology. This allows not only for more nuanced inter-individual comparisons but also intra-individual comparisons. In our view, the LPF does this more comprehensively than the maladaptive traits by offering a five-point Likert scale ranging from typical/healthy to atypical/unhealthy. Due to its coverage of the full range from typical to atypical, the LPF represents full dimensionality in the way that theoretical tenets of dimensionality prescribe (see, e.g., Cicchetti, 2006; Rutter & Rutter, 1993; Rutter & Sroufe, 2000). Moreover, LPF's severity index helpfully identifies when personality functioning crosses clinical threshold. For traits, at present, no guidance is provided for when a trait should be considered severe enough to cross clinical threshold. Given its maladaptive nature, perhaps it is the mere presence that warrants treatment? If so, traits operate relatively similar to traditional PD categories—individuals have them or they don't have them—just organized around five dimensions instead of 10 categories and allowing a severity rating similar to symptom count. We view this as a challenge for the trait perspective in personality pathology—as do some trait psychologists (e.g., Hopwood, Schwaba, Wright, Bleidorn, & Zanarini, 2022). Against this background, we ask the question: Does re-envisioning personality disorder traits as maladaptive or basic traits really improve the assessment, diagnosis, and treatment of personality disorders? In this chapter we argue that traits are not enough, and that the answer to a more precise and clinically useful diagnosis of personality disorder lies in the dimension of LPF—defined as an intrapsychic *capacity* for making sense of oneself and others. Traits remain useful—and we will explicate why. Before we elaborate this argument further, we present the current state of the science on the AMPD and ICD-11, with a special focus on the LPF.

The AMPD and ICD-11: State of the Science

The Validity, Reliability, and Clinical Utility of the AMPD

Since its publication in 2013, a substantial number of studies have evaluated various aspects of the validity and reliability of the AMPD and the ICD-11. This research was recently reviewed in a 10-year retrospective special issue of *Personality Disorders: Theory, Research and Treatment* (see editorial; Sharp & Miller, 2022), with empirical support for the AMPD organized in four papers to cover Criterion A (Level of Personality Functioning; Morey, McCredie, Bender, & Skodol, 2022), Criterion B (maladaptive trait domains; Clark & Watson, 2022), the full model (Widiger & Hines, 2022), as well as a paper specifically dedicated to the clinical utility of the AMPD (Bach & Tracy, 2022). Sharp and Miller (2022) concluded that the data of the last 10 years are sufficient to justify inclusion of the AMPD in Section II of the DSM-5, echoing the conclusions of other reviews on the empirical basis of the AMPD (Krueger & Hobbs, 2020; Milinkovic & Tiliopoulos, 2020; Morey, Benson, Busch, & Skodol, 2015; Rodriguez-Seijas, Ruggero, Eaton, & Krueger, 2019; Sharp & Wall, 2021; Waugh et al., 2017; Zimmermann, Kerber, Rek, Hopwood, & Krueger, 2019). Here, we provide a brief summary of this research, specifically with regard to LPF.

Factor structure. Factor analytic evidence by and large supports the proposed unidimensional factor structure of the LPF, both in adults, using the Level of Personality Functioning Scale-Self Report (LPFS-SR) (e.g. Hopwood, Good, & Morey, 2018; Morey, 2017), and in adolescents, using the Level of Personality Functioning Scale-Brief Form 2.0 (LPFS-BF 2.0), Semi-structured interview for Personality functioning DSM-5 (STiP-5.1), and Levels of

Personality Functioning Questionnaire (LoPF-Q 12–18) (Balzen et al., in press; Kerr et al., 2022; Wu, Allman, Balzen, Hutsebaut, & Sharp, 2024). While some studies found support for a two-factor structure (self and interpersonal) (e.g., Hutsebaut, Feenstra, & Kamphuis, 2016; Weekers, Hutsebaut, & Kamphuis, 2019), or a four-factor structure (identity, self-direction, empathy, and intimacy) (Goth, Birkhölzer, & Schmeck, 2018; Sleep et al., 2019) of LPF, factors appear to be so highly correlated that it justifies the use of a total score as a single indicator of personality disturbance. At the same time, research suggests that the consideration of individual LPF profiles across the four domains of identity, self-direction, intimacy, and empathy may provide clinically useful information (Thomson et al., 2024). Therefore, LPF is most likely best understood as consisting of both a general factor representing a single indicator of personality disturbance, and specific factors of identity, self-direction, intimacy, and empathy that can provide nuance in the description of an individual's personality functioning (Gamache, Savard, Leclerc, & Cote, 2019; Kerr et al., 2022; Siefert et al., 2020).

Reliability. Multiple studies have demonstrated excellent inter-rater reliability on interview-based measures of LPF including intra-class correlations of .98 for clinician-rated LPF (Morey, 2019a), up to .92 on the STiP-5.1 (Hutsebaut, Kamphuis, Feenstra, Weekers, & De Saeger, 2017), and up to .96 on the Structured Clinical interview for the DSM-5 Alternative Model for Personality Disorders (SCID-5-AMPD Module I) (Christensen et al., 2018). Test-retest reliability is equally strong with two-week interval reliability coefficient reported at .92 for the LPFS-SR and an average of .84 on the SCID-5-AMPD (Ohse et al., 2023). Internal consistency for all LPF measures is high, with studies showing excellent internal consistency for DSM ratings by both clinicians (Dereboy, Dereboy, & Eskin, 2018) and even by undergraduate student raters (Cruitt, Boudreaux, King, Oltmanns, & Oltmanns, 2019; Zimmermann et al., 2014).

Convergent validity. Multiple studies have demonstrated convergent validity of LPF measures with other LPF measures (e.g., McCabe, Oltmanns, & Widiger, 2021; Ohse et al., 2023), other measures of personality disorder (e.g., Eggermont et al., 2023; Morey, 2017; Paap, Pedersen, Kvarstein, & Hummelen, 2023; Wu et al., 2024), maladaptive traits (Widiger et al., 2019), basic personality traits (Biberdzic, Tang, & Tan, 2021), and conceptually related constructs such as identity disturbance (Gamache et al., 2019; Kerr et al., 2022; Morey, 2017; Paap et al., 2023; Wu et al., 2024). Convergent validity is further demonstrated in studies showing strong correlations between LPF and emotional and cognitive correlates that are expected to associate with personality disorder. For instance, Roche et al. (2016) showed prospective relations between LPF and cognitive distortions. Cognitive distortions also defined a latent class high in LPF impairment in adolescents (Eggermont et al., 2023). LPF has also been shown to associate with deficits in mentalizing (Zettl et al., 2020), as well as reduced affiliative behavior and more negative daily affect (Ringwald, Hopwood, Pilkonis, & Wright, 2021). LPF further associates with alterations in social (but not monetary) reward processing in adolescents (Babinski et al., 2023). In fact, LPF appears to outperform BPD features in predicting social reward alterations in adolescents (Boone et al., 2025).

Predictive validity. LPF appears to be clinically useful in predicting a range of clinical outcomes, including treatment participation and satisfaction with the provider (Papamalis, Kalyva, Teare, & Meier, 2020), treatment drop-out (Busmann et al., 2019), and general function (Roche, Jacobson, & Phillips, 2018). LPF furthermore appears to be able to detect change as a function of treatment in adults (Kvarstein et al., 2023) and in adolescents (Hessels, De Moor, Deutz, Laceulle, & VanAken, 2024; Sharp, Kulesz, & Kerr, 2024).

Head-to-head comparisons in predictive validity. The AMPD was designed to provide full coverage of the traditional categorical personality disorders. Indeed, research supports full coverage of the traditional categories, including schizotypal PD (Kwapil & Neus Barrantes-Vidal, 2022), antisocial PD (Anderson & Kelley, 2022), borderline PD (Vanwoerden & Stepp, 2022), narcissistic PD (Miller, Crowe, & Sharpe, 2022), avoidant PD (Hummelen, Ulltveit-Moe Eikenaes, & Wilberg, 2022); and partial coverage for obsessive-compulsive PD (Samuel, Balling, & Bucher, 2022). Thus, the AMPD and ICD-11 systems are supposed to measure the same constructs as the traditional PD categories, just better organized to reflect clinical realities and the empirical structure of psychopathology. Even so, several recent studies have demonstrated that AMPD measures perform as well or even outperform measures of traditional categories in predicting clinical outcomes. Sharp et al. (2024) found that combined LPF and trait self-report assessment was a better predictor of treatment outcome than BPD self-report in inpatient adolescents, mirroring the results of a similar study with adolescent outpatients (Hessels et al., 2024). Maffly-Kipp and Morey (2024) found that AMPD components (LPF and traits) consistently added unique variance beyond the Section II categorical PD diagnoses in predicting clinical outcome judgments, whereas the Section II diagnoses were rarely incremental above the AMPD. Further, the AMPD predicted clinical outcome judgments very consistently (98.3% of regressions) compared to the Section II predictors (70% of regressions), and the single Criterion A judgment (LPF) was the strongest overall predictor. The authors concluded that the AMPD is as—and by some measures more—effective than the DSM-5 categorical model at predicting clinician's judgment of outcomes in clinical cases.

Clinical utility. Several studies have shown that LPF assessment can distinguish individuals who have personality disorder from those who do not, using the LPFS-SR (e.g., Morey, 2018), the LPFS-BF 2.0 (e.g., Hutsebaut et al., 2016; Wu et al., 2024), the STiP-5.1 (e.g., Hutsebaut et al., 2017), and LoPF-Q (Kerr et al., 2022). Acceptability among clinicians has also been demonstrated (e.g., Heltne et al., 2022; Morey, 2018; Morey & Hopwood, 2019) as well as acceptance among patients and/or their families (Cano & Sharp, 2023). Finally, measures of LPF have been shown to be useful in identifying treatment targets (Bliton, Rosenstein, & Pincus, 2022; Skodol, Morey, Bender, & Oldham, 2015), and case conceptualization in adults (Waugh et al., 2017) and in adolescents (Schmeck, Schluter-Muller, Foelsch, & Doering, 2013).

The Validity, Reliability, and Clinical Utility of the ICD-11

With a shorter lifespan than the AMPD, fewer studies have been conducted directly evaluating the validity, reliability, and clinical utility of the ICD-11 system; however, due to its close resemblance to the AMPD, it is reasonable to expect that the AMPD's empirical foundation applies to the ICD-11 (Bach & Mulder, 2022b). In fact, it was the existing empirical basis of the AMPD that facilitated the transition from a categorical to a dimensional system for personality disorder diagnosis in the ICD-11 (Bach et al., 2022; Bach & Mulder, 2022a; Mulder, 2021). Studies are beginning to emerge that provide direct support for the ICD-11. For instance, a 14-item measure was developed to assess for ICD-11 PD (the Personality Disorder Severity ICD-11 [PDS-ICD-11]; Bach et al., 2021), showing evidence of a unidimensional factor structure, criterion validity, incremental validity, and the capacity to distinguish between individuals with and without personality disorder. In terms of clinical utility, Hansen et al. (2019) surveyed 163 mental health professionals' perceived clinical utility of the ICD-11 dimensional PD framework compared with the ICD-10 categorical PD framework. Results showed an advantage for ICD-11 system, specifically with regards to utility for treatment planning, communicating with patients, comprehensiveness, and ease of use. At present, a number of studies are underway to further establish the ICD-11 personality disorder system that will add to the existing shared empirical foundation of the AMPD (Bach & Mulder, 2022b).

Challenges to the Dimensionalization of Personality Disorder

Taken together, the current state of the science on the AMPD and ICD-11 clearly supports their validity, reliability, and clinical utility. As mentioned, the AMPD is, however, not yet recommended for the main section (Section II) of the DSM-5. Support continues to be expressed for a categorical approach, especially from those who work within a medical paradigm. Three main arguments are put forward. First, the criteria by which the decision is made to replace one diagnostic system (e.g., Section II PD) with an alternative (e.g., the AMPD in Section III) requires that the newly proposed diagnostic system shows superiority over the existing system in terms of key validators, such as the antecedents, correlates, and outcomes of the disorder, as well as superior reliability and clinical utility (https://www.psychiatry.org/psychiatrists/practice/dsm/submit-proposals). While a substantial number of studies have demonstrated support for the validity, reliability, and clinical utility of the AMPD, relatively fewer studies were designed and implemented to evaluate the superiority of the AMPD over any PD category, precisely because the AMPD was designed to provide coverage of the categories, but reorganized in such a way that it provides better structural integrity than the 10 categorical PDs. The idea is that PD can be assessed and diagnosed with a more parsimonious, less cumbersome diagnostic process by evaluating one simple indicator of personality dysfunction, instead of evaluating 10 separate (yet overlapping) personality disorders. Despite its promise, in the absence of data claiming superiority, categorical camps have expressed concerns regarding the effort it would take to overhaul existing diagnostic practices.

The second major concern in relinquishing the categorical approach is the belief that a robust treatment literature has developed especially around borderline personality disorder and that by eliminating it, this treatment literature, and the services organized around it, would be lost. Despite the advantages of a structurally more rigorous and parsimonious diagnostic system, critics argue that the overhaul of services organized around evidence-based treatment for borderline personality disorder would be to the detriment of patients (Gunderson, 2013).

Third, proponents of the categorical model argue that a strong literature base does indeed support several of the categories—most notably borderline personality disorder, antisocial personality disorder, schizotypical personality disorder, and avoidant personality disorder. Using the well-established Robins and Guze (1970) criteria for evaluating the validity and reliability of psychiatric disorders, these critics (who are less concerned about the structural integrity of psychopathology) argue that genetic, biological, and environmental antecedents, correlates, and outcomes have been described for these disorders, warranting their further use in psychiatric nomenclature.

The AMPD—LPF in particular—is also challenged from the opposite side of the categorical/dimensional divide. Proponents of what is termed the "personality-psychopathology spectrum" approach challenge the idea that there is something unique about personality pathology that can be distinguished from other psychopathology. Represented perhaps most strongly in the Hierarchical Taxonomy of Psychopathology (HiTOP) approach (Kotov et al., 2021), personality pathology is integrated into hierarchically organized spectra along with all other forms of psychopathology and/or is viewed to represent an overall severity score of psychopathology (the so-called p factor) (Caspi et al., 2014). In this view, internalizing, externalizing, and psychotic spectra dimensions are tethered to the temperamental dimensions that underlie them (Clark, 2005) and are seen as the basis of the organization of all psychopathology. The HiTOP consortium contends that their model finally assigns the prominent role to personality that it deserves in psychiatric nomenclature (Krueger et al., 2018). This is achieved by the fact that five of the major spectra dimensions in HiTOP (Internalizing, Thought Disorder, Disinhibited Externalizing, Antagonistic Externalizing, and Detachment) map onto the AMPD dimensional trait model (negative affectivity, psychoticism, disinhibition, antagonism, and detachment), which, as described earlier, map onto the Big Five trait dimensions. In this way, trait-defined personality is weaved into, or subserves, all manifestations of psychopathology. Should HiTOP be successful, there would be no need for separate diagnostic categories of personality, mood, anxiety, and schizophrenia disorders. There would also be no need for LPF—that is, a unique, distinct indicator of personality functioning that draws on an individual's capacity to reflect on and regulate the self in the context of interpersonal relationships. In this model, the general factor explaining co-variance of personality pathology (and all other psychopathology) symptoms is the p factor, and not a general personality disorder (gPD) factor as proposed by Sharp et al. (2015).

In the following section, we address the challenges raised from both sides of the categorical/dimensional continuum by emphasizing that to understand a phenomenon, it is helpful to consider its development.

The Development of Personality and Personality Disorder

What Is Personality and What Is Personality Disorder?

Ways in which individuals differ from one another are observable already in infancy. These individual differences are referred to as temperamental traits, specifically the early-emerging basic dispositions in the domains of activity, affectivity, attention, and self-regulation (Shiner et al., 2012). Over time, these dispositional traits interact with the environment to develop into broader, more inclusive higher-order personality traits that map onto the Big Five (Shiner, 2003). As mentioned before, Criterion B of the AMPD draws on this literature and represents the extreme (maladaptive) variants of these basic traits (De Clercq, De Fruyt, & Widiger, 2009; De Clercq, Decuyper, & De Caluwé, 2014; J. L. Shiner & Tackett, 2014; Tackett, 2006). As such, an individual with a personality disorder is therefore someone with excessively high levels of maladaptive traits.

In our view, traits—even maladaptive traits—are not enough to define personality (McAdams, 2015; McAdams & Olson, 2010) or personality disorder (Sharp & Wall, 2021). We can all think of individuals who are high in emotional sensitivity, impulsiveness, reactivity, and so on, who do not have personality disorder. High levels of traits in and of themselves do not indicate personality disorder (Clark, Nuzum, & Ro, 2017). To fully describe a person, McAdams (2015) suggests that a person's goals and values in addition to their narrative identity must also be considered. In so doing, we can imagine two individuals, both high in impulsivity, with one individual applying it productively in his work as a race car driver, describing himself as someone who had to learn to manage their impulsiveness to their advantage; while another is unable to productively manage their impulsivity, describing themselves as out of control, defective, and lost. McAdams' (2015) model clearly points to a definition of personality that goes beyond traits. It suggests a conceptualization of personhood that includes an active mind that interacts with the environment in decisions about goals and values, in addition to building a narrative about a past, present, and future self. We have argued that this view of personality maps on to LPF as defined in the AMPD, specifically "... a pattern of *inner experience* and behavior that leads to distress or impairment" (DSM-5, chapter II, page 645, emphasis added) (Sharp, 2020, 2022; Sharp, Vanwoerden, & Wall, 2018; Sharp & Wall, 2017, 2021). Consistent with early conceptualizations of personality (Freud, 1923; James, 1892; Mead, 1934) before the trait approach became dominant, as well as the intended meaning of LPF in the AMPD (Bender, Morey, & Skodol, 2011), we view the core of personality functioning as the capacity to make sense of one's own and others' minds and behaviors and to implement this knowledge in service of productive and mutually rewarding relationships (Sharp & Wall, 2021). This definition of personality was influenced by several psychodynamic views on personality (Blatt & Lerner, 1983; Fonagy, 1989; Fonagy, Gergely, Jurist, & Target, 2002; Kernberg, 1967; Kernberg, 1984; Livesley, 2003; Masterson, 1988). In these models, healthy personality functioning is indicated by a capacity to reflect (non-defensively) on one's characteristic ways of thinking, feeling, and behaving; to be able to describe one's inner experiences coherently; to make oneself understandable to others; to be aware of and employ one's agency, goals, and motives; and to be able to see oneself from the outside in, and from the inside out. In this sense, personality is no longer viewed as a passive set of dispositional traits, but has an organizing function (Kernberg & Caligor, 2005; Sharp & Oldham, 2022)—not only what the personality is, but also what the personality does (McAdams, 2015)—in particular, making sense of self and other in a relational context. Viewed through this lens, LPF, as a dimensional diagnosis, offers both the recognition of the disorder, while at the same time providing a more fluid account of problems in terms of malleable functioning, rather than fixed traits.

How Do Personality and Personality Disorder Develop?

McAdams's (2015) model of personality development integrates several decades of research in developmental psychology with research on personality change and continuity over time. He outlines three layers of personality development: (1) the self as actor (dispositional traits), (2) the self as agent (goals and values, characteristic adaptations), and (3) the self as author (narrative life story). Already in infancy, dispositional traits facilitate the observation of individual differences in personality, laying the foundation for the more biologically based aspects of personality. A second layer of personality emerges with the shift to a motivated agent around ages five to seven, marking a developing sense of agency and ability to establish goals. Now the child is no longer merely acting upon the world, but begins to take ownership of feelings, thoughts, and behaviors. During this shift, theory of mind (rudimentary mentalizing) also emerges as children begin to realize that humans have certain beliefs and desires underlying their behaviors, and that they themselves carry their own driving beliefs and desires (Balzen & Sharp, 2024). In adolescence, as metacognitive capacity increases, the third layer in personality development emerges: the self as author, constructing a life story by weaving together the personal past, present, and future in order to develop a deeper understanding of identity (McAdams & McLean, 2013). Though emerging at different developmental stages, these three layers continue to consolidate throughout the course of our lives, and personality "binds" with each ensuing layer (McAdams, 2015).

How does the binding of personality occur? We have argued that in order to successfully achieve the "binding" of personality at each stage, individuals mentalize self and others (Balzen & Sharp, under review; Sharp & Bevington, 2022; Sharp & Wall, 2021). Early indicators of mentalizing are, for instance, the social referencing that takes place between a caregiver and a child—that is, a child seeking out the caregiver's emotional reactions to gauge their own affective reactions (Vandivier & Hertenstein, 2013). Social referencing is an important building block for the emergence of mentalizing, because in paying attention to the same object or event, infants and caregivers begin to develop and communicate a shared understanding of the world. At this stage, caregivers mediate much of an infant's experiences through, for instance, naming things, including the infant's own emotions and behaviors as she acts upon the world. As infants become more verbal, they begin to take ownership of naming emotions, albeit in a very rudimentary way (Ruba & Pollak, 2020). During toddlerhood, the capacity for identifying emotions in self and others develops further. An important developmental milestone is the ability to engage in pretend play (Weisberg, 2015)—the ability to temporarily imagine an alternative reality, but recognizing the difference between reality and imagination. This is, for the toddler, the first indication that she has a mind that stands apart from reality. In addition, pretend play serves as the first "trying on" of different identities—a function young people return to in adolescence.

At the age of four, a further important milestone in the development of mentalizing occurs—that is, the development of theory of mind (Perner & Wimmer, 1985). Whereas toddlers are aware of and can name emotions in self and others, naming and thinking about thoughts only emerge at age four. At this age, children can officially mindread (imagine what others are thinking), but it is not until about ages six to eight that children are able to begin thinking about their own thoughts and the thoughts of others (Miller, 2009). Caregivers continue to play an important role in mediating the child's subjective (inner) experience by creating mediated learning experiences (Klein, Wieder, & Greenspan, 1987) that enhance learning about the self and others, facilitating the socialization of children's emotion and self-regulation, including emotion regulation (Eisenberg, Cumberland, & Spinrad, 1998).

During middle childhood there is a sharp increase in perspective-taking skills such that children are able to understand complex social interaction (Hollarek & Lee, 2022), which also brings a sharp increase in self-conscious emotions (shame, pride, embarrassment) (Lagattuta & Thompson, 2007). Children now have well-developed self-concepts, and individual differences in self-esteem are observable (Harter, 1982). However, the metacognitive (reflective) capacity is not quite there yet for children to form an integrated representation (sense) of self. This capacity develops only in adolescence, when adolescents are able to integrate multiple hypotheses about the self, beginning to commit to a particular identity and self-narrative (Ferrer-Wreder & Kroger, 2019). Described thus, the binding of personality is a cumulative developmental process characterized by the reciprocal interaction of self and interpersonal functioning subserved by the growing capacity to reflect on self and others. While caregivers mediate this reflective capacity almost entirely in infancy and toddlerhood, this important capacity becomes less and less mediated as children age into adulthood.

Personality disorder, then, is when personality fails to bind. For some reason mentalizing development has gone off course, reflective capacity is thwarted, the development of self has failed to move through the layers of personality development, personality is weakly bound, and an incoherent sense of self emerges (Sharp, 2020). This has serious implications for interpersonal functioning and intimacy in particular. Without a solid sense of a unique identity, and the capacity to flexibly adjust the self to a changing interpersonal context, navigating intimacy becomes challenging. Cogently described by Erikson (cited in Evans, 1967), mature intimacy is "the ability to fuse your identity with somebody else's without fear that you're going to lose something yourself." Conversely, intimacy is important for the continued growth of the self, as self and interpersonal function become inextricably linked:

> growth of the self requires meetings between I and Thou, in which each person recognizes the other as he is; each says what he means and means what he says; each values and contributes to the unfolding of the other without imposing or manipulating. And this always means some degree of distance and independence. It does not depend on one revealing to another

everything that exists within, but requires only that the person be who he is, genuinely present. (Moustakas, 1956)

Throughout the course of this development, traits remain relatively stable (Bridgett, Burt, Edwards, & Deater-Deckard, 2015; de Clercq, van Leeuwen, van den Noortgate, de Bolle, & de Fruyt, 2009), and are limited in their ability to explain diverging personality trajectories—why for some youth making sense of themselves in the context of their relationship with others proceeds along typical lines, while for others, it is a more complicated journey. Personality disorder therefore does not lie in maladaptive traits themselves, but in the human capacity to make sense of oneself—including one's traits, how to manage one's dispositions, and how to integrate them into a coherent and productive representation of self. Without this capacity, interpersonal relationships are hard to manage, and we see the dual, inextricably linked impairment in self and interpersonal functioning (LPF) emerge as a single indicator of personality functioning. It is for this reason that we have argued self-functioning to be the nexus of personality disorder (Sharp, 2020; Sharp & Wall, 2021).

In summary, the early precursors of personality disorder may be observable in extreme traits early on; however, it is not until adolescence that we can fully assess the presence of personality disorder. This is because the core domains of LPF—identity, self-directedness, empathy, and intimacy—are developmental tasks central to adolescence. That these combine into a unidimensional severity continuum of personality functioning makes possible inter- and intra-individual evaluation of differences in personality functioning cross-sectionally and over time. We consider this a substantial advancement in the field of personality disorder—a parsimonious, dimensional, single indicator of personality disorder that is malleable to treatment. It is in this malleability that the destigmatization of a dimensional approach to personality disorder lies.

Empirical Evidence

While McAdams' (2015) model of personality development is empirically grounded, research evaluating the extension of this model to the development of personality disorder is nascent. Here, we discuss some of the emerging literature supporting various aspects of this developmental pathway.

One of the first tasks in establishing an empirical basis for this pathway is to demonstrate a normative increase in personality dysfunction in adolescence in the same way that a normative increase has been shown for personality disorder (Cohen, Crawford, Johnson, & Kasen, 2005; de Clercq, van Leeuwen et al., 2009; Kaess, Brunner, & Chanen, 2014). Demonstrating a similar course in AMPD-defined personality disorder as previously identified for maladaptive traits (de Clercq, van Leeuwen et al., 2009) and borderline traits (Cohen et al., 2005) may be one indicator of validity (Robins & Guze, 1970). In a recent school-based study of over 2,000 young people (aged 12 to 18) using a latent mean difference approach, we showed a normative increase in identity diffusion from ages 12 to 16, thereafter decreasing at age 17 (Sharp et al., 2021). Bogaerts et al. (2021) similarly demonstrated mean increases in identity confusion from ages 12 to 15, thereafter decreasing from ages 15 to 23. Evaluating the prediction that two trajectories of personality pathology may be observed in adolescence (Sharp et al., 2018)—one in which youth follow a normative decline in personality pathology and one in which youth do not follow this normative decline—and using a measure of LPF, Eggermont et al. (2023) followed 1,480 community-based adolescents in a three-wave longitudinal study. Their data confirmed the normative increase and subsequent decrease in impairment of personality functioning found by Sharp et al. (2021) and Bogaerts et al. (2021). In addition, they showed that there were young people who by age 12 already showed high levels of personality dysfunction and that these levels increased even further throughout the course of adolescence. These young people were distinguishable from youth with lower levels of personality impairment in that the former evidenced higher levels of psychopathology, self-harm, emotion dysregulation and maladaptive traits. Eggermont et al. (2023) cogently described this group of young people as "having the feeling of drifting through life without a clear sense of direction, of not being in touch with their 'real' self and experiencing contradictory feelings about themselves; and these feelings only seemed to increase towards adulthood."

A second question to address is whether early maladaptive traits associate with later impairment in self-functioning as the model would prescribe. In a longitudinal follow-up study of 157 children first assessed at age 10, Vanwoerden et al. (2022) showed that high levels of emotional instability and disagreeableness predicted social problems in early adolescence and problems in self-functioning in early adulthood. An indirect effect of childhood narcissistic (antagonistic) traits on higher levels of self-functioning via lower levels of social problems was also found. This study provides preliminary evidence for the idea of layers of personality development that cumulatively binds together to impact a young adult's developing sense of self.

A third question to evaluate is whether there is indeed evidence of disturbances in identity function in adolescents with personality disorder. In the Sharp et al. (2021) study, age-varying associations between borderline personality disturbance and identity diffusion were evaluated. Results showed that throughout adolescence, identity diffusion is significantly associated with borderline personality features, and becomes more closely associated with increasing age. In this study, identity diffusion was assessed through self-report (the Assessment of Identity Development in Adolescence [AIDA]) (Goth et al., 2012; Sharp, McLaren et al., 2022). A more stringent, interview-based test of the association between identity and personality pathology was undertaken by Lind et al. (2019), who coded attachment interviews of 70 inpatient adolescents for narrative coherence. Consistent with expectations, results demonstrated a significant association between narrative incoherence and borderline features, mirroring findings in adults with borderline personality disorder (Lind, Adler, & Clark, 2020). In a follow-up study, associations between attachment coherence and narrative coherence were demonstrated (Lind, Vanwoerden, Penner, & Sharp, 2020), providing initial support for the idea that narrative coherence (an indicator of healthy self-functioning) may relate to the caregiving environment.

Building on these findings, Lind et al. (2022) further demonstrated in a sample of 174 adolescent inpatients that adolescents' narrative identity (i.e., themes/future wishes of agency and communion) associated with mentalizing. Specifically, themes of thwarted agency and communion were associated with lower capacity for mentalizing, as assessed with the Movie Assessment for Social Cognition (MASC; Dziobek et al., 2006), and with borderline pathology. That coded narrative identity was associated with an experimentally derived assessment of mentalizing is noteworthy, since this association cannot be explained by shared method variance. In another study using structural equation modeling with self-report measures, we showed that childhood emotional abuse was associated with identity diffusion through a mediated pathway of mentalizing (reflective capacity) (Penner, Gambin, & Sharp, 2019). More recently, we employed a self-report measure of awareness of narrative identity to evaluate its association with personality pathology. Beyond the typical dimensions of narrative coherence (temporal, thematic, and causal coherence), the Awareness of Narrative Identity Questionnaire (ANIQ; Hallford & Mellor, 2017) assesses individuals' recognition of having life stories and the perception of how these stories provide a sense of self-understanding. Mirroring the results of coded narrative identity, results showed a significant, albeit modest, correlation between borderline features and lower self-reported awareness of narrative identity in adolescents (Balzen, Blacutt, Lind, Penner, & Sharp, 2024).

A fourth question toward establishing the empirical basis for the role LPF plays in adolescent personality development relates to confusion about the meaning of LPF that arose after the publication of the AMPD in 2013 (Sharp & Wall, 2021). Specifically, LPF was suggested to merely reflect the functional consequence of high levels of maladaptive traits—that is, if an individual has high levels of maladaptive traits, their ability to carry out roles and perform activities in daily life (i.e., social, interpersonal, occupational, recreational, and basic functioning) would be impeded (Widiger & Trull, 2007). In this view, LPF could simply correspond to the number of co-occurring diagnoses or a general score on a measure of psychiatric symptoms (Tyrer & Johnson, 1996)—in essence, the p factor. However, empirical findings appear to suggest that LPF is more than simple disability or psychiatric severity. For instance, psychiatrist-rated LPF, but not general psychosocial disability scores, predicted treatment drop-out in adults (Busmann et al., 2019). Consistent with these findings, we showed that identity diffusion incremented general psychosocial disability in the association with borderline pathology in a Lithuanian community sample of 379 adolescents and a clinic sample of 74 adolescents (Sharp, Kerr, & Barkauskiene, 2022). Moreover, in a predominantly Hispanic community-based sample of 419 adolescents in the United States, LPF incremented general psychiatric severity in predicting personality pathology (Sharp & Cervantes, 2023). On the basis of these findings, and consistent with other recent attempts to clarify this conceptual confusion (Hopwood, 2024), we have argued that the definition of LPF should stay close to how it was originally intended—not as the functional consequence of high levels of traits, but as the source of personality disorder (see also Sharp & Wall, 2021).

A final question for establishing the model presented here is to ask if LPF is distinct from maladaptive traits. Indeed, several studies have demonstrated overlap in LPF and maladaptive traits (Sleep, Weiss, Lynam, & Miller, 2020; Widiger et al., 2019); others have demonstrated incremental value of LPF over maladaptive traits (J. L. Anderson & Sellbom, 2018; Bastiaansen, De Fruyt, Rossi, Schotte, & Hofmans, 2013; Berghuis, Kamphuis, & Verheul, 2014; Creswell, Bachrach, Wright, Pinto, & Ansell, 2016; Hentschel & Pukrop, 2014). Recently, the incremental value of LPF over traits was also demonstrated in adolescents (Barkauskiene et al., 2022). We have argued that the distinction between LPF and traits is enhanced through the self components of LPF rather than its interpersonal aspects. This is because maladaptive trait domains typically exclude traits explicitly related to self and identity function, while these are prominently represented in LPF (Sharp & Wall, 2021). Consistent with this notion, Zimmermann et al. (2015) showed that self pathology incremented traits (but not vice versa) in predicting the overall LPF rating. In addition, it appears that self pathology cannot be accounted for within a five-factor personality structure (Berghuis, Kamphuis, & Verheul, 2012) and that the self domain of LPF provides incremental value beyond the interpersonal domain of LPF and beyond Section II PD criteria in predicting psychosocial functioning and symptom severity (Christensen et al., 2020; Hutsebaut et al., 2017; Weekers et al., 2019).

Taken together, there is emerging evidence supporting the developmental relevance of maladaptive self- and interpersonal functioning for adolescence. While research continues to accumulate in this regard, several questions remain. Importantly, the pre-adolescent precursors to maladaptive LPF need to be identified. Our model and empirical evidence (Vanwoerden et al., 2022; De Clercq, Verbeke, De Caluwe, Vercruysse, & Hofmans, 2017) suggest high levels of maladaptive traits to be an important risk marker, but it is also likely that developmental precursors of self-function such as self-esteem or self-concept play a role. Describing the exact developmental trajectory of personality dysfunction along self- and interpersonal lines is important, as doing so would identify malleable preventative targets for intervention.

A Single Dimensional Indicator of Personality Pathology and the Structure of Psychopathology

If it is so that personality disorder is best represented by a single dimensional indicator of self- and interpersonal functioning, a critical question that remains is how best to integrate personality pathology into emerging models of general psychopathology. As noted in section "Problems with the Categorical System for the Diagnosis of Personality Disorder," one of the primary motivations for developing a new model of personality disorder was the recognition that the 10-category system of PDs results in substantial heterogeneity of symptom expression within PD categories and extensive comorbidity across PD categories (Clark, 2007; Sharp, 2016; Widiger & Trull, 2007), suggesting that the categorical system does not adequately capture the latent structure of PD symptoms. Over the last 10 years, investigations of bifactor models of PD symptoms have demonstrated support for an alternative structure as promoted by the AMPD—that is, the existence of a general factor of PD, *gPD*, representing a common core shared by PD categories that explains their frequent comorbidity (Sharp et al., 2015; Wright et al., 2016).

These "plate tectonics" in PD classification (Widiger & Trull, 2007) were part of a larger zeitgeist: a growing awareness of the need to restructure models of general psychopathology due to frequent transdiagnostic comorbidity, heterogeneity within disorder categories, and lack of support for conceptualizing psychopathology as distinct categories rather than dimensions (Kotov et al., 2021). Early investigations borne out of developmental psychopathology research had supported the grouping of commonly comorbid disorders into internalizing (i.e., anxiety and depressive disorders) and externalizing (i.e., substance use, antisocial PD) factors, in addition to thought disorder and somatoform factors (Achenbach, 1978; Kotov, 2011; Kotov et al., 2010; Krueger, 1999; Krueger et al., 1998). However, findings from factor analytic studies suggested substantial correlations between factors (Wright et al., 2013), and findings from cross-sectional and prospective studies indicated substantial rates of concurrent and sequential comorbidity across internalizing and externalizing disorders (Anderson, 1987; Angold et al., 1999; Copeland et al., 2013; Kim-Cohen et al., 2003; Mesman et al., 2001). As a result, around the same time that the latent structure of PDs was being investigated, factor analyses were undertaken to investigate the latent structure of psychopathology across internalizing, externalizing, and other disorders. In two seminal papers, Lahey et al. (2012) and Caspi et al. (2014) identified a general factor of psychopathology—termed the p factor—that explained co-variation among internalizing, externalizing, and other disorders. These models suggest that there is something common across all forms of psychopathology.

There is yet to be consensus on what this *something* is, as researchers have so far suggested that the p factor could reflect one or more of the following: neuroticism or negative emotionality (Brandes et al., 2019; Lahey et al., 2012; Southward et al., 2023); impulsive response to emotion (Carver et al., 2017; Southward et al., 2023); disordered thought (Caspi et al., 2014); common etiological factor(s) (Caspi et al., 2023; Lahey et al., 2012); or some combination of these, among other explanations. As has been debated with LPF, some have suggested that the p factor could reflect a consequence (rather than a cause) of psychopathology, such as functional impairment (Oltmanns et al., 2018; Southward et al., 2023). Others note that the p factor, *gPD*, and other general factors that emerge from factor analyses could reflect statistical artifacts rather than meaningful sources of variation (Van Bork et al., 2017). It is therefore critical to supplement factor analyses with theoretical interpretations and validity studies that elucidate the nomological net of these general factors and determine whether they aid in clinical decision-making (Bornovalova et al., 2020; Caspi et al., 2024; Levin-Aspenson et al., 2021; Southward et al., 2023). Watts et al. (2023) strongly urged researchers to move beyond unrestricted bifactor models of general factors, noting that these models tend to demonstrate good fit even when they don't accurately capture latent structure, and can be limited in interpretability due to poor replication across samples. They call on researchers to develop more precisely articulated, falsifiable theories about the meaning of general factors and to use more rigorous tests, such as by imposing constraints on bifactor models according to a priori theories (Watts et al., 2023).

Notwithstanding these criticisms, just as the identification of *gPD* corroborated the development of a new model for personality disorders (the AMPD), the identification of the p factor prompted the development of new models for general psychopathology, of which the most widely recognized is the empirically derived Hierarchical Taxonomy of Psychopathology (HiTOP) (Kotov et al., 2017). The HiTOP model posits a hierarchical structure of psychopathology with several levels of description, starting with the general p factor and moving down through other superspectra, spectra, subfactors, syndromes, and symptom components and maladaptive traits (Kotov et al., 2021). The contents of this model are continually refined as more data is collected, reflecting a data-driven approach. The primary aim of this model is to describe underlying relationships among different signs and symptoms of psychopathology in ways that will inform research (i.e., our understanding of etiology and developmental mechanisms) and clinical practice (i.e., prognosis and treatment planning) (DeYoung et al., 2022; Kotov et al., 2021).

Some attempts have been made to integrate PD into the HiTOP model. As reviewed by Kotov et al. (2017), investigations of the joint structure of PD and general psychopathology have focused primarily on maladaptive personality traits. In this literature, maladaptive traits are most often conceptualized according to the maladaptive trait domains used in AMPD Criterion B: negative affectivity, antagonism, disinhibition, detachment, and psychoticism, corresponding to the five-factor model (Watson & Clark, 2020). Factor analyses of the joint structure of maladaptive traits and categorical PD symptoms with general psychopathology supported a six-factor model in which five factors align with the maladaptive trait domains (Kotov, 2011; Røysamb et al., 2011; Wright & Simms, 2015). This resulted in the elaboration of six spectra in the HiTOP model: internalizing (related to negative affectivity), disinhibited externalizing, antagonistic externalizing, thought disorder (related to psychoticism), detachment, and a sixth somatoform factor without a clear maladaptive trait counterpart (Kotov et al., 2017). These spectra describe co-variation in lower-order subfactors (i.e., distress, antisocial behavior) and syndromes (i.e., social anxiety) (Kotov et al., 2017, 2021). When examining the placement of categorical PD *symptoms* in these models (Kotov, 2011; Røysamb et al., 2011; Wright & Simms, 2015), PD symptoms generally related to spectra in patterns that one would expect based on the typical and maladaptive traits associated with each PD category (i.e., narcissistic PD symptoms onto antagonistic externalizing, schizotypal PD symptoms onto thought disorder, borderline PD symptoms onto internalizing and antagonistic externalizing) (American Psychiatric Association, 2013; Samuel & Widiger, 2008). On the whole, then, maladaptive traits have been shown to bridge personality pathology and general psychopathology. These findings align with extensive past research suggesting that personality traits and psychopathology can influence the presentation of one another, play a causal role in the development of one another, and share common etiology (Kotov et al., 2010; Krueger & Tackett, 2003; Tackett, 2006; Widiger, 2011; Widiger, Sellbom et al., 2019).

However, with a dominant focus on maladaptive traits, self- and interpersonal functioning has been largely absent from efforts to place personality pathology in HiTOP. Despite the extensive work done to identify self- and interpersonal impairment as the core of PD (Sharp & Miller, 2022), so much so that it is conditional to PD diagnosis in the AMPD and the ICD-11, this common factor of PD is not represented in HiTOP. Instead, the meaning of personality pathology in HiTOP has largely been reduced to maladaptive traits. At the same time, though, maladaptive traits have been mapped onto spectra and therefore related to virtually all forms of psychopathology. This disperses PD across the HiTOP model, failing to designate a common core of PD, even though HiTOP's organization is expected to predict common etiology, risk factors, and treatment outcomes (DeYoung et al., 2022; Kotov et al., 2021). Thus, as Ringwald et al. (2019) note, relying solely on the HiTOP model to describe personality pathology "effectively eliminates personality pathology as a distinct construct."

Without considering a common *gPD* factor, PD starts to merge with the spectra, distinguished then only by severity (i.e., perhaps PD is just extreme internalizing/externalizing, or less extreme thought disorder). It has indeed been suggested that internalizing/externalizing, PD, and thought disorder form a spectrum of increasing severity (Kernberg, 1984; Sharp & Wall, 2018). However, critically, we have argued that there is also a qualitative difference between internalizing/externalizing and PD—namely, impairment in self and interpersonal functioning, driven by a failure to form a coherent sense of self in adolescence (Sharp & Wall, 2018). There is also empirical evidence supporting the consideration of a *gPD* factor. Wright et al. (2016) demonstrated that the *gPD* emerging from a bifactor model of PD was a stronger predictor of social and occupational functioning than specific factors of PDs, and that the *gPD* appeared to be more malleable than specific factors, exhibiting a substantially greater decline over the course of 10 years. The authors suggested that effective treatments of PD should thus target core features common to PDs (Wright et al., 2016).

Thus, we argue that models and theories of personality pathology must retain a description of the distinctive core of PD, self- and interpersonal impairment, and cannot rely solely on general models of psychopathology such as HiTOP. HiTOP still has clear utility regarding personality; indeed, integrating maladaptive traits into a model of general psychopathology will likely have substantial benefit in research and clinical practice by encouraging greater consideration of reciprocal relationships between traits and psychopathology (Mullins-Sweatt et al., 2020; Waszczuk et al., 2022; Widiger, Sellbom et al., 2019). But HiTOP can only tell half of the story about personality pathology. As noted by Ringwald et al. (2019), hierarchical models provide perspective on the relationship between traits and general psychopathology but lose focus on "foundational understandings of personality pathology," while bifactor models of personality pathology provide needed perspective on the common factor of personality pathology. These authors demonstrated that hierarchical models and bifactor models of DSM-IV PD criteria had equivalently good fits, providing empirical support that both models have their own utility. Of note, van Bork et al. (2017) demonstrated that hierarchical and bifactor models will almost always have nearly equivalent fit and should be interpreted using theory and validity studies; in this case, theory suggests the importance of retaining both models, and both models would benefit from continued validation.

Widiger, Bach et al. (2019) suggested that measures of self and interpersonal impairments be included in analyses of the HiTOP structure, to determine empirically whether these impairments might load on different spectra or form their own spectrum. We agree with these authors (Widiger, Bach et al. 2019) that because Criterion A and Criterion B have been shown to be significantly correlated, and Criterion B traits and categorical PD symptoms load onto several different HiTOP spectra, it seems likely that self- and interpersonal impairments would end up being similarly dispersed across the different spectra. However, we have argued that while impairment in self- and interpersonal functioning is evident in other psychopathology (i.e., anxiety and mood disorders), self- and interpersonal functioning in those disorders constitute the consequence of pathology in another system (e.g. the mood system) and not its source (Sharp & Wall, 2021). For personality disorder, self- and interpersonal functioning is the source of disorder. This distinction is important, because it implies different targets for intervention. Accordingly, HiTOP alone would not be informative for understanding the common core of PD and how PD is distinct from other disorders, even if self- and interpersonal impairments were added to the model. Of note, HiTOP doesn't purport to accomplish this, as the model is not meant to be used to classify people in such a way that a given person would be expected to have symptoms from only one spectrum (DeYoung et al., 2022). Instead, contributors to HiTOP envision that researchers and clinicians can use the model to understand the underlying structure connecting several symptom and trait dimensions and to describe a person's position on these dimensions (DeYoung et al., 2022). This is a critical distinction to make, given that other DSM-5 disorders (i.e., anxiety and depressive disorders) appear to "live" more comfortably within one HiTOP spectrum, which may lead clinicians to misinterpret spectra as diagnostic classes, while the core of PD appears to "live" outside the model.

In our view, a key focus for future research would be to merge the structure of psychopathology at the phenotypic level with structure at other levels of analysis. For instance, if we can imagine a representation of psychopathology that also includes a neurocognitive organization of psychopathology, we would likely see the internalizing spectrum represented in more basic mood- and reward systems, and personality functioning represented in higher-order networks (e.g., systems for social processes) that draw on basic mood- and reward systems. We are a long way away from this level of empirical integration across multiple levels of analysis; however, there is benefit in imagining it, as it may help us identify key treatment targets that would lead to the most effective outcomes for individuals with challenges in personality functioning.

Conclusion

In conclusion, without theories and models of a general factor of PD that can relate unitary self- and interpersonal impairment to a core PD construct suggestive of distinct developmental mechanisms and distinct functional outcomes, personality loses its original definition as described by William James, Sigmund Freud, Erik Erikson, and George Herbert Mead, who placed clear emphasis on the fact that humans actively contribute to building a representation of self and that this constitutes a core feature of personality. We have argued that the definition of PD in the AMPD and ICD-11 is consistent with these early definitions, specifically in its description of the entry criterion for diagnosis: maladaptive self- and interpersonal functioning. In our view, the assessment of maladaptive self- and interpersonal functioning is conditional to the diagnosis of PD. We further contend that in adults and adolescents, as per the ICD-11, the evaluation of traits should be optional, and may provide helpful additional information about how maladaptive self- and interpersonal dysfunction manifests in an individual. However, if we take seriously the developmental model put forward in this chapter, the evaluation of traits in children as a precursor to the later development of an incoherent sense of self is critical. Of course, high levels of maladaptive traits in pre-adolescent children may indicate a vulnerability for a variety of later psychopathology, but despite its non-specificity, the assessment of traits in pre-adolescents, especially in combination with an assessment of the child's developing mentalizing capacity, may be helpful in deciding the extent to which personality development should be a focus of treatment.

In conclusion, dimensional models as represented by the AMPD and ICD-11 are transformative in that they identify a single dimensional indicator of personality pathology that is distinct from other forms of psychopathology. Because of this categorical distinction, these models do not represent "full" dimensional models (like HiTOP), and we have presented evidence as to why we view this distinction as necessary. As evidence continues to accumulate on the equivalent and even superior validity of the AMPD and ICD-11 compared to the traditional categorical PD model, we look forward to the potential benefits that these dimensionally informed models could bring to PD assessment, diagnosis, and treatment. We hope to see that this new focus on self- and interpersonal functioning ultimately improves the lives of people with PDs and their families, not least by destigmatizing personality disorder by placing us all on a communal continuum of personality functioning; and sending the message that with the right support, people with PDs can grow to better understand and relate to themselves and others, find purpose and self-direction, and live fulfilling lives.

References

Achenbach, T. M. (1978). The child behavior profile: I. Boys aged 6–11. *Journal of Consulting and Clinical Psychology, 46*(3), 478–488. https://doi.org/10.1037/0022-006X.46.3.478

American Psychiatric Association. (2013). *Diagnostic and statistical manual of mental disorders* (Fifth Edition). American Psychiatric Association. https://doi.org/10.1176/appi.books.9780890425596

Anderson, J. C. (1987). DSM-III disorders in preadolescent children: Prevalence in a large sample from the general population. *Archives of General Psychiatry, 44*(1), 69. https://doi.org/10.1001/archpsyc.1987.01800130081010

Anderson, J., & Kelley, S. E. (2022). Antisocial personality disorder and psychopathy: The AMPD in review. *Personality Disorders: Theory, Research and Treatment, 13*(4), 397–401. https://doi.org/10.1037/per0000525

Anderson, J. L., & Sellbom, M. (2018). Evaluating the DSM-5 Section III personality disorder impairment criteria. *Personality Disorders: Theory, Research, and Treatment, 9*(1), 51–61. https://doi.org/10.1037/per0000217

Angold, A., Costello, E. J., & Erkanli, A. (1999). Comorbidity. *Journal of Child Psychology and Psychiatry, 40*(1), 57–87. https://doi.org/10.1111/1469-7610.00424

Babinski, D. E., Kujawa, A., Pegg, S., Leslie, J. M., Pothoven, C., Waschbusch, D. A., & Sharp, C. (2023). Social and monetary reward processing in youth with early emerging personality pathology: An RDoC-informed study. *Research on Child and Adolescent Psychopathology, 52*, 567–578. https://doi.org/10.1007/s10802-023-01147-9

Bach, B., Brown, T. A., Mulder, R. T., Newton-Howes, G., Simonsen, E., & Sellbom, M. (2021). Development and initial evaluation of the ICD-11 personality disorder severity scale: PDS-ICD-11. *Personality and Mental Health, 15*(3), 223–236. doi:10.1002/pmh.1510

Bach, B., Kramer, U., Doering, S., di Giacomo, E., Hutsebaut, J., Kaera, A., De Panfilis, C., Schmahl, C., Swales, M., Taubner, S., & Renneberg, B. (2022). The ICD-11 classification of personality disorders: a European perspective on challenges and opportunities. *Borderline Personality Disorder and Emotion Dysregulation, 9*(1), 12. https://doi.org/10.1186/s40479-022-00182-0

Bach, B., & Mulder, R. (2022a). Clinical implications of ICD-11 for diagnosing and treating personality disorders. *Current Psychiatry Reports, 24*(10), 553–563. http://doi.org/10.1007/s11920–022–01364-x

Bach, B., & Mulder, R. (2022b). Empirical foundation of the ICD-11 classification of personality disorders. In S. Huprich (Ed.), *Personality disorders and pathology: Integrating clinical assessment and practice in the DSM-5 and ICD-11* (pp. 27–52): American Psychological Association.

Bach, B., & Tracy, M. (2022). Clinical utility of the alternative model of personality disorders: A 10th year anniversary review. *Personality Disorders: Theory, Research, and Treatment, 13*(4), 369–379. https://doi.org/10.1037/per0000527

Balzen, K., & Sharp, C. (2024). The contribution of mentalization-based theory and practice to for understanding and treating self-injurious behavior in young people. *Journal of Infant, Child, and Adolescent Psychotherapy, 23*(1), 108–121. https://doi.org/10.1080/15289168.2024.2311555

Balzen, K. M., Blacutt, M., Lind, M., Penner, F., & Sharp, C. (2024). Awareness of narrative identity questionnaire (ANIQ) in early adolescents: Psychometric evaluation and association with features of personality disorder. *Journal of Personality Assessment, 106*(3), 337–346. https://doi.org/10.1080/00223891.2023.2258979

Balzen, K. M., Kerr, S., Gecha, T., Hutsebaut, J., Berghuis, H., & Sharp, C. (2025). First psychometric evaluation of the English version of the Semi-Structured Interview for Personality Functioning (STiP-5.1). *Journal of Personality Assessment*, *107*(1), 1–11. https://doi.org/10.1080/00223891.2024.2365325

Balzen, K. M., & Sharp, C. (2024). The contribution of mentalization-based theory and practice for understanding and treating self-injurious behavior in young people. *Journal of Infant, Child, and Adolescent Psychotherapy*, *23*(1), 108–121. https://doi.org/10.1080/15289168.2024.2311555

Barkauskiene, R., Gaudiesiute, E., Adler, A., Gervinskaite-Paulaitiene, L., Laurinavicius, A., & Skabeikyte-Norkiene, G. (2022). Criteria A and B of the Alternative DSM-5 Model for Personality Disorders (AMPD) capture borderline personality features among adolescents. *Front Psychiatry*, *13*, 828301. https://doi.org/10.3389/fpsyt.2022.828301

Bastiaansen, L., De Fruyt, F., Rossi, G., Schotte, C., & Hofmans, J. (2013). Personality disorder dysfunction versus traits: Structural and conceptual issues. *Personality Disorders: Theory, Research, and Treatment*, *4*(4), 293–303. https://doi.org/10.1037/per0000018

Bender, D. S., Morey, L. C., & Skodol, A. E. (2011). Toward a model for assessing level of personality functioning in DSM-5, part I: A review of theory and methods. *Journal of Personality Assessment*, *93*(4), 332–346. https://doi.org/10.1080/00223891.2011.583808

Berghuis, H., Kamphuis, J. H., & Verheul, R. (2012). Core features of personality disorder: Differentiating general personality dysfunctioning from personality traits. *Journal of Personality Disorders*, *26*(5), 704–716. https://doi.org/10.1521/pedi.2012.26.5.704

Berghuis, H., Kamphuis, J. H., & Verheul, R. (2014). Specific personality traits and general personality dysfunction as predictors of the presence and severity of personality disorders in a clinical sample. *Journal of Personality Assessment*, *96*(4), 410–416. https://doi.org/10.1080/00223891.2013.834825

Biberdzic, M., Tang, J., & Tan, J. H. (2021). Beyond difficulties in self-regulation: The role of identity integration and personality functioning in young women with disordered eating behaviours. *Journal of Eating Disorders*, *9*(1), 93. https://doi.org/ARTN 9310.1186/s40337-021-00398-5

Blatt, S. J., & Lerner, H. (1983). The psychological assessment of object representation. *Journal of Personality Assessment*, *47*(1), 7–28. https://doi.org/10.1207/s15327752jpa4701_2

Bliton, C. F., Rosenstein, L. K., & Pincus, A. L. (2022). Trading patients: Applying the alternative model for personality disorders to two cases of borderline personality disorder over time and across therapists. *Frontiers in Psychology*, *13*, 794624. https://doi.org/ARTN 79462410.3389/fpsyg.2022.794624

Bogaerts, A., Claes, L., Buelens, T., Verschueren, M., Palmeroni, N., Bastiaens, T., & Luyckx, K. (2021). Identity synthesis and confusion in early to late adolescents: Age trends, gender differences, and associations with depressive symptoms. *Journal of Adolescence*, *87*, 106–116. https://doi.org/10.1016/j.adolescence.2021.01.006

Bonnington, O., & Rose, D. (2014). Exploring stigmatisation among people diagnosed with either bipolar disorder or borderline personality disorder: A critical realist analysis. *Social Science & Medicine*, *123*, 7–17. https://doi.org/10.1016/j.socscimed.2014.10.048

Boone, K., Babinski, D., Kujawa, A., Pegg, S., & Sharp, C. (2025). The incremental validity of level of personality functioning over borderline personality features in associations with early adolescent social reward processing. *Personality and Mental Health*, *19*(1), e70000. https://doi.org/10.1002/pmh.70000

Bornovalova, M. A., Choate, A. M., Fatimah, H., Petersen, K. J., & Wiernik, B. M. (2020). Appropriate use of bifactor analysis in psychopathology research: Appreciating benefits and limitations. *Biological Psychiatry*, *88*(1), 18–27. https://doi.org/10.1016/j.biopsych.2020.01.013

Brandes, C. M., Herzhoff, K., Smack, A. J., & Tackett, J. L. (2019). The p Factor and the n Factor: Associations Between the General Factors of Psychopathology and Neuroticism in Children. *Clinical Psychological Science*, *7*(6), 1266–1284. https://doi.org/10.1177/2167702619859332

Bridgett, D. J., Burt, N. M., Edwards, E. S., & Deater-Deckard, K. (2015). Intergenerational transmission of self-regulation: A multidisciplinary review and integrative conceptual framework. *Psychological Bulletin*, *141*(3), 602–654. https://doi.org/10.1037/a0038662

Buer Christensen, T., Eikenaes, I., Hummelen, B., Pedersen, G., Nysæter, T. E., Bender, D. S., Skodol, A. E., & Selvik, S. G. (2020). Level of personality functioning as a predictor of psychosocial functioning-concurrent validity of Criterion A. *Personality Disorders-Theory Research and Treatment*, *11*(2), 79–90. https://doi.org/10.1037/per0000352

Buer Christensen, T., Paap, M. C. S., Arnesen, M., Koritzinsky, K., Nysaeter, T. E., Eikenaes, I., Germans Selvik, S., Walther, K., Torgersen, S., Bender, D. S., Skodol, A. E., Kvarstein, E., Pedersen, G., & Hummelen, B. (2018). Interrater reliability of the structured clinical interview for the DSM-5 alternative model of personality disorders module i: Level of personality functioning scale. *Journal of Personality Assessment*, *100*(6), 630–641. https://doi.org/10.1080/00223891.2018.1483377

Busmann, M., Wrege, J., Meyer, A. H., Ritzler, F., Schmidlin, M., Lang, U. E., Gaab, J., Walter, M., & Euler, S. (2019). Alternative Model of Personality Disorders (DSM-5) predicts dropout in inpatient psychotherapy for patients with personality disorder. *Frontiers in Psychology*, *10*, 952. https://doi.org/10.3389/fpsyg.2019.00952

Cano, K., & Sharp, C. (2023). A consumer perspective on personality diagnostic systems: One size does not fit all. *Journal of Personality Disorders*, *37*(3), 263–284. https://doi.org/10.1521/pedi.2023.37.3.263

Carver, C. S., Johnson, S. L., & Timpano, K. R. (2017). Toward a functional view of the p factor in psychopathology. *Clinical Psychological Science*, *5*(5), 880–889. https://doi.org/10.1177/2167702617710037

Caspi, A., Houts, R. M., Belsky, D. W., Goldman-Mellor, S. J., Harrington, H., Israel, S., Meier, M. H., Ramrakha, S., Shalev, I., Poulton, R., & Moffitt, T. E. (2014). The p factor: One general psychopathology factor in the structure of psychiatric disorders? *Clinical Psychological Science*, *2*(2), 119–137. https://doi.org/10.1177/2167702613497473

Caspi, A., Houts, R. M., Fisher, H. L., Danese, A., & Moffitt, T. E. (2024). The general factor of psychopathology (p): Choosing among competing models and interpreting p. *Clinical Psychological Science*, *12*(1), 53–82. https://doi.org/10.1177/21677026221147872

Chorpita, B. F., Daleiden, E. L., Ebesutani, C., Young, J., Becker, K. D., Nakamura, B. J., Phillips, L., Ward, A., Lynch, R., Trent, L., Smith, R. L., Okamura, K., & Starace, N. (2011). Evidence-based treatments for children and adolescents: An updated review of indicators of efficacy and effectiveness. *Clinical Psychology-Science and Practice*, *18*(2), 154–172. https://doi.org/10.1111/j.1468–2850.2011.01247.x

Cicchetti, D. (2006). Development and psychopathology. In D. Cicchetti & J. D. Cohen (Eds.), *Development and psychopathology* (2nd ed., pp. 1–23). Wiley.

Clark, L. A. (2005). Temperament as a unifying basis for personality and psychopathology. *Journal of Abnormal Psychology*, *114*(4), 505–521. https://doi.org/10.1037/0021-843x.114.4.505

Clark, L. A. (2007). Assessment and diagnosis of personality disorder: Perennial issues and an emerging reconceptualization. *Annual Review of Psychology*, *58*, 227–257. https://doi.org/DOI 10.1146/annurev.psych.57.102904.190200

Clark, L. A., Nuzum, H., & Ro, E. (2017). Manifestations of personality impairment severity: Comorbidity, course/prognosis, psychosocial dysfunction, and "borderline" personality features. *Current Opinion in Psychology*, *21*, 117–121. https://doi.org/10.1016/j.copsyc.2017.12.004

Clark, L. A., & Watson, D. (2022). The trait model of the DSM-5 alternative model of personality disorder (AMPD): A structural review. *Personality Disorders: Theory, Research, and Treatment*, *13*(4), 328–336. https://doi.org/10.1037/per0000568

Cohen, P., Crawford, T. N., Johnson, J. G., & Kasen, S. (2005). The children in the community study of developmental course of personality disorder. *Journal of Personality Disorders*, *19*(5), 466–486. https://doi.org/10.1521/pedi.2005.19.5.466

Copeland, W. E., Adair, C. E., Smetanin, P., Stiff, D., Briante, C., Colman, I., Fergusson, D., Horwood, J., Poulton, R., Jane Costello, E., & Angold, A. (2013). Diagnostic transitions from childhood to adolescence to early adulthood. *Journal of Child Psychology and Psychiatry*, *54*(7), 791–799. https://doi.org/10.1111/jcpp.12062

Creswell, K. G., Bachrach, R. L., Wright, A. G., Pinto, A., & Ansell, E. (2016). Predicting problematic alcohol use with the DSM-5 alternative model of personality pathology. *Personality Disorders: Theory, Research, and Treatment*, *7*(1), 103–111. https://doi.org/10.1037/per0000131

Cruitt, P. J., Boudreaux, M. J., King, H. R., Oltmanns, J. R., & Oltmanns, T. F. (2019). Examining criterion a: DSM-5 level of personality functioning as assessed through life story interviews. *Personality Disorders: Theory, Research, and Treatment*, *10*(3), 224–234. https://doi.org/10.1037/per0000321

De Clercq, B., De Fruyt, F., & Widiger, T. A. (2009). Integrating a developmental perspective in dimensional models of personality disorders. *Clinical Psychology Review*, *29*(2), 154–162. https://doi.org/10.1016/j.cpr.2008.12.002

De Clercq, B., Decuyper, M., & De Caluwé, E. (2014). Developmental manifestations of borderline personality pathology from and age-specific dimensional personality disorder trait framework. In C. Sharp & J. Tackett (Eds.), *Handbook of Borderline Personality Disorder in Children and Adolescents* (pp. 81–94). Springer.

de Clercq, B., van Leeuwen, K., van den Noortgate, W., de Bolle, M., & de Fruyt, F. (2009). Childhood personality pathology: dimensional stability and change. *Developmental Psychopathology*, *21*(3), 853–869. https://doi.org/10.1017/S0954579409000467

De Clercq, B., Verbeke, L., De Caluwe, E., Vercruysse, T., & Hofmans, J. (2017). Understanding adolescent personality pathology from growth trajectories of childhood oddity. *Developmental Psychopathology*, *29*(4), 1403–1411. https://doi.org/10.1017/S0954579417000347

Dereboy, F., Dereboy, C., & Eskin, M. (2018). Validation of the DSM-5 alternative model personality disorder diagnoses in Turkey, Part 1: LEAD validity and reliability of the personality functioning ratings. *Journal of Personality Assessment*, *100*(6), 603–611. https://doi.org/10.1080/00223891.2018.1423989

DeYoung, C. G., Kotov, R., Krueger, R. F., Cicero, D. C., Conway, C. C., Eaton, N. R., Forbes, M. K., Hallquist, M. N., Jonas, K. G., Latzman, R. D., Rodriguez-Seijas, C., Ruggero, C. J., Simms, L. J., Waldman, I. D., Waszczuk, M. A., Widiger, T. A., & Wright, A. G. C. (2022). Answering questions about the Hierarchical Taxonomy of Psychopathology (HiTOP): Analogies to whales and sharks miss the boat. *Clinical Psychological Science*, *10*(2), 279–284. https://doi.org/10.1177/21677026211049390

Dziobek, I., Fleck, S., Kalbe, E., Rogers, K., Hassenstab, J., Brand, M., Kessler, J., Woike, J. K., Wolf, O. T., & Convit, A. (2006). Introducing MASC: A movie for the assessment of social cognition. *Journal of Autism and Developmental Disorders*, *36*(5), 623–636. https://doi.org/10.1007/s10803-006-0107-0

Eaton, N. R., South, S. C., & Krueger, R. F. (2015). The meaning of comorbidity among common mental disorders. In T. Millon, R. F. Krueger, & E. Simonsen (Eds.), *Contemporary directions in psychopathology: Scientific foundations of the DSM-IV and ICD-11* (pp. 223–241). The Guilford Press.

Eggermont, K., Raymaekers, K., Claes, L., Buelens, T., Bogaerts, A., & Luyckx, K. (2023). Impairment in personality functioning throughout adolescence and co-development with personality traits, emotion regulation strategies, and psychopathology. *Journal of Research in Personality*, *104*, 1 –11. https://doi.org/104380 10.1016/j.jrp.2023.104380

Eisenberg, N., Cumberland, A., & Spinrad, T. L. (1998). Parental socialization of emotion. *Psychological Inquiry*, *9*(4), 241–273. https://doi.org/10.1207/s15327965pli0904_1

Evans, R. I. (1967). *Dialogue with Erik Erikson*: Harper & Row.

Ferrer-Wreder, L., & Kroger, J. (2019). *Identity in adolescence: The balance between self and other*. Routledge.

Fonagy, P. (1989). *On tolerating mental states: Theory of mind in borderline personality*. Bulletin of the Anna Freud Centre.

Fonagy, P., Gergely, G., Jurist, E. L., & Target, M. (2002). *Affect regulation, mentalization, and the development of self*. Other Press.

Frances, A. (1993). Dimensional diagnosis of personality: not whether, but when and which. *Psychological Inquiry*, *4*(2), 110–111. https://doi.org/10.1207/s15327965pli0402_7

Freud, S. (1923). *The ego and the id*.Hogarth.

Gamache, D., Savard, C., Leclerc, P., & Cote, A. (2019). Introducing a short self-report for the assessment of DSM-5 level of personality functioning for personality disorders: The self and interpersonal functioning scale. *Personality Disorders: Theory, Research, and Treatment*, *10*(5), 438–447. https://doi.org/10.1037/per0000335

Goth, K., Birkhölzer, M., & Schmeck, K. (2018). LoPF-Q 12-18 (levels of personality functioning questionnaire) German version: A self-report questionnaire for measuring personality functioning in adolescence—Short description. Retrieved from http://www.academic-tests.com

Goth, K., Foelsch, P., Schluter-Muller, S., Birkholzer, M., Jung, E., Pick, O., & Schmeck, K. (2012). Assessment of identity development and identity diffusion in adolescence—Theoretical basis and psychometric properties of the self-report questionnaire AIDA. *Child and Adolescent Psychiatry and Mental Health, 6*(1), 27. https://doi.org/10.1186/1753-2000-6-27

Gunderson, J. G. (2013). Seeking clarity for future revisions of the personality disorders in DSM-5. *Personality Disorders: Theory, Research, and Treatment. 4*(4), 368–376.

Hallford, D. J., & Mellor, D. (2017). Development and validation of the awareness of narrative identity questionnaire (ANIQ). *Assessment, 24*(3), 399–413. https://doi.org/10.1177/1073191115607046

Hansen, S. J., Christensen, S., Kongerslev, M. T., First, M. B., Widiger, T. A., Simonsen, E., & Bach, B. (2019). Mental health professionals' perceived clinical utility of the ICD-10 vs. ICD-11 classification of personality disorders. *Personality and Mental Health, 13*(2), 84–95. https://doi.org/10.1002/pmh.1442

Harter, S. (1982). The Perceived Competence Scale for Children. *Child Development, 53*(1), 87–97.

Heltne, A., Bode, C., Hummelen, B., Falkum, E., Selvik, S. G., & Paap, M. C. S. (2022). Norwegian clinicians' experiences of learnability and usability of SCID-II, SCID-5-PD and SCID-5-AMPD-I interviews: A sequential multi-group qualitative approach. *Journal of Personality Assessment, 104*(5), 599–612. https://doi.org/10.1080/00223891.2021.1975726

Hentschel, A. G., & Pukrop, R. (2014). The essential features of personality disorder in DSM-5: The relationship between criteria A and B. *Journal of Nervous and Mental Disease, 202*(5), 412–418. https://doi.org/10.1097/NMD.0000000000000129

Hessels, C. J., De Moor, E. L., Deutz, M. H. F., Laceulle, O. M., & VanAken, M. A. G. (2024). Personality pathology in youth: A comparison of the categorical and alternative model in relation to internalizing and externalizing pathology and age-adequate psychosocial functioning. *Personality Disorders: Theory, Research and Treatment, 15*(5), 293–303. https://doi.org/10.1037/per0000681

Hollarek, M., & Lee, N. C. (2022). Current understanding of developmental changes in adolescent perspective taking. *Current Opinion in Psychology, 45*, 101308. https://doi.org/10.1016/j.copsyc.2022.101308

Holzberg, J. D., & Wittenborn, J. R. (1953). The quantified multiple diagnostic procedure in psychiatric classification. *Journal of Clinical Psychology, 9*(2), 145–148. https://doi.org/10.1002/1097-4679(195304)9:2<145::aid-jclp2270090211>3.0.co;2-2

Hopwood, C. J. (2024). Personality functioning, problems in living, and personality traits. *Journal of Personality Assessment, 107*(2), 143–158. https://doi.org/10.1080/00223891.2024.2345880

Hopwood, C. J., Good, E. W., & Morey, L. C. (2018). Validity of the DSM-5 levels of personality functioning scale-self report. *Journal of Personality Assessment, 100*(6), 650–659. https://doi.org/10.1080/00223891.2017.1420660

Hopwood, C. J., Schwaba, T., Wright, A. G. C., Bleidorn, W., & Zanarini, M. C. (2022). Longitudinal associations between borderline personality disorder and five-factor model traits over 24 years. *European Journal of Personality, 36*(1), 72–90. https://doi.org/08902070211012918 10.1177/08902070211012918

Hummelen, B., Ulltveit-Moe Eikenaes, I., & Wilberg, T. (2022). Is the alternative model for personality disorders able to capture avoidant personality disorder according to Section II of the DSM-5? A systematic review. *Personality Disorders: Theory, Research, and Treatment, 13*(4), 412–417. https://doi.org/10.1037/per0000553

Hutsebaut, J., Feenstra, D. J., & Kamphuis, J. H. (2016). Development and preliminary psychometric evaluation of a brief self-report questionnaire for the assessment of the DSM-5 level of Personality Functioning Scale: The LPFS brief form (LPFS-BF). *Personality Disorders: Theory, Research, and Treatment, 7*(2), 192–197. https://doi.org/10.1037/per0000159

Hutsebaut, J., Kamphuis, J. H., Feenstra, D. J., Weekers, L. C., & De Saeger, H. (2017). Assessing DSM-5-oriented level of personality functioning: Development and psychometric evaluation of the Semi-Structured Interview for Personality Functioning DSM-5 (STiP-5.1). *Personality Disorders: Theory, Research, and Treatment, 8*(1), 94–101. https://doi.org/10.1037/per0000197

James, W. (1892). *Psychology*. Fawcett.

Kaess, M., Brunner, R., & Chanen, A. (2014). Borderline personality disorder in adolescence. *Pediatrics, 134*(4), 782–793. https://doi.org/10.1542/peds.2013-3677

Kernberg, O. (1967). Borderline personality organization. *Journal of the American Psychoanalytic Association, 15*(3), 641–685.

Kernberg, O. F. (1984). *Severe personality disorders: Psychotherapeutic strategies*. Yale University Press.

Kernberg, O. F., & Caligor, E. A. (2005). Psychoanalytic theory of personality disorders. In M. F. Lenzenweger & J. F. Clarkin (Eds.), *Major Theories of Personality Disorder* (2nd ed., pp. 114–156). Guilford Press.

Kerr, S., McLaren, V., Cano, K., Vanwoerden, S., Goth, K., & Sharp, C. (2022). Levels of Personality Functioning Questionnaire 12–18 (LoPF-Q 12-18): Factor structure, validity, and clinical cut-offs. *Assessment*, *30*(6), 1764–1776. https://doi.org/10.1177/10731911221124340

Kim-Cohen, J., Caspi, A., Moffitt, T. E., Harrington, H., Milne, B. J., & Poulton, R. (2003). Prior juvenile diagnoses in adults with mental disorder: Developmental follow-back of a prospective-longitudinal cohort. *Archives of General Psychiatry*, *60*(7), 709. https://doi.org/10.1001/archpsyc.60.7.709

Klein, P. S., Wieder, S., & Greenspan, S. I. (1987). A theoretical overview and empirical study of Mediated Learning Experience: Prediction of preschool performance from mother-infant interactions patterns. *Infant Mental Health Journal*, *8*(2), 110–129.

Kotov, R. (2011). New Dimensions in the Quantitative Classification of Mental Illness. *Archives of General Psychiatry*, *68*(10), 1003. https://doi.org/10.1001/archgenpsychiatry.2011.107

Kotov, R., Gamez, W., Schmidt, F., & Watson, D. (2010). Linking "big" personality traits to anxiety, depressive, and substance use disorders: A meta-analysis. *Psychological Bulletin*, *136*(5), 768–821. https://doi.org/10.1037/a0020327

Kotov, R., Krueger, R. F., Watson, D., Achenbach, T. M., Althoff, R. R., Bagby, R. M., Brown, T. A., Carpenter, W. T., Caspi, A., Clark, L. A., Eaton, N. R., Forbes, M. K., Forbush, K. T., Goldberg, D., Hasin, D., Hyman, S. E., Ivanova, M. Y., Lynam, D. R., Markon, K., . . . Zimmerman, M. (2017). The Hierarchical Taxonomy of Psychopathology (HiTOP): A dimensional alternative to traditional nosologies. *Journal of Abnormal Psychology*, *126*(4), 454–477. https://doi.org/10.1037/abn0000258

Kotov, R., Krueger, R. F., Watson, D., Cicero, D. C., Conway, C. C., DeYoung, C. G., Eaton, N. R., Forbes, M. K., Hallquist, M. N., Latzman, R. D., Mullins-Sweatt, S. N., Ruggero, C. J., Simms, L. J., Waldman, I. D., Waszczuk, M. A., & Wright, A. G. C. (2021). The Hierarchical Taxonomy of Psychopathology (HiTOP): A quantitative nosology based on consensus of evidence. *Annual Review of Clinical Psychology*, *17*(1), 83–108. https://doi.org/10.1146/annurev-clinpsy-081219-093304

Krueger, R. F. (1999). The structure of common mental disorders. *Archives of General Psychiatry*, *56*(10), 921. https://doi.org/10.1001/archpsyc.56.10.921

Krueger, R. F., Caspi, A., Moffitt, T. E., & Silva, P. A. (1998). The structure and stability of common mental disorders (DSM-III-R): A longitudinal-epidemiological study. *Journal of Abnormal Psychology*, *107*(2), 216–227. https://doi.org/10.1037/0021-843X.107.2.216

Krueger, R. F., Derringer, J., Markon, K. E., Watson, D., & Skodol, A. E. (2012). Initial construction of a maladaptive personality trait model and inventory for DSM-5. *Psychological Medicine*, *42*(9), 1879–1890. https://doi.org/10.1017/S0033291711002674

Krueger, R. F., & Eaton, N. R. (2010). Personality traits and the classification of mental disorders: Toward a more complete integration in DSM-5 and an empirical model of psychopathology. *Personality Disorders: Theory, Research, and Treatment*, *1*(2), 97–118. https://doi.org/10.1037/a0018990

Krueger, R. F., & Hobbs, K. A. (2020). An overview of the DSM-5 Alternative Model of Personality Disorders. *Psychopathology*, *53*(3–4), 126–132. https://doi.org/10.1159/000508538

Krueger, R. F., Kotov, R., Watson, D., Forbes, M. K., Eaton, N. R., Ruggero, C. J., Simms, L. J., Widiger, T. A., Achenbach, T. M., Bach, B., Bagby, R. M., Bornovalova, M. A., Carpenter, W. T., Chmielewski, M., Cicero, D. C., Clark, L. A., Conway, C., DeClercq, B., DeYoung, C. G., Docherty, A. R., . . . Zimmermann, J. (2018). Progress in achieving quantitative classification of psychopathology. *World Psychiatry*, *17*(3), 282–293. https://doi.org/10.1002/wps.20566

Krueger, R. F., & Tackett, J. L. (2003). Personality and psychopathology: working toward the bigger picture. *Journal of Personality Disorders*, *17*(2), 109–128. https://doi.org/10.1521/pedi.17.2.109.23986

Kvarstein, E. H., Frøyhaug, M., Pettersen, M. S., Carlsen, S., Ekberg, A., Fjermestad-Noll, J., Ulvestad, D. A., Gikling, E. L., Hjermann, E., Lindberget, K., Omvik, S., Eikenæs, I. U., Hummelen, B., Morken, K. T. E., Wilberg, T., & Pedersen, G. A. F (2023). Improvement of personality functioning among people treated within personality disorder mental health services. A longitudinal, observational study. *Front Psychiatry*, *14*, 1163347. https://doi.org/10.3389/fpsyt.2023.1163347

Kwapil, T., & Neus Barrantes-Vidal. (2022). Schizotypal personality disorder in the Alternative Model for Personality Disorders. *Personality Disorders: Theory, Research and Treatment*, *13*(4), 392–396. https://doi.org/10.1037/per0000538

Lagattuta, K. H., & Thompson, R. A. (2007). The development of self-conscious emotions: Cognitive processes and social influences. In J. L. Tracy, R. W. Robins, & J. P. Tangney (Eds.), *The self-conscious emotions: Theory and research* (pp. 91–113). The Guilford Press.

Lahey, B. B., Applegate, B., Hakes, J. K., Zald, D. H., Hariri, A. R., & Rathouz, P. J. (2012). Is there a general factor of prevalent psychopathology during adulthood? *Journal of Abnormal Psychology*, *121*(4), 971–977. https://doi.org/10.1037/a0028355

Levin-Aspenson, H. F., Watson, D., Clark, L. A., & Zimmerman, M. (2021). What is the general factor of psychopathology? Consistency of the p factor across samples. *Assessment*, *28*(4), 1035–1049. https://doi.org/10.1177/1073191120954921

Lind, M., Adler, J. M., & Clark, L. A. (2020). Narrative identity and personality disorder: An empirical and conceptual review. *Current Psychiatry Reports*, *22*(12), 67. https://doi.org/10.1007/s11920-020-01187-8

Lind, M., Vanwoerden, S., Bo, S., & Sharp, C. (2022). Borderline personality disorder in adolescence: The role of narrative identity in the intrapsychic reasoning system. *Personality Disorders: Theory, Research, and Treatment*, *13*(5), 451–459. https://doi.org/10.1037/per0000517

Lind, M., Vanwoerden, S., Penner, F., & Sharp, C. (2019). Inpatient adolescents with borderline personality disorder features: Identity diffusion and narrative incoherence. *Personality Disorders: Theory, Research, and Treatment*, *10*(4), 389–393. https://doi.org/10.1037/per0000338

Lind, M., Vanwoerden, S., Penner, F., & Sharp, C. (2020). Narrative coherence in adolescence: relations with attachment, mentalization, and psychopathology. *Journal of Personality Assessment*, *102*(3), 380–389. https://doi.org/10.1080/00223891.2019.1574805

Livesley, J. (2003). *Practical management of personality disorders*. Guilford.

Livesley, W. J. (1998). Suggestions for a framework for an empirically based classification of personality disorder. *Canadian Journal of Psychiatry*, *43*(2), 137–147.

Maffly-Kipp, J., & Morey, L. C. (2024). Comparing the DSM-5 categorical model of personality disorders and the Alternative Model of Personality Disorders regarding clinician judgments of risk and outcome. *Personality Disorders: Theory, Research and Treatment*, *15*(5), 315–321. https://doi.org/10.1037/per0000657

Masterson, J. F. (1988). *The search for the real self: Unmasking the personality disorders of our age*. The Free Press.

McAdams, D. P. (2015). *The art and science of personality development*. Guilford Press.

McAdams, D. P. (2015). Three lines of personality development: A conceptual itinerary. *European Psychologist*, *20*(4), 252–264. https://doi.org/10.1027/1016-9040/a000236

McAdams, D. P., & McLean, K. C. (2013). Narrative identity. *Current Directions in Psychological Science*, *22*(3), 233–238. https://doi.org/10.1177/0963721413475622

McAdams, D. P., & Olson, B. D. (2010). Personality development: Continuity and change over the Life Course. *Annual Review of Psychology*, *61*, 517–542. https://doi.org/10.1146/annurev.psych.093008.100507

McCabe, G. A., Oltmanns, J. R., & Widiger, T. A. (2021). Criterion A scales: Convergent, discriminant, and structural relationships. *Assessment*, *28*(3), 813–828. https://doi.org/10.1177/1073191120947160

Mead, G. H. (1934). *Mind, self, and Society from the standpoint of a social behaviorist*. University of Chicago Press.

Mesman, J., Bongers, I., & Koot, H. (2001). Preschool developmental pathways to preadolescent internalizing and externalizing problems. *Journal of Child Psychology and Psychiatry, and Allied Disciplines*, *42*(5), 679–689.

Milinkovic, M. S., & Tiliopoulos, N. (2020). A systematic review of the clinical utility of the DSM-5 Section III Alternative Model of Personality Disorder. *Personality Disorders: Theory, Research, and Treatment*, *11*(6), 377–397. https://doi.org/10.1037/per0000408

Miller, J. D., Crowe, M. L., & Sharpe, B. M. (2022). Narcissism and the DSM-5 Alternative Model of Personality Disorder. *Personality Disorders: Theory, Research, and Treatment*, *13*(4), 407–411. https://doi.org/10.1037/per0000534

Miller, S. A. (2009). Children's understanding of second-order mental states. *Psychological Bulletin, 135*(5), 749–773. https://doi.org/10.1037/a0016854

Morey, L. C. (2017). Development and initial evaluation of a self-report form of the DSM-5 Level of Personality Functioning Scale. *Psychological Assessment, 29*(10), 1302–1308. https://doi.org/10.1037/pas0000450

Morey, L. C. (2018). Application of the DSM-5 Level of Personality Functioning Scale by lay raters. *Journal of Personality Disorders, 32*(5), 709–720. https://doi.org/10.1521/pedi_2017_31_305

Morey, L. C. (2019a). Interdiagnostician reliability of the DSM-5 Section II and Section III alternative model criteria for borderline personality disorder. *Journal of Personality Disorders, 33*(6), 721–S718. https://doi.org/10.1521/pedi_2019_33_362

Morey, L. C. (2019b). On parsimony in personality disorder classification: Rejoinder to Sleep et al. (2019). *Psychological Assessment, 31*(10), 1206–1207. https://doi.org/10.1037/pas0000774

Morey, L. C. (2019c). Thoughts on the assessment of the DSM-5 Alternative Model for Personality Disorders: Comment on Sleep et al. *Psychological Assessment, 31*(10), 1192–1199. https://doi.org/10.1037/pas0000710

Morey, L. C., Benson, K. T., Busch, A. J., & Skodol, A. E. (2015). Personality disorders in DSM-5: Emerging research on the alternative model. *Current Psychiatry Reports, 17*(4), 558. https://doi.org/10.1007/s11920-015-0558-0

Morey, L. C., & Hopwood, C. J. (2019). Expert preferences for categorical, dimensional, and mixed/hybrid approaches to personality disorder diagnosis. *Journal of Personality Disorders, 34*(Suppl C), 124–131. https://doi.org/10.1521/pedi_2019_33_398

Morey, L. C., McCredie, M. N., Bender, D. S., & Skodol, A. E. (2022). Criterion A: Level of personality functioning in the Alternative DSM-5 Model for Personality Disorders. *Personality Disorders: Theory, Research and Treatment, 3*(4), 305–315. https://doi.org/10.1037/per0000551

Moustakas, C. E. (1956). *The self: Explorations in personal growth*. Harper & Brothers.

Mulder, R. T. (2021). ICD-11 Personality disorders: Utility and implications of the new model. *Frontiers in Psychiatry, 12*, 655548. https://doi.org/65554810.3389/fpsyt.2021.655548

Mullins-Sweatt, S. N., Hopwood, C. J., Chmielewski, M., Meyer, N. A., Min, J., Helle, A. C., & Walgren, M. D. (2020). Treatment of personality pathology through the lens of the hierarchical taxonomy of psychopathology: Developing a research agenda. *Personality and Mental Health, 14*(1), 123–141. https://doi.org/10.1002/pmh.1464

Ohse, L., Zimmermann, J., Kerber, A., Kampe, L., Mohr, J., Kendlbacher, J., Busch, O., Rentrop, M., & Hörz-Sagstetter, S. (2023). Reliability, structure, and validity of module I (personality functioning) of the Structured Clinical Interview for the Alternative DSM-5 Model for Personality Disorders (SCID-5-AMPD-I). *Personality Disorders: Theory, Research, and Treatment, 14*(3), 287–299. https://doi.org/10.1037/per0000576

Oldham, J. M., & Skodol, A. E. (2000). Charting the future of Axis II. *Journal of Personality Disorders, 14*(1), 17–29. https://doi.org/10.1521/pedi.2000.14.1.17

Oltmanns, J. R., Smith, G. T., Oltmanns, T. F., & Widiger, T. A. (2018). General factors of psychopathology, personality, and personality disorder: Across domain comparisons. *Clinical Psychological Science, 6*(4), 581–589. https://doi.org/10.1177/2167702617750150

Paap, M. C. S., Pedersen, G., Kvarstein, E., & Hummelen, B. (2023). Evaluating the construct validity of the Norwegian version of the level of personality functioning scale—Brief form 2.0 in a large clinical sample. *Journal of Personality Assessment, 106*(1), 49–59. https://doi.org/10.1080/00223891.2023.2182694

Papamalis, F. E., Kalyva, E., Teare, M. D., & Meier, P. S. (2020). The role of personality functioning in drug misuse treatment engagement. *Addiction, 115*(4), 726–739. https://doi.org/10.1111/add.14872

Penner, F., Gambin, M., & Sharp, C. (2019). Childhood maltreatment and identity diffusion among inpatient adolescents: The role of reflective function. *Journal of Adolescence, 76*, 65–74. https://doi.org/10.1016/j.adolescence.2019.08.002

Perner, J., & Wimmer, H. (1985). "John thinks that Mary thinks that . . .": Attribution of second-order beliefs by 5- to 10-year-old children. *Journal of Experimental Child Psychology, 39*(3), 437–471 URLJ: http://www academicpress com/jecp.

Ringwald, W. R., Hopwood, C. J., Pilkonis, P. A., & Wright, A. G. C. (2021). Dynamic features of affect and interpersonal behavior in relation to general and specific personality pathology. *Personality Disorders—Theory Research and Treatment*, *12*(4), 365–376. https://doi.org/10.1037/per0000469

Ringwald, W. R., Beeney, J. E., Pilkonis, P. A., & Wright, A. G. C. (2019). Comparing hierarchical models of personality pathology. *Journal of Research in Personality*, *81*, 98–107. https://doi.org/10.1016/j.jrp.2019.05.011

Robins, E., & Guze, S. B. (1970). Establishment of diagnostic validity in psychiatric illness—Its application to schizophrenia. *American Journal of Psychiatry*, *126*(7), 983–987.

Roche, M. J., Jacobson, N. C., & Phillips, J. J. (2018). Expanding the validity of the level of personality functioning scale observer report and self-report versions across psychodynamic and interpersonal paradigms. *Journal of Personality Assessment*, *100*(6), 571–580. https://doi.org/10.1080/00223891.2018.1475394

Roche, M. J., Jacobson, N. C., & Pincus, A. L. (2016). Using repeated daily assessments to uncover oscillating patterns and temporally-dynamic triggers in structures of psychopathology: Applications to the Alternative Model of Personality Disorders. *Journal of Abnormal Psychology*, *125*(8), 1090–1102. https://doi.org/10.1037/abn0000177

Rodriguez-Seijas, C., Ruggero, C., Eaton, N. R., & Krueger, R. F. (2019). The DSM-5 Alternative Model for Personality Disorders and clinical treatment: A review. *Current Treatment Options in Psychiatry*, *6*, 284–298. https://doi.org/10.1007/s40501-019-00187-7

Røysamb, E., Kendler, K. S., Tambs, K., Ørstavik, R. E., Neale, M. C., Aggen, S. H., Torgersen, S., & Reichborn-Kjennerud, T. (2011). The joint structure of DSM-IV Axis I and Axis II disorders. *Journal of Abnormal Psychology*, *120*(1), 198–209. https://doi.org/10.1037/a0021660

Ruba, A. L., & Pollak, S. D. (2020). Children's emotion inferences from masked faces: Implications for social interactions during COVID-19. *Public Library of Science One*, *15*(12), e0243708. https://doi.org/10.1371/journal.pone.0243708

Rutter, M., & Rutter, M. (1993). *Developing minds*. Basic Books.

Rutter, M., & Sroufe, L. A. (2000). Developmental psychopathology: Concepts and challenges. *Development and Psychopathology*, *12*, 265–296.

Samuel, D. B., Balling, C. E., & Bucher, M. A. (2022). The Alternative Model of Personality Disorder is inadequate for capturing obsessive-compulsive personality disorder. *Personality Disorders: Theory, Research, and Treatment*, *13*(4), 418–421. https://doi.org/10.1037/per0000544

Samuel, D., & Widiger, T. (2008). A meta-analytic review of the relationships between the five-factor model and DSM-IV-TR personality disorders: A facet level analysis. *Clinical Psychology Review*, *28*(8), 1326–1342. https://doi.org/10.1016/j.cpr.2008.07.002

Schmeck, K., Schluter-Muller, S., Foelsch, P. A., & Doering, S. (2013). The role of identity in the DSM-5 classification of personality disorders. *Child and Adolescent Psychiatry and Mental Health*, *7*(1), 27. https://doi.org/10.1186/1753-2000-7-27

Sharp, C. (2016). Current trends in BPD research as indicative of a broader sea-change in psychiatric nosology. *Personality Disorders: Theory, Research, and Treatment*, *7*(4), 334–343. https://doi.org/10.1037/per0000199

Sharp, C. (2020). Adolescent personality pathology and the Alternative Model for Personality Disorders: Self development as nexus. *Psychopathology*, *53*(3–4), 198–204. https://doi.org/10.1159/000507588

Sharp, C. (2022). Fulfilling the promise of the LPF: Commentary on Morey et al. *Personality Disorders: Theory, Research and Treatment*, *13*(4), 316–320. https://doi.org/10.1037/per0000567

Sharp, C., & Bevington, D. (2022). *The mentalizing therapist: A primer for clinicians*. The Guildford Press.

Sharp, C., & Cervantes, B. R. (2023). Maladaptive self- and interpersonal functioning increments general psychiatric severity in the association with adolescent personality pathology. *Children (Basel)*, *10*(1), 120. https://doi.org/10.3390/children10010120

Sharp, C., Kerr, S., & Barkauskiene, R. (2022). The incremental utility of maladaptive self and identity functioning over general functioning for borderline personality disorder features in adolescents.

Personality Disorders: Theory, Research, and Treatment, *13*(5), 474–481. https://doi.org/10.1037/per0000547

Sharp, C., Kulesz, P., & Kerr, S. (2024). Prospective prediction of treatment outcomes in adolescents: A head-to-head comparison of alternative model for personality disorder versus borderline personality disorder. *Personality Disorders: Theory, Research, and Treatment*, *15*(5), 379–385. https://doi.org/10.1037/per0000675

Sharp, C., McLaren, V., Musetti, A., Vanwoerden, S., Hernandez Ortiz, J., Schmeck, K., Birkhoelzer, M., & Goth, K. (2022). The Assessment of Identity Development in Adolescence (AIDA) Questionnaire: First psychometric evaluation in two North American samples of young people. *Journal of Personality Assessment*, *105*(4), 451–462. https://doi.org/10.1080/00223891.2022.2119860

Sharp, C., & Miller, J. D. (2022). 10-year retrospective on the DSM-5 Alternative Model of Personality Disorder: Seeing the forest for the trees. *Personality Disorders: Theory, Research and Treatment*, *13*(4), 301–304. https://doi.org/10.1037/per0000595

Sharp, C., & Oldham, J. (2022). Nature and assessment of personality pathology and diagnosis. *American Journal of Psychotherapy*, *76*(1), 3–8. https://doi.org/10.1176/appi.psychotherapy.20220016

Sharp, C., Vanwoerden, S., & Wall, K. (2018). Adolescence as a sensitive period for the development of personality disorder. *Psychiatric Clinics of North America*, *41*(4), 669–683. https://doi.org/10.1016/j.psc.2018.07.004

Sharp, C., & Wall, K. (2018). Personality pathology grows up: Adolescence as a sensitive period. *Current Opinion in Psychology*, *21*, 111–116. https://doi.org/10.1016/j.copsyc.2017.11.010

Sharp, C., & Wall, K. (2021). DSM-5 level of personality functioning: Refocusing personality disorder on what it means to be human. *Annual Review of Clinical Psychology*, *17*, 313–337. https://doi.org/10.1146/annurev-clinpsy-081219-105402

Sharp, C., Wright, A. G. C., Fowler, J. C., Frueh, B. C., Allen, J. G., Oldham, J., & Clark, L. A. (2015). The structure of personality pathology: Both general ('g') and specific ('s') factors? *Journal of Abnormal Psychology*, *124*(2), 387–398. https://doi.org/10.1037/abn0000033

Sheehan, L., Nieweglowski, K., & Corrigan, P. (2016). The stigma of personality disorders. *Current Psychiatry Reports*, *18*(1), 11. https://doi.org/1110.1007/s11920-015-0654-1

Sheets, E., & Craighead, W. E. (2007). Toward an empirically based classification of personality pathology. *Clinical Psychology—Science and Practice*, *14*(2), 77–93. https://doi.org/10.1111/j.1468-2850.2007.00065.x

Shiner, J. L., & Tackett, J. L. (2014). Personality disorders in children and adolescents. In E. J. Mash & R. A. Barkley (Eds.), *Child Psychopathology* (3rd ed., pp. 848–896). Guilford.

Shiner, R. C., A. (2003). Personality differences in childhood and adolescence: Measurement, development, and consequences. *Journal of Child Psychology and Psychiatry*, *44*(1), 2–32.

Shiner, R. L., Buss, K. A., McClowry, S. G., Putnam, S. P., Saudino, K. J., & Zentner, M. (2012). What is temperament now? Assessing progress in temperament research on the twenty-fifth anniversary of Goldsmith et al. *Child Development Perspectives*, *6*(4), 436–444. https://doi.org/10.1111/j.1750-8606.2012.00254.x

Siefert, C. J., Sexton, J., Meehan, K., Nelson, S., Haggerty, G., Dauphin, B., & Huprich, S. (2020). Development of a short form for the DSM-5 Levels of Personality Functioning Questionnaire. *Journal of Personality Assessment*, *102*(4), 516–526. https://doi.org/10.1080/00223891.2019.1594842

Skodol, A. E., Clark, L. A., Bender, D. S., Krueger, R. F., Morey, L. C., Verheul, R., Alarcon, R. D., Bell, C. C., Siever, L. J., & Oldham, J. M. (2011). Proposed changes in personality and personality disorder assessment and diagnosis for DSM-5 Part I: Description and rationale. *Personality Disorders-Theory Research and Treatment*, *2*(1), 4–22. https://doi.org/10.1037/a0021891

Skodol, A. E., Morey, L. C., Bender, D. S., & Oldham, J. M. (2015). The Alternative DSM-5 Model for Personality Disorders: A clinical application. *American Journal of Psychiatry*, *172*(7), 606–613. https://doi.org/10.1176/appi.ajp.2015.14101220

Sleep, C. E., Lynam, D. R., Widiger, T. A., Crowe, M. L., & Miller, J. D. (2019). An evaluation of DSM-5 Section III personality disorder Criterion A (impairment) in accounting for psychopathology. *Psychological Assessment*, *31*(10), 1181–1191. https://doi.org/10.1037/pas0000620

Sleep, C. E., Weiss, B., Lynam, D. R., & Miller, J. D. (2020). The DSM-5 Section III personality disorder criterion in relation to both pathological and general personality traits. *Personality Disorders: Theory, Research, and Treatment*, *11*(3), 202–212. https://doi.org/10.1037/per0000383

Southward, M. W., Cheavens, J. S., & Coccaro, E. F. (2023). Defining the *p* -factor: An empirical test of five leading theories. *Psychological Medicine*, *53*(7), 2732–2743. https://doi.org/10.1017/S003329172 2001635

Tackett, J. L. (2006). Evaluating models of the personality-psychopathology relationship in children and adolescents. *Clinical Psychology Review*, *26*(5), 584–599. https://doi.org/10.1016/j.cpr.2006.04.003

Thomson, M., Cavelti, M., Lerch, S., Koenig, J., Reichl, C., Mürner-Lavanchy, I., Wyssen, A., & Kaess, M. (2024). Clinical profiles of adolescent personality pathology: A latent structure examination of the Semi-Structured Interview for Personality Functioning DSM-5 (STiP-5.1) in a help-seeking sample. *Borderline Personality Disorder and Emotion Dysregulation*, *11*(1), 9. https://doi.org/10.1186/s40479-024-00252-5

Trull, T. J., & Durrett, C. A. (2005). Categorical and dimensional models of personality disorder. *Annual Review of Clinical Psychology*, *1*, 355–380. https://doi.org/10.1146/annurev.clinpsy.1.102803.144009

Tyrer, P., & Alexander, J. (1979). Classification of personality disorder. *British Journal of Psychiatry*, *135*, 163–167. https://doi.org/10.1192/bjp.135.2.163

Tyrer, P., & Johnson, T. (1996). Establishing the severity of personality disorder. *American Journal of Psychiatry*, *153*(12), 1593–1597. https://doi.org/10.1176/ajp.153.12.1593

Van Bork, R., Epskamp, S., Rhemtulla, M., Borsboom, D., & Van Der Maas, H. L. J. (2017). What is the *p* -factor of psychopathology? Some risks of general factor modeling. *Theory & Psychology*, *27*(6), 759–773. https://doi.org/10.1177/0959354317737185

Vandivier, L. E., & Hertenstein, M. J. (2013). Social referencing in infancy: Important findings and future directions. In C. Mohiyeddini, M. Eysenck, & S. Bauer (Eds.), *Handbook of psychology of emotions (Vol. 1): Recent theoretical perspectives and novel empirical findings* (pp. 81–85). Nova Science Publishers.

Vanwoerden, S., Franssens, R., Sharp, C., & De Clercq, B. (2022). The development of Criterion A personality pathology: The relevance of childhood social functioning for young adult daily self-functioning. *Child Psychiatry & Human Development*, *53*(6), 1148–1160. https://doi.org/10.1007/s10 578-021-01187-6

Vanwoerden, S., & Stepp, S. D. (2022). The DSM-5 alternative model conceptualization of borderline personality disorder: A review of the evidence. *Personality Disorders: Theory, Research and Treatment*, *13*(4), 402–406. https://doi.org/10.1037/per0000563

Verheul, R., Bartak, A., & Widiger, T. (2007). Prevalence and construct validity of personality disorder not otherwise specified (PDNOS). *Journal of Personality Disorders*, *21*(4), 359–370. https://doi.org/10.1521/pedi.2007.21.4.359

Wampold, B. E., & Imel, Z. E. (2015). *The great psychotherapy debate: The evidence for what makes psychotherapy work* (2nd ed.): Routledge/Taylor & Francis Group.

Waszczuk, M. A., Hopwood, C. J., Luft, B. J., Morey, L. C., Perlman, G., Ruggero, C. J., Skodol, A. E., & Kotov, R. (2022). The prognostic utility of personality traits versus past psychiatric diagnoses: Predicting future mental health and functioning. *Clinical Psychological Science*, *10*(4), 734–751. https://doi.org/10.1177/21677026211056596

Watson, D., & Clark, L. A. (2020). Personality traits as an organizing framework for personality pathology. *Personality and Mental Health*, *14*(1), 51–75. https://doi.org/10.1002/pmh.1458

Watts, A. L., Greene, A. L., Ringwald, W., Forbes, M. K., Brandes, C. M., Levin-Aspenson, H. F., & Delawalla, C. (2023). Factor analysis in personality disorders research: Modern issues and illustrations of practical recommendations. *Personality Disorders: Theory, Research, and Treatment*, *14*(1), 105–117. https://doi.org/10.1037/per0000581

Waugh, M. H., Hopwood, C. J., Krueger, R. F., Morey, L. C., Pincus, A. L., & Wright, A. G. C. (2017). Psychological assessment with the DSM-5 Alternative Model for Personality Disorders: Tradition and innovation. *Professional Psychology: Research and Practice*, *48*(2), 79–89. https://doi.org/10.1037/pro0000071

Weekers, L. C., Hutsebaut, J., & Kamphuis, J. H. (2019). The Level of Personality Functioning Scale-Brief Form 2.0: Update of a brief instrument for assessing level of personality functioning. *Personality and Mental Health*, *13*(1), 3–14. https://doi.org/10.1002/pmh.1434

Weisberg, D. S. (2015). Pretend play. *Wiley Interdisciplinary Reviews: Cognitive Science*, *6*(3), 249–261. https://doi.org/10.1002/wcs.1341

Widiger, T. A. (2011). Personality and psychopathology. *World Psychiatry*, *10*(2), 103–106. https://doi.org/10.1002/j.2051-5545.2011.tb00024.x

Widiger, T. A., Bach, B., Chmielewski, M., Clark, L. A., DeYoung, C., Hopwood, C. J., Kotov, R., Krueger, R. F., Miller, J. D., Morey, L. C., Mullins-Sweatt, S. N., Patrick, C. J., Pincus, A. L., Samuel, D. B., Sellbom, M., South, S. C., Tackett, J. L., Watson, D., Waugh, M. H., Wright, A. G. C., . . . Thomas, K. M. (2019). Criterion A of the AMPD in HiTOP. *Journal of Personality Assessment*, *101*(4), 345–355. https://doi.org/10.1080/00223891.2018.1465431

Widiger, T. A., & Clark, L. A. (2000). Toward DSM-V and the classification of psychopathology. *Psychological Bulletin*, *126*(6), 946–963. https://doi.org/10.1037//0033-2909.126.6.946

Widiger, T. A., & Frances, A. (1987). Interviews and inventories for the measurement of personality-disorders. *Clinical Psychology Review*, *7*(1), 49–75. https://doi.org/10.1016/0272-7358(87)90004-3

Widiger, T. A., & Hines, A. (2022). The Diagnostic and Statistical Manual of Mental Disorders, Fifth Edition Alternative Model of Personality Disorder. *Personality Disorders: Theory, Research, and Treatment*, *13*(4), 347–355. https://doi.org/10.1037/per0000524

Widiger, T. A., Sellbom, M., Chmielewski, M., Clark, L. A., DeYoung, C. G., Kotov, R., Krueger, R. F., Lynam, D. R., Miller, J. D., Mullins-Sweatt, S., Samuel, D. B., South, S. C., Tackett, J. L., Thomas, K. M., Watson, D., & Wright, A. G. C. (2019). Personality in a Hierarchical Model of Psychopathology. *Clinical Psychological Science*, *7*(1), 77–92. https://doi.org/10.1177/2167702618797105

Widiger, T. A., & Simonsen, E. (2005). Alternative Dimensional Models of Personality Disorder: Finding a common ground. *Journal of Personality Disorders*, *19*(2), 110–130. https://doi.org/10.1521/pedi.19.2.110.62628

Widiger, T. A., & Trull, T. J. (2007). Plate tectonics in the classification of personality disorder: Shifting to a dimensional model. *American Psychologist*, *62*(2), 71–83. https://doi.org/10.1037/0003-066X.62.2.71

Wittenborn, J. R., Holzberg, J. D., & Simon, B. (1953). Symptom correlates for descriptive diagnosis. *Genetic Psychology Monographs*, *47*(2), 237–302.

World Health Organization (2019). *ICD-11: International classification of diseases* (11th revision). Retrieved from https://icd.who.int/.

Wright, A. G. C., Hopwood, C. J., Skodol, A. E., & Morey, L. C. (2016). Longitudinal validation of general and specific structural features of personality pathology. *Journal of Abnormal Psychology*, *125*(8), 1120–1134. https://doi.org/10.1037/abn0000165

Wright, A. G. C., Krueger, R. F., Hobbs, M. J., Markon, K. E., Eaton, N. R., & Slade, T. (2013). The structure of psychopathology: Toward an expanded quantitative empirical model. *Journal of Abnormal Psychology*, *122*(1), 281–294. https://doi.org/10.1037/a0030133

Wright, A. G. C., & Simms, L. J. (2015). A metastructural model of mental disorders and pathological personality traits. *Psychological Medicine*, *45*(11), 2309–2319. https://doi.org/10.1017/S0033291715000252

Wu, J., Allman, M., Balzen, K., Hutsebaut, J., & Sharp, C. (2024). First psychometric evaluation of the Level of Personality Functioning Scale—Brief Form 2.0 in adolescents. *Personality Disorders: Theory, Research, and Treatment*, *15*(6), 492–503. https://doi.org/10.1037/per0000674

Zettl, M., Volkert, J., Vogele, C., Herpertz, S. C., Kubera, K. M., & Taubner, S. (2020). Mentalization and criterion a of the Alternative Model for Personality Disorders: Results from a clinical and nonclinical sample. *Personality Disorders: Theory, Research, and Treatment*, *11*(3), 191–201. https://doi.org/10.1037/per0000356

Zimmermann, J., Benecke, C., Bender, D. S., Skodol, A. E., Schauenburg, H., Cierpka, M., & Leising, D. (2014). Assessing DSM-5 level of personality functioning from videotaped clinical interviews: A pilot study with untrained and clinically inexperienced students. *Journal of Personality Assessment*, *96*(4), 397–409. https://doi.org/10.1080/00223891.2013.852563

Zimmermann, J., Bohnke, J. R., Eschstruth, R., Mathews, A., Wenzel, K., & Leising, D. (2015). The latent structure of personality functioning: Investigating Criterion A from the Alternative Model for Personality Disorders in DSM-5. *Journal of Abnormal Psychology*, *124*(3), 532–548. https://doi.org/10.1037/abn0000059

Zimmermann, J., Kerber, A., Rek, K., Hopwood, C. J., & Krueger, R. F. (2019). A brief but comprehensive review of research on the Alternative DSM-5 Model for Personality Disorders. *Current Psychiatry Reports*, *21*(9), 92. https://doi.org/10.1007/s11920-019-1079-z

CHAPTER 10

Dimensional Models of Temperament and Psychopathology

LINDSAY N. GABEL, HALEY E. GREEN, THOMAS M. OLINO, AND ELIZABETH P. HAYDEN

Introduction

INTEREST in the role of individual differences in the experience, expression, and self-regulation of emotion and behavior, and how these individual differences are associated with maladaptation, can be dated to antiquity. In contemporary psychological science, the study of early emerging trait-like variation in emotion and behavior and associated outcomes falls under the domain of *temperament*, defined as individual differences in heritable, early emerging reactive and regulatory traits. Of course, personality research is also concerned with heritable trait variation in emotionality and self-regulation and how these predispose to psychopathology. Nevertheless, there are important differences in how the fields of personality and temperament research have evolved, with strengths and weaknesses characterizing both research traditions.

Personality research has a strong tradition of addressing structural questions as they pertain to self-reported variation in individual differences, drawing upon relatively large samples of adults, oftentimes in cross-sectional data (Durbin & Hicks, 2014). The current understanding we have regarding the dimensional nature and structure of individual differences in adulthood is, accordingly, robust and data driven. In contrast, temperament researchers have traditionally used smaller samples of infants and children, richly characterized with diverse assessment methods and longitudinal approaches. In further contrast to the relatively agnostic, data-driven approach to characterizing adult personality, our understanding of the nature of early temperament is rooted in theory-driven models of children's individual differences, infrequently subjected to strict empirical tests. The oftentimes arbitrary distinctions between, and disparate approaches to, temperament and personality research have impeded progress in understanding individual differences from a lifespan perspective. Research on, and theories of, individual differences across the lifespan will benefit from greater integration of temperament and personality perspectives and methods, a point to which we return several times in this chapter.

Although progress has been made in terms of characterizing temperament-psychopathology associations in recent decades, foundational issues regarding the nature of early temperament and how it is best conceptualized and measured remain unclear. With these questions in mind, in the current chapter, our goal is to position what is currently known about temperament-psychopathology associations within a methodological perspective. We have chosen this orientation because we strongly agree with the recent assertion that psychological science "rests on the foundations of measurements" (Parsons et al., 2019). Indeed, any claims regarding temperament and its role in the development of psychopathology are constrained by methodological issues and must be contextualized accordingly.

For this reason, we first provide a critical overview of relevant methodologies for the study of temperament. Next, we briefly discuss models of individual differences and the need to develop integrated, dimensional frameworks of individual differences from a lifespan perspective. We then highlight frameworks for understanding the mechanisms through which temperament-psychopathology associations might emerge and summarize empirical support for these frameworks. Across these themes, we include discussion of key methodological considerations and approaches we deem important toward promoting a broad, robust literature on how early emerging individual differences eventuate in psychopathology.

Integrating Models and Measures of Individual Differences across the Lifespan

Assessment of Temperament

In early development, temperament dimensions are oftentimes assessed via self- or informant report, in which parents, teachers, or other knowledgeable informants rate the temperament of infants and young children who are unable to complete self-report measures. Questionnaire methods offer the advantages of being relatively economical and efficient, and different informants potentially provide critical information about how traits are expressed in different contexts (e.g., home, school) and have unique predictive power (Clark et al., 2017; Luan et al., 2018). For instance, some research shows that youths report trait-related changes during adolescence (i.e., increases in agreeableness and conscientiousness) that are not captured in reports completed by their parents, who report decreases in youths' neuroticism (Luan et al., 2017).

The "flip side" of the coin of unique predictive power is limited convergence of different informants, the rule of measures of individual differences, not the exception (Durbin & Wilson, 2012). Importantly, there is no consensus regarding which types of informants (e.g., mothers, teachers) yield the most valid information on youth temperament, and informant factors, such as the informant's own traits, psychopathology, or their knowledge of normative development, influence temperament ratings. For example, mothers' history of psychopathology and personality traits have been associated with ratings of their children's temperament (Durbin & Wilson, 2012; Forman et al., 2003; but see Olino et al., 2020), and maternal negative emotionality (NE) may moderate the convergence between observer versus maternal ratings of children's temperament, such that greater convergence with observational measures was found for mothers with higher NE (Hayden et al., 2010). For older youth and adults, self-report ratings may be more efficiently obtained than informant reports, yet may also be subject to biases (e.g., social desirability; Pedregon et al., 2012); further, shared method variance inflates associations among temperament ratings and other constructs (e.g., psychopathology) assessed via questionnaire (Cole, 1987; Spector et al., 2019). This results in potentially spurious associations among temperament dimensions and symptoms of psychopathology and impedes a clear understanding of how temperament and psychopathology become associated (Durbin & Hicks, 2014). For these reasons, researchers are encouraged to include multiple informants and methods to elucidate patterns of temperament-psychopathology associations. Although there is no agreed-upon method for integrating different sources of information on temperament, researchers should attend to the relevant literature highlighting developmental shifts in the differential predictive validity of different informants (e.g., parent versus child self-report) and outcomes (e.g., internalizing versus externalizing psychopathology).

Historically, observational measures of temperament are considered the "gold standard" approach for assessing infants and young children (e.g., Hawes et al., 2021; Liu et al., 2020; Martin-Storey et al., 2009). These approaches overcome some of the limitations of questionnaire approaches by relying on trained raters to score relevant behaviors during either standardized tasks or more naturalistic settings (e.g., a child playing with a parent at home). As an example of the former, in the Laboratory Temperament Assessment Battery (LAB Tab; Goldsmith et al., 1995), young children complete a series of standardized tasks (e.g., experiencing a stranger enter the room, having to wait to receive rewards, etc.) designed to elicit a range of individual differences in temperament dimensions, and trained raters score behavioral indicators of temperament traits according to a coding manual. Standardized observational methods bolster the validity of comparisons of differences in temperament across individuals by minimizing variation in context but may have lower ecological validity compared to observations in more naturalistic settings (Karp et al., 2004; Robbins et al., 2024). Notably, observational measures of temperament typically show modest convergence with questionnaire ratings of temperament (Goldsmith et al., 2012), suggesting that these measures may reflect different temperamental processes, tap different aspects of overlapping constructs, and/or have unique sources of measurement error (e.g., observational temperament measures collected in laboratory settings may be influenced by the novel laboratory environment; Barrett et al., 2007; Hayden, 2022; Saudino, 2009).

Despite their advantages, observational measures of temperament are typically costly and time-consuming compared to self- and informant reports, and few observational measures of temperament in older youths and adults have been validated (with the notable exceptions of Borkenau et al., 2001 and Durbin et al., 2009, whose observational measures of adult temperament were associated with self- and informant reports of temperament). However, alternative observational methods have recently been developed to address these limitations. These include "thin slice" approaches, in which observers rate children's temperament after exposure to brief behavioral samples (Tackett et al., 2019). Compared to traditional observational paradigms, such as the Lab-TAB, thin-slice approaches are highly versatile (i.e., can be used with any videotaped or observed interaction) and require significantly less time and training (Whalen et al., 2020). In addition, in recent studies of adults, researchers have begun to use ambulatory assessment tools, such as the Electronically Activated Recorder (EAR; Mehl, 2017), a wearable device that repeatedly captures brief audio recordings, to derive indices of adults' personality (Sun & Vazire, 2019; Tackman et al., 2020). Although still time-consuming for researchers and less frequently used with youth to date, ambulatory assessment methods reduce participant burden and may facilitate the collection of observational measures of temperament. In adults, personality ratings derived from EAR recordings have converged with in-the-moment self-ratings of some Big Five traits, including extraversion, conscientiousness, and neuroticism (Sun & Vazire, 2019; Tackman et al., 2020), highlighting the potential of these methods for future research as relevant technologies become more affordable and available.

Models of Individual Differences in Temperament

Dimensional models of temperament in youth have been developed over the last several decades (Buss & Plomin, 1975; Rothbart, 1981; Thomas & Chess, 1977), laying the groundwork for contemporary approaches to child temperament. In early work, Thomas and Chess (1977) performed inductive content analysis on observations of young children and interviews with parents from the New York Longitudinal Study (NYLS), positing a model comprised of nine temperament dimensions reflecting early emerging variation across a range of behaviors:

activity level, rhythmicity (the regularity of biological functions, such as sleeping and eating), approach versus withdrawal (the tendency to approach or withdraw from novel stimuli), adaptability (capacity to adapt to change in the environment), intensity (how strongly the child reacts to the environment, whether positively or negatively), sensitivity to stimuli, mood, distractibility, and attention span/persistence. Using these nine dimensions, Thomas and Chess classified children in the NYLS as "difficult" (crying frequently, difficulty adapting to changes in environment and following routines), "easy" (ease adapting to new situations and following routines, generally positive affect), and "slow to warm up" (comparatively slow to adapt to novelty with low-intensity emotional affect; Thomas & Chess, 1977). However, subsequent factor analyses did not replicate the original nine-factor structure posited by Thomas and Chess (Bohlin et al., 1981; Presley & Martin, 1994), raising questions about the validity of this older conceptualization of temperament.

Buss and Plomin (1975, 1984) developed an alternative four-factor model of temperament based on contemporaneous models of animal temperament, which identified fearfulness, aggression, affiliativeness, and impulsivity as core temperament dimensions in primates (Diamond, 1957). Known as the EASI model, this alternative model of human temperament comprised emotionality (the tendency to experience negative emotions), activity (amount of energy put forth), sociability (tendency to prefer being with others), and impulsivity (disinhibition). These temperament dimensions overlap conceptually with several of those proposed by Thomas and Chess; for instance, the activity dimension overlaps with Thomas and Chess' activity and impulsivity dimensions, and the emotionality dimension overlaps with Thomas and Chess' intensity and mood dimensions. In conceptualizing temperament with far fewer dimensions than Thomas and Chess, however, the EASI model is more parsimonious. Nevertheless, the significant contrast between these two early models ostensibly both capturing early individual differences is striking, a point to which we return later in this chapter. Further, the lack of a distinct dimension characterizing positive emotionality is potentially problematic, given theory positing its relatively specific role in depression and related conditions (Clark & Watson, 1991).

In contemporary research on temperament, Rothbart's biobehavioral model of temperament (Rothbart et al., 2001) is likely the most influential and widely used framework. This model defines temperament as individual differences in reactivity (i.e., physiological sensitivity and intensity of reactions to internal and external changes in the environment) and self-regulation (i.e., processes that moderate responses to the environment) and comprises three broad domains: extraversion/surgency (which includes positive emotionality as a core feature), negative affectivity (NA), and effortful control (EC), with extraversion/surgency and NA reflecting positive and negative emotional reactivity and EC reflecting self-regulation. Each domain includes unique lower-order facets (e.g., fear, anger, and sadness are facets of NA; Rothbart & Bates, 2006). This model was informed by the temperament dimensions described by Thomas and Chess (1977) and was originally developed to capture infants' individual differences, but was later extended to children, adolescents, and adults, with corresponding measures designed to capture homotypic continuity across development.

Rothbart's temperament dimensions of extraversion/surgency, NA, and EC resemble the Big Five personality dimensions of extraversion, neuroticism, and conscientiousness, as well as the Big Three personality dimensions of PE, NE, and constraint (Clark et al., 2017; Clark & Watson, 2008; Zuckerman et al., 1993). This high face validity and conceptual overlap with models of adult personality fosters the examination of temperament across the lifespan and comparison with models of adult personality; further, distinct factors reflecting positive and negative emotionality facilitates integration of this temperament framework in causal models of psychopathology that posit divergent roles of trait emotionality. However, extant factor analytic work often fails to support Rothbart's hypothesized temperament structures (e.g., Kim et al., 2003; Kotelnikova et al., 2016; Kotelnikova et al., 2017). Thus, although Rothbart's framework offers advantages over other classic dimensional temperament frameworks, additional validation of the framework and measurement development is likely needed.

Integrating Theoretical Models of Temperament

In contrast to the adult personality literature, which has converged on the Big Five model as a unifying framework, the temperament literature remains fragmented due to variations in the way temperament is conceptualized. Though supporting evidence can be mustered for different models (De Pauw et al., 2009), this variation has hindered research progress (Shiner et al., 2012). A universal model of temperament is the critical foundation underlying work on associations between temperament and psychopathology (Tackett, 2006). We therefore highlight issues arising from the fragmented state of the temperament literature and discuss how prominent models of temperament might be integrated.

"Jingle-jangle" issues have long been identified as a source of fragmentation within the temperament literature (e.g., Tackett, 2006) and remain an ongoing problem nearly two decades later. Briefly, "jingle" issues refer to cases where the same term is used to refer to different constructs; "jangle" issues refer to cases where different terms are used to refer to the same construct. To illustrate, the temperament dimensions of effortful control and conscientiousness have often been used interchangeably with "executive functioning," "self-regulation," "self-control," "inhibition," and "impulsivity," despite arguments that these constructs are at least theoretically distinct from one another (Nigg et al., 2017; Shields et al., 2022). This imprecision in terminology has significant consequences for the cumulative science of temperament and its associations with psychopathology (Hayden, 2022). For example, in one study examining the structure of youth personality pathology, two different measures purporting to measure the trait of impulsivity both loaded onto a higher-order disagreeableness dimension, but in opposite directions (Kushner et al., 2013). Such findings point to flaws in the conceptualization and measurement of individual traits that then obscure relationships between traits and broader dimensions of temperament.

Jingle-jangle issues similarly muddy the literature on relationships between temperament traits and psychopathology, as relationships between psychopathology and theoretically similar (but empirically distinct) temperament constructs may be quite different. For example, evidence suggests that variance specific to attentional problems is strongly associated with measures of executive functioning, but not conscientiousness (Shields et al., 2022). Based on these findings, researchers seeking to explore how individual differences in traits shape attentional problems should select a measure that assesses executive functioning rather than conscientiousness. Despite this, measures designed to assess the temperamental equivalent of conscientiousness (i.e., the Effortful Control subscales of the Adult Temperament Questionnaire [ATQ; Evans & Rothbart, 2007] and Child Behavior Questionnaire [CBQ; Rothbart et al., 2001]) are presented as measures of executive functioning in the Research Domain Criteria (RDoC) framework (NIMH, 2024). In this way, the "conceptual clutter" introduced by imprecise terminology and varying definitions of constructs impedes the study of relationships between temperament traits and psychopathology (Morrison et al., 2016). Its consequences can be readily seen in failures to replicate findings and reduced precision in meta-analyses of associations between temperament and psychopathology (Kostyrka-Allchorne et al., 2020).

It is therefore critical that temperament researchers work toward establishing a united, common language with which to refer to various constructs. Echoing others, we call for explicit definitions of constructs and demarcation of the boundaries between them (Hayden, 2022). Recent review papers dedicated to this purpose, such as those on self-regulation (Nigg, 2017) and behavioral inhibition (Fox et al., 2023), are useful exemplars. In addition, rigorous validity studies of temperament constructs are needed. Specifically, where boundaries between theoretically similar constructs remain blurred, gaining extrinsic convergent validity evidence to untangle construct overlap may be helpful (Gonzalez et al., 2021). However, following the recommendations of Flake and colleagues (2017), we caution that efforts to improve the external validity of constructs be undertaken only after first improving temperament measures at the structural level (e.g., item functioning, factor structure, reliability, measurement invariance).

Despite outstanding measurement issues, researchers have attempted to integrate various models of temperament with the goal of establishing a unifying framework. Notable reviews have converged on similar sets of overarching dimensions. For instance, Soto and Tackett (2015) identified four core temperament domains: persistence, negative emotionality, activity level, and sociability. More recently, in a meta-review, Kostyrka-Allchorne and colleagues (2020) identified four similar domains: attention/regulatory behavior, emotionality, activity, and surgency/extraversion. Finally, the Little Six model, comprising the Big Five factors plus a sixth factor representing activity level, represents a blend of the most prominent temperament and personality traits in the youth and adult literatures (Shiner & DeYoung, 2013).

Although these reviews differ in the labels ascribed to different domains of temperament, possibly reflecting jingle-jangle issues, they suggest four viable overarching domains of temperament reflecting individual differences in regulatory, emotional, activity, and social domains. However, the nature and number of facets comprising these domains remains unclear, and current measures seem ill-equipped to elucidate these concerns. At present, the number of facets assessed by different temperament measures varies widely, ranging from none (Emotion, Activity, and Sociability (EAS) Scale; Buss & Plomin, 1984) to 30 (NEO-3; Shiner et al., 2012), and empirical support for facets is often poor (Kotelnikova et al., 2016, 2017). For instance, on the widely used Early Adolescent Temperament Questionnaire—Revised (EATQ-R; Capaldi & Rothbart, 1992), facets under the broader effortful control and negative emotionality dimensions form cohesive domains; however, facets under positive emotionality do not (Lawson et al., 2021), rendering facet-level scores for this dimension unusable.

The hazy construct validity of trait facets and limitations in their measurement are concerning given the important role that facets may play in understanding the development of temperament/personality and its links with psychopathology. For instance, facets (and even narrower levels of abstraction, such as nuances, which are indexed by little more than a few items) capture more age-specific information than broad traits, including the Big Five dimensions (Hang et al., 2021). Specifically, in lifespan studies where personality measures have been used to predict respondents' ages, facets allow for 36% more accurate prediction of respondents' ages compared to domains (Hang et al., 2021). Although additional developmentally informed work is needed, current findings suggest that broad domains, such as extraversion, may have less utility than their facets, such as warmth and assertiveness, for understanding individual differences across the lifespan.

Facets may also have greater predictive value in studies of associations between temperament and psychopathology dimensions. Recent meta-analytic work linking temperament traits to childhood adjustment showed that, akin to research on adult personality, negative emotionality is a strong predictor of both internalizing and externalizing psychopathology and thus may be a transdiagnostic risk factor (Kostyrka-Allchorne et al., 2020). At the same time, NE showed low specificity, which the authors attributed to the dimension capturing a wide range of negative emotions, including fear, sadness, and anger (Kostyrka-Allchorne et al., 2020). To capture specific trait-disorder pathways, temperament may need to be assessed at the level of facets rather than broad dimensions. Indeed, whereas certain facets (e.g., low attention to larger goals, a facet of conscientiousness) are associated with many disorders, some (e.g., high temperamental fear) appear to shape the *manifestation* of disorder that develops (i.e., pathoplasticity; Rettew, 2019). Thus, although temperament/personality at the domain level may be most useful for understanding comorbidity between different forms of psychopathology, lower-order elements of temperament may contribute to a more nuanced understanding of which aspects of temperament/personality drive associations with psychopathology (Conway et al., 2019; Ka et al., 2021). For example, venturesomeness and dominance are the facets of extraversion most strongly related to mania (Watson et al., 2019). Research examining which, and how many, facets best represent the higher- and lower-order dimensions of temperament, and whether these change across development, is an important area for further research.

Linking Dimensional Models of Temperament and Personality

For decades, temperament and personality research have largely proceeded independently, such that researchers align their work with either the "youth" or "adult" literatures and rarely cross the no-man's-land of emerging adulthood. Further, self-described "temperament" and "personality" researchers have historically used different sets of dimensions to characterize the traits of individuals, precluding comparisons across developmental stages. The separation of temperament and personality may stem in part from differences in research traditions, as described earlier in this chapter, but may also reflect outdated perceptions that temperament and personality differ on important conceptual or theoretical grounds. In contemporary psychological science, models of temperament and personality in fact show strong conceptual overlap (Shiner et al., 2012), perhaps most notably between Rothbart's temperament dimensions and the Big Five and Big Three models of adult personality (Clark et al., 2017; Clark & Watson, 2008; Zuckerman et al., 1993). Specifically, Rothbart's five-factor model of adult temperament, which consists of orienting sensitivity, effortful control, extraversion, affiliativeness, and negative affect (Evans & Rothbart, 2007), closely corresponds to the Big Five dimensions of openness, conscientiousness, extraversion, agreeableness, and neuroticism. This conceptual overlap is further reflected in the newer Little Six model of children's temperament proposed by Shiner and DeYoung (2013) and Soto and John (2014), which includes the Big Five traits plus an additional dimension capturing activity level. The Little Six model has been supported by studies investigating the combined structure of temperament and personality measures (De Pauw et al., 2009; Soto, 2016).

Indeed, there are clear parallels between the dimensions used to characterize temperament and personality. Why, then, does the tendency to treat temperament and personality as distinct constructs persist? Despite the substantial overlap between models of temperament and personality, empirical support for a single set of dimensions that characterize individual differences in traits across the lifespan continues to elude researchers. Developmental scientists have posited that temperament captures the earliest emerging individual differences in traits that are strongly influenced by biological and heritable factors, whereas personality reflects these foundational individual differences as shaped by processes of normative developmental change and through interactions with environmental phenomena and psychopathology. For instance, temperament/personality traits are potentially more easily differentiated from psychopathology symptoms very early in life, when psychopathology is relatively rare;

once psychopathology onsets, however, personality traits and symptoms co-evolve over time and development (Wilson & Olino, 2022). Thus, temperament and personality are perhaps best conceptualized as two manifestations of the same latent construct. Much as depression in childhood presents differently than depression in adulthood (Klein et al., 2005), individual differences in heritable reactive and regulatory traits also present differently across development. This brings us to the most challenging barrier to uniting the temperament, personality, and psychopathology literatures: the heterotypic continuity of traits.

Navigating Heterotypic Continuity of Traits

It is unclear how best to conceptualize temperament/personality as manifestations of the same latent construct while also accommodating developmental change. Not only do developmental researchers study the interplay of temperament and psychopathology over time, but they do so amid the "moving ground" of development (Shiner et al., 2012; Tackett & Durbin, 2017). As social and cognitive demands evolve across development, the same temperament trait may manifest as different behaviors as children age (Shiner et al., 2012; Tackett & Durbin, 2017). For example, in toddlerhood, conscientiousness (or effortful control) may manifest as waiting one's turn in a game with peers; in adolescence, it may be expressed as deciding to study for an upcoming test instead of spending time with friends. Thus, temperament researchers are faced with the challenge of balancing continuity of measurement with developmental sensitivity. On the one hand, measures must be different enough to be developmentally appropriate for infants, toddlers, children, adolescents, and adults; on the other hand, measures that are too different may no longer capture the same construct.

The potential differentiation of traits as individuals mature is a related challenge associated with heterotypic continuity. For instance, some aspects of temperament may either not exist or not be readily observable in early life, and only "come online" as individuals enter later developmental stages. For instance, regulatory traits (e.g., effortful control) may subsume agreeableness and openness in childhood, only differentiating into meaningfully distinct dimensions in adulthood (Rothbart et al., 2001; Soto & Tackett, 2015). This is supported by findings that agreeableness and openness are more strongly and positively related to conscientiousness in childhood and adolescence than in adulthood (Soto & Tackett, 2015), as well as studies showing strong associations between regulatory deficits in childhood and low agreeableness in mid-adolescence (Baardstu et al., 2017). Thus, it may be that aspects of effortful control in childhood are precursors to agreeableness and openness traits later in life, rendering individual differences in effortful control particularly important for study. The point in development at which effortful control can be reliably assessed is almost certainly an important individual difference in its own right; however, certain aspects of regulatory behavior cannot be assessed in infancy, given that the cognitive faculties required to monitor and modulate behavior do not begin developing until toddlerhood (Kostyrka-Allchorne et al., 2020). Longitudinal research that examines the structure of temperament/personality across a variety of ages to map the emergence of traits from infancy to adulthood is needed (Wilson & Olino, 2022). Structural studies focusing on single-year increments, particularly between ages two and eight, during which rapid personality development takes place (Caspi et al., 2005), would be particularly informative. We encourage researchers to capitalize on existing longitudinal datasets in conducting this important work.

The issue of heterotypic continuity also has important implications for investigations of predictive validity. For example, recent large-scale longitudinal work suggests that temperament measures administered in infancy show predictive validity above and beyond personality measures for adult outcomes (Wright & Jackson, 2022); however, this finding may simply reflect differences in structural conceptualizations, given that infant temperament was assessed using dimensions based on Rothbart and Campos' traditional temperament models (i.e., activity, fearfulness, positive affect, predictability, and compliance), whereas adolescent and adult personality was assessed using the Big Five dimensions. Surprisingly, when including temperament and personality measures together in regression analyses, trait compliance, which has no clear analog among the Big Five dimensions, emerged as the most frequent predictor of adjustment in adulthood. However, the predictive value of compliance may appear greater simply because less of its variance is accounted for by adult personality measures. This example highlights the challenge of comparing the predictive validity of temperament and personality dimensions when the measures used to assess these constructs derive from different conceptual models. Ultimately, it shows how the dichotomization of temperament and personality hinders our understanding of how enduring characteristics and behaviors of individuals shape psychopathology outcomes across development.

Greater recognition of the conceptual overlap between temperament and personality models has led to the development of measures that directly assess the Big Five in youth (e.g., the Hierarchical Personality Inventory for Children—HiPIC; Mervielde & De Fruyt, 1999, the Inventory of Child Individual Differences—ICID; Halverson et al., 2003). We encourage increased integration of these models and measures in future research on children's individual differences toward facilitating a better understanding of the development of individual differences across the lifespan. In addition, developmental scaling is a promising approach for navigating heterotypic continuity when assessing temperament/personality (Petersen et al., 2020). In this approach, different measures that assess the same construct at different ages, but contain at least some overlapping content, are placed on the same scale (Petersen et al., 2020). Critically, this approach permits the study of developmental change in temperament traits while still using developmentally sensitive measures. Moreover, developmental scaling is compatible with data obtained from multiple informants (Petersen & LeBeau, 2022) and multiple methods, including questionnaire-based and observational approaches (Hosch et al., 2022). Further, it is easily implemented with existing temperament measures, such as the Rothbart questionnaires (e.g., IBQ-R, ECBQ, TMCQ, EATQ-R, and ATQ), which assess content specific to each developmental stage (i.e., infancy, early childhood, middle childhood, adolescence, and adulthood) but also contain content that overlaps with preceding and subsequent stages. However, we reiterate the importance of improving temperament measures before using them in developmental scaling designs. We refer readers to recent work by Hosch and colleagues (2022) on children's self-regulation for an example of how developmental scaling can be used to assess developmental change in temperament traits and encourage the use of such approaches toward understanding associations between the development of traits and psychopathology.

Temperament and Psychopathology across the Lifespan

Classical Models of Temperament and Psychopathology

Linking individual differences in temperament traits to psychopathology outcomes remains a core goal of temperament and developmental psychopathology research. Several influential models have been developed to explain associations and conceptual boundaries between temperament/personality and psychopathology, including the common cause, spectrum, precursor, predisposition, pathoplasticity/exacerbation, concomitants, and consequences/scar models (Durbin & Hicks, 2014; Klein et al., 2018; Klein et al., 2011). Although these classical models initially emphasized personality and psychopathology linkages, given evidence showing that personality and temperament dimensions have comparably strong heritability and stability across development (Watson et al., 2006) and the ample conceptual overlap between leading models of temperament and personality (Clark et al., 2017; De Pauw et al., 2009), they have been extended to temperament domains (Klein et al., 2011). We acknowledge that these models have considerable conceptual overlap with one another, and the same findings can often be interpreted as support for multiple models. Further, multiple models may be necessary to fully account for the diverse processes that underlie the development of associations between temperament and psychopathology within and between individuals. We provide a brief description of each model and related research below.

The common cause, spectrum, and precursor models assert that temperament/personality and psychopathology share causal factors but do not influence one another. The common cause model holds that the same or converging causal influences give rise to both psychopathology and personality. In the strictest versions of this model, temperament/personality and psychopathology are distinct entities that are no longer associated with one another after overlapping etiological factors are accounted for (Durbin & Hicks, 2014). High genetic correlations between neuroticism and psychopathology support the common cause model, but also the continuum/spectrum and precursor models (described in the next section; Hettema et al., 2006; Kendler et al., 2006; Kendler & Myers, 2010).

The continuum/spectrum model identifies psychopathology and temperament as existing on the same spectrum, with psychopathology viewed as elevated expressions of relevant temperament dimensions (e.g., depression is characterized as elevated NE and low PE). The Hierarchical Taxonomy of Psychopathology (HiTOP; Kotov et al., 2022) is a comprehensive model of psychopathology aimed at providing a dimensional framework to describe all manifestations of psychopathology. The HiTOP framework also includes maladaptive traits and has been interpreted as a spectrum model viewing psychopathology and temperament/personality on the same dimension, with temperament/personality variables defined as consistent vulnerabilities toward psychopathology symptoms (DeYoung et al., 2022). The precursor model also views psychopathology and personality as existing on the same spectrum but asserts that the development of temperament/personality traits precedes the development of psychopathology. The tripartite model of depression and anxiety (Clark & Watson, 1991), initially developed as a structural model to explain covariation between depression and anxiety, was extended to a precursor model that holds that negative emotionality (NE) is a precursor of both depression and anxiety, whereas low positive emotionality (PE) is a precursor of depression (Clark et al., 1994; Khazanov & Ruscio, 2016). Notably, however, the tripartite model does not specify the developmental timing of when NE and PE vulnerabilities are likely to contribute to depressive or anxious symptoms. Associations between psychopathology and NE are unsurprising, given that virtually all forms of psychopathology are at least partly characterized by negative emotional states (Kotov et al., 2010; Stanton & Watson, 2014; Widiger et al., 2019); in this respect, rather than NE being useful as a marker of risk for specific forms of psychopathology, elevated NE is likely most useful in differentiating those with disorder from those without. In contrast, low PE is a relatively more specific precursor of certain forms of psychopathology, including depression, social anxiety, and schizotypy (Kendall et al., 2015; Watson, 2016; Watson & Naragon-Gainey, 2010).

In predisposition and pathoplasticity models, psychopathology and temperament/personality influence one another. As in the precursor model, the predisposition model posits that temperament/personality dimensions develop prior to psychopathology, but where the precursor model views psychopathology and temperament/personality as arising from shared causal processes but not influencing one another, the predisposition model views temperament/personality and psychopathology as having distinct etiologies and influencing one another. Diathesis-stress models of psychopathology, in which a vulnerability (e.g., high trait neuroticism) gives rise to psychopathology in the context of environmental stress, are predisposition models. Researchers have used predisposition models to examine associations among a variety of temperament dimensions and forms of psychopathology, including behavioral inhibition (BI) and anxiety, and NE (or neuroticism) and PE (or extraversion) and depression and anxiety (Andrews et al., 2024; Hengartner et al., 2016; Klein & Mumper, 2018; Shokrkon & Nicoladis, 2021; Williams et al., 2021). However, most studies focus on NE or neuroticism, and prospective associations between other temperament/personality dimensions and later psychopathology, especially in conjunction with other risk factors (e.g., stressful life events), have been examined much less frequently (Lavender et al., 2015). Further work is therefore needed to elucidate links between temperament/personality dimensions other than NE and psychopathology.

Pathoplasticity models hold that temperament/personality dimensions contribute to the expression, severity, duration, and treatment response of psychopathology after onset, potentially explaining the heterogeneity in symptom presentations often observed across individuals with the same condition. This model has received mixed research support; for example, underregulated and overregulated presentations of eating disorders have been identified based on high scores on oppositionality and self-harm dimensions (conceptually similar to the Big Five dimensions of (low) agreeableness and neuroticism, respectively) and high scores on compulsivity (Farstad et al., 2016; Lavender et al., 2015). Similarly, early "difficult" temperament per Thomas and Chess' model (Thomas & Chess, 1977), which overlaps with NE, predicts the course of later depressive episodes (Sherman et al., 2016). In contrast, Olino and colleagues (2024) examined pathoplastic influences of temperament/personality on expression of depressive symptomatology across those five samples and found minimal evidence that temperament/personality influenced depressive symptoms. As with the predisposition model, much of the work examining the contribution of temperament/personality to the course of psychopathology has focused on NE, with fewer studies examining the influence of other temperament/personality traits on the course of psychopathology.

In contrast, in concomitants and consequences/scar models, psychopathology permanently or temporarily influences temperament/personality dimensions. The concomitants model asserts that an individual's temperament/personality is influenced by contemporaneous symptoms of psychopathology, but that temperament/personality returns to presymptomatic levels when symptoms improve. Using longitudinal designs with assessments during and after participants experienced major depressive episodes (MDEs) to rule out potential state effects of depression on participants' self-reported temperament (e.g., Karsten et al., 2012), Ormel and colleagues (2004) and Jylhä and colleagues (2009) found that NE increased during MDEs but returned to pre-episode levels after remission. In consequences/scar models, psychopathology has a lasting impact on temperament/personality dimensions. Some findings support this phenomenon; for example, harm avoidance, an aspect of NE, was increased at long-term follow-up assessments following remission of depressive episodes (Rosenström et al., 2015). In addition, De Bolle and colleagues (2016) found positive associations between youths' internalizing behaviors and later trait emotional instability, introversion, disagreeableness, and compulsivity. Similarly, externalizing behaviors contributed to subsequent increases in disagreeableness (De Bolle et al., 2016). However, other studies have failed to detect long-term changes in temperament/personality following depressive episodes (Jylhä et al., 2009; Williams et al., 2021). Longitudinal research with long-term follow-up assessments is needed to investigate the scar model, particularly in forms of psychopathology other than depression.

To date, research has yet to identify which of these models most accurately describe(s) the complex links between temperament/personality and psychopathology (Durbin & Hicks, 2014; Klein et al., 2011). This may be because research findings are often consistent with multiple models (e.g., all models predict associations between temperament/personality and psychopathology); further, it is unclear what the appropriate statistical models are to test competing frameworks of associations between temperament/personality and psychopathology. Additionally, classical models of temperament/personality and psychopathology associations are imprecise; for example, scar models do not specify the time course over which psychopathology is hypothesized to change temperament/personality. Lastly, as these models are not mutually exclusive, complex combinations of the associations described in multiple models are possible. Nevertheless, recent studies comparing these models in referred and non-referred youth tend to support the continuum/spectrum model, with minor support for the pathoplasticity/exacerbation and vulnerability models (De Bolle et al., 2016; Brandes, 2023; but see Olino et al., 2024).

Before reviewing broader issues in the study of dimensional models of temperament and psychopathology, we note that the time course for the development of temperament relative to typical age of onset and chronicity of specific forms of psychopathology are key considerations for researchers interested in investigating associations between temperament and psychopathology (Durbin & Hicks, 2014). Importantly, temperament dimensions emerge early and become more stable from youth through young adulthood (Bleidorn et al., 2022; Roberts & DelVecchio, 2000). In contrast, different forms of psychopathology tend to onset at different developmental stages and vary in chronicity or stability. For example, psychosis typically emerges in adolescence or early adulthood, and many individuals go on to experience multiple episodes of psychosis across the lifespan (Amminger et al., 2011), whereas separation anxiety onsets in childhood (Costello et al., 2003) and typically remits by adolescence (Costello et al., 2011). Accordingly, researchers seeking to study associations between psychopathology and temperament should select developmental periods in which the form of psychopathology under study will be expressed to capture complex associations between temperament and psychopathology. This is no small task, given that pathoplastic effects may apply such that traits differentially influence the manifestation of psychopathology during different developmental stages.

Linking Dimensional Models of Temperament and Psychopathology

Developing a unified taxonomy encompassing both traits and psychopathology dimensions is a goal for many temperament and personality researchers alike (Chetcuti et al., 2019; Gjerde et al., 2023; Mervielde et al., 2005; Ostlund et al., 2021; Shields et al., 2021). Within the temperament literature, recent efforts have focused on integrating temperament dimensions into prevailing dimensional frameworks of psychopathology and personality, such as the RDoC framework (National Institute of Mental Health, 2024; see Sanislow et al., this volume) and HiTOP (Kotov et al., 2022; see Pham and Forbes, this volume).

It has been said that temperament research "implemented an RDoC approach even before there was an RDoC" (Ostlund et al., 2021). Indeed, like RDoC, temperament research is grounded in a dimensional, transdiagnostic approach to individual differences in behavior and emphasizes the biological and heritable underpinnings of these differences. Despite these similarities, however, temperament traits are largely absent from the RDoC framework. Some developmental researchers have situated higher-order temperament factors within current RDoC domains of function, with negative emotionality falling under negative valence systems, sociability (comprising activity level, surgency, etc.) under positive valence systems and social processes, and self-regulation under cognitive systems (Chetcuti et al., 2019). Others have proposed modifications to the RDoC framework that would allow temperament research to be better integrated. For instance, to better incorporate trait-based emotional processes, Franklin and colleagues (2015) proposed adding a "motivation" domain as well as combining the positive and negative valence domains into a dimensional "valence" domain (Franklin et al., 2015). Similarly, Ostlund and colleagues (2021) discussed the advantages of adding a "life span considerations" subsection to the RDoC matrix. Within this subsection, researchers could use developmental qualifiers to provide information on how RDoC constructs, including traits, might manifest and change over the course of development (Ostlund et al., 2021). These proposed modifications would infuse a much-needed developmental perspective to the mostly static RDoC matrix.

Building on research with adults, evidence suggests that youth temperament/personality and psychopathology are best conceptualized as overlapping hierarchical models (Brandes, 2023; De Bolle et al., 2016; Tackett & Hallquist, 2022). That is, like personality, temperament and psychopathology likely share the same empirical space, such that individual differences in both typical functioning (i.e., temperament) and maladaptive functioning (i.e., psychopathology) can be described by the same dimensions or domains (Wright & Hopwood, 2022). Thus, falling in the maladaptive ranges of dimensional temperament/personality traits may foreshadow the development of psychopathology (Tackett & Hallquist, 2022), consistent with several models of temperament-psychopathology associations (see the previous section). This provides support for a joint taxonomy of temperament and psychopathology dimensions. Further, recent work indicates that youth psychopathology can be organized in a hierarchical, dimensional structure similar to the HiTOP model of adult psychopathology (Forbes et al., 2025). Thus, integrating dimensional models of temperament and youth psychopathology into the HiTOP framework is a logical next step (Gjerde et al., 2023; Shields et al., 2021). Indeed, the ways in which relationships between temperament/personality and psychopathology dimensions change over the course of development is an explicit goal of the HiTOP model (Tackett & Hallquist, 2022).

Although HiTOP provides a theoretical basis for integrating development (i.e., temperament dimensions) into taxonomies of personality and psychopathology, empirical work in this area is in its infancy. Findings of strong associations between temperament dimensions and symptoms of psychopathology (e.g., Hayne et al., 2023; Wiltink et al., 2015) are consistent with the HiTOP assertion that temperament and psychopathology are likely the same construct (Widiger et al., 2019). That is, psychopathology may represent the extreme end of a continuum on which both temperament and psychopathology reside, with psychopathology being associated with impairment (Widiger et al., 2019). However, cross-sectional studies finding associations between temperament and psychopathology could also be interpreted as consistent with other models of temperament and psychopathology (e.g., predisposition and pathoplasticity models or precursor models; described in previous sections), as cross-sectional designs do not speak to prospective associations between temperament and psychopathology or vice versa. Finally, researchers have struggled to replicate structures of temperament and psychopathology proposed by hierarchical models such as HiTOP, even at the broadest levels of the hierarchy (Hawes et al., 2023; Watts et al., 2022). For instance, the first factorial study of the joint structure of personality and psychopathology in childhood found that the p factor—a construct thought to underlie all variation in psychopathology—in children comprises high scores on inattention, oppositional defiant behavior, and hyperactivity, as well as low scores on conscientiousness and agreeableness (Gjerde et al., 2023). In addition, three group factors representing negative affectivity, positive affectivity, and antagonism emerged in a second bifactor model (Gjerde et al., 2023). However, the dimensions that comprise the p factor appear to vary widely across samples (Hawes et al., 2023; Watts et al., 2022; Watts et al., 2024), such that the p factor may simply reflect variations in the measures and dimensions of temperament and psychopathology that are modeled across studies. These idiosyncrasies are likely to be even more pronounced when attempting to replicate the structure of the p factor across youth and adult samples, due to the heterotypic continuity of traits across development (see earlier discussions of this issue). In summary, the chimeric nature of the p factor remains a significant barrier to the development of valid and reliable joint taxonomies of temperament, personality, and psychopathology.

Implications for Prevention and Treatment

Empirical findings that individual differences in temperament traits are associated with the development of psychopathology have prompted the development of temperament-based preventative efforts and interventions. Such interventions often have the joint goals of promoting goodness-of-fit between the child's environment and his or her temperamental traits as well as expanding the child's behavioral repertoire to better adapt to his or her environment (Iverson & Gartstein, 2018; McClowry & Collins, 2012; Shiner et al., 2012). We briefly touch upon these programs here, given their potential utility for enhancing our understanding of temperament-psychopathology relationships.

Of these approaches, some cater to youth with specific temperament traits, such as the Cool Little Kids program (Dodd et al., 2017; Rapee et al., 2005), a six-session intervention for behaviorally inhibited children designed to prevent later anxiety problems. Meta-analytic analyses of 16 studies examining the Cool Little Kids program found medium (Hedge's $g = .54$) and large (Hedge's $g = .84$) effect sizes when comparing intervention and control groups for child- and parent-reported decreases in children's anxiety symptoms, respectively (Mychailyszyn, 2017). Further, treatment gains were sustained up to 12 months post-intervention (Mychailyszyn, 2017, although see more recent work concerning longer-term outcomes [Bayer et al., 2022]).

Other interventions are suitable for diverse temperament traits, such as the INSIGHTS into Children's Temperament program (McClowry et al., 2005), which can be implemented with children who are shy as well as children who show temperament traits characterized by low persistence, high motor activity, and high negative emotionality, termed "high-maintenance" temperament traits (Iverson & Gartstein, 2018). This 10-session program provides children, caregivers, and teachers with psychoeducation concerning child temperament and equips them with behavior change strategies designed to be responsive to children's individual differences. A review of six RCTs found that the INSIGHTS program reduced children's behavior problems at home and school with small to medium effect sizes (Iverson & Gartstein, 2018). Treatment effects estimated from growth models were greatest for children exhibiting "high-maintenance" temperament traits, with these children showing reduced disruptive (standardized effect size [ES] = .42) and off-task-behaviors (ES = .33) as well as increased behavioral engagement (ES = .35) (McCormick et al., 2015). In addition, shy children receiving the INSIGHTS intervention program showed increases in academic achievement compared to shy peers in a control program (ES = .36 to .40), with effects mediated by increases in behavioral engagement (O'Connor et al., 2014).

Finally, other temperament-based interventions integrate temperament concepts into existing therapeutic approaches. For instance, the Tuning in to Toddlers (TOTS) program (Pade et al., 2006) promotes goodness-of-fit between children's temperament traits and caregivers' parenting styles within a parent-child interaction protocol. Similarly, the Unified Protocol (UP; Barlow et al., 2017) targets negative emotionality within a cognitive-behavioral therapy

(CBT) framework for youths and adults with emotional disorders. Both the TOTS program and the UP have been found to be effective for improving child adjustment outcomes. For instance, the largest RCT of the TOTS program to date showed small-to-medium effect sizes for decreases in child behavior problems, increases in child competence, and decreases in child stress as measured by hair cortisol (Cohen's d = .27 to .35) compared to waitlist controls (Havighurst et al., 2022). In addition, the UP is supported by a robust evidence base comprising several meta-analytic reviews reporting large effect sizes for treating emotional disorders across the lifespan (Farchione et al., 2024).

Temperament-based interventions present several advantages over traditional treatment approaches, such as their transdiagnostic approach and potential to disrupt risk trajectories before psychological disorders emerge by targeting trait-based risk factors. However, questions remain regarding the conditions under which these interventions are most effective. Chief among these are questions regarding the mechanism(s) by which temperament-psychopathology associations emerge. For example, precursor and predisposition models suggest that temperament traits precede the development of symptoms (Andrews et al., 2024; Clark & Watson, 1991; Hengartner et al., 2016; Klein & Mumper, 2018; Lavender et al., 2015; Shokrkon & Nicoladis, 2021; Williams et al., 2021). Based on these models, interventions that modify maladaptive temperament traits could prevent the development of psychopathology. In contrast, consequences/scar models suggest that experiencing psychopathology symptoms can lead to lasting changes in youths' temperament traits (De Bolle et al., 2016; Rosenström et al., 2015). Based on these models, resources invested in temperament-based interventions may be better spent on treatments that target psychopathology symptoms directly. Thus, further naturalistic and treatment research on temperament and psychopathology is needed, as these approaches can inform one another.

Presupposing the verity of mechanistic models in which temperament influences psychopathology, when and to whom should temperament-based interventions be administered? With respect to timing, it is unclear when in development traits should be assessed to maximize their predictive validity for adjustment outcomes. For instance, certain frameworks (e.g., precursor and predisposition models) suggest that interventions for maladaptive traits should be administered in the earliest stages of development to prevent psychopathology before it typically onsets. However, meta-analytic evidence suggests that infancy is too early to identify children who may benefit from preventative programs based on their temperament traits, as traits assessed in infancy only modestly predict variance in psychopathology later in childhood (Kostyrka-Allchorne et al., 2020). Researchers have similarly sought to address the question of to whom temperament-based interventions should be administered through identifying characteristics of youth at greatest temperamental risk for psychopathology. For instance, recent findings indicate that children showing elevated daring and emotional dysregulation are at greater risk for aggressive behavior (Ostrov et al., 2023). Thus, in contrast to existing interventions for aggression, which focus primarily on modifying social cognitions, alternative interventions that reduce temperament traits, such as emotion dysregulation and daring, may be more effective for children who score highly on these traits (Ostrov et al., 2023).

Further, interactions between traits—particularly between reactivity and regulatory traits—may amplify risk for psychopathology (Gjerde et al., 2023; Nielsen et al., 2019; Shiner et al., 2012). For example, attention and self-regulation moderate associations between reactivity and adjustment outcomes, such that children who exhibit both low conscientiousness and high neuroticism may be particularly vulnerable to poor adjustment (Gjerde et al., 2023; Shiner et al., 2012). Similarly, among toddlers showing low PE traits, having higher effortful control was associated with greater reductions in internalizing and externalizing symptoms over the course of childhood (Nielsen et al., 2019). Isolated studies have also explored moderators of treatment response for temperament-based interventions. For instance, children exhibiting higher surgency and higher negative emotionality show fewer gains in treatment for disruptive and inattentive symptoms (Hare & Graziano, 2020). In addition, a longitudinal RCT of the Cool Little Kids program (described earlier in this section) found that risk for internalizing problems in middle childhood was attenuated only for children with anxious parents (Bayer et al., 2022). Similarly, RCTs from the INSIGHTS program (described previously) suggest that this intervention is most beneficial for boys and children with relatively severe behavioral problems (Iverson & Gartstein, 2018). Lastly, caregivers with lower education and who rate their children as more temperamentally "difficult" tend to find the psychoeducational components of temperament-based interventions more useful compared to other caregivers (Iverson & Gartstein, 2018).

Identifying at what stage and which youths would benefit most from temperament-based intervention hinges on valid assessments of temperament traits. To date, virtually all measures of temperament have been developed for use in research contexts; thus, their utility in clinical settings is unknown (Gartstein et al., 2016). Furthermore, large epidemiological studies have yet to be conducted for any measure of temperament (Rettew, 2019; Gartstein et al., 2012). As a result, there are no standardized norms to contextualize empirical observations of individual differences in temperament traits (Tackett & Durbin, 2017) and when trait elevations are associated with adverse outcomes, rendering it difficult to reliably identify children at temperamental risk for psychopathology. As a result, idiosyncratic methods for identifying children in need of intervention have been used (e.g., one standard deviation above the mean of a sample on a given trait according to parent-report measures; Rapee et al., 2005). Thus, mapping the ranges of temperament traits associated with increased risk for symptoms remains an important goal for improving the effectiveness of temperament-based approaches to intervention.

Using latent profile analysis (LPA) to map trait-symptom associations is one means of achieving this goal. LPA is a statistical approach that identifies subgroups within a population based on shared characteristics. Far from a new approach, LPA has been regularly used within the temperament literature to identify subpopulations of children who score highly on certain traits according to questionnaire or observational measures of temperament (e.g., Beekman et al., 2015; Buss, 2011; Gartstein et al., 2017; Loken, 2004; van den Akker, 2010). Often, these subgroups are then further characterized by examining patterns of symptomatology shared by group members. For instance, toddlers showing a temperament profile characterized by "dysregulated fear" (i.e., high temperamental fear in low-threat situations) have been found to exhibit more anxious symptoms (Buss, 2011).

At first blush, clustering approaches such as LPA may seem antithetical to dimensional models of temperament, because these approaches generate discontinuous categories of temperament "profiles" (e.g., "slow-to-warm-up" infants, "difficult" toddlers; Beekman et al., 2015; Thomas & Chess, 1977). However, we argue that clustering techniques can be a useful addition to the statistical toolbox of the dimensional temperament researcher. Notably, these techniques can augment dimensional models by permitting the identification and characterization of specific ranges of a dimensional trait that may be closely tied to psychopathology symptoms. For instance, identifying the range of scores on a measure of dysregulated fear that are most predictive of anxiety problems would help clinicians select children who are most likely to benefit from temperament-based interventions for anxiety. Work such as this could identify any potential discontinuities between elevations in traits and expressions of psychopathology reliably associated with impairment. Despite its potential for informing theory and intervention targets, however, LPA has yet to be deployed in this way with large-scale, representative samples conducive to establishing norms for a measure of temperament. In addition, there are substantial psychometric concerns with several temperament measures which limit their use as valid research and clinical tools (e.g., Clark et al., 2016; Enlow et al., 2016; Gartstein et al., 2012; Lawson et al., 2021).

Conclusion

As it stands, the future of research on dimensional models of temperament and psychopathology holds both promise and formidable challenges. Temperament is a complex construct, as is psychopathology; studying the relationships between these constructs is, ipso facto, a complex endeavor. In this chapter, we have highlighted several overarching issues that pose formidable challenges to the field. These are: integrating dimensional models of temperament, navigating the heterotypic continuity of traits across development, linking dimensional models of temperament and psychopathology, and evaluating temperament-based approaches to intervention. Failure to prioritize these issues will cause research on associations between temperament and psychopathology to stagnate (Durbin & Hicks, 2014). However, what has been, need not always be (DeMayo et al., 2021), and the recent revitalization of foundational measurement work is indeed cause for optimism. We eagerly anticipate future research on temperament-psychopathology associations grounded in this revitalization.

References

Amminger, G. P., Henry, L. P., Harrigan, S. M., Harris, M. G., Alvarez-Jimenez, M., Herrman, H., Jackson, H. J., & McGorry, P. D. (2011). Outcome in early-onset schizophrenia revisited: Findings from the Early Psychosis Prevention and Intervention Centre long-term follow-up study. *Schizophrenia Research*, *131*(1), 112–119. https://doi.org/10.1016/j.schres.2011.06.009

Andrews, K. L., Jamshidi, L., Nisbet, J., Afifi, T. O., Sauer-Zavala, S., Kratzig, G. P., Teckchandani, T. A., Neary, J. P., & Carleton, R. N. (2024). Associations between personality and mental health among Royal Canadian Mounted Police cadets. *Journal of Police and Criminal Psychology*, *39*(1), 213–226. https://doi.org/10.1007/s11896-023-09639-6

Baardstu, S., Karevold, E. B., & von Soest, T. (2017). Childhood antecedents of agreeableness: A longitudinal study from preschool to late adolescence. *Journal of Research in Personality*, *67*, 202–214. https://doi.org/10.1016/j.jrp.2016.10.007

Barlow, D. H., Farchione, T. J., Bullis, J. R., Gallagher, M. W., Murray-Latin, H., Sauer-Zavala, S., Bentley, K. H., Thompson-Hollands, J., Conklin, L. R., Boswell, J. F., Ametaj, A., Carl, J. R., Boettcher, H. T., & Cassiello-Robbins, C. (2017). The unified protocol for transdiagnostic treatment of emotional disorders compared with diagnosis-specific protocols for anxiety disorders. *JAMA Psychiatry*, *74*(9), 875. https://doi.org/10.1001/jamapsychiatry.2017.2164

Barrett, L. F., Mesquita, B., Ochsner, K. N., & Gross, J. J. (2007). The experience of emotion. *Annual Review of Psychology*, *58*, 373–403. https://doi.org/10.1146/annurev.psych.58.110405.085709

Bayer, J. K., Brown, A., Prendergast, L. A., Bretherton, L., Hiscock, H., Mihalopoulos, C., Nelson-Lowe, M., Gilbertson, T., Noone, K., Bischof, N., Beechey, C., Muliadi, F., & Rapee, R. M. (2022). Follow-up of the *Cool Little Kids* translational trial into middle childhood. *Journal of Child Psychology and Psychiatry*, *63*(1), 88–98. https://doi.org/10.1111/jcpp.13464

Beekman, C., Neiderhiser, J. M., Buss, K. A., Loken, E., Moore, G. A., Leve, L. D., Ganiban, J. M., Shaw, D. S., & Reiss, D. (2015). The development of early profiles of temperament: Characterization, continuity, and etiology. *Child Development*, *86*(6), 1794–1811. https://doi.org/10.1111/cdev.12417

Bleidorn, W., Schwaba, T., Zheng, A., Hopwood, C. J., Sosa, S. S., Roberts, B. W., & Briley, D. A. (2022). Personality stability and change: A meta-analysis of longitudinal studies. *Psychological Bulletin*, *148*(7–8), 588–619. https://doi.org/10.1037/bul0000365

Bohlin, G., Hagekül, B., & Lindhagen, K. (1981). Dimensions of infant behavior. *Infant Behavior and Development*, *4*, 83–96. https://doi.org/10.1016/S0163-6383(81)80011-2

Borkenau, P., Riemann, R., Angleitner, A., & Spinath, F. M. (2001). Genetic and environmental influences on observed personality: Evidence from the German Observational Study of Adult Twins. *Journal of Personality and Social Psychology*, 80(4), 655–668. https://doi.org/10.1037/0022-3514.80.4.655

Brandes, C. M. (2023). *Personality in a hierarchical and dimensional model of youth psychopathology* (pp. 1–146) [Dissertation]

Buss, A. H., & Plomin, R. (1975). *A temperament theory of personality development* (p. 256). Wiley-Interscience.

Buss, A., & Plomin, R. (1984). *Temperament: Early developing personality traits*. Lawrence Erlbaum.

Buss, K. A. (2011). Which fearful toddlers should we worry about? Context, fear regulation, and anxiety risk. *Developmental Psychology*, 47(3), 804–819. https://doi.org/10.1037/a0023227.

Capaldi, D. M., & Rothbart, M. K. (1992). Development and validation of an early adolescent temperament measure. *The Journal of Early Adolescence*, *12*(2), 153–173. https://doi.org/10.1177/027243169201 2002002

Caspi, A., Roberts, B. W., & Shiner, R. L. (2005). Personality development: Stability and change. *Annual Review of Psychology*, *56*(1), 453–484. https://doi.org/10.1146/annurev.psych.55.090902.141913

Chetcuti, L., Uljarević, M., & Hudry, K. (2019). Editorial perspective: Furthering research on temperament in autism spectrum disorder. *Journal of Child Psychology and Psychiatry*, *60*(2), 225–228. https://doi.org/10.1111/jcpp.12957

Clark, D. A., Durbin, C. E., Hicks, B. M., Iacono, W. G., & McGue, M. (2017). Personality in the age of industry: Structure, heritability and correlates of personality in middle childhood from the perspective of parents, teachers, and children. *Journal of Research in Personality*, *67*, 132–143.

Clark, D. A., Listro, C. J., Lo, S. L., Durbin, C. E., Donnellan, M. B., & Neppl, T. K. (2016). Measurement invariance and child temperament: An evaluation of sex and informant differences on the Child Behavior Questionnaire. *Psychological Assessment*, *28*(12), 1646–1662. https://doi.org/10.1037/pas0000299

Clark, L. A., & Watson, D. (1991). Tripartite model of anxiety and depression: Psychometric evidence and taxonomic implications. *Journal of Abnormal Psychology*, *100*(3), 316–336.

Clark, L. A., & Watson, D. (2008). Temperament: An organizing paradigm for trait psychology. In O. P. John, R. W. Robins, & L. A. Pervin (Eds.), *Handbook of personality: Theory and research* (3rd ed., pp. 265–286). The Guilford Press.

Clark, L. A., Watson, D., & Mineka, S. (1994). Temperament, personality, and the mood and anxiety disorders. *Journal of Abnormal Psychology*, *103*(1), 103–116. https://doi.org/10.1037//0021-843X.103.1.103

Cole, D. A. (1987). Utility of confirmatory factor analysis in test validation research. *Journal of Consulting and Clinical Psychology*, 55(4), 584–594. https://doi.org/10.1037/0022-006X.55.4.584

Conway, C. C., Li, Y. I., & Starr, L. R. (2019). Trait anhedonia is a transdiagnostic correlate of internalizing problems during adolescence. *Journal of Research in Personality*, *81*, 56–63. https://doi.org/10.1016/j.jrp.2019.05.004

Costello, E. J., Copeland, W., & Angold, A. (2011). Trends in psychopathology across the adolescent years: What changes when children become adolescents, and when adolescents become adults? *Journal of Child Psychology and Psychiatry*, 52(10), 1015–1025. https://doi.org/10.1111/j.1469-7610.2011.02446.x

Costello, E. J., Mustillo, S., Erkanli, A., Keeler, G., & Angold, A. (2003). Prevalence and development of psychiatric disorders in childhood and adolescence. *Archives of General Psychiatry*, *60*(8), 837. https://doi.org/10.1001/archpsyc.60.8.837

De Bolle, M., De Clercq, B., De Caluwé, E., & Verbeke, L. (2016). Exploring the complexity of the childhood trait-psychopathology association: Continuity, pathoplasty, and complication effects. *Development and Psychopathology*, 28(1), 139–148. https://doi.org/10.1017/s0954579415000346

DeMayo, B. (Writer), & Surjik, S. (Director). (2021, December 17). Kaer Morhen (Season 2, Episode 10) [TV series episode]. In L. Schmidt Hissrich, S. Emaneul, A. Sakharov, T. Bagiński, J. Sawko, P. Sikora, J. F. Brown, S. Daniel, S. Gaub, M. O'Toole, M. Ostrowski, & K. Żbikowski (Executive Producers), *The Witcher*. Little Schmidt Productions, Hivemind, Platige Image.

De Pauw, S. S. W., Mervielde, I., & Van Leeuwen, K. G. (2009). How are traits related to problem behavior in preschoolers? Similarities and contrasts between temperament and personality. *Journal of Abnormal Child Psychology*, 37(3), 309–325. https://doi.org/10.1007/s10802-008-9290-0

DeYoung, C. G., Chmielewski, M., Clark, L. A., Condon, D. M., Kotov, R., Krueger, R. F., Lynam, D. R., Markon, K. E., Miller, J. D., Mullins-Sweatt, S. N., Samuel, D. B., Sellbom, M., South, S. C., Thomas, K. M., Watson, D., Watts, A. L., Widiger, T. A., Wright, A. G. C., & Workgroup, the H. N. P. (2022). The distinction between symptoms and traits in the Hierarchical Taxonomy of Psychopathology (HiTOP). *Journal of Personality*, *90*(1), 20–33. https://doi.org/10.1111/jopy.12593

Diamond, S. (1957). *Personality and temperament.* Harper & Brothers.

Dodd, H. F., Hudson, J. L., & Rapee, R. M. (2017). Temperament in youth internalizing disorders. In D. McKay, J. S. Abramowitz, & E. A. Storch (Eds.), *Treatments for psychological problems and syndromes* (pp. 504–524). John Wiley & Sons Ltd.

Durbin, C. E., & Hicks, B. M. (2014). Personality and psychopathology: A stagnant field in need of development. *European Journal of Personality*, *28*(4), 362–386. https://doi.org/10.1002/per.1962

Durbin, C. E., Schalet, B. D., Hayden, E. P., Simpson, J., & Jordan, P. L. (2009). Hypomanic personality traits: A multi-method exploration of their association with normal and abnormal dimensions of personality. *Journal of Research in Personality*, 43(5), 898–905. https://doi.org/10.1016/j.jrp.2009.04.010

Durbin, C. E., & Wilson, S. (2012). Convergent validity of and bias in maternal reports of child emotion. *Psychological Assessment*, *24*(3), 647–660. https://doi.org/10.1037/a0026607

Enlow, M. B., White, M. T., Hails, K., Cabrera, I., & Wright, R. J. (2016). The Infant Behavior Questionnaire–Revised: Factor structure in a culturally and sociodemographically diverse sample in the United States. *Infant Behavior and Development*, *43*, 24–35. https://doi.org/10.1016/j.infbeh.2016.04.001

Farchione, T. J., Long, L. J., Spencer-Laitt, D., Moreno, J., & Barlow, D. H. (2024). State of the science: The Unified Protocol for transdiagnostic treatment of emotional disorders. *Behavior Therapy*, *55*(6), 1189–1204.

Farstad, S. M., McGeown, L. M., & von Ranson, K. M. (2016). Eating disorders and personality, 2004–2016: A systematic review and meta-analysis. *Clinical Psychology Review*, *46*, 91–105. https://doi.org/10.1016/j.cpr.2016.04.005

Flake, J. K., Pek, J., & Hehman, E. (2017). Construct validation in social and personality research. *Social Psychological and Personality Science*, *8*(4), 370–378. https://doi.org/10.1177/1948550617693063

Forbes, M. K., Watts, A. L., Twose, M., Barrett, A., Hudson, J., Lyneham, H., McLellan, L., Newton, N., Sicouri, G., Chapman, C., McKinnon, A., Rapee, R., Slade, T., Teesson, M., Markon, K. E., & Sunderland, M. (2025). A hierarchical model of the symptom-level structure of psychopathology in youth. *Clinical Psychological Science*, *13*(2), 278–300. https://doi.org/10.1177/21677026241257852

Forman, D. R., O'Hara, M. W., Larsen, K., Coy, K. C., Gorman, L. L., & Stuart, S. (2003). Infant emotionality: Observational methods and the validity of maternal reports. *Infancy*, *4*(4), 541–565. https://doi.org/10.1207/S15327078IN0404_08

Fox, N. A., Zeytinoglu, S., Valadez, E. A., Buzzell, G. A., Morales, S., & Henderson, H. A. (2022). Annual research review: Developmental pathways linking early behavioral inhibition to later anxiety. *Journal of Child Psychology and Psychiatry*, *64*(4), 537–561. https://doi.org/10.1111/jcpp.13702

Franklin, J. C., Jamieson, J. P., Glenn, C. R., & Nock, M. K. (2015). How developmental psychopathology theory and research can inform the Research Domain Criteria (RDoC) project. *Journal of Clinical Child & Adolescent Psychology*, *44*(2), 280–290. https://doi.org/10.1080/15374416.2013.873981

Gartstein, M. A., Bridgett, D. J., & Low, C. M. (2012). Asking questions about temperament: Self- and other-report measures across the lifespan. In M. Zentner & R. L. Shiner (Eds.), *Handbook of temperament* (pp. 183–208). Guilford Publications.

Gartstein, M. A., Prokasky, A., Bell, M. A., Calkins, S., Bridgett, D. J., Braungart-Rieker, J., Leerkes, E., Cheatham, C. L., Eiden, R. D., Mize, K. D., Jones, N. A., Mireault, G., & Seamon, E. (2017). Latent profile and cluster analysis of infant temperament: Comparisons across person-centered approaches. *Developmental Psychology*, *52*(10), 1811–1825. https://doi.org/10.1037/dev0000382

Gartstein, M. A., Putnam, S. P., Aron, E. N., & Rothbart, M. K. (2016). Temperament and personality. In S. Maltzman (Ed.), *The Oxford handbook of treatment processes and outcomes in psychology: A multidisciplinary, biopsychosocial approach* (pp. 11–41). Oxford University Press.

Gjerde, L. C., Eilertsen, E. M., McAdams, T. A., Cheesman, R., Moffitt, T. E., Caspi, A., Eley, T. C., Røysamb, E., Rosenström, T. H., & Ystrom, E. (2023). The *p* factor of psychopathology and personality in middle childhood: Genetic and gestational risk factors. *Psychological Medicine*, *53*(9), 4275–4285. https://doi.org/10.1017/s0033291723000077

Goldsmith, H. H., & Gagne, J. R. (2012). Behavioral assessment of temperament. In M. Zentner & R. L. Shiner (Eds.), *Handbook of temperament* (pp. 209–228). The Guilford Press.

Goldsmith, H. H., Reilly, J., Lemery, K. S., Longley, S., & Prescott, A. (1995). Laboratory Temperament Assessment Battery: Preschool version. Unpublished manuscript.

Gonzalez, O., MacKinnon, D. P., & Muniz, F. B. (2021). Extrinsic convergent validity evidence to prevent jingle and jangle fallacies. *Multivariate Behavioral Research*, *56*(1), 1–17. https://doi.org/10.1080/00273171.2019.1707061

Halverson, C. F., Havill, V. L., Deal, J., Baker, S. R., Victor, J. B., Pavlopoulos, V., Besevegis, E., & Wen, L. (2003). Personality structure as derived from parental ratings of free descriptions of children: The Inventory of Child Individual Differences. *Journal of Personality*, *71*(6), 995–1026. https://doi.org/10.1111/1467-6494.7106005

Hang, Y., Soto, C. J., Speyer, L. G., Haring, L., Lee, B., Ostendorf, F., & Mõttus, R. (2021). Age differences in the big five personality domains, facets and nuances: A replication across the life span. *PsyArXiv Preprints* . https://doi.org/10.31234/osf.io/bzkwd

Hare, M. M., & Graziano, P. A. (2020). Treatment response among preschoolers with disruptive behavior disorders: The role of temperament and parenting. *Journal of Clinical Child & Adolescent Psychology*, *50*(6), 950–965. https://doi.org/10.1080/15374416.2020.1846540

Havighurst, S. S., Kehoe, C. E., Harley, A. E., Radovini, A., & Thomas, R. (2022). A randomized controlled trial of an emotion socialization parenting program and its impact on parenting, children's behavior and parent and child stress cortisol: *Tuning in to Toddlers*. *Behavior Research and Therapy*, *149*, 104016. https://doi.org/10.1016/j.brat.2021.104016

Hawes, M. T., Farrell, M. R., Cannone, J. L., Finsaas, M. C., Olino, T. M., & Klein, D. N. (2021). Early childhood temperament predicts intolerance of uncertainty in adolescence. *Journal of Anxiety Disorders*, *80*, 102390. https://doi.org/10.1016/j.janxdis.2021.102390

Hawes, M. T., Klein, D. N., Olino, T. M., & Kotov, R. (2023). Multi-method longitudinal investigation of the general factor of child temperament (GFT): Substantive phenomenon or methodological artifact? *Journal of Research in Personality*, *104*, 104375. https://doi.org/10.1016/j.jrp.2023.104375

Hayden, E. P. (2022). A call for renewed attention to construct validity and measurement in psychopathology research. *Psychological Medicine*, *52*(14), 2930–2936. https://doi.org/10.1017/s0033291722003221

Hayden, E. P., Durbin, C. E., Klein, D. N., & Olino, T. M. (2010). Maternal personality influences the relationship between maternal reports and laboratory measures of child temperament. *Journal of Personality Assessment*, *92*(6), 586–593. https://doi.org/10.1080/00223891.2010.513308

Hayne, D. P., Phillips, W., Cosh, S. M., & Price, I. (2023). Examining personality trait patterns in transdiagnostic dimensions of psychopathology. *Current Psychology*, *42*(22), 18524–18538. https://doi.org/10.1007/s12144-022-03028-8

Hengartner, M. P., Ajdacic-Gross, V., Wyss, C., Angst, J., & Rössler, W. (2016). Relationship between personality and psychopathology in a longitudinal community study: A test of the predisposition model. *Psychological Medicine*, *46*(8), 1693–1705. https://doi.org/10.1017/S0033291716000210

Hettema, J. M., Neale, M. C., Myers, J. M., Prescott, C. A., & Kendler, K. S. (2006). A population-based twin study of the relationship between neuroticism and internalizing disorders. *American Journal of Psychiatry*, *163*(5), 857–864. https://doi.org/10.1176/ajp.2006.163.5.857

Hosch, A., Oleson, J. J., Harris, J. L., Goeltz, M. T., Neumann, T., LeBeau, B., Hazeltine, E., & Petersen, I. T. (2022). Studying children's growth in self-regulation using changing measures to account for heterotypic continuity: A Bayesian approach to developmental scaling. *Developmental Science*, *25*(6), e13280. https://doi.org/10.1111/desc.13280

Iverson, S. L., & Gartstein, M. A. (2018). Applications of temperament: A review of caregiver-focused temperament-driven interventions. *Early Education and Development*, *29*(1), 31–52. https://doi.org/10.1080/10409289.2017.1341805

Jylhä, P., Melartin, T., Rytsälä, H., & Isometsä, E. (2009). Neuroticism, introversion, and major depressive disorder—Traits, states, or scars? *Depression and Anxiety*, *26*(4), 325–334. https://doi.org/10.1002/da.20385

Ka, L., R, E., K, W., G, J., & Lje, B. (2021). Associations between facets and aspects of Big Five personality and affective disorders: A systematic review and best evidence synthesis. *Journal of Affective Disorders*, *288*, 175–188. https://doi.org/10.1016/j.jad.2021.03.061

Karp, J., Serbin, L. A., Stack, D. M., & Schwartzman, A. E. (2004). An observational measure of children's behavioural style: Evidence supporting a multi-method approach to studying temperament. *Infant and Child Development*, *13*(2), 135–158. https://doi.org/10.1002/icd.346

Karsten, J., Penninx, B. W., Riese, H., Ormel, J., Nolen, W. A., & Hartman, C. A. (2012). The state effect of depressive and anxiety disorders on big five personality traits. *Journal of psychiatric research*, *46*(5), 644–650.

Kendall, A. D., Zinbarg, R. E., Mineka, S., Bobova, L., Prenoveau, J. M., Revelle, W., & Craske, M. G. (2015). Prospective associations of low positive emotionality with first onsets of depressive and anxiety disorders: Results from a 10-wave latent trait-state modeling study. *Journal of Abnormal Psychology*, *124*(4), 933–943. https://doi.org/10.1037/abn0000105

Kendler, K. S., Gatz, M., Gardner, C. O., & Pedersen, N. L. (2006). Personality and major depression: A Swedish longitudinal, population-based twin study. *Archives of General Psychiatry*, *63*(10), 1113. https://doi.org/10.1001/archpsyc.63.10.1113

Kendler, K. S., & Myers, J. (2010). The genetic and environmental relationship between major depression and the five-factor model of personality. *Psychological Medicine*, *40*(5), 801–806. https://doi.org/10.1017/S0033291709991140

Khazanov, G. K., & Ruscio, A. M. (2016). Is low positive emotionality a specific risk factor for depression? A meta-analysis of longitudinal studies. *Psychological Bulletin*, *142*(9), 991–1015. https://doi.org/10.1037/bul0000059

Kim, S., Brody, G. H., & Murry, V. M. (2003). Factor structure of the Early Adolescent Temperament Questionnaire and measurement invariance across gender. *The Journal of Early Adolescence*, *23*(3), 268–294. https://doi.org/10.1177/0272431603254178

Klein, D. N., Dougherty, L. R., & Olino, T. M. (2005). Toward guidelines for evidence-based assessment of depression in children and adolescents. *Journal of Clinical Child & Adolescent Psychology*, *34*(3), 412–432. https://doi.org/10.1207/s15374424jccp3403_3

Klein, D. N., Finsaas, M. C., Goldstein, B. L., Kessel, E. M., Kopala-Sibley, D. C., & Kotov, R. (2018). Personality and depression. In The SAGE handbook of personality and individual differences: Applications of personality and individual differences (pp. 36–62). SAGE Publications.

Klein, D. N., Kotov, R., & Bufferd, S. J. (2011). Personality and depression: Explanatory models and review of the evidence. *Annual Review of Clinical Psychology*, *7*(1), 269–295. https://doi.org/10.1146/annurev-clinpsy-032210-104540

Klein, D. N., & Mumper, E. E. (2018). Behavioral inhibition as a precursor to psychopathology. In K. Pérez-Edgar & N. A. Fox (Eds.), *Behavioral inhibition: Integrating theory, research, and clinical perspectives* (pp. 283–307). Springer International Publishing. https://doi.org/10.1007/978-3-319-98077-5_13

Kostyrka-Allchorne, K., Wass, S. V., & Sonuga-Barke, E. J. S. (2020). Research review: Do parent ratings of infant negative emotionality and self-regulation predict psychopathology in childhood and adolescence? A systematic review and meta-analysis of prospective longitudinal studies. *Journal of Child Psychology and Psychiatry*, *61*(4), 401–416. https://doi.org/10.1111/jcpp.13144

Kotelnikova, Y., Olino, T. M., Klein, D. N., Kryski, K. R., & Hayden, E. P. (2016). Higher- and lower-order factor analyses of the Children's Behavior Questionnaire in early and middle childhood. *Psychological Assessment*, *28*(1), 92–108. https://doi.org/10.1037/pas0000153

Kotelnikova, Y., Olino, T. M., Klein, D. N., Mackrell, S. V. M., & Hayden, E. P. (2017). Higher- and lower-order factor analyses of the Temperament in Middle Childhood Questionnaire. *Assessment*, *24*(8), 1050–1061. https://doi.org/10.1177/1073191116639376

Kotov, R., Cicero, D. C., Conway, C. C., DeYoung, C. G., Dombrovski, A., Eaton, N. R., First, M. B., Forbes, M. K., Hyman, S. E., Jonas, K. G., Krueger, R. F., Latzman, R. D., Li, J. J., Nelson, B. D., Regier, D. A., Rodriguez-Seijas, C., Ruggero, C. J., Simms, L. J., Skodol, A. E., . . . Wright, A. G. C. (2022). The Hierarchical Taxonomy of Psychopathology (HiTOP) in psychiatric practice and research. *Psychological Medicine*, *52*(9), 1666–1678. https://doi.org/10.1017/S0033291722001301

Kotov, R., Gamez, W., Schmidt, F., & Watson, D. (2010). Linking "big" personality traits to anxiety, depressive, and substance use disorders: A meta-analysis. *Psychological Bulletin, 136*(5), 768–821. https://doi.org/10.1037/a0020327

Kushner, S. C., Tackett, J. L., & Barbara De Clercq. (2013). The joint hierarchical structure of adolescent personality pathology: Converging evidence from two approaches to measurement. *The Journal of the Canadian Academy of Child and Adolescent Psychiatry, 22*(3), 199–205.

Lavender, J. M., De Young, K. P., & Wonderlich, S. A. (2015). Personality as a risk factor for eating disorders. In *The Wiley handbook of eating disorders* (pp. 418–429). John Wiley & Sons, Ltd. https://doi.org/10.1002/9781118574089.ch32

Lawson, K. M., Atherton, O. E., & Robins, R. W. (2021). The structure of adolescent temperament and associations with psychological functioning: A replication and extension of Snyder et al. (2015). *Journal of Personality and Social Psychology, 121*(5), e19–e39. https://doi.org/10.1037/pspp0000380

Liu, P., Kryski, K. R., Smith, H. J., Joanisse, M. F., & Hayden, E. P. (2020). Transactional relations between early child temperament, structured parenting, and child outcomes: A three-wave longitudinal study. *Development and Psychopathology, 32*(3), 923–933. https://doi.org/10.1017/S0954579419000841

Loken, E. (2004). Using latent class analysis to model temperament types. *Multivariate Behavioral Research, 39*, 625–652. https://doi.org/10.1207/s15327906mbr3904_3

Luan, Z., Hutteman, R., Denissen, J. J. A., Asendorpf, J. B., & van Aken, M. A. G. (2017). Do you see my growth? Two longitudinal studies on personality development from childhood to young adulthood from multiple perspectives. *Journal of Research in Personality, 67*, 44–60. https://doi.org/10.1016/j.jrp.2016.03.004

Luan, Z., Poorthuis, A. M. G., Hutteman, R., Denissen, J. J. A., Asendorpf, J. B., & van Aken, M. A. G. (2018). Unique predictive power of other-rated personality: An 18-year longitudinal study. *Journal of Personality, 87*(3), 532–545. https://doi.org/10.1111/jopy.12413

Martin-Storey, A., Serbin, L. A., Stack, D. M., & Schwartzman, A. E. (2009). The behaviour style observation system for young children predicts teacher-reported externalizing behaviour in middle childhood. *Infant and Child Development, 18*(4), 337–350. https://doi.org/10.1002/icd.601

McClowry, S. G., & Collins, A. (2012). Temperament-based intervention: Reconceptualized from a response-to-intervention framework. In M. Zentner & R. L. Shiner (Eds.), *Handbook of temperament* (pp. 607–626). Guilford Publications.

McClowry, S. G., Snow, D. L., & Tamis-LeMonda, C. S. (2005). An evaluation of the effects of INSIGHTS on the behavior of inner city primary school children. *The Journal of Primary Prevention, 26*(6), 567–584. https://doi.org/10.1007/s10935-005-0015-7

McCormick, M. P., O'Connor, E. E., Cappella, E., & McClowry, S. G. (2015). Getting a good start in school: Effects of INSIGHTS on children with high maintenance temperaments. *Early Childhood Research Quarterly, 30*, 128–139. https://doi.org/10.1016/j.ecresq.2014.10.006

Mehl, M. R. (2017). The Electronically Activated Recorder (EAR): A Method for the naturalistic observation of daily social behavior. *Current Directions in Psychological Science, 26*(2), 184–190. https://doi.org/10.1177/0963721416680611

Mervielde, I., De Clercq, B., De Fruyt, F., & Van Leeuwen, K. (2005). Temperament, personality, and developmental psychopathology as childhood antecedents of personality disorders. *Journal of Personality Disorders, 19*(2), 171–201. https://doi.org/10.1521/pedi.19.2.171.62627

Mervielde, I., & De Fruyt, F. (1999). Construction of the Hierarchical Personality Inventory for Children (HiPIC). In I. J. Deary, F. De Fruyt, & F. Ostendorf (Eds). *Personality psychology in Europe* (Vol. 7, pp. 107–127). Tilburg University Press.

Morrison, F. J., & Grammer, J. K. (2016). Conceptual clutter and measurement mayhem: Proposals for cross-disciplinary integration in conceptualizing and measuring executive function. In J. A. Griffin, P. McCardle, & L. S. Freund (Eds.), *Executive function in preschool-age children: Integrating measurement, neurodevelopment, and translational research* (pp. 327–348). American Psychological Association. https://doi.org/10.1037/14797-015

Mychailyszyn, M. P. (2017). "Cool" youth: A systematic review and comprehensive meta-analytic synthesis of data from the *Cool Kids* family of intervention programs. *Canadian Psychology, 58*(2), 105–115. http://dx.doi.org/10.1037/cap0000101

National Institute of Mental Health. (2024). *RDoC Matrix*. Www.nimh.nih.gov. https://www.nimh.nih.gov/research/research-funded-by-nimh/rdoc/constructs/rdoc-matrix

Nielsen, J. D., Olino, T. M., Dyson, M. W., & Klein, D. N. (2019). Reactive and regulatory temperament: Longitudinal associations with internalizing and externalizing symptoms through childhood. *Journal of Abnormal Child Psychology*, *47*(11), 1771–1784. https://doi.org/10.1007/s10802-019-00555-0

Nigg, J. T. (2017). Annual Research Review: On the relations among self-regulation, self-control, executive functioning, effortful control, cognitive control, impulsivity, risk-taking, and inhibition for developmental psychopathology. *Journal of Child Psychology and Psychiatry*, *58*(4), 361–383. https://doi.org/10.1111/jcpp.12675

O'Connor, E. E., Cappella, E., McCormick, M. P., & McClowry, S. G. (2014). Enhancing the academic development of shy children: A test of the efficacy of INSIGHTS. *School Psychology Review*, *43*(3), 239–259. https://doi.org/10.1080/02796015.2014.12087426

Olino, T. M., Guerra-Guzman, K., Hayden, E. P., & Klein, D. N. (2020). Evaluating maternal psychopathology biases in reports of child temperament: An investigation of measurement invariance. *Psychological Assessment*, *32*(11), 1037–1046. https://doi.org/10.1037/pas0000945

Olino, T. M., Schlechter, P., Klein, D. N., Kotov, R., & Seeley, J. R. (2024). Personality and presentation of depression symptoms: A preliminary examination of the pathoplasticity model. *Clinical Psychological Science*, *13*(3), 506–519. https://doi.org/10.1177/21677026241283401

Ormel, J., Oldehinkel, A. J., & Vollebergh, W. (2004). Vulnerability before, during, and after a major depressive episode: A 3-wave population-based study. *Archives of General Psychiatry*, *61*(10), 990–996. https://doi.org/10.1001/archpsyc.61.10.990

Ostlund, B., Myruski, S., Buss, K., & Pérez-Edgar, K. E. (2021). The centrality of temperament to the Research Domain Criteria (RDoC): The earliest building blocks of psychopathology. *Development and Psychopathology*, *33*(5), 1584–1598. https://doi.org/10.1017/s0954579421000511

Ostrov, J. M., Murray-Close, D., Perry, K. J., Blakely-McClure, S. J., Perhamus, G. R., Mutignani, L. M., Kesselring, S., Memba, G. V., & Probst, S. (2022). The development of forms and functions of aggression during early childhood: A temperament-based approach. *Development and Psychopathology*, *35*(2), 941–957. pahttps://doi.org/10.1017/s0954579422000177

Pade, H., Taube, D. O., Aalborg, A. E., & Reiser, P. J. (2006). An immediate and long-term study of a temperament and parent-child interaction therapy based community program for preschoolers with behavior problems. *Child & Family Behavior Therapy*, *28*(3), 1–28. https://doi.org/10.1300/J019v28n03_01

Parsons, S., Kruijt, A.-W., & Fox, E. (2019). Psychological science needs a standard practice of reporting the reliability of cognitive-behavioral measurements. *Advances in Methods and Practices in Psychological Science*, *2*(4), 378–395.

Pedregon, C. A., Farley, R. L., Davis, A., Wood, J. M., & Clark, R. D. (2012). Social desirability, personality questionnaires, and the "better than average" effect. *Personality and Individual Differences*, *52*(2), 213–217. https://doi.org/10.1016/j.paid.2011.10.022

Petersen, I. T., Choe, D. E., & LeBeau, B. (2020). Studying a moving target in development: The challenge and opportunity of heterotypic continuity. *Developmental Review*, *58*, 100935. https://doi.org/10.1016/j.dr.2020.100935

Petersen, I. T., & LeBeau, B. (2022). Creating a developmental scale to chart the development of psychopathology with different informants and measures across time. *Journal of Psychopathology and Clinical Science*, *131*(6), 611–625. https://doi.org/10.1037/abn0000649

Presley, R., & Martin, R. P. (1994). Toward a structure of preschool temperament: Factor structure of the Temperament Assessment Battery for Children. *Journal of Personality*, *62*(3), 415–448. https://doi.org/10.1111/j.1467-6494.1994.tb00304.x

Rapee, R. M., Kennedy, S., Ingram, M., Edwards, S., & Sweeney, L. (2005). Prevention and early intervention of anxiety disorders in inhibited preschool children. *Journal of Consulting and Clinical Psychology*, *73*(3), 488–497.

Rettew, D. C. (2019). Distinguishing temperament from psychopathology. In R. DelCarmen-Wiggins & A. S. Carter (Eds.), *The Oxford handbook of infant, toddler, and preschool mental health assessment*

(2nd edn) (pp. 157–174). Oxford University Press. https://doi.org/10.1093/oxfordhb/9780199837182.013.7

Robbins, M. L., Jonnalagadda, P., & Spahr, C. M. (2024). Rebalancing social & personality psychology methods: The case for naturalistic observation. *Social and Personality Psychology Compass*, *18*(1), e12917. https://doi.org/10.1111/spc3.12917

Roberts, B. W., & DelVecchio, W. F. (2000). The rank-order consistency of personality traits from childhood to old age: A quantitative review of longitudinal studies. *Psychological Bulletin*, *126*(1), 3–25. https://doi.org/10.1037/0033-2909.126.1.3

Rosenström, T., Jylhä, P., Pulkki-Råback, L., Holma, M., Raitakari, O. T., Isometsä, E., & Keltikangas-Järvinen, L. (2015). Long-term personality changes and predictive adaptive responses after depressive episodes. *Evolution and Human Behavior*, *36*(5), 337–344. https://doi.org/10.1016/j.evolhumbehav.2015.01.005

Rothbart, M. K. (1981). Measurement of temperament in infancy. *Child Development*, *52*(2), 569–578. https://doi.org/10.2307/1129176

Rothbart, M. K., Ahadi, S. A., Hershey, K. L., & Fisher, P. (2001). Investigations of temperament at three to seven years: The Children's Behavior Questionnaire. *Child Development*, *72*(5), 1394–1408. https://doi.org/10.1111/1467-8624.00355

Rothbart, M. K., & Bates, J. E. (2006). Temperament. In W. Damon, R. Lerner, & N. Eisenberg (Eds.), *Handbook of child psychology: Vol. 3. Social, emotional, and personality development* (6th ed., pp. 99–166). New York: Wiley.

Saudino, K. J. (2009). Do different measures tap the same genetic influences? A multi-method study of activity level in young twins. *Developmental Science*, *12*(4), 626–633. https://doi.org/10.1111/j.1467-7687.2008.00801.x

Sherman, B. J., Vousoura, E., Wickramaratne, P., Warner, V., & Verdeli, H. (2016). Temperament and major depression: How does difficult temperament affect frequency, severity, and duration of major depressive episodes among offspring of parents with or without depression? *Journal of Affective Disorders*, *200*, 82–88. https://doi.org/10.1016/j.jad.2016.04.033

Shields, A. N., Giljen, M., España, R. A., & Tackett, J. L. (2021). The p factor and dimensional structural models of youth personality pathology and psychopathology. *Current Opinion in Psychology*, *37*, 21–25. https://doi.org/10.1016/j.copsyc.2020.06.005

Shields, A. N., Malanchini, M., Vinnik, L., Tucker-Drob, E. M., Harden, K. P., & Tackett, J. L. (2022). Genetic variance in conscientiousness relates to youth psychopathology beyond executive functions. *Journal of Psychopathology and Clinical Science*, *131*(8), 830–846. https://doi.org/10.1037/abn0000781

Shiner, R. L., Buss, K. A., McClowry, S. G., Putnam, S. P., Saudino, K. J., & Zentner, M. (2012). What is temperament *now*? Assessing progress in temperament research on the twenty-fifth anniversary of Goldsmith et al. (1987). *Child Development Perspectives*, *6*(4), 436–444. https://doi.org/10.1111/j.1750-8606.2012.00254.x

Shiner, R. L., & DeYoung, C. G. (2013). The structure of temperament and personality traits: A developmental perspective. In P. D. Zelazo (Ed.), *The Oxford handbook of developmental psychology, Vol. 2. Self and other* (pp. 113–141). Oxford University Press.

Shokrkon, A., & Nicoladis, E. (2021). How personality traits of neuroticism and extroversion predict the effects of the COVID-19 on the mental health of Canadians. *PLOS ONE*, *16*(5), e0251097. https://doi.org/10.1371/journal.pone.0251097

Soto, C. J. (2016). The little six personality dimensions from early childhood to early adulthood: Mean-level age and gender differences in parents' reports. *Journal of Personality*, *84*(4), 409–422.

Soto, C. J., & John, O. P. (2014). Traits in transition: the structure of parent-reported personality traits from early childhood to early adulthood. *Journal of Personality*, *82*(3), 182–199.

Soto, C. J., & Tackett, J. L. (2015). Personality traits in childhood and adolescence. *Current Directions in Psychological Science*, *24*(5), 358–362. https://doi.org/10.1177/0963721415589345

Spector, P. E., Rosen, C. C., Richardson, H. A., Williams, L. J., & Johnson, R. E. (2019). A new perspective on method variance: A measure-centric approach. *Journal of Management*, *45*(3), 855–880. https://doi.org/10.1177/0149206316687295

Stanton, K., & Watson, D. (2014). Positive and negative affective dysfunction in psychopathology. *Social and Personality Psychology Compass*, *8*(9), 555–567. https://doi.org/10.1111/spc3.12132

Sun, J., & Vazire, S. (2019). Do people know what they're like in the moment? *Psychological Science*, *30*(3), 405–414. https://doi.org/10.1177/0956797618818476

Tackett, J. L. (2006). Evaluating models of the personality-psychopathology relationship in children and adolescents. *Clinical Psychology Review*, *26*(5), 584–599. https://doi.org/10.1016/j.cpr.2006.04.003

Tackett, J. L., & Durbin, C. E. (2017). Advances in research on youth personality: Introduction to the special issue. *Journal of Research in Personality*, *67*, 1–2. https://doi.org/10.1016/j.jrp.2017.03.004

Tackett, J. L., & Hallquist, M. (2022). The need to grow: Developmental considerations and challenges for modern psychiatric taxonomies. *Journal of Psychopathology and Clinical Science*, *131*(6), 660–663. https://doi.org/10.1037/abn0000751

Tackett, J. L., Lang, J. W. B., Markon, K. E., & Herzhoff, K. (2019). A correlated traits, correlated methods model for thin-slice child personality assessment. *Psychological Assessment*, *31*(4), 545–556. https://doi.org/10.1037/pas0000635

Tackman, A. M., Baranski, E. N., Danvers, A. F., Sbarra, D. A., Raison, C. L., Moseley, S. A., Polsinelli, A. J., & Mehl, M. R. (2020). "Personality in its natural habitat" revisited: A pooled, multi-sample examination of the relationships between the Big Five personality traits and daily behaviour and language use. *European Journal of Personality*, *34*(5), 753–776. https://doi.org/10.1002/per.2283

Thomas, A., & Chess, S. (1977). *Temperament and development* (pp. xv, 270). Brunner/Mazel.

van den Akker, A. L., Dekovic, M., Prinzie, P., & Asscher, J. J. (2010). Toddlers' temperament profiles: Stability and relations to negative and positive parenting. *Journal of Abnormal Child Psychology*, *38*, 485–495. https://doi.org/10.1007/s10802-009-9379-0

Watson, D. (2016). Positive mood dysfunction in psychopathology. In *The Wiley handbook of positive clinical psychology* (pp. 57–71). John Wiley & Sons, Ltd. https://doi.org/10.1002/9781118468197.ch5

Watson, D., Kotov, R., & Gamez, W. (2006). Basic dimensions of temperament in relation to personality and psychopathology. In *Personality and psychopathology* (pp. 7–38). The Guilford Press.

Watson, D., & Naragon-Gainey, K. (2010). On the specificity of positive emotional dysfunction in psychopathology: Evidence from the mood and anxiety disorders and schizophrenia/schizotypy. *Clinical Psychology Review*, *30*(7), 839–848. https://doi.org/10.1016/j.cpr.2009.11.002

Watson, D., Stanton, K., Khoo, S., Ellickson-Larew, S., & Stasik-O'Brien, S. M. (2019). Extraversion and psychopathology: A multilevel hierarchical review. *Journal of Research in Personality*, *81*, 1–10. https://doi.org/10.1016/j.jrp.2019.04.009

Watts, A. L., Greene, A. L., Bonifay, W., & Fried, E. I. (2024). A critical evaluation of the *p*-factor literature. *Nature Reviews Psychology*, *3*, 108–122.

Watts, A. L., Makol, B. A., Palumbo, I. M., De Los Reyes, A., Olino, T. M., Latzman, R. D., DeYoung, C. G., Wood, P. K., & Sher, K. J. (2022). How robust is the p factor? Using multitrait-multimethod modeling to inform the meaning of general factors of youth psychopathology. *Clinical Psychological Science*, *10*(4), 640–661. https://doi.org/10.1177/21677026211055170

Whalen, D. J., Gilbert, K. E., Jackson, J. J., Barch, D. M., & Luby, J. L. (2020). Using a thin slice coding approach to assess preschool personality dimensions. *Journal of Personality Assessment*, *103*(2), 214–223. https://doi.org/10.1080/00223891.2020.1722140

Widiger, T. A., Sellbom, M., Chmielewski, M., Clark, L. A., DeYoung, C. G., Kotov, R., Krueger, R. F., Lynam, D. R., Miller, J. D., Mullins-Sweatt, S., Samuel, D. B., South, S. C., Tackett, J. L., Thomas, K. M., Watson, D., & Wright, A. G. C. (2019). Personality in a hierarchical model of psychopathology. *Clinical Psychological Science*, *7*(1), 77–92. https://doi.org/10.1177/2167702618797105

Williams, A. L., Craske, M. G., Mineka, S., & Zinbarg, R. E. (2021). Reciprocal effects of personality and general distress: Neuroticism vulnerability is stronger than scarring. *Journal of Abnormal Psychology*, *130*(1), 34–46. https://doi.org/10.1037/abn0000635

Wilson, S., & Olino, T. M. (2022). A developmental perspective on personality and psychopathology across the life span. *Journal of Personality*, *89*(5), 915–932. https://doi.org/10.1111/jopy.12623

Wiltink, S., Nelson, B., Velthorst, E., Wigman, J. T. W., Lin, A., Baksheev, G., Cosgrave, E., Ross, M., Ryan, J., & Yung, A. R. (2015). The relationship between personality traits and psychotic like experiences in a large non-clinical adolescent sample. *Personality and Individual Differences*, *73*, 92–97. https://doi.org/10.1016/j.paid.2014.09.030

Wright, A. G. C., & Hopwood, C. J. (2022). Integrating and distinguishing personality and psychopathology. *Journal of Pesronality*, *90*, 5–19. https://doi.org/10.1111/jopy.12671

Wright, A. J., & Jackson, J. J. (2022). Childhood temperament and adulthood personality differentially predict life outcomes. *Scientific Reports*, *12*(1), 10286. https://doi.org/10.1038/s41598-022-14666-0

Zuckerman, M., Kuhlman, D. M., Joireman, J., Teta, P., & Kraft, M. (1993). A comparison of three structural models for personality: The Big Three, the Big Five, and the Alternative Five. *Journal of Personality and Social Psychology*, *65*(4), 757–768. https://doi.org/10.1037/0022-3514.65.4.757

CHAPTER 11

The Achenbach System for Empirically Based Assessment

WILLIAM E. COPELAND

Introduction

THIS chapter provides an updated review of one of the first empirically based systems of psychopathology. This system was developed by a singular figure within developmental psychopathology, Dr. Thomas Achenbach. Dr. Achenbach first developed this system as part of his work for his doctoral thesis at the University of Minnesota. His project was simple: to develop a system of child psychopathology from bottom-up observations of children's behavior rather than from top-down conceptualization and theories about the nature and structure of psychopathology. It is difficult to put this insight into proper focus from a 21st-century perspective in which big data and analytics have become dominant lenses for scientific inquiry. In the middle part of the 20th century, child psychiatry and psychology were dominated by expert-based top-down theories that generally resisted empirical validation or testing. Dr. Achenbach's doctoral thesis launched a career that lasted more than five decades, expanding on this system to describe psychopathology across the lifespan and, indeed, across innumerable countries and cultures around the world.

Dr. Achenbach died in late 2023. To the end, he was a champion for empiricism as the foundation for mental health research. Empiricism relies on what is observed rather than what is supposed. In one of his last publications, he stated it thusly: "To advance knowledge that can be used to help people, it is important to prevent conceptual paradigms from impeding the quest for data regarding how people actually function" (T. M. Achenbach, 2020, p. 20). Put differently, Dr. Achenbach always preferred to listen to the data, rather than to the experts. What follows is an attempt to introduce this system of developmental psychopathology and the associated assessment measures to the next generation of researchers and clinicians. The interested reader is encouraged to look to other in-depth reviews of Dr. Achenbach's work from the man himself (T. M. Achenbach, 2020; T. M. Achenbach et al., 2017; Achenbach et al., 2016). Rather than trying to replicate those efforts, the focus of this chapter is to distill the essential features of Dr. Achenbach's work that continues to allow the Achenbach System of Empirically Based Assessment (ASEBA) to be distinguished from other taxonomic efforts and assessment measures. Thus, we start with a description of the pillars of ASEBA, then we describe the measures themselves and the model of psychopathology derived from these measures. Finally, we discuss its application to clinical work, research, and training.

Pillars of the ASEBA System

The measures that make up the ASEBA system may seem rather familiar. Each of the measures consists of a long list of problem behavior (~100 to 120 items) that are rated on a three-point scale from "not true" to "somewhat or sometimes true" to "very true or often true." The respondent is asked to endorse items based on the prior two-month period. In addition to problem items, the instruments include items for assessing competencies, adaptive functioning, and personal strengths; plus open-ended items for reporting the best things about the person being assessed, what concerns the respondent most about the person being assessed, and other clinically useful information. Respondents are encouraged to add comments on either paper or online versions of the instruments, which take about 10 to 20 minutes to complete. For respondents who cannot complete assessment instruments independently, an interviewer with no specialized training can read the items aloud and enter the responses. **Table 11.1** lists the instruments by age range. Information about obtaining these measures is available at https://store.aseba.org/.

While familiar, the ASEBA system represents a substantial break from traditional approaches to mental health assessment and taxonomy. This contrast was perhaps most stark when the system was introduced 50 years ago, but a combination of four features makes this system distinctive—even unique—to this day. To make this more salient for the reader, the first part of this chapter will review the core pillars of the ASEBA system: empirically based taxonomy, multi-informant assessment, norm-based comparisons, and multicultural validation. At this point, the ASEBA encompasses over 20 measures of behavioral and emotional functioning across four distinct age ranges across the lifespan. All of these measures without exception conform to the following ASEBA pillars. ASEBA measures support data collection from all available sources (multi-informant assessment) to inform identification of emotional and behavioral functioning constructs derived from how the items cluster with one another (empirically based) that are then compared to typical levels of functioning within one's community (norm-based comparisons and multicultural validation). Together, these pillars ensure that ASEBA measures and the information derived from them have the strongest empirical foundation from which to inform clinical care as well as efforts to understand psychopathology across the lifespan.

Empirically Based Taxonomy

From its inception, the ASEBA was intended by Dr. Achenbach to be strongly rooted in objective empiricism about the nature of psychopathology. This paradigm prioritizes analysis of observable data from which the constructs of psychopathology are derived. The observable data in this case are provided by all informed eyewitnesses. For children, questionnaires are completed by parents, a teacher, other caregivers, and the children themselves. The questionnaires assess a broad range of behavioral, emotional, and cognitive items. This information is collected for a large group of children. Next, these items are tested to see how they statistically co-vary or cluster with one another to understand how the items should be grouped. The role of the client is to report on what they observe, the role of the scientist is to analyze the observational data to derive constructs, and the role of the clinician is to report back on their client's scores on the derived constructs. In each case, the goal is to maximize the impact of observation and minimize the role of interpretation. That is not to say, of course, that this approach—or any approach—is or can be free of interpretation, but with the "bottom-up" or data-driven paradigm the role of interpretation is minimized to allow—as much as it is possible—the data "to speak for themselves." This approach is best understood as a corrective effort to the predominant "top-down" paradigms at the time the ASEBA was originally developed. Such "top-down" paradigms are still, arguably, the dominant approach to psychopathology taxonomy.

"Top-down" paradigms prioritize conceptualizations about the nature and structure of psychopathology that are derived from the mind of the researcher. As such, these paradigms may

TABLE 11.1 Achenbach System of Empirically Based Assessment (ASEBA) Instruments for Ages 1½–90+ Years

Ages	Informants	Normative Sample N[a]	Psychopathology Scales	Strengths Scales
1½ 5 Years				
CBCL/1½-5	Parent figures	19,806	Syndromes, *DSM*, Int, Ext, Total, Stress	Language Development
C-TRF	Daycare providers, preschool teachers	8,974	Syndromes, *DSM*, Int, Ext, Total, Stress	NA
6–18 Years				
CBCL/6-18	Parent figures	59,804	Syndromes, *DSM*, Int, Ext, Total, OCP[b], SCT[c], Stress	Activities, Social, School, Total Competence
TRF	Teachers, school staff	32,349	Syndromes, *DSM*, Int, Ext, Total, OCP[b], SCT[c], Stress	Academic, Adaptive
YSR	Youths	31,300	Syndromes, *DSM*, Int, Ext, Total, OCP[b], SCT[c], Stress	Activities, Social, Total Competence, Positive Qualities
18–59 Years				
ABCL	Collaterals	8,322	Syndromes, *DSM*, Int, Ext, Total, OCP[b], SCT[c], Substance Use	Friends, Spouse/Partner, Personal Strengths
ASR	Adults	11,790	Syndromes, *DSM*, Int, Ext, Total, OCP[b], SCT[c], Substance Use	Friends, Spouse/Partner, Family, Job, Education, Personal Strengths
60–90+ Years				
OABCL	Collaterals	6,105	Syndromes, *DSM*, Total, Substance Use	Friends, Spouse/Partner, Personal Strengths
OASR	Older adults	10,049	Syndromes, *DSM*, Total, Substance Use	Friends, Spouse/Partner, Personal Strengths

CBCL/1½-5 = Child Behavior Checklist for Ages 1½–5; C-TRF = Caregiver-Teacher Report Form; CBCL/6-18 = Child Behavior Checklist for Ages 6–18; TRF = Teacher Report Form; YSR = Youth Self-Report; BPM/6-18 = Brief Problem Monitor for Ages 6–18; ABCL = Adult Behavior Checklist; ASR = Adult Self-Report; BPM/18-59 = Brief Problem Monitor for Ages 18–59; OABCL = Older Adult Behavior Checklist; OASR = Older Adult Self-Report.

[a] Multicultural samples from dozens of societies.

[b] Obsessive-Compulsive Problems scale.

[c] Sluggish Cognitive Tempo scale.

also incorporate empirical data, but it is the conceptualizations or categories themselves that become the primary focus of research and clinical applications. In this paradigm, the role of the client may still be to report observations, but the scope of the observations may be limited by the conceptual model. The role of the scientist is not merely to analyze the data, but also to use the data to update and inform the existing conceptual model. The role of the clinician is then not to just report back on the client's observations but also to interpret the data in the context of the conceptual model. In each case, the goal is to maximize the impact of interpretation as it relates to the original model of psychopathology. Such approaches go back to (and even predate) Freud's psychoanalytic theory and continue to impact psychopathology today through the focus on constructs included in the *Diagnostic and Statistical Manual of Mental Disorders* (DSM) and the International Classification of Disorders (ICD).

Until 1968, the first edition of the *Diagnostic and Statistical Manual* (DSM-I)—which embodied the official American psychiatric nosology—contained only the following two categories for child psychopathology: adjustment reaction of childhood, and schizophrenic reaction, childhood type (American Psychiatric Association, 1952). Neither of these diagnostic categories was derived from empirical assessment of children's problems, and neither one provided explicit criteria for deciding which children qualified for which diagnosis. The understanding of childhood mental health problems was severely wanting.

In providing a justification for his alternative approach, Dr. Achenbach suggested, "The isolation of clusters of empirical attributes is a logical first step" (Achenbach, 1966, p. 2). He was not the first to apply factor analytic approaches to potential symptoms or even the first to apply such methods to the study of child psychopathology. That distinction applies to work by Hewitt and Jenkins in 1946 (Hewitt & Jenkins, 1946). They recorded the presence of 94 problems in 500 child guidance clinic case histories. Chosen on the basis of high frequency or "obvious clinical importance," 45 of the problem items were analyzed to identify three clusters hypothesized by the authors and designated as the overinhibited child, the unsocialized aggressive child, and the socialized delinquent child. Any experienced clinician or researcher will immediately see in these clusters some of the same dimensions of psychopathology used to this day. This work set a foundation for Dr. Achenbach's efforts, which broadened the domains of items under study.

In his initial study (Achenbach, 1966), Dr. Achenbach mined case histories of 300 males and 300 females in a child psychiatry clinic with an equal number of participants in middle childhood and adolescence to study patterns of co-variation on 74 problem items. The problem items were amassed from review of intake notes for clinical cases at psychiatric clinics. These problem items were then subjected to exploratory factor analysis to explore relations between broad- and narrow-spectrum groupings of problems. Principal factor analyses yielded a bipolar first factor comprising problem items at one pole that were designated as "Externalizing," because they involved conflict with others and with social mores (aggressive and rule-breaking behaviors). Items comprising the other pole of the first factor were designated as "Internalizing," because they involved problems within the self (anxiety, depression, social withdrawal, and somatic complaints without apparent medical cause). The unipolar second factor was designated as "Severe and Diffuse Psychopathology," because its high-loading items included such problems as bizarre behavior, hallucinations, delusions, feeling of persecution, being confused, fearing one's own impulses, compulsions, and obsessions. Matrices including numerous principal factors beyond the first two were rotated to several criteria for orthogonal and oblique simple structure. Sets of problem items found to have high loadings on factors identified in multiple rotations were designated with descriptive labels for their content, such as "Aggressive Behavior," "Attention Problems," and "Somatic Complaints."

With the advancement of electronic computers, many such multivariate analyses of associations among problem items soon followed. These typically involved factor-analytic or cluster-analytic approaches of large problem sets reported by parents, teachers, mental health workers, and case histories. Prominent efforts included those of Conners (1969), Miller (1967), Quay (1964), and others. Despite the great variety of assessment instruments, samples, sources of data, analytic methods, and labels for the findings, reviews of the multivariate studies revealed convergence on two broad-spectrum groupings of children's problems designated as internalizing (or "overcontrolled") and externalizing (or "undercontrolled"), plus more numerous narrow-spectrum syndromes (Achenbach, 1966, 1978; Quay, 1977). Dr. Achenbach preferred that term "syndrome" to designate a set of problems found to co-occur, rather than the term "disorder." The internalizing grouping comprises narrow-spectrum syndromes of anxiety, depression, social withdrawal, and somatic complaints without apparent medical cause. The externalizing grouping, by contrast, comprises narrow-spectrum syndromes of aggressive and rule-breaking behavior. The broad-spectrum internalizing/externalizing distinction has since been employed in over 75,000 published studies (Achenbach et al., 2016). No similar data on use of this broad spectrum is available for its use in clinical practice.

For each ASEBA instrument, data from clinical and nonclinical samples have been subjected to exploratory factor analyses (EFAs) and confirmatory factor analyses (CFAs) to derive first-order or broad-band syndromes. Scores on these syndromes have then been subjected to second-order factor analyses to identify narrow-band syndromes. There are commonalities and differences across the lifespan. **Table 11.2** lists the syndromes derived from the assessment instruments for each age range.

TABLE 11.2 ASEBA Syndromes Listed by Internalizing and Externalizing Groupings

Ages	Internalizing	Neither Int nor Ext	Externalizing
1½–5 Years			
CBCL/1½-5, C-TRF	Anxious/Depressed Emotionally Reactive Somatic Complaints Withdrawn	Sleep Problems	Aggressive Behavior Attention Problems
6–18 Years			
CBCL/6-18, TRF, YSR	Anxious/Depressed Somatic Complaints Withdrawn/Depressed	Attention Problems Social Problems Thought Problems	Aggressive Behavior Rule-Breaking Behavior
18–59 Years			
ABCL, ASR	Anxious/Depressed Somatic Complaints Withdrawn	Attention Problems Thought Problems	Aggressive Behavior Intrusive Rule-Breaking Behavior
60–90+ Years	No Internalizing vs. Externalizing groupings		
OABCL, OASR	Anxious/Depressed, Functional Impairment, Irritable/Disinhibited, Memory/Cognition Problems, Somatic Complaints, Thought Problems, Worries		

Note: A Total Problems (General Psychopathology) scale is also scored on all instruments. CBCL/1½-5 = Child Behavior Checklist for Ages 11½–5; C-TRF = Caregiver-Teacher Report Form; CBCL/6-18 = Child Behavior Checklist for Ages 6–18; TRF = Teacher Report Form; YSR = Youth Self-Report; ABCL = Adult Behavior Checklist; ASR = Adult Self-Report; OABCL = Older Adult Behavior Checklist; OASR = Older Adult Self-Report.

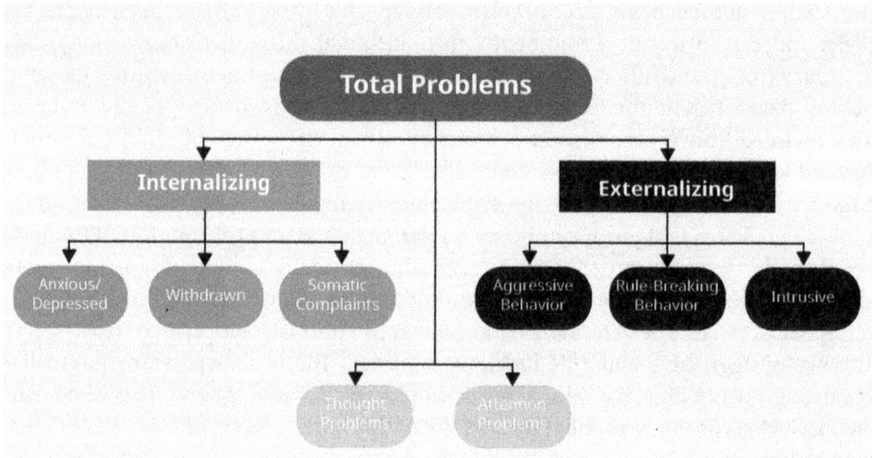

FIGURE 11.1 Hierarchy of empirically derived problem scales for ages 18–59. Figure adapted from https.//aseba.org/wp-content/uploads/2019/04/catalog.pdf: copyright 2019 T.M. Achenbach

Notably, the broad-spectrum internalizing/externalizing distinction is observed in preschool, school-aged, and adult forms. It is not observed in the older adult forms. Likewise, second-order syndromes within internalizing and externalizing scales are similar within these early age groups with a few exceptions (e.g., emotionally reactive syndrome in preschool-age measures, intrusive problems in adult-age measures). A few syndromes do not load on either the internalizing or the externalizing scale. In preschool age, this includes only the sleep problems syndrome. In school-age and adult forms, this includes attention problems and thought problems. **Figure 11.1** displays a hierarchical model of factor-analytically derived syndromes, internalizing and externalizing groupings of syndromes, and the Total Problems scale scored from the ASR and ABCL for ages 18 to 59.

Multi-formant Assessment

A "bottom-up approach" described above is only as strong as the information that is then studied empirically. As such, the second pillar of ASEBA is one that is focused on rigorous assessment by collecting relevant information from as many informants as might have relevant information. In adulthood, it is common—indeed, the norm—to rely on the individual themselves as the only source for information on their behavior and functioning. This practice is directly related to referral practices: adults presenting for mental health care are typically self-referred. As such, it is presumed that they will be best suited to characterizing their functioning. Children, however, rarely self-refer. Children typically present for mental health services because either their parent is concerned about their functioning at home or school personnel are concerned about their functioning at school. As such, it is not only reasonable but preferable to obtain information about the child's functioning from multiple sources that may have relevant information. Put simply, no single person is privy to all the variations in the child's functioning that commonly occur in interactions with different people in different settings (e.g., home and school). The goal of multi-informant assessment, therefore, is to give all individuals who observe the child/adolescent an opportunity to report on their observations and inform clinical decision-making.

The strength of multi-informant assessment is that it provides multiple sources of information about the child/adolescent. The challenge of multi-informant assessment is that it provides multiple sources of information about the child—and, of course, the informants may not agree perfectly. At this point, we have decades of evidence about such cross-informant agreement (and disagreement). Meta-analyses of *r*s between ratings of children's problems by people who play similar roles and see children in similar contexts (pairs of parents, teachers, mental health workers, observers) have yielded mean cross-informant *r*s around 60 (Achenbach et al., 1987; De Los Reyes et al., 2015). Among people who play different roles and see children in different contexts (e.g., parents vs. teachers), cross-informant *r*s have averaged around .30. And among self-ratings by children versus ratings by others, the cross-informant *r*s have ranged from the .20s to the .40s, depending on the children's ages and on who rated the children. Even the *r*s around .60 for pairs of similar informants mean that each informant may provide different information about an assessed child, and even more so for pairs of informants whose roles differ in relation to an assessed child. Dr. Achenbach's 1987 meta-analyses have now been cited in over 8,348 publications (Google Scholar, May 17, 2024), and their modest cross-informant correlations have been cited as being among "the most robust findings in child clinical research" (De Los Reyes & Kazdin, 2005).

The traditional interpretation of these inter-correlations is that they are more modest than one would expect given that each informant is rating the same child on the same set of behaviors. This apparent discrepancy could even be interpreted as casting doubt on the validity of a given informant. That was not the view of Dr. Achenbach. In his seminal 1987 review of this work, he stated, "This [interpretation] neglects another possibility that different informants contribute different information. Because we lack definitive criteria against which to validate measures of childhood problems, it is essential to preserve the contributions of different informants even if they do not correlate well with each other. Low correlations between informants may indicate that the target variables differ from one situation to another, rather than that the informants' reports are invalid or unreliable" (Achenbach et al., 1987, p. 213). Dr. Achenbach's interpretation is consistent with the ancient wisdom of the parable of the blind men and an elephant, in which each of the blind men's descriptions of the elephant is subjective, incomplete, and, yet, still true.

The importance of considering such situational specificity and therefore the value of multiple informants has not yet been similarly appreciated in assessment of adult psychopathology (Achenbach, 2006). While there have been many fewer studies of cross-informant agreement regarding adult rather than child psychopathology, meta-analyses of cross-informant *r*s among self- and collateral-ratings of adult psychopathology have found a mean *r* of 0.44 for externalizing problems and 0.43 for internalizing problems (Achenbach et al., 2005). Interestingly, correlations between self-reports and collateral reports of substance use were higher at 0.68, suggesting such observations may be less inferential. Similarly, DSM diagnoses based only on adult self-reports have also been found to differ substantially from diagnoses for the same individual based on data from other informants (Meyer et al., 2001). Again, this suggests that information from multiple informants is not redundant and may be similarly complementary (or even contradictory), as has been observed in childhood assessment. Consequently, the ASEBA assessment of adults as well as children include measures to support data from informants who know the assessed person, as well as data from self-reports. While this approach is the norm in childhood assessment, the ASEBA system is still distinctive in this regard among other assessment measures in adults.

Visual comparisons of multi-informant data help users quickly spot agreements and disagreements between self- and other reports on individual items as well as scale scores. See **Figure 11.2** for an example of the profiles produced by a multi-informant comparison.

In addition, ASEBA profiles provide measures of agreement between each pair of informants as well as the 25th percentile, mean, and 75th percentile for such correlations to

Multi-Informant Comparison - Syndrome Scale T Scores

Form	Eval ID	Assessed Person	Age	Informant	Relation	Society	Date
ABC1	01	Cross, Lana	39	Cross, Martin	Spouse	Group 1	02/01/2014
ASR2	02	Cross, Lana	39		Self	Group 1	02/01/2014
ABC3	01	Cross, Martin	40	Cross, Lana	Spouse	Group 1	02/02/2014
ASR4	02	Cross, Martin	40		Self	Group 1	01/31/2014
CBC5	01	Cross, Robert	11	Cross, Martin	Parent	Group 1	01/03/2014
CBC6	02	Cross, Robert	11	Cross, Lana	Parent	Group 1	02/01/2014
TRF7	03	Cross, Robert	11	Hotchkiss, Mary	Teacher	Group 1	01/01/2014
YSR8	04	Cross, Robert	11		Self	Group 1	02/02/2014

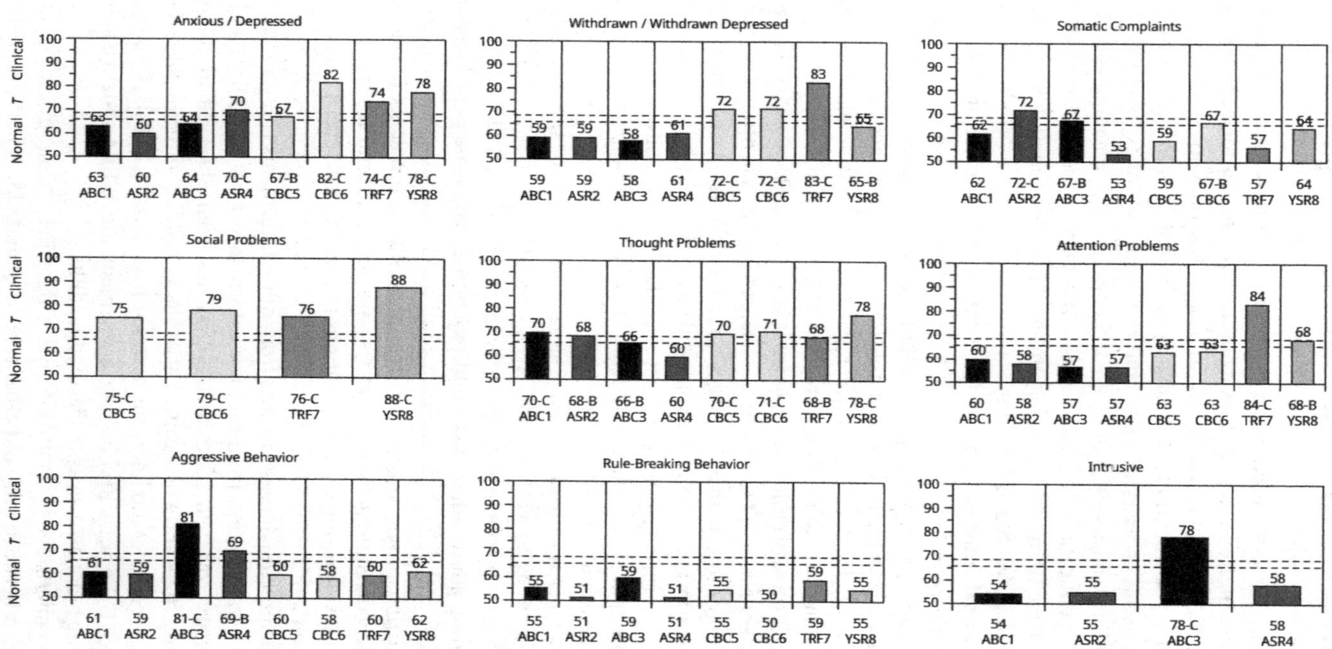

B = Borderline clinical range; C = Clinical range; Broken Lines = Borderline clinical range
**nc = The scores are not computed due to missing data.*

FIGURE 11.2 Bar graphs produced by the Multicultural Family Assessment Module displaying syndrome scores for multiple family measures (Copyright Achenbach and Rescorla, 2015)

identify if the pattern of agreement is average, above, or below. For both clinical and research purposes, computerized multi-informant data can also be aggregated in various ways. For example, self- and other ratings can be averaged to identify scales on which individuals are most and least deviant. Patterns of partial agreement may also be important. For example, ratings by three of a boy's teachers may be elevated on the DSM-oriented Attention-Deficit Hyperactivity Problems scale, whereas ratings by the boy's parents are in the normal range on this scale. Although the teachers view the boy as having attention-deficit/hyperactivity disorder (ADHD), the parents say that he cannot have ADHD, because he spends hours engrossed in video games. The elevated scores on the ADH Problems scale scored from TRFs completed by the boy's teachers provide detailed documentation of the teachers' perceptions of the boy's problems in three different classrooms, but the normal-range scores on the ADH Problems scale scored from the CBCLs completed by the boy's parents and their reports of his engrossment in video games indicate that interventions for ADHD problems should focus on the boy's functioning in school rather than being based on the assumption that he has an inherent attention deficit that affects his functioning at home as well as at school.

Norm-based Comparisons

Empirical "bottom-up" taxonomy coupled with multi-informant assessment provides a strong foundation for ASEBA. The remaining pillars provide the appropriate context for nuanced interpretation of the information collected. The third pillar of the ASEBA is norm-based comparisons. Norms allow users to see where a given individuals' scores fall in relation to distributions of scores for relevant comparison groups. This is a particularly important consideration for mental health problems as compared to other health concerns.

With psychopathology, there are some problems that in and of themselves provide evidence that clinical care is needed. If a child presents with plans to hurt themselves imminently or an adult reports seeing things that aren't there, then clinical intervention is likely to be provided immediately. This is not the case, however, for many mental health problems that tend to be viewed in terms of broader patterns or syndromes rather than isolated entities. Consider a child who presents to a clinician as restless, high-energy, and often climbing on furniture. To determine if intervention is merited, the clinician must first reference this cluster of symptoms with some external standard. In the case of the DSM, the consideration is whether the child displays six of nine symptoms of attention-deficit hyperactivity disorder and these symptoms also meet additional DSM criteria related to duration of symptoms, onset before a certain age, and evidence that the symptoms are present across contexts. These criteria apply whether the child is 7 or 17, a male or a female, despite significant differences in the frequency of these behaviors by age and gender. The ASEBA approach, in contrast, will interpret this cluster of behaviors in comparison to norms obtained from peers who are of the same age and gender as the presenting child. Thus, the clinical interpretation of the same cluster of symptoms will vary substantively if our presenting child is a 17-year old that identifies as female versus a 3-year old boy.

Norms based on distributions of scale scores obtained by population samples of people provide metrics for gauging whether an assessed individual's score is sufficiently elevated—compared to scores for a population sample of peers—to warrant clinical concern. Norms for specific scales can help providers decide whether an individual needs services and which problems should be targeted first. Norms can be used by the clinician to explain their rationale for treatment to the child and their family using an easily interpretable metric. In the DSM approach, the assessment information is interpreted dichotomously as to whether or not the patient/individual meets criteria for a diagnosis. In the ASEBA approach, the child's score will be interpreted continuously based on its percentile relative to the normative population and whether or not it meets some threshold for statistical deviance (e.g., 90th or 95th percentile). This is the same type of interpretation that is provided for other continuously distributed traits like scores on standardized academic tests or body mass index. After an intervention begins, norms continue to be useful for evaluating whether progress assessments indicate adequate movement from the clinical to the normal range, and for determining the favorability of outcomes in relation to normative levels.

Norm-based comparisons are useful for clinicians, intuitive to families, and flexible to accommodate the full range of mental health problems. At the same time, the process of obtaining population-based norms is intensive and costly. For example, the 1999 National Survey of Children, Youths, and Adults to renorm the ASEBA instruments was conducted in conjunction with Temple University's Institute for Survey Research from February 1999 through January 2000 (Achenbach & Rescorla, 2003; Achenbach & Rescorla, 2001b). The goal was to obtain data on mental health problems for a national probability sample of children and adults. The sampling procedure required sampling households within 100 primary sampling units chosen to be collectively representative of the 48 contiguous United States. After eligible households were identified within these sampling units, candidate participants were selected by stratified randomized procedures to produce the overall age distribution sought for the entire National Survey, with similar proportions of participants at each gender and age group. Parents of youth were asked for permission to interview their child to complete the Youth Self-Report and also asked to provide contact information for Teacher Report Forms to be sent out to the child's teachers. This information was necessary to obtain distributions of scores for all relevant items and scales across all age and gender groups covered by ASEBA instruments as well as multiple informants. Norms for ASEBA instruments were constructed from distributions of scores obtained for regional nonclinical population samples in the 1970s and 1980s (Achenbach & Edelbrock, 1986; Achenbach & Edelbrock, 1983). Norms were obtained for national U.S. nonclinical population samples via home interview surveys in 1989 and 1999–2000 (Achenbach et al., 2004; Achenbach & Rescorla, 2000, 2001a, 2003). The processing for renorming the ASEBA family of measures is currently ongoing. The fees associated with use of these measures are used to fund this effort, to insure that the norms continue to be available.

Multicultural Validation

Like norm-based comparison, multicultural validation is based on the fundamental idea that mental health problems typically need to be understood in their appropriate context. Norm-based comparisons typically put scores within a particular developmental context (e.g., preschool-age female or school-age male); multicultural validation considers common patterns of mental problems within a broader societal context. While the previous observation may seem simplistic and self-evident, almost all the research base for our understanding of psychopathology is based on work in a few, rather similar, Western societies. It should not be assumed, however, that the models and methodologies originating from those few societies automatically apply to people in all other societies. This is a similar point as was made earlier for norm-based assessment. What is an appropriate interpretation for one individual at one point in development may not apply to someone at a different point in the development. Models and methodology developed in a particular society should be empirically tested within other societies.

This is not a new observation. Arthur Kleinman (Kleinman, 1977) described this concern over forty years ago when he questioned research that uncritically exported mental health constructs from one society or culture to another. The application of the same standardized research methods to people in different societies is known as "etic" research. The term "etic" was derived by the linguist Kenneth Pike (Pike, 1967) from the word "phonetic," that is, linguists' systems for standardized representations of speech sounds that are meaningful in any of the world's languages. Etic research differs from emic research (Pike, 1967, derived from the term "phonemic," that is, linguists' systems for representing sounds that are meaningful in a particular language. Whereas etic research uses the same standardized methods to assess people in many societies (with translations, if needed), emic research uses methods tailored to a particular society. This tension between these approaches spurred the rise of transcultural psychiatry, the landmark 2001 WHO Report on Mental Health, and the burgeoning field of global mental health (Prince et al., 2007; World Health Organization, 2001).

There is a long history of cross-cultural research in psychology that compares two or three societies and draws inferences about all members of each society from differences on measures applied to samples from each society (see in-depth description of this issue by (Hermans & Kempen, 1998)). This type of piecemeal cross-cultural work is often the norm in studies of psychopathology because of the costs and logistical challenges of conducting large-scale data collection in many societies. By contrast, the ASEBA program of multicultural research on psychopathology has assessed population samples in many societies using the same standardized assessment methods to obtain distributions of quantitative scores, both within and between societies. To facilitate such research, ASEBA instruments are available in 113 languages. Published reports of use of ASEBA instruments in over 100 societies and cultural groups are also available (Pascal, 2021). This provides a strong foundation from which to assess the following aspects of multicultural validity of ASEBA: (1) generalizability of the syndromic structure; (2) generalizability of item structures; and (3) mean levels of syndromes and items.

The first step in testing multicultural validity is to determine whether the syndromic structure of the ASEBA instruments derived from factor analyses of primarily U.S. ASEBA data applies to other societies. Confirmatory factor analyses (CFAs) have been performed on data from population samples in over 50 societies. Separate CFAs have been performed on the ratings of problem items on each ASEBA instrument in population samples for ages 1½–5, 6–18, 18–59, and 60–90+ (Ivanova, Achenbach, Dumenci et al., 2007; Ivanova et al., 2011; Ivanova, Achenbach, Rescorla, Dumenci, Almqvist, Bathiche et al., 2007; Ivanova, Achenbach, Rescorla, Dumenci, Almqvist, Bilenberg et al., 2007; Ivanova et al., 2010; Ivanova, Achenbach, Rescorla, Turner, Ahmeti-Pronaj, et al., 2015; Achenbach, Rescorla, Turner, Árnadóttir, et al., 2015; Ivanova et al., 2020, 2021). Fit indices from these CFAs suggest that the ASEBA syndrome structures obtained in the United States also provide a good fit to the clustering of problem items in other cultures and societies as well. Thus, despite vast differences in languages, cultures, gene pools, political and economic systems, geographical locations, etc., people's ratings of ASEBA problem items yielded similar syndrome structures within age ranges 1½–5, 6–18, 18–59, and 60–90+.

The next step is to test whether the relative rank orderings of individual items were similar or different across different societies. To do this, the mean of the 0-1-2 ratings was computed for each problem item on each ASEBA instrument in each sample. *Q* correlations were computed between the mean of the ratings on each item of a particular instrument for Society A versus Society B, Society A versus Society C, and so on for all pairs of societies. The *Q* correlations computed between every pair of societies in which ratings for a particular instrument (e.g., the ASR) were obtained were then averaged to compute the omnicultural mean *Q* correlation between rankings of item ratings for that particular instrument. The omnicultural mean *Q* correlation for every instrument across samples from many different societies for ages 1½–5, 6–18, 18–59, and 60–90+ was in the .70s (Rescorla, Achenbach, et al., 2012; Rescorla, Ivanova, et al., 2012; Rescorla et al., 2011; Rescorla, Achenbach, Ivanova, Turner, Althoff, et al., 2016; Rescorla,

Achenbach, Ivanova, Turner, Árnadóttir, et al., 2016; Rescorla et al., 2020). These large omnicultural mean *Q* correlations indicate considerable similarity in the problem items that tended to receive relatively low, medium, or high ratings from different kinds of informants rating individuals of different ages across many different societies on every inhabited continent. Moreover, the finding that the omnicultural mean *Q* correlation for every instrument was in the .70s, despite differences among the instruments, societies, samples, age ranges, and raters, indicates a striking degree of uniformity in the quantitative measurement of item structures across populations around the world.

The multicultural work presented to this point suggests similarities in the factor and item structure of the ASEBA instruments across societies around the world, however, these findings do not necessarily mean that scale scores were similar in different societies, nor for different genders, nor for different ages within the age ranges for which each instrument was designed. To test possible societal, gender, and age differences in the magnitudes of problem scale scores, analyses of variance (ANOVAs) were used to compare scores on all scales of each instrument for the societies from which population samples were assessed with each instrument (Rescorla, Achenbach, et al., 2012; Rescorla, Ivanova, et al., 2012; Rescorla et al., 2011; Rescorla, Achenbach, Ivanova, Turner, Althoff, et al., 2016; Rescorla, Achenbach, Ivanova, Turner, Árnadóttir, et al., 2016; Rescorla et al., 2020). For each instrument, the effects of gender, age, and interactions on problem scales ranged from nonsignificant to very small, according to Cohen's (Cohen, 1988) criteria for effect sizes (ESs) in ANOVAs. The effects of differences among societies were significant for all problem scales scored from all ASEBA instruments for ages 1½–90+ years, with ESs ranging from very small to large, according to Cohen's criteria. Interestingly, when the largest societal ESs were identified for each instrument, 27 of the 33 largest ESs were for internalizing scales. This suggests that societal differences affect the actual prevalence of internalizing problems more than other problems and/or that societal differences affect self- and informant perceptions of internalizing problems more than other problems. The other problems that show smaller societal differences than internalizing problems include not only problems scored on externalizing scales but also problems assessed by scales for attention problems and scales designated as functional impairment, memory/cognition problems, dementia problems, and psychotic problems scored from both the OASR and OABCL.

These results provide some of the strongest evidence of differences in levels of mental health problems across different societies. On most ASEBA instruments, the means of the problem scale scores were distributed approximately normally around the average of the mean problem scale scores for all the societies, that is, around the omnicultural mean. For example, for the mean CBCL/6-18 Total Problems scores were compared for 42 societies. Mean raw scores ranged from just over a mean score of 13 for Japan to near 40 for Brazil with an omnicultural mean of 24.0 (SD=6.74). Twenty-six of the counties were within one standard deviation of the omnicultural mean. This held across measures with approximately two-thirds of the societies' mean Total Problems scores on a particular measure being within $\pm$1 *SD* of the omnicultural mean. These results suggest that application of norms derived in the United States to a child in Japan or Brazil would not be appropriate. To allow this information to inform clinical practice in societies around the world, multicultural norms were constructed for ASEBA instruments (Achenbach & Rescorla, 2007, 2010, 2015, 2019).

The steps for deriving multicultural norms were as follows. First, the mean Total Problems scores were computed for a particular instrument (e.g., the Child Behavior Checklist for children ages 6 to 18) for the normative sample from each available society. Next, societies having mean Total Problems scores >1 *SD* below the omnicultural mean were designated as Group 1, that is, societies having relatively low problem scores on that instrument. Societies having mean Total Problems scores ± 1 *SD* from the omnicultural mean were designated as Group 2, that is, societies having intermediate problem scores on that instrument. And societies having mean Total Problems scores >1 *SD* above the omnicultural mean were designated as Group 3, that is, societies having relatively high problem scores. Next, a cumulative frequency distribution of scores on a given problem scale were computed in a given society's sample, separately for each gender within each age range for which the instrument was normed (e.g., the CBCL/6-18 has separate norms for each gender at ages 6–11 and 12–18). The cumulative frequency distribution generated a percentile for each raw scale score. The percentiles obtained for scores in all a particular group's samples for a particular problem scale were then averaged to form a multicultural cumulative frequency distribution for that scale. Normalized *T* scores were then assigned on the basis of the averaged percentiles. This process allows for clinicians in societies around the world to immediately obtain norms that are relevant for their society rather than relying on thresholds and expectations from the limited set of countries in which most mental health research is done. There are no other measures of psychopathology for which such information is widely available.

Summary

The pillars reviewed in this chapter provide the basis for an assessment approach that is based on observations from all informants with potentially useful information, a taxonomy of psychopathology that is grounded in empirical constructs of psychopathology, and data-informed interpretation of assessment results based on one's developmental stage and societal context. It is also the only assessment system within psychopathology that is so closely tied to a single researcher. At the same time, the system was constructed at each step to minimize the importance of the beliefs, theories, biases, hypotheses, and notions of researchers and clinicians alike. Dr. Achenbach's role was to step out of the way and to allow the data to speak for itself. This approach has allowed the ASEBA system to be a robust tool for all of those who are interested in lifespan psychopathology. The sections below review the applications of this system to clinicians, researchers, and trainees.

Application to Clinical Practice

The system is first and foremost a set of tools for the rigorous assessment of developmental psychopathology. As such, ASEBA instruments continue to be among the most widely used assessment measures for psychopathology in the world, particularly for the assessment of mental health problems in childhood and adolescence. This is not an accident. Dr. Achenbach designed the measures with a focus on early-life psychopathology and with the goal to maximize their usefulness for clinicians.

ASEBA instruments can be used in many settings with many service models and requiring little clinician time or cost. The full-length instruments described can be completed in about 10 to 20 minutes on paper or online. Briefer instruments are available for follow-up assessments. Instruments completed on paper can be scored by clerical workers on hand-scored profiles or can be entered into computers for scoring and storing data. Instruments can be completed online using desktops, laptops, tablets, and smart phones. When entered online, the data are scored automatically for access by clinicians. For informants who cannot complete the instruments independently, interviewers with no specialized training—such as receptionists—can read the items aloud and enter the responses. PC and Web versions of ASEBA can immediately generate profiles of scale scores displayed in relation to multicultural norms appropriate for each informant, comparisons of item ratings by different informants, and *Q* correlations among 0-1-2 ratings of problem items by different informants. This information and their graphical output provide a set of tools for explaining the assessment results and rationale for treatment plans with individuals and their families in a manner that can be easily understood.

Dr. Achenbach's goal was not only to create a set of tools to meet clinicians' current needs, but he often talked about creating tools that could also *improve* clinical practice. Below are three examples of these efforts.

Family-based Assessment. It is a truism of child psychology and psychiatry that all clinicians aspire to care that is family based. For this aspiration to be realized, however, it is necessary to have assessment tools that integrate information obtained *from* and *about* different family members. ASEBA accomplishes this, in part, through its suite of multi-informant instruments that cover the lifespan. ASEBA instruments allow for each member of the family to provide information about themselves as well as on multiple other family members using a harmonized set of instruments. But this is often not sufficient. To facilitate family-based assessment and treatment, results from these assessments need to be integrated on the family level. Dr. Achenbach and colleagues developed the Multicultural Family Assessment Module (MFAM; Achenbach et al., 2015) to meet this goal. The MFAM can be used to display bar graphs of problem scale scores obtained from ratings of a child by multiple informants on side-by-side bar graphs (as seen in **Figure 11.2**), but the MFAM also displays bar graphs of problem scales scored from forms completed by each parent about themselves or other family members about each parent. Furthermore, the MFAM generates bar graphs that *compare* child and adult scale scores on syndromes that have counterparts for ages 6–18 and 18–59.

This tool can be used to facilitate family-based feedback on the assessment process. Clinicians can show MFAM bar graphs to family members and encourage them to point out similarities and differences between magnitudes of scores obtained from different informants' ratings. The MFAM can also reveal similarities and differences between child and parent scores on counterpart scales. For example, if a mother and daughter both have elevated scores on the Anxious/Depressed syndrome scale, this suggests that they may both need help in this area. Even when a child is the identified client, elevated problem scale scores for parents and marked discrepancies between parents' ratings of themselves and their partner may provide a basis for interventions to help the parents. This process of reviewing results for multiple family members at the same time shifts the focus on treatment from a single identified patient to a more accurate picture of how each family member is functioning and how their functioning may affect one another. Recent work suggests that this process of reviewing assessment results for the family, rather than just a given child, improves parental mental health literacy and increases parental attitudinal engagement with health supports and services (Ivanova et al., 2024).

Measurement-based Care. Repeated assessment of key clinical targets through care has been identified as an evidence-based tool to improve clinical outcomes (Bickman, 2008; Bickman et al., 2016; Garland et al., 2010; Weisz et al., 2015;, 2017). This process typically involves assessing mental health problems over intervals of days or weeks. The full-length ASEBA forms discussed thus far may provide a broad assessment of functioning initially, but the length of such forms may not be well-suited to a frequent reassessment schedule. To address this concern, Dr. Achenbach developed the Brief Problem Monitor (BPM; (Achenbach & Ivanova, 2018; Achenbach et al., 2011, 2017)).

The BPM measures can be filled out online or on paper in one to two minutes to assess internalizing, externalizing, attention problems, and Total Problems over a period specified by the clinician (e.g., seven days). The BPM measure changes occur in relation to interventions rendered over limited time intervals, such as contingency management to reduce a child's disruptive behavior in a classroom. Separate versions of the BPM are designed for completion by parents and teachers of 6 to 18-year-olds, for completion by 11 to 18-year-old youths to describe themselves, and for completion by 18 to 59-year-olds and their collaterals. Software for scoring the various versions of the BPM generates bar graphs comparing scale scores obtained from multiple informants on multiple occasions, plus line graphs comparing trajectories of scores over 2 to 10 occasions. Like the other instruments described in this chapter, the scale scores are standardized for the gender and age of the person being assessed, the type of informant (parent, teacher, youth, adult, adult collateral), and the appropriate multicultural norm group.

Outcome-based Care. It is increasingly recognized that evidence-based assessments of progress and outcomes are essential for optimizing and evaluating mental health and related services. It is also rarely practiced. This process involves comparing data from standardized intake assessments with the same measures administered during and/or at the end of the service. This can be accomplished with ASEBA forms as well as other assessment instruments. It is not always possible, however, to be sure whether these changes meet a reasonable standard to indicate improvement. To address this concern, Dr. Achenbach developed the Progress & Outcomes App (P&O; T. Achenbach, 2020).

The P&O app generates bar graphs of ASEBA problems and strengths scale scores obtained for individual clients on two or more occasions. In order to determine whether changes in scale scores exceed chance expectations, the P&O app does statistical computations based on the standard error of measurement. Without the clinician doing any statistics, the P&O app's output displays asterisks with bars for scale scores that show changes exceeding chance expectations from one assessment to another. Data from multiple informants can be included in the output, which clinicians can show clients for discussion of the evidence for improvement and/or possible needs for changes in services. The manual provides details of various ways to evaluate progress and outcomes for groups as well as for individual clients.

Application to Research

Many of the features that make ASEBA instruments attractive for clinical care also make them well-suited to research. These instruments have been used in over 11,000 publications from over 100 societies and cultural groups to address the full breadth of research topics related to mental health (Pascal, 2021). The following sections provide illustrations of a few research applications of the empirically based assessment instruments and constructs derived from them that were the focus of Dr. Achenbach during his career.

Societal and Cultural Contributions to Mental Health. It is unknown how much variation in mental health problems is associated with differences between societal and cultural groups, over and above differences among individuals. "Societies" refer to geopolitically demarcated populations having a dominant language, including countries but also populations that are not countries, such as Puerto Rico. "Culture" is defined as an accumulated set of beliefs, values, and social norms that impact the behavior of a relatively large group of people (Lustig et al., 2006). To identify major cultural groups around the world, the Global Leadership and Organizational Effectiveness (GLOBE) study obtained measures of attitudes and other characteristics of people in 62 societies (Hofstede, 1984; House et al., 2004). Using these international data plus previous research and theory, over 200 scholars from 69 societies classified societies into 10 culture clusters designated as Anglo, Confucian Asia, Eastern Europe, Germanic Europe, Latin America, Latin Europe, Middle East, Nordic Europe, and Southern Asia.

Because of the broad range of societies in which the ASEBA instruments have been studied, it is possible to leverage these samples to test the effects of culture cluster, society, and individual differences on mental health problems. Rescorla et al. (Rescorla et al., 2019) applied this approach to CBCL/6-18 ratings of problems for 72,493 children from 45 societies. They then used hierarchical linear modeling (HLM) to estimate the percentage of variance in 17 CBCL problem scale scores accounted for by culture cluster, society, and individual differences. Averaged across all 17 problem scale scores, Rescorla et al. found that a mean of 4.2% of variance was accounted for by culture cluster, 6.1% of variance was accounted for by society, and 89.8% of variance was accounted for by individual differences and variables not measured in the HLM model. Although the effects of society and culture cluster were each significant at $p<.001$, together they accounted for a mean of only 10.3% of the variance in scale scores. In a subsequent study, Ivanova et al. (Ivanova et al., 2022) applied similar HLM analyses to scores obtained on 17 YSR problem scales paralleling the 17 CBCL scales. The scores were obtained by 39,849 youths who completed YSRs in 38 societies from the 10 GLOBE culture clusters. Averaged across all 17 problem scales, Ivanova et al. found that a mean of 1.5% of variance was accounted for by culture cluster, 6.0% of variance was accounted for by society, and 92.5% of variance was accounted for by individual differences. Compared to the 4.2% for the CBCL/6-18, less variance in the YSR was accounted for by culture cluster (1.5%) and about the same amount of variance (6.1% vs. 6.0%) was accounted for by society.

Continuity of Mental Health Problems. The U.S. National Longitudinal Study initially assessed a nationally representative sample of 2,734 4–16-year-olds on the basis of home interviews in which parents rated their children's problems and competencies and reported on many child and family variables. Subsequent assessments three, six, and nine years later included parent, teacher, and self-ratings on instruments that assessed ASEBA models for psychopathology, plus reports of signs of disturbance, such as suicidal behavior, receipt of mental health services, trouble with the law, substance abuse, and being fired from a job.

Scores on scales for empirically based syndromes significantly predicted scores on the corresponding syndrome scales and various signs of disturbance at three-, six-, and nine-year intervals, after controlling for numerous demographic and other variables (Achenbach et al., 1995a, 1995b, 1995c, 1998). The empirically based syndrome models for psychopathology and the assessment procedures for operationalizing them thus revealed considerable continuity in patterns of problems from early childhood to adolescence and from adolescence to young adulthood. In a comparison of syndrome scores across a 23-year period, overall total problem scores increased by two points with only a modest increase in the levels of service use (Achenbach et al., 2003). Interestingly, the relative rank ordering of items across 23 years was stable with Q correlations of 0.94. The findings also showed that the empirically based competence scores could predict signs of disturbance that were not included in the syndrome models. Parent, teacher, and self-ratings on competence and adaptive strengths scales added significantly to the prediction of signs of disturbance, especially to the prediction of total disturbance scores, which aggregated the different signs of disturbance.

Interplay between SES and Psychopathology. Wadsworth and Achenbach (Wadsworth & Achenbach, 2005) tested the hypothesis that factors associated with SES contribute to differences in levels of psychopathology in the U.S. National Longitudinal Study. Early cross-sectional studies had found that psychopathology is more prevalent among lower SES than upper SES adults (e.g., Hollingshead & Redlich, 1958). However, cross-sectional studies of adults cannot test the extent to which the higher prevalence results from "downward drift" in SES among adults whose psychopathology impairs their ability to maintain higher SES or instead results from a higher initial incidence of psychopathology among lower SES people. To prevent the possible contribution of downward drift from confounding research on relations between SES and psychopathology, it is necessary to compare the developmental courses of psychopathology for children whose families differ in SES. This excludes downward drift as an explanation, because children's psychopathology is not apt to cause their families' SES to drift downward.

Over the nine years of the U.S. National Longitudinal Study, it was found that the scores of significantly more children from low SES than high SES families increased from the normal to the clinical range on the ASEBA anxious/depressed, somatic complaints, thought problems, rule-breaking behavior, and aggressive behavior syndromes. These findings supported the hypothesis that low SES predicts developmental increases in the problems modeled by these syndromes. However, it was also found that, among children who initially obtained clinically elevated scores on the withdrawn/depressed and somatic complaints syndromes, fewer from low SES than higher SES families subsequently obtained scores in the normal range. For these particular kinds of problems, the evidence thus indicated a greater "cumulative prevalence" of elevated problem scores among lower than higher SES children. In other words, there was a greater developmental accumulation of (i.e., less remission of) elevated scores among children from lower than higher SES families. Both the greater incidence and greater cumulative prevalence of particular kinds of problems thus contributed to the higher prevalence of psychopathology among those born into lower than higher SES families.

Application to Training

It is still the case that there are substantial gaps between research and practice in the field of mental health (Weisz et al., 2005, 2015). While the evidence base for empirically supported treatments for child mental health concerns is promising (Weisz et al., 2013), the vast majority of such studies involve children who have not been referred for care, therapists who are not active practitioners but trainees, and situations in which the care is not provided in community settings (Weisz et al., 2014). When mental health treatments are studied in "real world" settings, the results are not as encouraging (Copeland et al., 2022; Jörg et al., 2012). In response to this gap, it is essential that training be structured around evidence-based assessment and follow-up (in addition to the long-time focus on evidence-based interventions).

Empirically based instruments serve as tools for obtaining multi-informant evidence regarding the problems and strengths of clients across the lifespan. For trainees who are new to clinical care, the broad-based perspective enabled by the ASEBA instruments helps to ensure that clinical "tunnel vision" does not result in incomplete treatment-planning. By routinely using developmentally appropriate ASEBA instruments, trainees can obtain well-differentiated pictures of clients' specific problems and strengths, as seen from multiple perspectives. The multiple informant comparisons highlighted in the ASEBA results provide an "ice breaker" for new clinicians to start often challenging conversations with families on their different perspectives on the child's/patient's functioning as well as why problems may vary from context to context. These conversations are challenging to new clinicians, as they can be viewed (incorrectly) as questioning a given informant's perspective rather than an opportunity to better understand the family's particular profile of challenges. Trainees can also compare aggregations of problems and strengths to norms based on population samples of peers in terms of standardized scale scores for empirically based constructs. Rather than getting caught up in unhelpful conversations about whether the youth meets criteria for a diagnosis (with all of its attendant stigma), the clinician can focus the conversation on how the level of problems compares to peers in a manner similar to how physicians deal with challenging conversations related to BMI and obesity. Trainees can structure conversations with clients by asking clients whether they have questions about the forms and can then ask them about items they endorsed and comments they entered. For example, if a youth endorsed the

YSR item "I can't get my mind off certain thoughts" and entered "death" in the space for a description, the trainee can say, "I see that you can't get your mind off death. Please tell me more about that." Finally, the BPM forms provide a quick and easy way for clinicians to return to these empirical anchors throughout the treatment process to evaluate progress and improvement based on external standards.

Conclusion

Dr. Achenbach began work on understanding patterns of mental health problems close to 60 years ago in graduate school in Minnesota. His doctoral dissertation, a factor analytic study of children's psychiatric symptoms, laid the groundwork for the ASEBA instruments and established the first principle of listening to the data. His program of research closely hewed to the content of that early work as well as to its empirical approach. I had the honor of working with Dr. Achenbach during his last few years. I remember a particular publication in which a coauthor and collaborator of Dr. Achenbach and me noted that the results turned out exactly as he expected they would have, given his theoretical background. In reply, Dr. Achenbach noted that as an empiricist he had no expectations that the analysis would turn out one way or the other. He went on to explain that the most important research questions are those whose findings are interesting regardless of the result. It is this clear-eyed empiricism and single-minded focus on only the most important questions that is Dr. Achenbach's greatest legacy. They enabled the great contributions to developmental science that have been recounted in this chapter. But most important, they provide a template for how to carry on his work and to advance the science of developmental psychopathology.

References

Achenbach, T. (2020). *ASEBA manual for assessing progress and outcomes of problems and strengths.* University of Vermont Research Center for Children, Youth, & Families.

Achenbach, T., & Ivanova, M. (2018). *Manual for the ASEBA® Brief Problem Monitor™ for ages 18–59.* University of Vermont, Research Center for Children, Youth, and Families.

Achenbach, T., McConaughy, S., Ivanova, M., & Rescorla, L. (2011). *Manual for the ASEBA Brief Problem Monitor (BPM).* ASEBA, 1–33.

Achenbach, T., McConaughy, S., Ivanova, M., & Rescorla, L. (2017). *Manual for the ASEBA Brief Problem Monitor for ages 6–18 (BPM/6–18).* University of Vermont Research Center for Children, Youth, and Families.

Achenbach, T., & Rescorla, L. (2007). *Multicultural supplement to the manual for the ASEBA school-age forms & profiles.* University of Vermont Research Center for Children, Youth, & Families.

Achenbach, T., & Rescorla, L. (2015). *Multicultural supplement to the manual for the ASEBA adult forms & profiles.* University of Vermont Research Center for Children, Youth, and Families.

Achenbach, T., & Rescorla, L. (2019). *Multicultural supplement to the manual for the ASEBA older adult forms & profiles.* University of Vermont Research Center for Children, Youth, and Families.

Achenbach, T., Rescorla, L., & Ivanova, M. (2015). *Guide to family assessment using the ASEBA.* University of Vermont Research Center for Children, Youth, and Families.

Achenbach, T. M. (1966). The classification of children's psychiatric symptoms: A factor-analytic study. *Psychological Monographs, 80*, 1–37.

Achenbach, T. M. (1978). Psychopathology in childhood: Research problems and issues. *Journal of Consulting and Clinical Psychology, 46*, 759–776.

Achenbach, T. M. (2006). As others see us: Clinical and research implications of cross-informant correlations for psychopathology. *Current Directions in Psychological Science, 15*(2), 94–98.

Achenbach, T. M. (2020). Bottom-up and top-down paradigms for psychopathology: A half-century odyssey. *Annual Review of Clinical Psychology, 16*, 1–24.

Achenbach, T. M., Dumenci, L., & Rescorla, L. A. (2003). Are American children's problems still getting worse? A 23-year comparison. *Journal of Abnormal Child Psychology*, *31*(1), 1–11.

Achenbach, T. M., & Edelbrock, C. S. (1986). *Manual for the Teacher's Report Form and Teacher Version of the Child Behavior Profile*. University of Vermonrt Department of Psychiatry.

Achenbach, T. M., Howell, C. T., McConaughy, S. H., & Stanger, C. (1995a). Six-year predictors of problems in a national sample of children and youth: II. Signs of disturbance. *Journal of the American Academy of Child and Adolescent Psychiatry*, *34*, 488–498.

Achenbach, T. M., Howell, C. T., McConaughy, S. H., & Stanger, C. (1995b). Six-year predictors of problems in a national sample of children and youth: I. Cross-informant syndromes. *Journal of the American Academy of Child and Adolescent Psychiatry*, *34*, 336–347.

Achenbach, T. M., Howell, C. T., McConaughy, S. H., & Stanger, C. (1995c). Six-year predictors of problems in a national sample: III. Transitions to young adult syndromes. *Journal of the American Academy of Child and Adolescent Psychiatry*, *34*, 658–669.

Achenbach, T. M., Howell, C. T., McConaughy, S. H., & Stanger, C. (1998). Six-year predictors of problems in a national sample: IV. Young adult signs of disturbance. *Journal of the American Academy of Child & Adolescent Psychiatry*, *37*(7), 718–727.

Achenbach, T. M., Ivanova, M. Y., & Rescorla, L. A. (2017). Empirically based assessment and taxonomy of psychopathology for ages 1½–90+ years: Developmental, multi-informant, and multicultural findings. *Comprehensive Psychiatry*, *79*, 4–18. https://doi.org/https://doi.org/10.1016/j.comppsych.2017.03.006

Achenbach, T. M., Ivanova, M. Y., Rescorla, L. A., Turner, L. V., & Althoff, R. R. (2016). Internalizing/externalizing problems: Review and recommendations for clinical and research applications. *Journal of the American Academy of Child & Adolescent Psychiatry*, *55*(8), 647–656. https://doi.org/https://doi.org/10.1016/j.jaac.2016.05.012

Achenbach, T. M., Krukowski, R. A., Dumenci, L., & Ivanova, M. Y. (2005). Assessment of adult psychopathology: Meta-analyses and implications of cross-informant correlations. *Psychological Bulletin*, *131*(3), 361–382.

Achenbach, T. M., McConaughy, S. H., & Howell, C. T. (1987). Child/adolescent behavioral and emotional problems: Implications of cross-informant correlations for situational specificity. *Psychological Bulletin*, *101*, 213–232.

Achenbach, T. M., Newhouse, P. A., & Rescorla, L. A. (2004). *Manual for the ASEBA Older Adult: Forms and Profiles: For Ages 60-90+: An integrated system of multi-informant assessment*. ASEBA.

Achenbach, T. M., & Rescorla, L. A. (2000). *Manual for the ASEBA Preschool Forms and Profiles: An integrated system of multi-informant assessment*. University of Vermont Department of Psychiatry.

Achenbach, T. M., & Rescorla, L. A. (2001a). *Manual for the ASEBA school-age forms & profiles: An integrated system of multi-informant assessment. University of Vermont*. Research Center for Children, Youth, & Families.

Achenbach, T. M., & Rescorla, L. A. (2001b). *Manual for the ASEBA School-Age Forms and Profiles*. University of Vermont Research Center for Children, Youth, & Families.

Achenbach, T. M., & Rescorla, L. A. (2003). *Manual for the ASEBA Adult Forms and Profiles*. University of Vermont Research Center for Children, Youth, & Families.

Achenbach, T. M., & Rescorla, L. A. (2010). *Multicultural supplement to the manual for the ASEBA preschool forms & profiles: Child behavior checklist for ages 1 ½–5, language development survey, caregiver-teacher report form; an integrated system of multi-informant assessment*. University of Vermont, Research Center for Children Youth, & Families.

Achenbach, T. N., & Edelbrock, C. S. (1983). *Manual for the child behavior checklist and revised profile*. University of Vermont.

American Psychiatric Association. (1952). *Diagnostic and statistical manual of mental disorders—DSM-I* (1 ed.). American Psychiatric Association.

Bickman, L. (2008). A measurement feedback system (MFS) is necessary to improve mental health outcomes. *Journal of the American Academy of Child and Adolescent Psychiatry*, *47*(10), 1114.

Bickman, L., Douglas, S. R., De Andrade, A. R. V., Tomlinson, M., Gleacher, A., Olin, S., & Hoagwood, K. (2016). Implementing a measurement feedback system: A tale of two sites. *Administration and*

Policy in Mental Health and Mental Health Services Research, *43*(3), 410–425. https://doi.org/10.1007/s10488-015-0647-8

Cohen, J. (1988). *Statistical power analysis for the behavioral sciences*. Erlbaum.

Conners, C. K. (1969). A teacher rating scale for use in drug studies with children. *American Journal of Psychiatry*, *126*, 884–888.

Copeland, W. E., Tong, G., & Shanahan, L. (2022). Do "real world" childhood mental health services reduce risk for adult psychiatric disorders? *Journal of the American Academy of Child & Adolescent Psychiatry*, *61*(8), 1041–1049.e1047. https://doi.org/https://doi.org/10.1016/j.jaac.2021.12.014

De Los Reyes, A., Augenstein, T. M., Wang, M., Thomas, S. A., Drabick, D. A., Burgers, D. E., & Rabinowitz, J. (2015). The validity of the multi-informant approach to assessing child and adolescent mental health. *Psychological Bulletin*, *141*(4), 858.

De Los Reyes, A., & Kazdin, A. E. (2005). Informant discrepancies in the assessment of childhood psychopathology: A critical review, theoretical framework, and recommendations for further study. *Psychological Bulletin*, *131*(4), 483.

Garland, A. F., Bickman, L., & Chorpita, B. F. (2010). Change what? Identifying quality improvement targets by investigating usual mental health care. *Administration and Policy in Mental Health and Mental Health Services Research*, *37*, 15–26.

Hermans, H. J., & Kempen, H. J. (1998). Moving cultures: The perilous problems of cultural dichotomies in a globalizing society. *American Psychologist*, *53*(10), 1111.

Hewitt, L. E., & Jenkins, R. L. (1946). Fundamental patterns of maladjustment; the dynamics of their origin; a statistical analysis based upon five hundred case records of children examined at the Michigan Child Guidance Institute.

Hofstede, G. (1984). *Culture's consequences: International differences in work-related values* (Vol. 5). Sage Publications.

Hollingshead, A. B., & Redlich, F. C. (1958). *Social class and mental illness*. John Wiley & Sons, Inc.

House, R. J., Hanges, P. J., Javidan, M., Dorfman, P. W., & Gupta, V. (2004). *Culture, leadership, and organizations: The GLOBE study of 62 societies*. Sage publications.

Ivanova, M. Y., Achenbach, T. M., Dumenci, L., Rescorla, L. A., Almqvist, F., Weintraub, S., Bilenberg, N., Bird, H., Chen, W. J., Dobrean, A., Döpfner, M., Erol, N., Fombonne, E., Fonseca, A. C., Frigerio, A., Grietens, H., Hannesdóttir, H., Kanbayashi, Y., Lambert, M., . . . Verhulst, F. C. (2007). Testing the 8-syndrome structure of the Child Behavior Checklist in 30 societies. *Journal of Clinical Child & Adolescent Psychology*, *36*(3), 405–417. https://doi.org/10.1080/15374410701444363

Ivanova, M. Y., Achenbach, T. M., Rescorla, L. A., Bilenberg, N., Bjarnadottir, G., Denner, S., Dias, P., Dobrean, A., Doepfner, M., Esmaeili, E. M., Frigerio, A., Gudmundsson, H. S., Jusiene, R., Kristensen, S., Lecannelier, F., Leung, P. W. L., Lima, V. S., Liu, J., Lobel, S. P., . . . Verhulst, F. C. (2011). Syndromes of preschool psychopathology reported by teachers and caregivers in 14 societies using the Caregiver-Teacher Report Form (C-TRF). *Journal of Early Childhood and Infant Psychology*, *7*, 87–103. https://www.proquest.com/scholarly-journals/syndromes-preschool-psychopathology-reported/docview/1461359982/se-2

Ivanova, M. Y., Achenbach, T. M., Rescorla, L. A., Dumenci, L., Almqvist, F., Bathiche, M., Bilenberg, N., Bird, H., Domuta, A., Erol, N., Fombonne, E., Fonseca, A., Frigerio, A., Kanbayashi, Y., Lambert, M. C., Leung, P., Liu, X., Minaei, A., Roussos, A., . . . Verhulst, F. C. (2007). Testing the Teacher's Report Form syndromes in 20 societies. *School Psychology Review*, *36*(3), 468–483. https://doi.org/10.1080/02796015.2007.12087934

Ivanova, M. Y., Achenbach, T. M., Rescorla, L. A., Dumenci, L., Almqvist, F., Bilenberg, N., Bird, H., Broberg, A. G., Dobrean, A., Döpfner, M., Erol, N., Forns, M., Hannesdottir, H., Kanbayashi, Y., Lambert, M. C., Leung, P., Minaei, A., Mulatu, M. S., Novik, T., . . . Verhulst, F. C. (2007). The generalizability of the Youth Self-Report syndrome structure in 23 societies. *Journal of Consulting and Clinical Psychology*, *75*(5), 729–738. https://doi.org/10.1037/0022-006X.75.5.729

Ivanova, M. Y., Achenbach, T. M., Rescorla, L. A., Harder, V. S., Ang, R. P., Bilenberg, N., Bjarnadottir, G., Capron, C., De Pauw, S. S. W., Dias, P., Dobrean, A., Doepfner, M., Duyme, M., Eapen, V., Erol, N., Esmaeili, E. M., Ezpeleta, L., Frigerio, A., Gonçalves, M. M., . . . Verhulst, F. C. (2010). Preschool psychopathology reported by parents in 23 societies: Testing the seven-syndrome model of the Child

Behavior Checklist for ages 1.5–5. *Journal of the American Academy of Child & Adolescent Psychiatry*, *49*(12), 1215–1224. https://doi.org/https://doi.org/10.1016/j.jaac.2010.08.019

Ivanova, M. Y., Achenbach, T. M., Rescorla, L. A., Turner, L. V., Ahmeti-Pronaj, A., Au, A., Maese, C. A., Bellina, M., Caldas, J. C., & Chen, Y.-C. (2015). Syndromes of self-reported psychopathology for ages 18–59 in 29 societies. *Journal of Psychopathology and Behavioral Assessment*, *37*(2), 171–183.

Ivanova, M. Y., Achenbach, T. M., Rescorla, L. A., Turner, L. V., Árnadóttir, H. A., Au, A., Caldas, J. C., Chaalal, N., Chen, Y. C., da Rocha, M. M., Decoster, J., Fontaine, J. R. J., Funabiki, Y., Guðmundsson, H. S., Kim, Y. A., Leung, P., Liu, J., Malykh, S., Marković, J., . . . Zasępa, E. (2015). Syndromes of collateral-reported psychopathology for ages 18–59 in 18 societies. *International Journal of Clinical and Health Psychology*, *15*(1), 18–28. https://doi.org/https://doi.org/10.1016/j.ijchp.2014.07.001

Ivanova, M. Y., Achenbach, T. M., Rescorla, L. A., Turner, L. V., Dumas, J. A., Almeida, V., Anafarta-Sendag, M., Bite, I., Boomsma, D. I., Caldas, J. C., Capps, J. W., Chen, Y.-C., Colombo, P., da Silva Oliveira, M., Dobrean, A., Erol, N., Frigerio, A., Funabiki, Y., Gedutienė, R., . . . Zasępa, E. (2020). The generalizability of Older Adult Self-Report (OASR) syndromes of psychopathology across 20 societies. *International Journal of Geriatric Psychiatry*, *35*(5), 525–536. https://doi.org/https://doi.org/10.1002/gps.5268

Ivanova, M. Y., Achenbach, T. M., Rescorla, L. A., Turner, L. V., Dumas, J. A., Almeida, V., Anafarta-Sendag, M., Carlos Caldas, J., Chen, Y.-C., da Silva Oliveira, M., Erol, N., Funabiki, Y., Guðmundsson, H. S., Kim, Y. A., Leite, M., Liu, J., Markovic, J., Misiec, M., Oh, K. J., . . . Zasępa, E. (2021). The generalizability of empirically derived syndromes of collateral-reported elder psychopathology across 11 societies. *Research in Nursing & Health*, *44*(4), 681–691. https://doi.org/https://doi.org/10.1002/nur.22161

Ivanova, M. Y., Achenbach, T. M., Turner, L., Almqvist, F., Begovac, I., Bilenberg, N., Bird, H., Broberg, A. G., Cordova Calderon, M. A., & Chahed, M. (2022). Effects of individual differences, society, and culture on youth-rated problems and strengths in 38 societies. *Journal of Child Psychology and Psychiatry*.

Ivanova, M. Y., Hall, A., Weinberger, S., Buckingham, S. L., Copeland, W. E., Crockett, P., Dainer-Best, J., D'Alberto, C., Dewey, L., Foret, D., Galano, M., Goodrich, L., Holly, L., Lane, N. E., Leahy, M., Lerner, M., Marsh, J., McGinnis, E. W., Paiva-Salisbury, M., . . . Hudziak, J. J. (2024). A pilot randomized controlled trial of the Family Assessment and Feedback Intervention (FAFI): Effects on mental health literacy and attitudinal engagement with health supports and services. *Child Psychiatry & Human Development*. https://doi.org/10.1007/s10578-024-01707-0

Jörg, F., Ormel, J., Reijneveld, S. A., Jansen, D. E., Verhulst, F. C., & Oldehinkel, A. J. (2012). Puzzling findings in studying the outcome of "real world" adolescent mental health services: The TRAILS study. *PLoS ONE*, *7*(9), e44704.

Kleinman, A. M. (1977). Depression, somatization and the "new cross-cultural psychiatry." *Social Science & Medicine (1967)*, *11*(1), 3–9.

Lustig, M. W., Koester, J., & Halualani, R. (2006). *Intercultural competence: Interpersonal communication across cultures*. Pearson/A and B.

Meyer, G. J., Finn, S. E., Eyde, L. D., Kay, G. G., Moreland, K. L., Dies, R. R., Eisman, E. J., Kubiszyn, T. W., & Reed, G. M. (2001). Psychological testing and psychological assessment: A review of evidence and issues. *American Psychologist*, *56*(2), 128.

Miller, L. C. (1967). Louisville Behavior Check List for males, 6–12 years of age. *Psychological Reports*, *21*(3), 885–896.

Pascal, J. A., T. M. (2021). *Bibliography of published studies using the ASEBA*. University of Vermont, Research Center for Children, Youth, and Families

Pike, K. L. (1967). Language in relation to a unified theory of the structure of human *behavior*. Walter de Gruyter.

Prince, M., Patel, V., Saxena, S., Maj, M., Maselko, J., Phillips, M. R., & Rahman, A. (2007). No health without mental health. *The Lancet*, *370*(9590), 859–877.

Quay, H. C. (1964). Dimensions of personality in delinquent boys as inferred from the factor analysis of case history data. *Child Development*, 479–484.

Quay, H. C. (1977). Measuring dimensions of deviant behavior: The Behavior Problem Checklist. *Journal of Abnormal Child Psychology*, *5*, 277–287.

Rescorla, L., Ivanova, M. Y., Achenbach, T. M., Begovac, I., Chahed, M., Drugli, M. B., Emerich, D. R., Fung, D. S. S., Haider, M., Hansson, K., Hewitt, N., Jaimes, S., Larsson, B., Maggiolini, A., Marković, J., Mitrović, D., Moreira, P., Oliveira, J. T., Olsson, M., . . . Zhang, E. Y. (2012). International Epidemiology of Child and Adolescent Psychopathology II: Integration and applications of dimensional findings from 44 societies. *Journal of the American Academy of Child & Adolescent Psychiatry*, *51*(12), 1273–1283.e1278. https://doi.org/https://doi.org/10.1016/j.jaac.2012.09.012

Rescorla, L. A., Achenbach, T. M., Ivanova, M. Y., Bilenberg, N., Bjarnadottir, G., Denner, S., Dias, P., Dobrean, A., Döpfner, M., Frigerio, A., Gonçalves, M., Guðmundsson, H., Jusiene, R., Kristensen, S., Lecannelier, F., Leung, P. W. L., Liu, J., Löbel, S. P., Machado, B. C., . . . Verhulst, F. C. (2012). Behavioral/emotional problems of preschoolers: Caregiver/teacher reports from 15 societies. *Journal of Emotional and Behavioral Disorders*, *20*(2), 68–81. https://doi.org/10.1177/1063426611434158

Rescorla, L. A., Achenbach, T. M., Ivanova, M. Y., Harder, V. S., Otten, L., Bilenberg, N., Bjarnadottir, G., Capron, C., De Pauw, S. S. W., Dias, P., Dobrean, A., Döpfner, M., Duyme, M., Eapen, V., Erol, N., Esmaeili, E. M., Ezpeleta, L., Frigerio, A., Fung, D. S. S., . . . Verhulst, F. C. (2011). International comparisons of behavioral and emotional problems in preschool children: Parents' reports from 24 societies. *Journal of Clinical Child & Adolescent Psychology*, *40*(3), 456–467. https://doi.org/10.1080/15374416.2011.563472

Rescorla, L. A., Achenbach, T. M., Ivanova, M. Y., Turner, L. V., Althoff, R. R., Árnadóttir, H. A., Au, A., Bellina, M., Caldas, J., & Chen, Y.-C. (2016). Problems and adaptive functioning reported by adults in 17 societies. *International Perspectives in Psychology*, *5*(2), 91–109.

Rescorla, L. A., Achenbach, T. M., Ivanova, M. Y., Turner, L. V., Árnadóttir, H., Au, A., Caldas, J. C., Chen, Y.-C., Decoster, J., Fontaine, J., Funabiki, Y., Guðmundsson, H. S., Leung, P., Liu, J., Maraš, J. S., Marković, J., Oh, K. J., da Rocha, M. M., Samaniego, V. C., . . . Zasepa, E. (2016). Collateral reports and cross-informant agreement about adult psychopathology in 14 societies. *Journal of Psychopathology and Behavioral Assessment*, *38*(3), 381–397. https://doi.org/10.1007/s10862-016-9541-2

Rescorla, L. A., Althoff, R. R., Ivanova, M. Y., & Achenbach, T. M. (2019). Effects of society and culture on parents' ratings of children's mental health problems in 45 societies. *European Child & Adolescent Psychiatry*, *28*(8), 1107–1115.

Rescorla, L. A., Genaro, B., Ivanova, M. Y., & International, A. C. (2020). International comparisons of emotionally reactive problems in preschoolers: CBCL/1½–5 findings from 21 societies. *Journal of Clinical Child & Adolescent Psychology*, *49*(6), 773–786. https://doi.org/10.1080/15374416.2019.1650366

Wadsworth, M. E., & Achenbach, T. M. (2005). Explaining the link between low socioeconomic status and psychopathology: Testing two mechanisms of the social causation hypothesis. *Journal of Consulting and Clinical Psychology*, *73*(6), 1146.

Weisz, J. R., Doss, A. J., & Hawley, K. M. (2005). Youth psychotherapy outcome research: A review and critique of the evidence base. *Annual Review of Psychology*, *56*, 337–363.

Weisz, J. R., Krumholz, L. S., Santucci, L., Thomassin, K., & Ng, M. Y. (2015). Shrinking the gap between research and practice: Tailoring and testing youth psychotherapies in clinical care contexts. *Annual Review of Clinical Psychology*, *11*, 139–163.

Weisz, J. R., Kuppens, S., Eckshtain, D., Ugueto, A. M., Hawley, K. M., & Jensen-Doss, A. (2013). Performance of evidence-based youth psychotherapies compared with usual clinical care: A multilevel meta-analysis. *JAMA Psychiatry*, *70*(7), 750–761.

Weisz, J. R., Kuppens, S., Ng, M. Y., Eckshtain, D., Ugueto, A. M., Vaughn-Coaxum, R., Jensen-Doss, A., Hawley, K. M., Krumholz Marchette, L. S., & Chu, B. C. (2017). What five decades of research tells us about the effects of youth psychological therapy: A multilevel meta-analysis and implications for science and practice. *American Psychologist*, *72*(2), 79.

Weisz, J. R., Ng, M. Y., & Bearman, S. K. (2014). Odd couple? Reenvisioning the relation between science and practice in the dissemination-implementation era. *Clinical Psychological Science*, *2*(1), 58–74.

World Health Organization. (2001). The World Health Report 2001: Mental health: new understanding, new hope.

CHAPTER 12

Clinical Staging

A Bridge between Categories and Dimensions

CRISTINA MEI, BARNABY NELSON, DOMINIC DWYER, AND PATRICK D. MCGORRY*

Overview

THE concept of staging was conceived in the early 20th century as a method to enhance patient outcomes and improve the utility of diagnosis in medicine. Its success as a classification system has seen it widely used in many medical disciplines (e.g., oncology, diabetes, and rheumatology) where distinct clinical stages along illness continua have been defined with therapeutic and prognostic implications. In psychiatry, the utility of diagnosis in guiding clinical decision-making (e.g., selecting a treatment approach, predicting course or prognosis) has been largely absent in conventional diagnostic systems (DSM and ICD), especially in young people with emerging disorders. These systems have not sufficiently optimized early detection, intervention, and prevention, owing to their emphasis on relatively late-stage disorders that fail to capture emerging and early stages of illness and their patterns of progression and comorbidity. The adjunct use of clinical staging in psychiatry to improve the utility of diagnosis across the full spectrum of clinical need, including presentations that have a need for care but fall below diagnostic thresholds, represents a major diagnostic advance. We describe the conceptual basis of clinical staging, the progress achieved in establishing its validity, and its implications for treatment.

Current Diagnostic Systems

For four decades, diagnosis in psychiatry has been dominated by expert-derived categories that have limited clinical utility and have failed to sufficiently enhance treatment selection, prognostication, and the linking of discrete diagnostic entities to their underlying mechanisms (First et al., 2018; Hickie et al., 2013b; Maj, 2020; McGorry & van Os 2013). The validity of these categories, which is grounded on the assumption that disparate diagnoses arise from independent pathways (McGorry, 2013), is challenged by the fact that they have not adequately facilitated attempts to identify disorder-specific markers of pathophysiology and treatment response, despite intense research efforts (Abi-Dargham et al., 2023; Stephan et al., 2016). These

* Reproduced and adapted with permission from C. Mei, B. Nelson, A. Giersch, P. D. McGorry (2023). Classification en stades cliniques (staging) des troubles mentaux [clinical staging of mental disorders]. EMC—Psychiatrie. France: Elsevier. We thank Anne Giersch, who contributed to the previous version of this chapter.

diagnostic categories largely represent fully established adult-type mental disorders (McGorry et al., 2007), a focus that neglects key differences in clinical presentations associated with stage of illness and age of onset. This has delayed and impeded early detection and intervention of less specific early clinical phenotypes or warning signs of specific syndromes. Most mental disorders have their onset between childhood and early adulthood (Caspi et al., 2020; Kessler et al., 2005; McGrath et al., 2023; Solmi et al., 2022), with early stages or subthreshold states largely characterized by transdiagnostic and fluctuating non-specific symptoms (Hartmann et al., 2019) that may potentially develop into clear and more stable syndromes (McGorry & van Os, 2013). This process is marked by substantial comorbidity (Caspi et al., 2020; Plana-Ripoll et al., 2019) and both homotypic (i.e., a subthreshold state preceding its corresponding syndrome) and heterotypic continuity (i.e., symptoms of one disorder evolving into another disorder) (Destrée et al., 2024; Hartmann et al., 2021; Lahey et al., 2014; Scott et al., 2021). These patterns of emergence highlight a fundamental weakness of siloed and static diagnostic approaches and point to the need for transdiagnostic systems with a developmental perspective (McGorry & Nelson, 2016; Poletti & Raballo 2021; Shah et al., 2020).

Clinical Staging

Clinical staging in psychiatry has been proposed as a more refined form of diagnosis that can complement traditional diagnostic systems, bridging the current disconnect among diagnosis, treatment, and prognosis (McGorry & Hickie 2019; McGorry et al., 2006). Since the initial proposal of staging for affective disorders (Fava & Kellner, 1993), clinical staging in psychiatry has been extensively refined to incorporate a range of mental disorders in a single model in line with their transdiagnostic and pluripotent nature—that is, the potential for symptoms to develop into different syndromes (Hickie et al., 2019; Hickie et al., 2013a; McGorry & Hickie 2019; McGorry et al., 2006; Shah et al., 2020). This all-encompassing approach is supported by evidence of shared etiological mechanisms across mental disorders (Gandal et al., 2018; Goodkind et al., 2015; Hollander et al., 2020; Hyman, 2019; Romer et al., 2021), and the existence of a general psychopathology factor ("*p*" factor) that cuts across major psychiatric syndromes (Caspi & Moffitt, 2018). It is also supported by key learnings from the early psychosis paradigm. First, full-threshold psychosis may not necessarily be preceded by attenuated psychotic symptoms (i.e., progression may follow a homotypic or heterotypic course) (Lee et al., 2018; Shah et al., 2017), making the detection of individuals at risk of developing psychosis more complex, especially as there is currently no specific predictive biomarker. Second, several studies have identified that rates of transition to psychosis in high-risk cohorts are declining (Simon et al., 2014; Yung et al., 2007) and that substantial proportions of ultra high risk for psychosis cohorts may have incident or persistent non-psychotic disorders (Beck et al., 2019; Lin et al., 2015; Spiteri-Staines et al., in press). Thus, prevention will be severely limited if it exclusively adopts a single disorder approach (McGorry et al., 2018). While separate staging models have been proposed for individual diagnoses, for example, depression, bipolar disorder, and psychosis (Berk et al., 2007; Carrión et al., 2017; Hetrick et al., 2008), transdiagnostic clinical staging can fully accommodate heterotypic continuity, unlike approaches confined to diagnostic siloes.

Clinical staging in psychiatry adds a longitudinal and developmental approach to diagnosis. It aims to determine where an individual lies along the potential evolution of illness: asymptomatic but at risk (Stage 0), help-seeking with distress (Stage 1a), attenuated syndromes (Stage 1b), first treated episode (Stage 2), persistence or recurrence (Stage 3), and treatment resistance (Stage 4) (Figure 12.1) (McGorry & Hickie, 2019). While this approach incorporates a dimensional model of mental illness, it retains a categorical framework that can be linked to

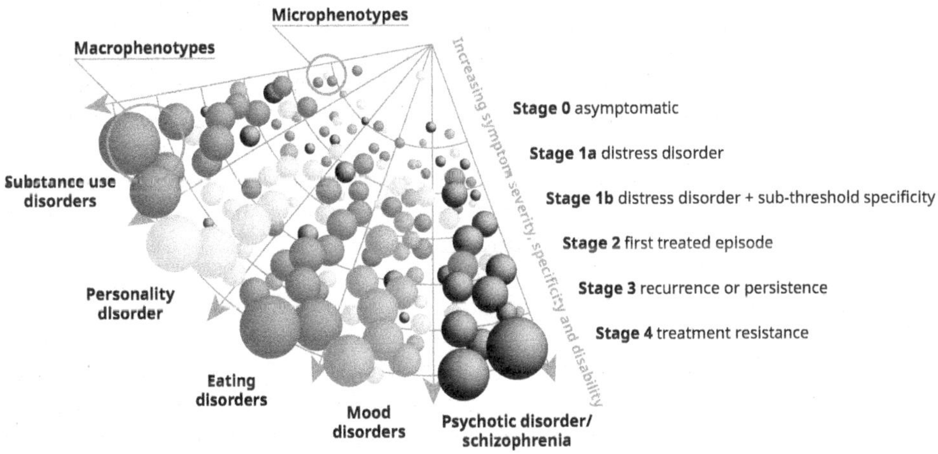

FIGURE 12.1 Clinical staging model illustrating clusters of early and overlapping symptoms (microphenotypes) and their potential progression into clear, and often comorbid, syndromes (macrophenotypes). Reproduced and adapted from McGorry and Mei (2021) with permission.

underlying neurobiological changes and treatment needs. The advantage of adopting a hybrid model is that it may increase the clinical utility of dimensional approaches (e.g., as seen in other medical areas such as the management of hypertension), since clinical decision-making is a largely binary process (Kendler, 2018). This requires that dimensional approaches have identifiable and meaningful thresholds that create categories, which are then linked to the potential benefits and risks of available therapeutic approaches. Within a clinical staging model, these categories or boundaries between stages also create a heuristic framework to research and clarify stage-specific neurobiological markers, which has the potential to inform the development of novel stage-based interventions (McGorry et al., 2014; McGorry & Mei, 2021).

Unlike traditional diagnostic frameworks, clinical staging in psychiatry captures the early manifestations of mental ill-health—that is, mixed and fluid symptomatology that do not meet threshold-level criteria, particularly seen in young people. As these early manifestations are often not recognized by conventional diagnostic systems, they have traditionally been excluded from care, where service eligibility remains largely based on meeting criteria for caseness (Hickie et al., 2013a; McGorry & Nelson, 2016). Transdiagnostic staging acknowledges that these early overlapping and non-specific symptoms may, over time, evolve into traditional syndromes while recognizing their extensive comorbidity and their dynamic trajectories that often traverse diagnostic boundaries (Caspi et al., 2020; McGrath et al., 2020; Plana-Ripoll et al., 2019). While staging can accommodate the inclusion of traditional diagnostic labels, particularly for the late stages of illness, this is dependent on their capacity and utility in guiding treatment selection (e.g., clozapine, lithium) (McGorry & van Os, 2013).

While staging places emphasis on the evolution of illness, the model fully recognizes that mental disorders are not invariably progressive; progression across stages is avertable and recovery at any stage of illness is possible. However, there is an underlying assumption that earlier clinical stages are associated with a lower risk of transition to later stages and less severe clinical and functional outcomes. These assumptions have been validated: help-seeking young people at Stage 1b (27.6%) are more likely to transition to a full-threshold disorder (Stage 2) than those at Stage 1a (8.5%) by 12-month follow-up (Destrée et al., 2024); and individuals at Stage 1b are more likely to disengage from education/employment and develop suicidal ideations and circadian disturbances than Stage 1a, while those at Stage 2+ are at higher risk of circadian disturbances than Stage 1b (Capon et al., 2022). Also, the prospect of recovery increases when treatment is delivered during early clinical stages that are marked by less severe symptomatic and functional impairment and have not reached neurobiological thresholds associated with later stages (Carpenter et al., 2019; McGorry et al., 2014; McGorry & Hickie, 2019; McGorry & Mei, 2021). The model is unidirectional; even if symptomatic and functional recovery is achieved, an individual is not reassigned to an earlier stage, as the underlying illness mechanisms may not have reversed, though they are plastic and dynamic in many respects (Hickie et al., 2013a; Shah et al., 2020).

Stage 0: Asymptomatic

Individuals at Stage 0 are asymptomatic and non-help-seeking, but are considered at risk of developing a mental disorder due to factors such as history of serious mental illness in a first-degree relative or exposure to trauma during childhood or adolescence. Individuals classified as being at Stage 0 may show subtle structural changes within the body of the hippocampus compared to healthy controls with no family history of serious mental illness (Nogovitsyn et al., 2020) and small deficits in IQ, verbal knowledge, and working memory (Velthorst et al., 2021).

Stages 1a and 1b: Distress Disorder with or without Subthreshold Specificity

Stage 1 encompasses the early phases of illness associated with professional help-seeking. Stages 1a and 1b each constitutes approximately 30–60% of young people who seek help at primary care youth mental health services (Filia et al., 2021; Iorfino et al., 2019; Purcell et al., 2015). Stage 1a is generally characterized by distress and non-specific symptoms, while features of Stage 1b include attenuated syndromes with increased symptom severity and functional impairment (Hickie et al., 2013a; Iorfino et al., 2019; Romanowska et al., 2020). Presenting clinical features may include anxiety and depressive symptoms, subthreshold manic and psychotic experiences, or other signs of more specific syndromes (Carpenter et al., 2019; Hickie et al., 2013a; Iorfino et al., 2019). A subset of young people at Stage 1a (approximately 37%) may present with complex clinical presentations (e.g., subthreshold manic and psychotic experiences, self-harm, low social and occupational functioning) and may be at high risk of progression to Stage 1b (Iorfino et al., 2019). Individuals at Stage 1b may meet criteria for DSM or ICD diagnoses; however, presenting symptoms have not reached the threshold of a Stage 2 disorder, which prompts a change in the type or intensity of treatment (Hickie et al., 2013a). Stage 1b cases are at risk of developing a range of mental disorders, even when specific syndromal at-risk criteria are met (e.g., psychosis risk, borderline personality disorder risk), supporting the conceptual foundation of transdiagnostic staging (Destrée et al., 2024; Hartmann et al., 2021). For example, Scott et al. (2021) found that individuals with self-reported subthreshold psychotic experiences were 17.3 times as likely to meet criteria for psychosis (homotypic evolution) and 5.8 times as likely to meet criteria for hypo/mania (heterotypic evolution) than individuals who did not meet "at risk" criteria for mood or psychotic syndromes. For those with self-reported subthreshold depression, they were more than three times as likely to develop depression (homotypic evolution) or hypo/mania and approximately twice as likely to develop psychosis (heterotypic evolution) than those without a subthreshold syndrome.

In addition to differential rates of progression to Stage 2, the distinction between Stages 1a and 1b is supported at a neurobiological level. While young people at Stage 1a demonstrate volume reductions in the limbic system that are largely within hippocampal subregions, those at Stage 1b show more extensive volume reductions across the hippocampal, amygdala, and thalamus subregions (Nogovitsyn et al., 2020). The authors concluded that differential patterns of volume deficits within the limbic system may be indicative of progression across early clinical stages in individuals at risk of serious mental illness (Nogovitsyn et al., 2020). In terms of neurocognition, Stage 1b is associated with lower composite scores than Stage 1a (Romanowska et al., 2018) and an intermediate profile between healthy controls and Stage 2/3 (i.e., Stages 2 and 3 pooled together) (Hermens et al., 2013). While Stages 1a and 1b are both associated with significantly worse sleep outcomes than are healthy controls (including reductions in sleep latency and subjective sleep quality, and greater daytime dysfunction and use of sleep medications), those in Stage 1b show the highest levels of overall sleep dysfunction than do healthy controls and Stages 0 and 1a (Stowkowy et al., 2020). Furthermore, transition from Stage 1b to Stage 2 has been associated with increased sleep-wake disturbances at baseline (Iorfino et al., 2019).

Stage 2: First Treated Episode

Approximately 13–28% of young people at Stage 1b transition to Stage 2 (Cross et al., 2017, Destrée et al., 2024; Hickie et al., 2013a; Iorfino et al., 2019). The risk of transition is greater for those presenting with an array of symptomatology across syndromes (i.e., meeting criteria for three or more at-risk groups—psychosis, bipolar disorder, major depressive disorder, and borderline personality disorder) (Destrée et al., 2024). Individuals at Stage 1a are at lower risk of progression to full-threshold Stage 2 disorder, occurring in 3–9% of cases (Destrée et al., 2024; Iorfino et al., 2019). This progression across clinical stages signifies the need for a change in treatment approach (e.g., the commencement of antidepressant or antipsychotic medication). At this stage, individuals present with clear and sustained features of, for example, psychotic, manic, depressive, or borderline disorders, with comorbidity being common.

Validation of the clinical high at-risk mental state (CHARMS) criteria, which aim to identify help-seeking young people at transdiagnostic risk for Stage 2 psychosis, bipolar disorder, major depressive disorder, and borderline personality disorder, indicates that 96% of transitions from Stage 1b to Stage 2 are initially to severe depression (Destrée et al., 2024). This is despite the sample (n=121) meeting at-risk criteria for a range of conditions. While this confirms both heterotypic and homotypic progression, it also suggests that severe depression may be an initial "gateway" to Stage 2 as subsequent transitions to other disorders (psychosis and borderline personality disorder) occurred in a subset of participants after the onset of severe depression over the 12-month follow-up period. However, larger studies with a longer follow-up period are required to confirm findings.

The boundary between Stages 1 and 2 has been evaluated in neurobiological studies, with findings indicating discernible patterns of neurobiological change between help-seeking individuals/attenuated syndromes and established disorders (Carpenter et al., 2019; McGorry et al., 2014; McGorry & Hickie, 2019; McGorry & Mei, 2021). With regard to neuroimaging, key findings for Stage 2/3 participants include significantly decreased frontal gray matter volume compared to Stage 1a/b (Lagopoulos et al., 2012), greater disruptions in white matter integrity than Stage 1b in the left anterior corona radiata and the body of the corpus callosum (Lagopoulos et al., 2013; Sacks et al., 2021), and increased radial diffusivity in the left anterior corona radiata (Lagopoulos et al., 2013). Neurocognitive studies indicate that Stage 2/3 is associated with greater levels of impairment compared to Stage 1b (Hermens et al., 2013). However, both groups (Stages 1b and 2/3) show similar improvement over time except in the domain of verbal memory, which has been shown to decline in individuals at Stage 2/3 and may represent a stage-specific marker (Tickell et al., 2019). Regarding circadian profiles, those classified at Stage 2 and above have significantly reduced levels of melatonin secretion and shorter phase angles (corresponding to the time difference between melatonin onset and sleep onset) compared to Stage 1b, with lower levels of melatonin associated with reduced performance on verbal memory tasks (Naismith et al., 2012).

Stages 3 and 4: Recurrence, Persistence, or Treatment Resistance

Stages 3 and 4 represent the late or end stages of an established illness, often resembling traditional diagnostic categories (e.g., schizophrenia, personality disorder, bipolar disorder), with progression to these stages largely reflecting illness recurrence or persistence (Carpenter et al., 2019; McGorry & Hickie, 2019). By definition, individuals assigned to Stage 3 have experienced Stage 2 syndromes with persistence or incomplete remission at 12 months after service entry or recurrence of illness following three months of complete recovery (Carpenter et al., 2019; Hickie et al., 2013a). Substages of Stage 3 may include an incomplete remission from a first episode (3a), recurrence or relapse that stabilizes with treatment (3b), and multiple relapses (3c) (McGorry et al., 2010). Some individuals may transition directly from Stage 2 to Stage 4, bypassing Stage 3. At Stage 4, individuals present with chronic and unremitting illness after receiving relevant services for at least two years (Carpenter et al., 2019; Hickie et al., 2013a). Prevention and treatment of comorbidity, including alcohol and other substance misuse, remain a key focus. At Stages 3 and 4, individuals often experience marked functional limitations and may demonstrate stable or progressive neurocognitive impairment (Allott, 2019). While there are neuroimaging findings related to this established stage of illness, including reduced hippocampal volume and enlarged ventricles for schizophrenia and white matter hyperintensities for major depressive and bipolar disorders, there is considerable overlap across diagnostic groupings in terms of brain regions implicated, with no conclusive neural markers for specific disorders (Bartholomeusz & Pantelis 2019). This supports the agnostic approach of transdiagnostic clinical staging.

Treatment Implications

While clinical staging has potential to guide mental health service delivery across the life span (Sawrikar et al., 2021), it is especially relevant to the care of young people (Shah et al., 2022) given that the majority of high-prevalence mental disorders have their onset by young adulthood (Caspi et al., 2020; Kessler et al., 2005; McGrath et al., 2023; Solmi et al., 2022) and that affected young people have the poorest access to professional care (de Girolamo et al., 2012). Clinical staging is developmentally sensitive in that it can distinguish early phases of illness (Stages 1a/1b), which typically emerge in younger age groups, from established illness (Stage 2 or later) often seen in young adults (Hickie et al., 2013a; Iorfino et al., 2019). Unlike current diagnostic approaches, clinical staging provides an early intervention and preventive framework that can adequately respond to subthreshold or emerging mental disorders, including presentations characterized by non-specific, mixed, and fluctuating symptoms, and heterotypic continuity (McGorry & Hickie, 2019). The application of staging to youth mental health has been found to be a good fit (i.e., stages can be differentiated based on clinical measures and risk of transition to later stages) (Addington et al., 2019; Iorfino et al., 2019), indicating its potential to support the allocation of care that is matched to current level of need and risk of illness progression. Clinical staging has been increasingly applied to youth mental health services to identify stage-specific treatment needs and outcomes, as outlined in this section. While improved outcomes have been achieved when applying a staged approach to psychotic disorders (Correll et al., 2018; Fusar-Poli et al., 2017; Mei et al., 2021), the clinical utility of staging for other presentations is an emerging area, and further research is needed examining its ability to enhance patient outcomes, the selection and personalization of treatments, and the prediction of prognosis (Shah et al., 2020).

A key principle of clinical staging is that mental health care, particularly for young people, is provided at the right time in a manner that is safe and effective, meaning, that it is proportionate to the presenting clinical picture (McGorry & Hickie, 2019). Interventions are stage-specific, targeting an individual's current mental health needs in addition to their risk of illness progression. The choice of intervention approach is guided by risk/benefit considerations and shared decision-making to ensure that the type, intensity, and duration of the intervention is matched to the individual's stage of illness, their risk profile, and their needs and preferences (McGorry & Hickie, 2019; McGorry et al., 2006). The staging model proposes that treatment delivered earlier in the illness course is more likely to be simple, benign, and effective than is treatment delivered at a later stage. This is in accordance with the differential patterns of impairment, risk of illness progression, and neurobiological changes across stages, as outlined in this chapter.

At Stage 0, universal (targeting the entire population) or selective (targeting subgroups at greater risk) prevention strategies are indicated to prevent the onset of anxiety, mood, psychotic, or other mental disorders. Potential strategies include mental health literacy interventions, family education, drug education, and brief cognitive skills training (McGorry et al., 2010).

Treatment at Stage 1 is often focused on alleviating distressing symptoms, reducing the risk of suicidality or self-harm, and preventing progression to Stage 2 disorders and the development of comorbidity. Here, a careful balance between overtreatment and undertreatment is required, although the latter is more typically the norm, as individuals experiencing the early stages of illness are regularly excluded from mental health care until criteria for a full-threshold disorder is met. Determining this balance may be best guided by data from sequential clinical trials, particularly those that involve transdiagnostic samples, which could assist in the identification of subgroups of individuals who require more or less intensive intervention (McGorry et al., 2023).

For Stage 1a, individuals generally benefit from brief low-intensity psychosocial interventions (Cross et al., 2016). Support may be provided via online platforms for individuals with low needs and clinical risks (e.g., very mild or mild symptoms and functional impairment, low risk of self-harm), allowing greater service resources to be directed toward individuals at later stages who present with greater complexity and require more intensive intervention (Davenport et al., 2020). An uncontrolled pilot study of young people accessing a digital mental health platform at headspace in Australia (a youth mental health service where the majority of users are at Stage 1) found that the platform was associated with high satisfaction, safety, and perceived helpfulness, as well as significant improvements in psychological distress and well-being, perceived stress, depression, loneliness, social support, autonomy, and self-competence (Alvarez-Jimenez et al., 2020).

Patients at Stage 1b generally require combinations of treatment (e.g., CBT and psychotropic medication) and prolonged care (>12 months), reflecting their more pronounced impairment at service entry, their greater risk of progression to severe mental illness, and their pattern of recovery (Cross et al., 2016). Transdiagnostic treatments have been developed, such as the Unified Protocol (Barlow et al., 2017), and may be suitable as a Stage 1b intervention. This is an area for future research, although recent evidence suggests that a transdiagnostic, digital, and clinically and peer-moderated treatment platform targeting psychological distress and psychosocial functioning may be a promising intervention for individuals at

Stage 1b (van Doorn et al., 2023). While the first 12 months of service contact represents the highest risk of transition (Hickie et al., 2013a), individuals at risk of psychosis may remain at long-term risk (up to 10 years) and may require ongoing monitoring (Nelson et al., 2013). Treatment outcomes for individuals at Stage 1b are diverse, with 23–33% showing reliable improvement and 5–13% showing reliable deterioration by six months on measures of distress, symptomatology, and functioning (Cross et al., 2018), highlighting the need for regular outcome monitoring (across all clinical stages) to ensure that the type and intensity of treatment is matched to an individual's evolving needs (Cross et al., 2019). At Stages 1a and 1b, a strong focus should be placed on targeting functional outcomes (Bowman et al., 2020), with transition to a subsequent stage predicted by poor social functioning and tenuous engagement with education and employment (Cross et al., 2017; Iorfino et al., 2019). Other key treatment targets, which are also predictors of transition to Stage 1b or Stage 2, include subthreshold manic and psychotic experiences, negative symptoms, self-harm, and circadian disturbances (Cross et al., 2017; Iorfino et al., 2019). These predictive factors are largely transdiagnostic, that is, they predict evolution to a range of discrete disorders.

Progression to Stage 2 signifies that an individual has reached a threshold that requires more intensive and specific care for a period of two to five years (Cross et al., 2019). Approaches may include psychotropic medication, intensive psychosocial interventions, and vocational and educational support. Reducing the duration of untreated illness is critical for improving treatment response. Individuals who have a shorter duration of illness may constitute a specific subgroup within Stage 2, with implications for treatment selection (Maj et al., 2021). For example, findings from a randomized controlled trial indicate that among the clinical population of patients with first episode psychosis, a small and highly selective subgroup who present with a short duration of untreated psychosis (less than six months) and low risk of self-harm or aggression (<5 on the Brief Psychiatric Rating Scale-4 Suicidality and Hostility subscales) may benefit from intensive psychosocial intervention and close monitoring without antipsychotic medication within the first six months of treatment engagement (Francey et al., 2020). While these results are promising, the long-term outcomes are unclear, as it was not established that psychosocial treatment was non-inferior to antipsychotic medication at 12 and 24 months (Francey et al., 2020). Individuals with persistent or recurrent illness (Stages 3 and 4) will require a longer duration of care, that is, at least several years, with a focus on treating comorbidity and persistent symptoms, functional recovery, quality of life, and relapse prevention.

Future Directions and Conclusions

Recognizing the limited utility of traditional silo-based and static diagnostic systems, transdiagnostic clinical staging offers an early detection, early intervention, and preventive framework. The model incorporates the earliest stages of illness evolution, bracketing concepts of threshold caseness or diagnostic labels. Unlike existing systems, staging recognizes the dynamic nature of mental disorders and actively facilities the delivery of effective and safe intervention at the right time, with a pre-emptive focus. To this end, methodologically sophisticated trials are needed to enhance the selection of stage-specific and patient-matched interventions. The recently proposed international consensus statement and clinical research agenda for staging may further advance the knowledge base and potentially refine the boundaries between stages (Shah et al., 2020). Future research may also be guided by recommendations that aim to improve the reporting and quality of transdiagnostic research more broadly (Fusar-Poli et al., 2019). While early research findings support the validity of staging mental disorders, it is an evolving approach and, as new evidence emerges, it has potential to be refined and enhanced. For example, a limitation of the current staging model, which ultimately reflects the field more broadly, is the lack of validated biomarkers of illness onset and progression. However, a strength of the model is that it provides a transdiagnostic framework that can be used to evaluate the pathophysiology of mental disorders and biomarkers for stage of illness. Extension of the staging model to include validated biomarkers or pathophysiological mechanisms that are linked to treatment decisions and prognostication is the ultimate aspiration, which would have considerable implications for personalized care.

References

Abi-Dargham, A., Moeller, S. J., Ali, F., DeLorenzo, C., Domschke, K., Horga, G., Jutla, A., Kotov, R., Paulus, M. P., Rubio, J. M., Sanacora, G., Veenstra-VanderWeele, J., & Krystal, J. H. (2023). Candidate biomarkers in psychiatric disorders: State of the field. *World Psychiatry, 22*: 236–262.

Addington, J., Liu, L., Goldstein, B.I., Wang, J., Kennedy, S. H., Bray, S., Lebel, C., Stowkowy, J., & MacQueen, G. (2019). Clinical staging for youth at-risk for serious mental illness. *Early Intervention in Psychiatry, 13*: 1416–1423.

Allott K. (2019). Staging of cognition in psychiatric illness. In P. D. McGorry & I. B. Hickie (Eds.), *Clinical staging in psychiatry: Making diagnosis work for research and treatment* (pp. 140–171). Cambridge University Press.

Alvarez-Jimenez, M., Rice, S., D'Alfonso, S., Leicester, S., Bendall, S., Pryor, I., Russon, P., McEnery, C., Santesteban-Echarri, O., Da Costa, G., Gilbertson, T., Valentine, L., Solves, L., Ratheesh, A., McGorry, P. D., & Gleeson, J. (2020). A novel multimodal digital service (moderated online social therapy+) for help-seeking young people experiencing mental ill-health: Pilot evaluation within a national youth E-mental health service. *Journal of Medical Internet Research* 22: e17155.

Barlow, D. H., Farchione, T. J., Bullis, J. R., Gallagher, M. W., Murray-Latin, H., Sauer-Zavala, S., Bentley, K. H., Thompson-Hollands, J., Conklin, L. R., Boswell, J. F., Ametaj, A., Carl, J. R., Boettcher, H. T., & Cassiello-Robbins, C. (2017). The Unified Protocol for Transdiagnostic Treatment of Emotional Disorders compared with diagnosis-specific protocols for anxiety disorders: A randomized clinical trial. *JAMA Psychiatry* 74: 875–884.

Bartholomeusz, C. F., & Pantelis, C. (2019). Neuroimaging and staging: Do disparate mental illnesses have distinct neurobiological trajectories? In P. D. McGorry & I. B. Hickie (Eds.), *Clinical staging in psychiatry: Making diagnosis work for research and treatment* (pp. 103–139). Cambridge University Press.

Beck, K., Andreou, C., Studerus, E., Heitz, U., Ittig, S., Leanza, L., & Riecher-Rossler, A. (2019). Clinical and functional long-term outcome of patients at clinical high risk (CHR) for psychosis without transition to psychosis: A systematic review. *Schizophrenia Research 210*: 39–47.

Berk, M., Conus, P., Lucas, N., Hallam, K., Malhi, G. S., Dodd, S., Yatham, L. N., Yung, A., & McGorry P. (2007). Setting the stage: From prodrome to treatment resistance in bipolar disorder. *Bipolar Disorders*, *9*: 671–678.

Bowman, S., McKinstry, C., Howie, L., McGorry, P. (2020). Expanding the search for emerging mental ill health to safeguard student potential and vocational success in high school: A narrative review. *Early Intervention in Psychiatry, 14*: 655–676.

Capon, W., Hickie, I. B., Varidel, M., Prodan, A., Crouse, J. J., Carpenter, J. S., Cross, S. P., Nichles, A., Zmicerevska, N., Guastella, A. J., Scott, E. M., Scott, J., Shah, J., & Iorfino, F. (2022). Clinical staging and the differential risks for clinical and functional outcomes in young people presenting for youth mental health care. *BMC Medicine* 20: 479.

Carpenter, J. S., Iorfino, F., Cross, S. P., Davenport, T. A., Hermens, D. F., Rohleder, C., Crouse, J. J., Leweke, F. M., Koethe, D., Guastella, A. J., Naismith, S. L., Scott, J., Scott, E. M., & Hickie, I. B. (2019). Combining clinical stage and pathophysiological mechanisms to understand illness trajectories in young people with emerging mood and psychotic syndromes. *Medical Journal of Australia* 211: S12–22.

Carrión, R. E., Correll, C. U., Auther, A. M., & Cornblatt, B. A. (2017). A severity-based clinical staging model for the psychosis prodrome: Longitudinal findings from the New York recognition and prevention program. *Schizophrenia Bulletin*, *43*: 64–74.

Caspi, A., Houts, R. M., Ambler, A., Danese, A., Elliott, M. L., Hariri, A., Harrington, H., Hogan, S., Poulton, R., Ramrakha, S., Rasmussen, L. J. H., Reuben, A., Richmond-Rakerd, L., Sugden, K., Wertz, J., Williams, B. S., & Moffitt, T. E. (2020). Longitudinal assessment of mental health disorders and comorbidities across 4 decades among participants in the Dunedin birth cohort study. *JAMA Network Open* 3: e203221.

Caspi, A., & Moffitt, T. E. (2018). All for one and one for all: Mental disorders in one dimension. *American Journal of Psychiatry* 175: 831–844.

Correll, C. U., Galling, B., Pawar, A., Krivko, A., Bonetto, C., Ruggeri, M., Craig, T. J., Nordentoft, M., Srihari, V. H., Guloksuz, S., Hui, C. L. M., Chen, E. Y. H., Valencia, M., Juarez, F., Robinson, D. G., Schooler, N. R., Brunette, M. F., Mueser, K. T., Rosenheck, R. A., . . . Kane, J. M. (2018). Comparison of early intervention services vs treatment as usual for early-phase psychosis: A systematic review, meta-analysis, and meta-regression. *JAMA Psychiatry* 75: 555–565.

Cross, S. P., Davenport, T. A., Scott, E. M., Iorfino, F., Sawrikar, V., & Hickie, I. B. (2019). A service delivery model to support highly personalised and measurement-based care in youth mental health. *Medical Journal of Australia*, *211*: S42–S46.

Cross, S. P., Scott, J. L., Hermens, D. F., & Hickie, I. B. (2018). Variability in clinical outcomes for youths treated for subthreshold severe mental disorders at an early intervention service. *Psychiatric Services*, *69*: 555–561.

Cross, S. P. M., Hermens, D. F., & Hickie, I. B. (2016). Treatment patterns and short-term outcomes in an early intervention youth mental health service. *Early Intervention in Psychiatry*, *10*: 88–97.

Cross, S. P. M., Scott, J., & Hickie, I. B. (2017). Predicting early transition from sub-syndromal presentations to major mental disorders. *BJPsych Open*, *3*: 223–227.

Davenport, T. A., Cheng, V. W. S., Iorfino, F., Hamilton, B., Castaldi, E., Burton, A., Scott, E. M., & Hickie, I. B. (2020). Flip the clinic: A digital health approach to youth mental health service delivery. *JMIR Mental Health*, *7*: e24578.

de Girolamo, G., Dagani, J., Purcell, R., Cocchi, A., & McGorry, P. D. (2012). Age of onset of mental disorders and use of mental health services: Needs, opportunities and obstacles. *Epidemiology and Psychiatric Sciences*, *21*: 47–57.

Destrée, L., McGorry, P., Chanen, A., Ratheesh, A., Davey, C., Polari, A., Amminger, P., Yuen, H. P., Hartmann, J., Dwyer, D., Spooner, R., & Nelson, B. (2024). Transdiagnostic risk identification: A validation study of the Clinical High At Risk Mental State (CHARMS) criteria. *Psychiatry Research*, *333*: 115745.

Fava, G. A., & Kellner, R. (1993). Staging: A neglected dimension in psychiatric classification. *Acta Psychiatr Scand*, *87*: 225–230.

Filia, K., Rickwood, D., Menssink, J., Gao, C. X., Hetrick, S., Parker, A., Hamilton, M., Hickie, I., Herrman, H., Telford, N., Sharmin, S., McGorry, P., & Cotton, S. (2021). Clinical and functional characteristics of a subsample of young people presenting for primary mental healthcare at headspace services across Australia. *Social Psychiatry and Psychiatric Epidemiology*, *56*: 1311–1323.

First, M. B., Rebello, T. J., Keeley, J. W., Bhargava, R., Dai, Y., Kulygina, M., Matsumoto, C., Robles, R., Stona, A.-C., & Reed, G. M. (2018). Do mental health professionals use diagnostic classifications the way we think they do? A global survey. *World Psychiatry*, *17*: 187–195.

Francey, S. M., O'Donoghue, B., Nelson, B., Graham, J., Baldwin, L., Yuen, H. P., Kerr, M. J., Ratheesh, A., Allott, K., Alvarez-Jimenez, M., Fornito, A., Harrigan, S., Thompson, A. D., Wood, S., Berk, M., & McGorry, P. D. (2020). Psychosocial intervention with or without antipsychotic medication for first-episode psychosis: A randomized noninferiority clinical trial. *Schizophrenia Bulletin Open*, *1*: sgaa015.

Fusar-Poli, P., McGorry, P. D., & Kane, J. M. (2017). Improving outcomes of first-episode psychosis: An overview. *World Psychiatry*, *16*: 251–265.

Fusar-Poli, P., Solmi, M., Brondino, N., Davies, C., Chae, C., Politi, P., Borgwardt, S., Lawrie, S. M., Parnas, J., & McGuire, P. (2019). Transdiagnostic psychiatry: A systematic review. *World Psychiatry*, *18*: 192–207.

Gandal, M. J., Haney, J. R., Parikshak, N. N., Leppa, V., Ramaswami, G., Hartl, C., Schork, A. J., Appadurai, V., Buil, A., Werge, T. M., Liu, C., White, K. P., Horvath, S., & Geschwind, D. H. (2018). Shared molecular neuropathology across major psychiatric disorders parallels polygenic overlap. *Science, 359*: 693.

Goodkind, M., Eickhoff, S. B., Oathes, D. J., Jiang, Y., Chang, A., Jones-Hagata, L. B., Ortega, B. N., Zaiko, Y. V., Roach, E. L., Korgaonkar, M. S., Grieve, S. M., Galatzer-Levy, I., Fox, P. T., & Etkin, A. (2015). Identification of a common neurobiological substrate for mental Illness. *JAMA Psychiatry, 72*: 305–315.

Hartmann, J. A., McGorry, P. D., Destree, L., Amminger, G. P., Chanen, A. M., Davey, C. G., Ghieh, R., Polari, A., Ratheesh, A., Yuen, H. P., & Nelson, B. (2021). Pluripotential risk and clinical staging: theoretical considerations and preliminary data from a transdiagnostic risk identification approach. *Frontiers in Psychiatry, 11*: 553578.

Hartmann, J. A., Nelson, B., Ratheesh, A., Treen, D., & McGorry, P. D. (2019). At-risk studies and clinical antecedents of psychosis, bipolar disorder and depression: A scoping review in the context of clinical staging. *Psychological Medicine, 49*: 177–189.

Hermens, D. F., Naismith, S. L., Lagopoulos, J., Lee, R. S. C., Guastella, A. J., Scott, E. M., & Hickie, I. B. (2013). Neuropsychological profile according to the clinical stage of young persons presenting for mental health care. *BMC Psychology, 1*: 8.

Hetrick, S. E., Parker, A. G., Hickie, I. B., Purcell, R., Yung, A. R., & McGorry, P. D. (2008). Early identification and intervention in depressive disorders towards a clinical staging model. *Psychotherapy and Psychosomatics, 77*: 263–270.

Hickie, I. B., Scott, E. M., Cross, S. P., Iorfino, F., Davenport, T. A., Guastella, A. J., Naismith, S. L., Carpenter, J. S., Rohleder, C., Crouse, J. J., Hermens, D. F., Koethe, D., Markus Leweke, F., Tickell, A. M., Sawrikar, V., & Scott, J. (2019). Right care, first time: A highly personalised and measurement-based care model to manage youth mental health. *Medical Journal of Australia, 211*: S3–S46.

Hickie, I. B., Scott, E. M., Hermens, D. F., Naismith, S. L., Guastella, A. J., Kaur, M., Sidis, A., Whitwell, B., Glozier, N., Davenport, T., Pantelis, C., Wood, S. J., & McGorry, P. D. (2013a). Applying clinical staging to young people who present for mental health care. *Early Intervention in Psychiatry, 7*: 31–43.

Hickie, I. B., Scott, J., Hermens, D. F., Scott, E. M., Naismith, S. L., Guastella, A. J., Glozier, N., & McGorry, P. D. (2013b). Clinical classification in mental health at the cross-roads: Which direction next? *BMC Medicine, 11*: 125.

Hollander, J. A., Cory-Slechta, D. A., Jacka, F. N., Szabo, S. T., Guilarte, T. R., Bilbo, S. D., Mattingly, C. J., Moy, S. S., Haroon, E., Hornig, M., Levin, E. D., Pletnikov, M. V., Zehr, J. L., McAllister, K. A., Dzierlenga, A. L., Garton, A. E., Lawler, C. P., & Ladd-Acosta, C. (2020). Beyond the looking glass: Recent advances in understanding the impact of environmental exposures on neuropsychiatric disease. *Neuropsychopharmacology, 45*: 1086–1096.

Hyman. S. E. (2019). New evidence for shared risk architecture of mental disorders. *JAMA Psychiatry, 76*: 235–236.

Iorfino, F., Scott, E. M., Carpenter, J. S., Cross, S. P., Hermens, D. F., Killedar, M., Nichles, A., Zmicerevska, N., White, D., Guastella, A. J., Scott, J., McGorry, P. D., & Hickie, I. B. (2019). Clinical stage transitions in persons aged 12 to 25 years presenting to early intervention mental health services with anxiety, mood, and psychotic disorders. *JAMA Psychiatry, 76*: 1167–1175.

Kendler, K. S. (2018). Classification of psychopathology: Conceptual and historical background. *World Psychiatry, 17*: 241–242.

Kessler, R. C., Berglund, P., Demler, O., Jin, R., Merikangas, K. R., & Walters, E. E. (2005). Lifetime prevalence and age-of-onset distributions of DSM-IV disorders in the national comorbidity survey replication. *Archives of General Psychiatry, 62*: 593–602.

Lagopoulos, J., Hermens, D. F., Hatton, S. N., Battisti, R. A., Tobias-Webb, J., White, D., Naismith, S. L., Scott, E. M., Ryder, W. J., Bennett, M. R., & Hickie, I. B. (2013). Microstructural white matter changes are correlated with the stage of psychiatric illness. *Translational Psychiatry, 3*: e248.

Lagopoulos, J., Hermens, D. F., Naismith, S. L., Scott, E. M., & Hickie, I. B. (2012). Frontal lobe changes occur early in the course of affective disorders in young people. *BMC Psychiatry, 12*: 4.

Lahey, B. B., Zald, D. H., Hakes, J. K., Krueger, R. F., & Rathouz, P. J. (2014). Patterns of heterotypic continuity associated with the cross-sectional correlational structure of prevalent mental disorders in adults. *JAMA Psychiatry*, *71*: 989–996.

Lee, T. Y., Lee, J., Kim, M., Choe, E., & Kwon, J. S. (2018). Can we predict psychosis outside the clinical high-risk state? A systematic review of non-psychotic risk syndromes for mental disorders. *Schizophrenia Bulletin*, *44*: 276–285.

Lin, A., Wood, S. J., Nelson, B., Beavan, A., McGorry, P., & Yung, A. R. (2015). Outcomes of nontransitioned cases in a sample at ultra-high risk for psychosis. *American Journal of Psychiatry*, *172*: 249–258.

Maj, M. (2020). Beyond diagnosis in psychiatric practice. *Annals of General Psychiatry*, *19*: 27.

Maj, M., van Os, J., De Hert, M., Gaebel, W., Galderisi, S., Green, M. F., Guloksuz, S., Harvey, P. D., Jones, P. B., Malaspina, D., McGorry, P., Miettunen, J., Murray, R. M., Nuechterlein, K. H., Peralta, V., Thornicroft, G., van Winkel, R., & Ventura, J. (2021). The clinical characterization of the patient with primary psychosis aimed at personalization of management. *World Psychiatry*, *20*: 4–33.

McGorry, P., Keshavan, M., Goldstone, S., Amminger, P., Allott, K., Berk, M., Lavoie, S., Pantelis, C., Yung, A., Wood, S., & Hickie, I. (2014). Biomarkers and clinical staging in psychiatry. *World Psychiatry*, *13*: 211–223.

McGorry, P., & Nelson, B. (2016). Why we need a transdiagnostic staging approach to emerging psychopathology, early diagnosis, and treatment. *JAMA Psychiatry*, *73*: 191–192.

McGorry, P., & van Os, J. (2013). Redeeming diagnosis in psychiatry: Timing versus specificity. *Lancet*, *381*: 343–345.

McGorry, P. D. (2013). The next stage for diagnosis: Validity through utility. *World Psychiatry*, *12*: 213–215.

McGorry, P. D., Hartmann, J. A., Spooner, R., & Nelson, B. (2018). Beyond the "at risk mental state" concept: Transitioning to transdiagnostic psychiatry. *World Psychiatry*, *17*: 133–142.

McGorry, P. D., & Hickie, I. B. (Eds.). (2019). *Clinical staging in psychiatry: Making diagnosis work for research and treatment*.Cambridge University Press.

McGorry, P. D., Hickie, I. B., Yung, A. R., Pantelis, C., & Jackson, H. J. (2006). Clinical staging of psychiatric disorders: A heuristic framework for choosing earlier, safe and more effective interventions. *Australian and New Zealand Journal of Psychiatry*, *40*: 616–622.

McGorry, P. D., & Mei, C. (2021). Clinical staging for youth mental disorders: Progress in reforming diagnosis and clinical care. *Annual Review of Developmental Psychology*, *3*: 15–39.

McGorry, P. D., Mei, C., Amminger, G. P., Yuen, H. P., Kerr, M., Spark, J., Wallis, N., Polari, A., Baird, S., Buccilli, K., Dempsey, S.-J. A., Ferguson, N., Formica, M., Krcmar, M., Quinn, A. L., Mebrahtu, Y., Ruslins, A., Street, R., Wannan, C., . . . Nelson, B. (2023). A sequential adaptive intervention strategy targeting remission and functional recovery in young people at ultrahigh risk of psychosis: The staged treatment in early psychosis (STEP) sequential multiple assignment randomized trial. *JAMA Psychiatry*, *80*: 875–885.

McGorry, P. D., Nelson, B., Goldstone, S., & Yung, A. R. (2010). Clinical staging: A heuristic and practical strategy for new research and better health and social outcomes for psychotic and related mood disorders. *Canadian Journal of Psychiatry*, *55*: 486–497.

McGorry, P. D., Purcell, R., Hickie, I. B., Yung, A. R., Pantelis, C., & Jackson, H. J. (2007). Clinical staging: A heuristic model for psychiatry and youth mental health. *Medical Journal of Australia*, *187*: S40–42.

McGrath, J. J., Al-Hamzawi, A., Alonso, J., Altwaijri, Y., Andrade, L. H., Bromet, E. J., Bruffaerts, R., de Almeida, J. M. C., Chardoul, S., Chiu, W. T., Degenhardt, L., Demler, O. V., Ferry, F., Gureje, O., Haro, J. M., Karam, E. G., Karam, G., Khaled, S. M., Kovess-Masfety, V., . . . Zaslavsky, A. M. (2023). Age of onset and cumulative risk of mental disorders: A cross-national analysis of population surveys from 29 countries. *The Lancet Psychiatry*, *10*: 668–681.

McGrath, J. J., Lim, C. C. W., Plana-Ripoll, O., Holtz, Y., Agerbo, E., Momen, N. C., Mortensen, P. B., Pedersen, C. B., Abdulmalik, J., Aguilar-Gaxiola, S., Al-Hamzawi, A., Alonso, J., Bromet, E. J., Bruffaerts, R., Bunting, B., de Almeida, J. M. C., de Girolamo, G., De Vries, Y. A., Florescu, S., . . . de Jonge, P. (2020). Comorbidity within mental disorders: A comprehensive analysis based on 145 990 survey respondents from 27 countries. *Epidemiology and Psychiatric Sciences*, *29*: e153.

Mei, C., van der Gaag, M., Nelson, B., Smit, F., Yuen, H. P., Berger, M., Krcmar, M., French, P., Amminger, G. P., Bechdolf, A., Cuijpers, P., Yung, A. R., & McGorry, P. D. (2021). Preventive interventions for individuals at ultra high risk for psychosis: An updated and extended meta-analysis. *Clinical Psychology Review*, *86*: 102005.

Naismith, S. L., Hermens, D. F., Ip, T. K. C., Bolitho, S., Scott, E., Rogers, N. L., & Hickie, I. B. (2012). Circadian profiles in young people during the early stages of affective disorder. *Translational Psychiatry*, *2*: e123.

Nelson, B., Yuen, H. P., Wood, S. J., Lin, A., Spiliotacopoulos, D., Bruxner, A., Broussard, C., Simmons, M., Foley, D. L., Brewer, W. J., Francey, S. M., Amminger, G. P., Thompson, A., McGorry, P. D., & Yung, A. R. (2013). Long-term follow-up of a group at ultra high risk ("prodromal") for psychosis: The PACE 400 study. *JAMA Psychiatry*, *70*: 793–802.

Nogovitsyn, N., Souza, R., Muller, M., Srajer, A., Metzak, P. D., Hassel, S., Ismail, Z., Protzner, A., Bray, S. L., Lebel, C., MacIntosh, B. J., Goldstein, B. I., Wang, J., Kennedy, S. H., Addington, J., & MacQueen, G. M. (2020). Aberrant limbic brain structures in young individuals at risk for mental illness. *Psychiatry and Clinical Neurosciences*, *74*: 294–302.

Plana-Ripoll, O., Pedersen, C. B., Holtz, Y., Benros, M. E., Dalsgaard, S., De Jonge, P., Fan, C. C., Degenhardt, L., Ganna, A., Greve, A. N., Gunn, J., Iburg, K. M., Kessing, L. V., Lee, B. K., Lim, C. C. W., Mors, O., Nordentoft, M., Prior, A., Roest, A. M., . . . McGrath, J. J. (2019). Exploring comorbidity within mental disorders among a Danish national population. *JAMA Psychiatry*, *76*: 259–270.

Poletti, M., & Raballo, A. (2021). Early intervention in psychiatry through a developmental perspective. *npj Schizophrenia*, *7*: 8.

Purcell, R., Jorm, A. F., Hickie, I. B., Yung, A. R., Pantelis, C., Amminger, G. P., Glozier, N., Killackey, E., Phillips, L. J., Wood, S. J., Harrigan, S., Mackinnon, A., Scott, E., Hermens, D. F., Guastella, A. J., Kenyon, A., Mundy, L., Nichles, A., Scaffidi, A., . . . McGorry, P. D. (2015). Demographic and clinical characteristics of young people seeking help at youth mental health services: Baseline findings of the Transitions Study. *Early Intervention in Psychiatry*, *9*: 487–497.

Romanowska, S., MacQueen, G., Goldstein, B. I., Wang, J., Kennedy, S. H., Bray, S., Lebel, C., & Addington, J. (2018). Neurocognitive deficits in a transdiagnostic clinical staging model. *Psychiatry Research*, *270*: 1137–1142.

Romanowska, S., MacQueen, G., Goldstein, B. I., Wang, J., Kennedy, S. H., Bray, S., Lebel, C., & Addington, J. (2020). Social and role functioning in youth at risk of serious mental illness. *Early Intervention in Psychiatry*, *14*: 463–469.

Romer, A. L., Elliott, M. L., Knodt, A. R., Sison, M. L., Ireland, D., Houts, R., Ramrakha, S., Poulton, R., Keenan, R., Melzer, T. R., Moffitt, T. E., Caspi, A., & Hariri, A. R. (2021). Pervasively thinner neocortex as a transdiagnostic feature of general psychopathology. *American Journal of Psychiatry*, *178*: 174–182.

Sacks, D. D., Lagopoulos, J., Hatton, S. N., Iorfino, F., Carpenter, J. S., Crouse, J. J., Naismith, S. L., Scott, E. M., Hickie, I. B., & Hermens, D. F. (2021). White matter integrity according to the stage of mental disorder in youth. *Psychiatry Research: Neuroimaging*, *307*: 111218.

Sawrikar, V., Stewart, E., LaMonica, H. M., Iorfino, F., Davenport, T. A., Cross, S., Scott, E., Naismith, S. L., Mowszowski, L., Guastella, A., & Hickie, I. B. (2021). Using staged care to provide "right care first time" to people with common affective disorders. *Psychiatric Services*, *72*: 691–703.

Scott, J., Martin, N. G., Parker, R., Couvy-Duchesne, B., Medland, S. E., & Hickie, I. (2021). Prevalence of self-reported subthreshold phenotypes of major mental disorders and their association with functional impairment, treatment and full-threshold syndromes in a community-residing cohort of young adults. *Early Intervention in Psychiatry*, *15*: 306–313.

Shah, J. L., Crawford, A., Mustafa, S. S., Iyer, S. N., Joober, R., & Malla, A. K. (2017). Is the clinical high-risk state a valid concept? Retrospective examination in a first-episode psychosis sample. *Psychiatric Services*, *68*: 1046–1052.

Shah, J. L., Jones, N., van Os, J., McGorry, P. D., & Gülöksüz, S. (2022). Early intervention service systems for youth mental health: Integrating pluripotentiality, clinical staging, and transdiagnostic lessons from early psychosis. *Lancet Psychiatry*, *9*: 413–422.

Shah, J. L., Scott, J., McGorry, P. D., Cross, S. P. M., Keshavan, M. S., Nelson, B., Wood, S. J., Marwaha, S., Yung, A. R., Scott, E. M., Öngür, D., Conus, P., Henry, C., & Hickie, I. B., for the

International Working Group on Transdiagnostic Clinical Staging in Youth Mental Health. (2020). Transdiagnostic clinical staging in youth mental health: A first international consensus statement. *World Psychiatry*, *19*: 233–242.

Simon, A. E., Umbricht, D., Lang, U. E., & Borgwardt, S. (2014). Declining transition rates to psychosis: The role of diagnostic spectra and symptom overlaps in individuals with attenuated psychosis syndrome. *Schizophrenia Research*, *159*: 292–298.

Solmi, M., Radua, J., Olivola, M., Croce, E., Soardo, L., Salazar de Pablo, G., Il Shin, J., Kirkbride, J. B., Jones, P., Kim, J. H., Kim, J. Y., Carvalho, A. F., Seeman, M. V., Correll, C. U., & Fusar-Poli, P. (2022). Age at onset of mental disorders worldwide: Large-scale meta-analysis of 192 epidemiological studies. *Molecular Psychiatry*, *27*: 281–295.

Spiteri-Staines, A. E., Yung, A. R., Lin, A., Hartmann, J. A., Amminger, P., McGorry, P. D., Thompson, A., Wood, S. J., & Nelson, B. (2024). Non-psychotic outcomes in young people at ultra-high risk of developing a psychotic disorder: A long-term follow-up study. *Schizophrenia Bulletin*, *50*, 1279–1286.

Stephan, K. E., Bach, D. R., Fletcher, P. C., Flint, J., Frank, M. J., Friston, K. J., Heinz, A., Huys, Q. J. M., Owen, M. J., Binder, E. B., Dayan, P., Johnstone, E. C., Meyer-Lindenberg, A., Montague, P. R., Schnyder, U., Wang, X. J., & Breakspear, M. (2016). Charting the landscape of priority problems in psychiatry, part 1: Classification and diagnosis. *Lancet Psychiatry*, *3*: 77–83.

Stowkowy, J., Brummitt, K., Bonneville, D., Goldstein, B. I., Wang, J., Kennedy, S. H., Bray, S., Lebel, C., MacQueen, G., & Addington, J. (2020). Sleep disturbances in youth at-risk for serious mental illness. *Early Intervention in Psychiatry*, *14*: 373–378.

Tickell, A. M., Lee, R. S. C., Hickie, I. B., & Hermens, D. F. (2019). The course of neuropsychological functioning in young people with attenuated vs discrete mental disorders. *Early Intervention in Psychiatry*, *13*: 425–433.

van Doorn, M., Monsanto, A., Wang, C. L., Verfaillie, S. C. J., van Amelsvoort, T., Popma, A., Jaspers, M. W. M., Öry, F., Alvarez-Jimenez, M., Gleeson, J. F., & Nieman, D. H. (2023). The effects of a digital, transdiagnostic, clinically and peer-moderated treatment platform for young people with emerging mental health complaints: Repeated measures within-subjects study. *JMIR Mhealth Uhealth*, *11*: e50636.

Velthorst, E., Mollon, J., Murray, R. M., de Haan, L., Germeys, I. M., Glahn, D. C., Arango, C., van der Ven, E., Di Forti, M., Bernardo, M., Guloksuz, S., Delespaul, P., Mezquida, G., Amoretti, S., Bobes, J., Saiz, P. A., García-Portilla, M. P., Santos, J. L., Jiménez-López, E., . . . Reichenberg, A. (2021). Cognitive functioning throughout adulthood and illness stages in individuals with psychotic disorders and their unaffected siblings. *Molecular Psychiatry*, *26*: 4529–4543.

Yung, A. R., Yuen, H. P., Berger, G., Francey, S., Hung, T.-C., Nelson, B., Phillips, L., & McGorry, P. (2007). Declining transition rate in ultra high risk (prodromal) services: Dilution or reduction of risk? *Schizophrenia Bulletin*, *33*: 673–681.

CHAPTER 13

Psychopathology through the Lens of Contemporary Integrative Interpersonal Theory

AARON L. PINCUS, AIDAN G. C. WRIGHT, AND CHRISTOPHER J. HOPWOOD

Introduction

We anticipate this chapter will be different from most of the others in this handbook, because Contemporary Integrative Interpersonal Theory (CIIT: Dawood et al., 2018; Hopwood et al., 2021; Pincus, 2005; Pincus & Ansell, 2013) is unlike many contemporary dimensional models of psychopathology such as the Hierarchical Taxonomy of Psychopathology (HiTOP; Kotov et al., 2021). For example, CIIT does not focus exclusively on structure; does not prioritize factor analytic logic, that is, every indicator falls on a dimension; nor does it have the same foci, emphases, or goals as do multivariate dimensional models of individual differences (Wiggins, 2003). CIIT is not a descriptive model of all possible psychiatric symptoms and how they are organized, and it does not aim to serve as an alternative diagnostic nosology. In fact, because CIIT focuses on adaptive and maladaptive patterns of functioning, it is agnostic about the best way to organize a descriptive diagnostic manual. CIIT is a model of how a highly social species engages in its social world, how that can go wrong, and what can be done about it. CIIT is not focused on which dimension or category a symptom belongs to, nor on dimension elevations or diagnostic thresholds. CIIT aims to articulate how a pattern of dynamic social-cognitive, affective, and behavioral processes within an interpersonal situation forms a gestalt that is socially reinforced over time, leading to adaptive or maladaptive functioning.

Harry Stack Sullivan's (1953a, 1953b, 1954, 1956, 1962, 1964) interpersonal theory of psychiatry was an early contribution to the relational psychoanalytic movement (Wake et al., 2022), and it also catalyzed a distinct and vital interpersonal paradigm (Wiggins, 2003) for clinical science and practice, advanced by the seminal efforts of several founding contributors (e.g., Benjamin, 1974; Carson, 1969; Kiesler, 1983, 1996; Leary, 1957; Wiggins, 1982). This evolving theory of personality and psychopathology has also kept pace with major empirical advances in psychological science over the past 70 years, leading to CIIT.

To articulate cause and effect models of psychopathology, CIIT combines empirically validated structural models with temporally dynamic momentary and developmental social-cognitive, affective, and behavioral processes across levels of analysis to articulate adaptive and maladaptive patterns of functioning (Hopwood et al., 2019; Pincus, Hopwood, & Wright, 2020; Pincus & Wright, 2011; Wright et al., 2023). This integration of structure and process offers an empirically supported and testable meta-theory to study personality (e.g., Dunlop et al., 2023; Halberstadt et al., 2023), psychopathology (e.g., Asan et al., 2023; Pincus et al., 2010), assessment (e.g., Pincus, Sadler, et al., 2014; Pincus, Hopwood, & Dawood, 2020), and psychotherapy (e.g., Anchin & Pincus, 2010; Cain et al., 2024) in a unified way (Pincus & Hopwood, 2025).

In this chapter, we review conceptualization of psychopathology through the lens of CIIT. We begin with a review of the CIIT's major assumptions, followed by an articulation of CIIT's definition of psychopathology in terms of distortion and dysregulation in interpersonal situations. We then discuss interpersonal case conceptualization, an approach that can be applied to dimensions of psychopathology, diagnostic categories of psychopathology, individual symptoms, general problems in living, and other clinically relevant constructs. Regardless of the nosological model, interpersonal case conceptualization can include interpersonal antecedents of psychopathology, interpersonal consequences of psychopathology, interpersonal pathoplasticity of psychopathology, and interpersonal disorders themselves. We conclude with a discussion of the role of interpersonal dynamics in dimensional models of psychopathology.

Contemporary Integrative Interpersonal Theory: 6 Foundational Assumptions

The six foundational assumptions of CIIT articulate the core interpersonal structures, systems, and processes; their organization and linkages; and their adaptive and maladaptive manifestations. These are summarized in Table 13.1 and reviewed in what follows.

> ***Assumption 1, The focus:*** *Fundamentally important functional expressions of personality and psychopathology typically occur in interpersonal situations.*

CIIT asserts that personality, psychopathology, and psychotherapy are best understood as dynamic interactions between self and other (Pincus, Cain, & Halberstadt, 2020), and these involve the integration of stable individual differences and recurrent temporally dynamic self-other patterns within interpersonal situations. The interpersonal situation (Figure 13.1) is the fundamental unit of analysis, offering a dyadic framework of self and other to systematically organize and describe CIIT's core structures and processes (Hopwood et al., 2019; Pincus, Hopwood, & Wright, 2020). Interpersonal situations characterize both immediate proximal interpersonal interactions, as well as mental representations of interpersonal interactions (e.g., schemas, expectancies, internal working models, object relations, memories, fantasies, dreams, etc.). Interpersonal situations are dynamically unfolding contexts in which important

TABLE 13.1 Assumptions of Contemporary Integrative Interpersonal Theory

1	Fundamental expressions of personality and psychopathology occur in interpersonal situations.
2	Interpersonal functioning can be organized by the dimensions of agency and communion.
3	Agency and communion manifest in multiple ways across functional domains
4	Satisfying agentic and communal motives drives interpersonal behavior.
5	Interpersonal transaction cycles describe and predict interpersonal patterns and sequences linking the component systems of the interpersonal situation.
6	Sustained deviations from developmentally and socioculturally expected interpersonal patterns (likely) reflect psychopathology.

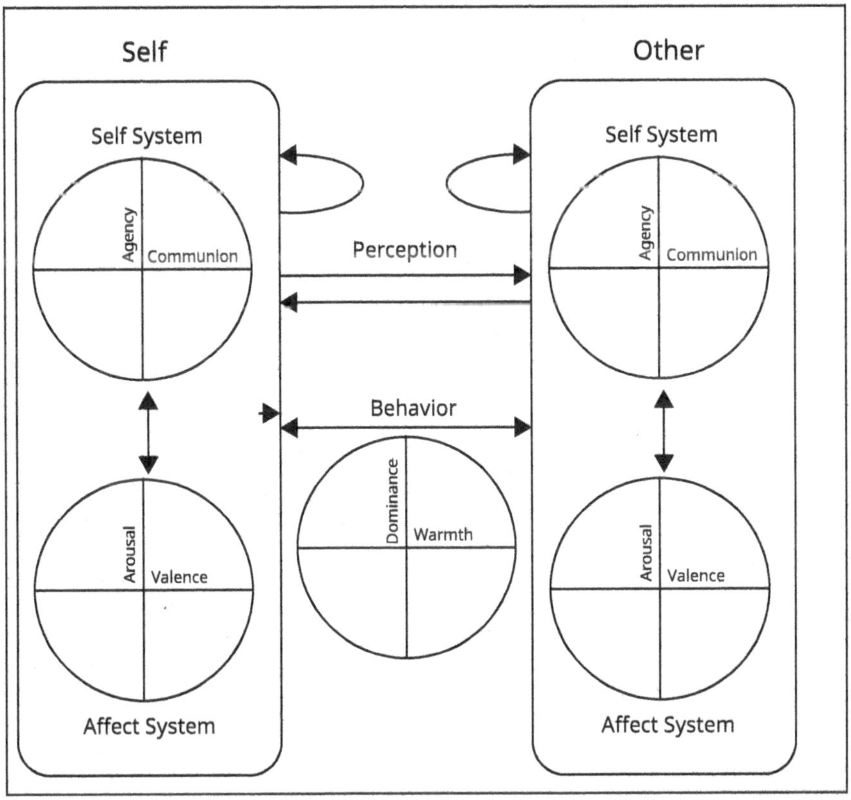

FIGURE 13.1 The interpersonal situation. From Hopwood, C.J, Wright, A.G.C., & Pincus, A.L. (2018). The Interpersonal Situation. DOI: 10.17605/OSF.IO/QJSCD.

social learning occurs across the lifespan, promoting personality organization, development, and adjustment/maladjustment through continuous patterning of self-other experiences.

Figure 13.1 characterizes the key components of interpersonal situations, including the self and other, both of which have self- and affect-systems. The self-system is organized by an individual's agentic and communal motives and self-concept, which reflect socially learned and reinforced interpersonal behaviors and dispositions (e.g., traits, values, efficacies, sensitivities and aversions, and problems). An individual's self-concept, self-esteem, and felt security shift as their agentic and communal motives are satisfied or frustrated. The affect-system, based on the dimensions of affective arousal and valence (Posner et al., 2005), is closely linked with the self-system (bidirectional arrows connecting the self- and affect-systems for both self and other). Positive emotions are a sign of motive satisfaction, while negative emotions are a sign of motive frustration, and emotional experience can impact the style and intensity of interpersonal behavior. As interactions cycle forward, interpersonal behavior further regulates emotional experiences through the satisfaction and frustration of interpersonal motives.

The box outlining self and other demarcates the interpersonal field (Wiggins & Trobst, 1999) in which interpersonal exchanges take place. Each person's perceptions and construals of self (curved unidirectional arrows) and other (straight unidirectional arrows) can be understood in terms of agency and communion. Perception refers to the identification of an observed act (i.e., what I perceived happened), while construal is the interpretation of the interpersonal communication conveyed by the act (i.e., intentions, needs, attitudes, impacts, etc.) and their influences.[1] Dominant (agentic) and warm (communal) behaviors are indicated by the bidirectional arrow between self and other. Within the interpersonal field, ongoing construal processes continuously modulate and regulate the functioning of the self-system, affect-system, and behavior. Research on the interpersonal situation framework suggests that correlations among variables in its component systems reflect clinically important inputs, mediators, and outputs (e.g., Asan et al., 2024; Edershile & Wright, 2025; Halberstadt et al., 2023; Kaurin, Pilkonis, & Wright, 2022; Wright et al., 2017). The interpersonal situation therefore offers an orderly language to apply to objective and subjective perspectives on social exchanges and relationships. Within the interpersonal field, individuals' self-concepts and motivations, perceptions and construals of self and other, and behaviors are characterized by agency and communion, while affect is organized by valence and arousal. Temporally dynamic links between these interpenetrating component systems (e.g., other behavior → self behavior, other behavior → self affect, self-affect → self behavior, self affect → self motivation) can characterize adaptive and psychopathological interpersonal patterns as interpersonal transactions unfold over time. The structural (i.e., interpersonal motives and dispositions) and process (i.e., patterns of interpersonal perception, construal, affect, and behavior) aspects of CIIT have been empirically investigated across the spectra of psychopathology.[2]

Assumption 2, The structure: *Interpersonal functioning can be organized using the dimensions of agency and communion.*

CIIT combines a dimensional model of interpersonal dispositions with temporally dynamic interpersonal processes to describe interpersonal functioning at multiple levels. The "metaconcepts" of agency and communion underlie an empirically validated two-dimensional structure referred to as the interpersonal circumplex (IPC; Fournier et al., 2011; Wiggins, 1996), which is used to derive explanatory and descriptive concepts at different levels of specificity (Figure 13.2—Top).

Agency and communion link CIIT to enormous literatures spanning the social and behavioral social sciences (Bakan, 1966; Baumeister & Leary, 1995; Helgeson, 1994; Johnson et al., 2012; Wiggins, 1991). In CIIT, agency refers to individuation and self-differentiation, and motives to get ahead and be in control versus motives to be passive and seek guidance from others. Communion refers to connection of self and others, and motives to get along and be close to others versus motives to be socially cold and distant from others. Interpersonal dispositions imply enduring patterns of perceiving, thinking, feeling, and behaving aggregated across time, place, and relationships. The IPC also identifies lower-order facets (or octants) describing specific interpersonal dispositions reflecting all possible blends of agency and communion (Figure 13.2—Bottom). Finally, the IPC also describes specific behaviors enacted within interpersonal situations (Moskowitz, 2005; Sadler et al., 2009; Woods et al., 2023).

Agentic and communal motives, dispositions, and behaviors are empirically related to contemporary dimensional models of personality and psychopathology such as the Five-factor Model (Ansell & Pincus, 2004; Du et al., 2021), the DSM-5 AMPD maladaptive trait model (Wright et al., 2012), the Hierarchical Taxonomy of Psychopathology, (Girard et al., 2017), and

[1] People can often, but not always, agree with one another's perception of an interpersonal act (e.g., interrupting someone who is talking is perceived as a dominant behavior). However, people can more often disagree with one another's construal of the interpersonal communication (e.g., the interrupter construes their dominant behavior as helpful and guiding, but the interrupted construes the other's dominant behavior as judgmental and controlling).

[2] Reviewed in later sections of the chapter.

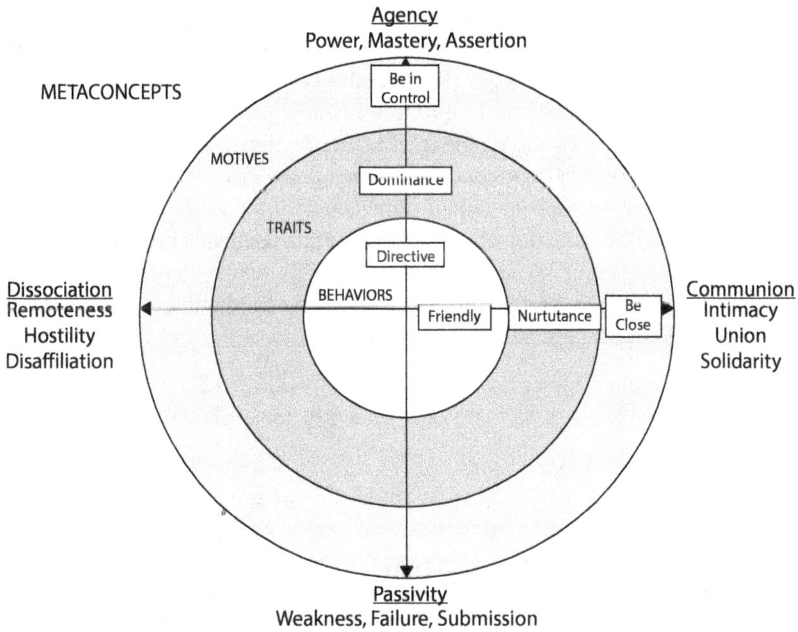

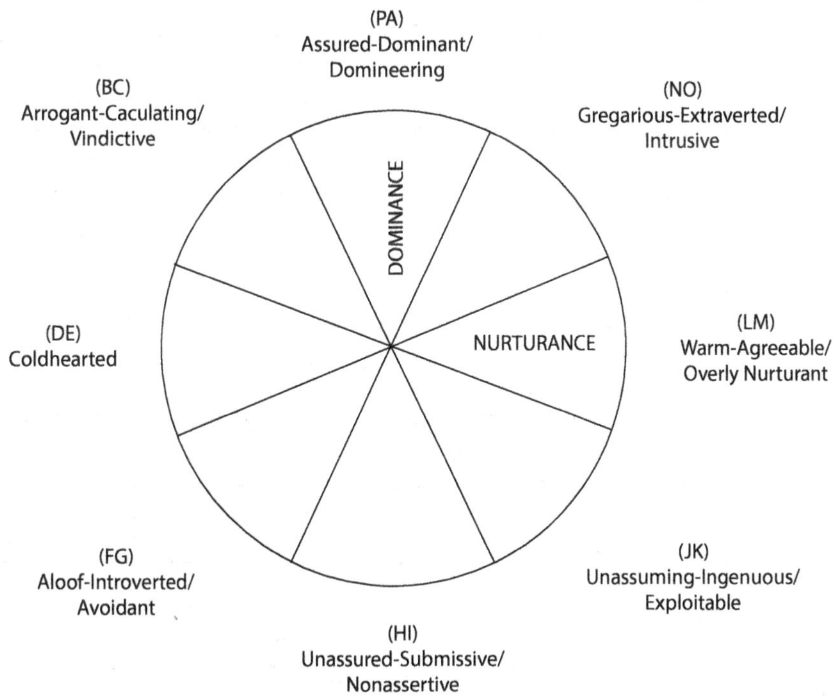

FIGURE 13.2 Agency and communion meta-concepts (Top). The Interpersonal Circumplex (Bottom). From, Cain, N. M., & Pincus, A. L. (2016). Treating maladaptive interpersonal signatures. In W. J. Livesley, G. S. Dimaggio, & J. F. Clarkin (Eds.), *Integrated treatment for personality disorder: A modular approach* (p. 307). Guilford Press. Reprinted with permission of Guilford Press.

the Dark Triad (Dowgwillo & Pincus, 2017). Our view is that agentic and communal motives, dispositions, and behaviors, and their associated dynamic processes, are highly relevant for any dimensional model of psychopathology (Hopwood et al., 2023).

The empirically supported agency and communion meta-framework and IPC structure serve as a "key conceptual map" (Kiesler, 1996, p. 172) for an interpersonal description of personality structures and personality processes. As a formal geometric model, the IPC identifies and operationalizes the primary interpersonal dimensions of focus, and how they relate to one another based on the trigonometry of a circle to generate falsifiable inferences (Gurtman & Pincus, 2003; Zimmermann & Wright, 2017). Importantly, agency and communion, and the IPC, are used to organize and describe both adaptive and maladaptive functioning (Leary, 1957; Pincus & Hopwood, 2012; Pincus & Wright, 2011).

> ***Assumption 3, The domains:*** *Agency and communion are critical features of personality and psychopathology that manifest in multiple ways across interpenetrating functional domains from brain to behavior.*

CIIT is an integrative and holistic theory about the nature of human interpersonal functioning. Agency and communion are attributes of human evolutionary architecture, naturally selected for their contributions to achieving the major life tasks of getting ahead and getting along (Hogan & Roberts, 2000). CIIT uses agency and communion to conceptualize core aspects of personality and psychopathology across multiple interpenetrating functional domains to generate actionable clinical conceptualizations of psychopathology (Hopwood et al., 2019). These domains include motivation (Horowitz et al., 2006), dispositions making up the self-concept (Wiggins, 1979), perception and construal of self and other (e.g., Kiesler et al., 1997; Pincus, Cain, & Halberstadt, 2020; Woods et al., 2023), mental representations (Heck & Pincus, 2001; Lukowitsky & Pincus, 2011), behaviors (Moskowitz, 2005), and neurobehavioral reward systems (Allen & DeYoung, 2017; Depue, 2006; Waller & Wagner, 2019). Human social goals, social information processing, social communication, and social schemas can all be characterized in agentic and communal terms. People even have neurobiologically based responses to agentic and communal experiences (Phalip et al., 2024).

From the outset, interpersonal theory has emphasized a multi-level understanding of personality and psychopathology (Leary, 1957). Unlike dimensional models of personality and psychopathology that emphasize structure, the aim was to find a structure capable of organizing both individual differences and temporally dynamic processes of human experience and functioning across interpenetrating levels and domains. This approach to articulation of human functioning was quite farsighted, as it addresses a major challenge facing the field—developing models that can both describe and explain personality and psychopathology (Allen et al., 2020; Baumert et al., 2019; Bornstein, 2019; Dalgleish et al., 2020; Sanislow, 2016).

> ***Assumption 4, What gets us moving:*** *Satisfying agentic and communal motives drives interpersonal behavior.*

Interpersonal behavior aims to satisfy agentic and communal motives (Grosse-Holtforth et al., 2011; Horowitz et al., 2006; Sullivan, 1953a; Trapnell & Paulhus, 2012), which can reflect specific short-term agentic and communal goals in a particular interpersonal situation (e.g., to control what happens), long-term agentic and communal strivings (e.g., to get ahead in life), and agentic and communal self-protective (defensive) strategies (e.g., to restore felt security and self-esteem in relation to others). CIIT asserts that satisfaction of agentic and communal motives increases positive affect, felt security, and self-esteem, and decreases negative affect and insecurity, while frustration of agentic and communal motives increases negative affect and insecurity and decreases positive affect, felt security, and self-esteem (Horowitz et al., 2006; Leary et al., 1995; Mahadevan et al., 2019, 2020; Pincus & Hopwood, 2012). This assumption explicitly links the self- and affect-systems in interpersonal situations (Halberstadt et al., 2023). Across short and long timescales, the link between motives and emotions can reinforce, shape, and maintain or punish and constrain interpersonal behaviors. People differ in the intensity and importance of agentic and communal motives due to their differences in biology and differences in their history of social learning in interpersonal situations experienced over the lifespan. Additionally, the intensity and importance of an individual's agentic and communal motives will fluctuate over time and across situations as the circumstances and the possibilities to satisfy agentic and communal motives change. Successful navigation of short- and long-term dynamic timescales involves flexible adaptation and reconciliation of one's motives with the demands of one's developmental stage, social roles, and specific interpersonal contexts (Wright et al., 2023).

Assumption 5, How we move: *Interpersonal transaction cycles describe and predict interpersonal patterns and sequences linking the component systems of the interpersonal situation.*

Interpersonal case conceptualization of psychopathology focuses on relatively stable individual differences in temporally dynamic patterns of self-other functioning in interpersonal situations to describe personality and psychopathology (Pincus & Wright, 2011). CIIT examines the links between the component systems of the interpersonal situation to identify the key processes of interpersonal transaction cycles. For example, when linking self and others' behavior in the interpersonal situation, CIIT refers to the normative, empirically supported social exchange patterns of interpersonal complementarity (Sadler et al., 2011) reflecting oppositeness on agency (dominance pulls for submission, submission pulls for dominance) and sameness on communion (warmth pulls for warmth, coldness pulls for coldness), as well as unique patterns and chronic deviations from what is expected. When linking the behavior of the other with the affective experience of the self, CIIT refers to interpersonal triggers. For example, numerous studies find reliable associations between one person's coldness or dominance and another's negative affect (Edershile & Wright, 2025; Kaurin, Dombrovski, Hallquist, & Wright, 2022; Sadikaj et al., 2011, 2013; Vize et al., 2024; Wright et al., 2017).

Importantly, the nature of the interpersonal situation itself contextualizes a given transaction cycle. For example, there is empirical evidence that differences in interpersonal situations (including settings, interaction partners, topics, etc.) influence patterns of interpersonal behavior (e.g., Hopwood et al., 2020; Moskowitz et al., 2007; Stadel et al., 2024) and that individual differences in personality and psychopathology further moderate these contextualized self-other patterns of interpersonal functioning (e.g., Dowgwillo et al., 2019; Roche et al., 2013a, 2013b; Sadikaj et al., 2010; Wang et al., 2014).

CIIT integrates all relevant psychological domains from Assumption 3 (e.g., motivation, perception, construal, affect, behavior) to fully describe interpersonal transaction cycles (Figure 13.3) relevant for human development, personality, psychopathology, and psychotherapy. An interpersonal transaction cycle can be described beginning with Person A's behavior (Box 1), which is perceived by Person B (Path 1). Person B construes Person A's interpersonal communications, motives, and intentions and notes their own evoked emotions (i.e., Person B's covert reaction—Box 2). Based on Person B's construal, emotions, and interpersonal motives, they choose a behavioral response toward Person A (Path 2), which is perceived and construed by Person A. As the transaction cycle continues, the meaning of behaviors, how they are perceived, the impacts they have, and what drives them can all be understood as variation in different levels of agency and communion (Pincus & Wright, 2011; Wright et al., 2023). Interpersonal transaction cycles describe an individual's notable adaptive and maladaptive

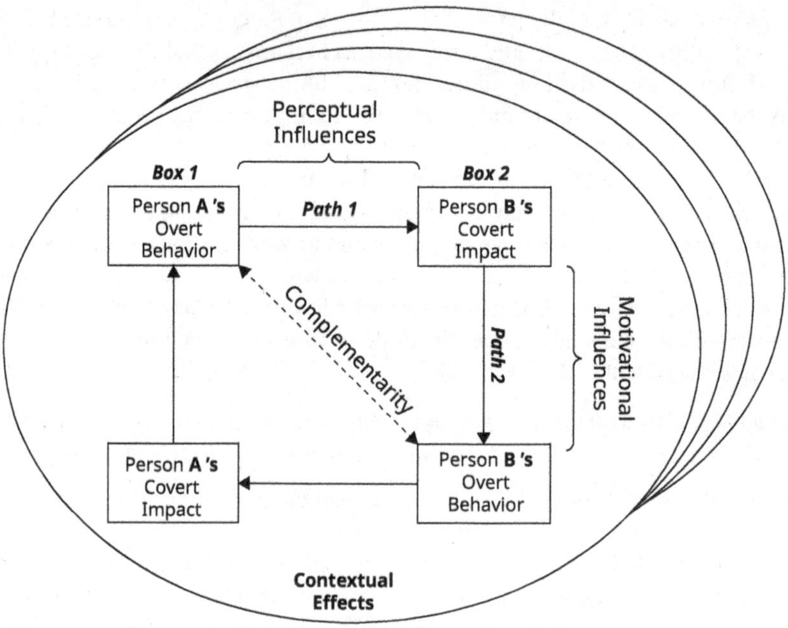

FIGURE 13.3 Interpersonal transaction cycle.

patterns of perception → construal → affect → motivation → behavior across contexts and situations, and research supports the assumption of reliable, developmentally, and culturally normative patterns of interpersonal transaction, as well as patterns that are characteristic of client difficulties and psychopathology (Cain & Pincus, 2016; Fournier et al., 2008; Hopwood, 2018; Skowron et al., 2010). Over the lifespan, repeated social learning experiences in interpersonal situations give rise to more stable, dispositional trends in interpersonal behavior (Wright et al., 2023).

> **Assumption 6, How we know we're moving in the right direction (or not):** *Sustained deviations from developmentally and socioculturally expected interpersonal patterns (likely) reflect psychopathology.*

Chronic deviations from normative social processes likely reflect psychopathology (Pincus et al., 2009), because they imply impaired comprehension of the consensual understanding of interpersonal situations, impaired communication of one's own interpersonal needs and motives, and impaired comprehension of the needs and intentions of others as conveyed by their interpersonal behavior (Cain et al., 2024). Between-person comparisons of interpersonal dispositions and patterns can characterize how a person is different from others, such as behaving in a more or less agentic and/or communal manner than the typical person or deviating from expected patterns of interpersonal complementarity across social exchanges. Within-person comparisons can identify important contexts, such as when there is a particularly strong interpersonal trigger like the association between other peoples' interpersonal behavior and an individual's angry affect (Lewis & Ridenour, 2020; Roche et al., 2014) or feelings of rejection (Meehan et al., 2018, 2019). Empirical studies consistently link psychopathology with higher levels of dispositional interpersonal problems (e.g., Girard et al., 2017; Monteleone et al., 2023; Wilson et al., 2017), distinct patterns of perception and behavior in interpersonal situations (e.g., Ambwani et al., 2015; Dowgwillo et al., 2019; Rappaport et al. 2014; Sadikaj et al., 2010; Wright et al., 2017), deviation from expected patterns of interpersonal complementarity across social exchanges (e.g., Ansell et al., 2008; Asan et al., 2024; Meisel et al., 2022; Roche, 2022; Roche et al., 2013a), and excessive variability in interpersonal behavior (e.g., Clegg et al., 2021; Côté et al., 2012; Moskowitz et al., 2011; Ringwald et al., 2021, 2022; Russell et al., 2007).

Definition of Psychopathology: Distortion and Dysregulation in the Interpersonal Situation

In CIIT, adaptive functioning is not characterized by how agentic or communal the person is, rather by the ability to mutually satisfy self and others' interpersonal motives consistently yet flexibly within the consensual understanding of contextual demands (Pincus & Hopwood, 2012). This reflects accurate perception and construal of self and other, and flexible and effective self-, affect-, and behavioral (field) regulation. Adaptive functioning is reflected in the capacity to enter varied interpersonal situations with a sense of security (i.e., feeling connected to others with little anxiety and low demand for emotion regulation) and self-esteem (i.e., feeling accepted and approved of by others with little threat to the self and low demand for self-regulation). This allows the individual to focus on the immediate situation, encode self and others' interpersonal behaviors accurately, and generate mutually satisfying responses. In such circumstances, self and others' behaviors will be relatively contingent with each other (i.e., complementarity) and culturally normative situational demands.

Thus, dysfunction is characterized by consistent inability to relate to others in a coordinated fashion that mutually satisfies the agentic and communal needs of self and other within the consensual understanding of contextual demands (Hopwood et al., 2013, 2015; Pincus & Hopwood, 2012). These impairments can stem from: (1) *distortion* in perception and construal of self and others, (2) self-, affect-, and/or behavioral (field) *dysregulation*, and (3) a secondary form of self-dysregulation referred to as "self-protective motives" that distortion and dysregulation often evoke.[3] Individuals with psychopathology enter a wide range of interpersonal situations with a sense of insecurity and threatened self-esteem. Hence the person focuses on self-protective agentic and communal motives rather than the immediate interpersonal situation and often does not respond to others in mutually satisfying ways. This is because the goal of their enacted agentic and communal behavior is to protect the self (i.e., restore felt security and self-esteem), and it is typically not contingent with the behavior of others and culturally normative contextual demands. Such interpersonal impairments are the result of both heritable biological temperaments and maladaptive social learning histories in atypical and traumatic developmental environments.[4] This is reflected in consistent impairment in accurately perceiving and construing self and others' behaviors, intentions, and needs (i.e., send and encode interpersonal communications) and the chronic engagement in agentic and communal behaviors aimed at satisfying self-protective motives to restore security and esteem. In sum, CIIT defines psychopathology in terms of chronic distortion and dysregulation in relation to others, which is operationalized by the interpersonal situation's component systems and their links (Figure 13.4).

[3] Sullivan (1953b) referred to these as "security operations," and they can also be conceptualized as psychological defenses.

[4] For full discussions of CIIT's developmental principles, see Dawood et al. (2018); Pincus, (2005); Pincus & Ansell, (2013).

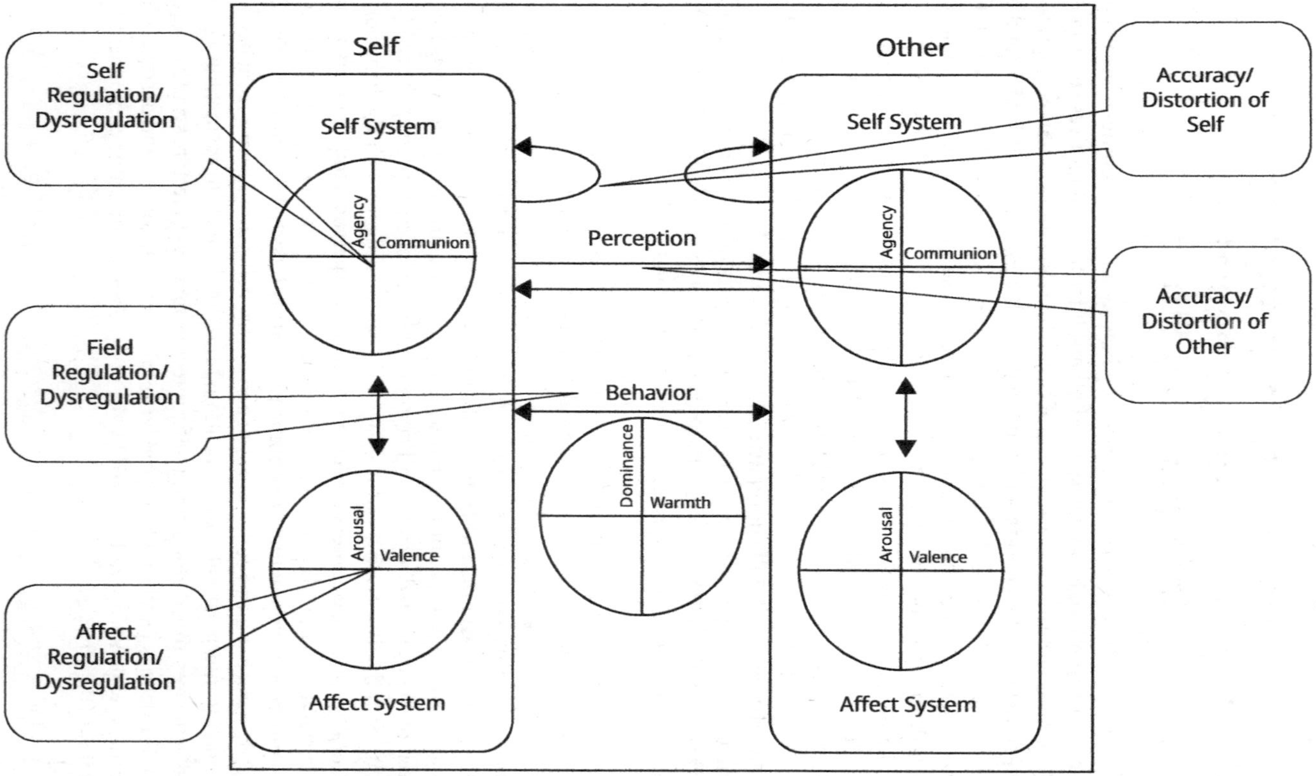

FIGURE 13.4 Distortion and dysregulation in interpersonal situations. From Pincus, A.L., Hopwood, C.J., & Wright, A.G.C. (2020). The interpersonal situation: An integrative framework for the study of personality, psychopathology, and psychotherapy. In D. Funder, J. F. Rauthmann, & R. Sherman (Eds.), *Oxford handbook of psychological situations* (p. 130). Oxford University Press. Reprinted with permission of Oxford University Press.

Distortion

Distortions reflect a discrepancy between perception and construal of an interpersonal situation and an objective understanding of the interpersonal situation. Sullivan (1953b) offered the term "parataxic distortion" to describe the misreading of self and others' interpersonal communications, intentions, needs, and emotions due to the influence of internal mental representations (e.g., cognitive schemas, internal working models, internal object relations). Parataxic distortions of interpersonal situations are often automatically or unconsciously triggered, leading to the experience of influential alternative and conflictual schemas that are often threatening or painful. Parataxic distortions trigger experiences of insecurity, shame, and low self-esteem or idealized views of self and others and unrealistically inflated security and self-esteem. In psychopathology, parataxic distortions can be rigid and regularly lead the person to experience objectively different interpersonal situations (i.e., different others, different contexts) as functionally equivalent. For example, a person with paranoid psychosis may experience most (if not all) interpersonal situations as threatening due to distorted construals of others' malevolent intentions, regardless of how others might view it. Alternatively, parataxic distortions can be chaotic or unstable, leading to highly inconsistent ways of experiencing objectively similar interpersonal situations (i.e., same others, same contexts). For example, a client diagnosed with personality pathology with prominent splitting may oscillate between seeing others as ideal caretakers and as uncaring abandoners, resulting in inconsistent and unpredictable relational behavior.

Dysregulation

Distorted perceptions and construals in interpersonal situations drive self-dysregulation (e.g., self-criticality/hatred, ego/status threat, self-protective motives), affect-dysregulation (e.g., dysphoria, shame, fear, anger), and behavioral dysregulation in the interpersonal field (e.g., aggression, withdrawal, intrusiveness, passivity) (Hopwood et al., 2019; Pincus, Hopwood, & Wright, 2020; Wright et al. 2023). Self-dysregulation reflects rigid or unstable ways of thinking about self and others in interpersonal situations typically giving rise to a negative, threatened, and/or inflated self-concept, as well as self-protective motives (Horowitz et al., 2006). Affect-dysregulation reflects how people feel about self and others in interpersonal situations and impairments in modulating emotional states and emotional expression. Behavioral (field) dysregulation reflects how people behave and affect others' thoughts, feelings, and behaviors in interpersonal situations, giving rise to rigid, extreme, and/or chaotic agentic and communal behaviors aimed at restoring security and self-esteem and influencing others.

Self-protective Motives. Distorted perceptions and construals of self and other often lead to experiencing interpersonal situations as threatening and/or painful (e.g., insecurity, shame), evoking dysregulation. Such experiences trigger an additional form of self-dysregulation referred to as self-protective motives that take precedence. These are motives to behave in particular ways that defend the self against the threat, insecurity, and shame, and are manifested in extreme, rigid, and/or chaotic agentic and communal behaviors (i.e., over-learned or impulsive maladaptive interpersonal patterns) that are not contingent on objective context or the other's motives, goals, and behaviors in the interpersonal situation. This catalyzes vicious circles (Millon, 2011; Vize et al., 2024) and self-fulfilling prophecies (Carson, 1982) via social reinforcement, and negatively impacts relationship quality and satisfaction (Gibson et al., 2024; Kurzius et al., 2022; Slotter et al., 2023). CIIT views maladaptive interpersonal patterns associated with psychopathology as logical responses to deeply entrenched distorted perceptions and construals, and subsequent dysregulation. The particular agentic and communal forms this takes for any given individual is a product of their heritable biological temperaments and history of social learning in interpersonal situations (Benjamin, 2003; Hopwood et al. 2019; Pincus & Hopwood, 2012).

Case Examples

We briefly provide two case examples of distortion and dysregulation in interpersonal situations, one reflecting psychosis and one reflecting personality pathology.

Psychosis. Diego is a 40-year-old heterosexual Mexican American male. He came from a large family for whom he reported ambivalent feelings. He lived in the same small town where he grew up, as did several brothers and sisters. Three generations of Diego's family owned and worked at a local restaurant that, over the years, attracted a large clientele of regulars. However, Diego was not involved with the restaurant, which upset his family. Diego struggled to obtain a culinary degree but developed transient paranoid concerns about the restaurant business, culinary instructors, restaurant customers, and even his family members. Over time Diego's symptoms worsened, leaving him unable to work, and he would not leave the house unless a trusted family member accompanied him. At times, his paranoia required brief inpatient treatment, and he was diagnosed with a delusional disorder. Diego's psychopathology contributed to a mistrustful and isolating interpersonal style, and he preferred being alone most of the time, because he feared others would humiliate or harm him.

Diego is chronically suspicious of others and experiences transient referential thinking that might be caused by a biologically based psychotic illness. In most interpersonal situations his perception and construal of others' intentions and behaviors is distorted as potentially judgmental and malignant, and himself as endangered. For example, he started to feel as though restaurant customers and culinary instructors were judging him as incompetent and family members and other employees were blaming him for any problems that arose in the restaurant. Diego experienced self- (experience of self as inadequate) and affective dysregulation (fear, shame, etc.), which evoked a self-protective motive and, with no explanation to others, he stopped going to the restaurant and culinary school. When others reached out, the cycle of distortion, dysregulation, and self-protective motives recurred. Diego distorted his construal of others' caring inquiries as humiliating angry reprimands that he again protected himself from via further withdrawal. This confused those who approached Diego. Some became anxious, some became frustrated, and most decided to keep their distance. Over time, all but Diego's closest family lost interest, leaving him more insular and distrustful. This maladaptive pattern of perceived threat (distortion), increased insecurity and decreased self-esteem (dysregulation), followed by detachment from others (self-protection) and eventual relationship dissolution is a socially reinforced vicious circle represented in Figure 13.5.

Personality Pathology. Erica is a 27-year-old heterosexual European American female. Her parents divorced when she was three years old, and Erica described them as self-absorbed, hostile to each other, and neglectful toward her except when they punished her. Erica moved away to go to college but dropped out after her freshman year because she found it boring. After dropping out of college, Erica worked as a bartender in a number of restaurants, hotels, and clubs. She did not have her own apartment, but stayed with friends or boyfriends if she was currently involved with someone. She had a large but superficial social network. Erica was a regular drinker and user of various street drugs, and frequently engaged in one-night sexual encounters. Several times she had agreed to more committed romantic relationships, but they did not last very long due to her infidelity. Erica was attractive and extraverted, and easily made friends. However, these relationships were often tumultuous and chaotic because

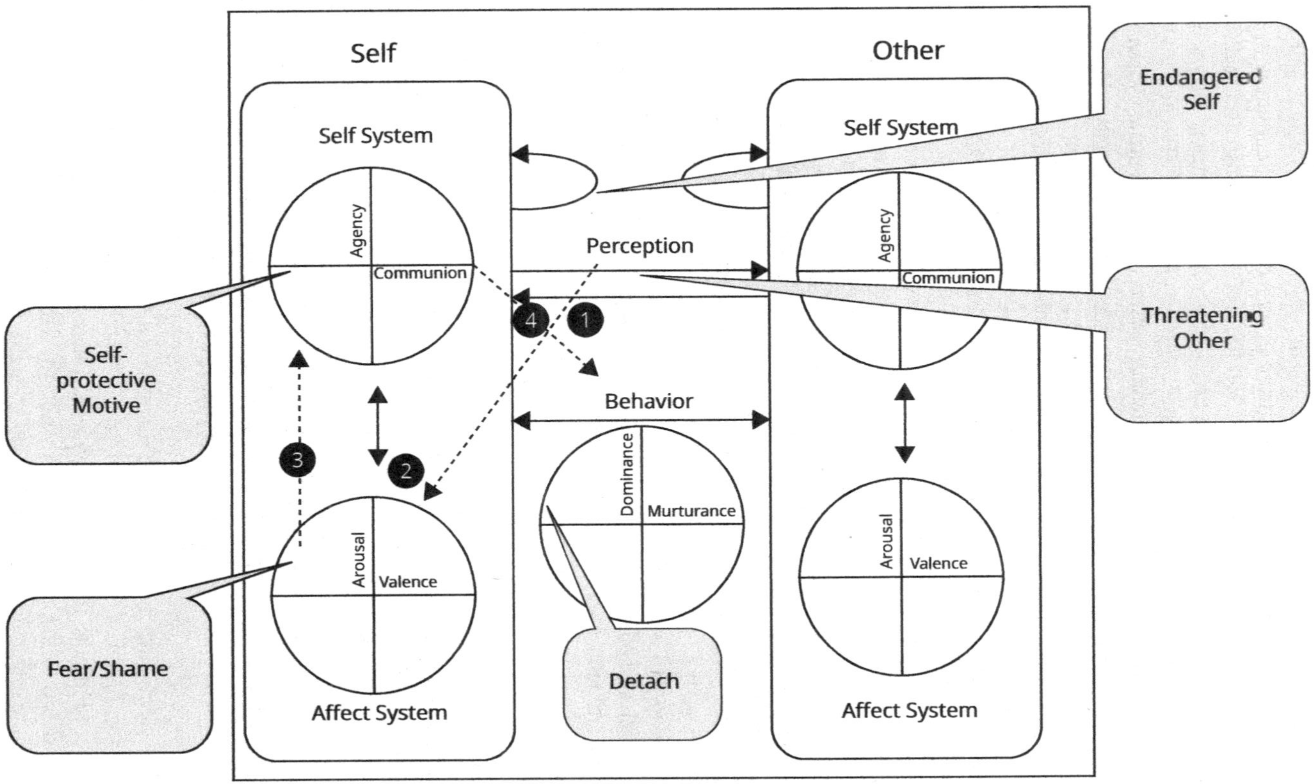

FIGURE 13.5 Diego's Suspicious Pattern of Distortion (1), Affect Dysregulation (2), Self-dysregulation (3), and Self-protection (4).

of her mood swings, self-absorption, occasionally aggressive behavior, and willingness to be dishonest and exploit others to get what she wanted.

Erica experienced identity diffusion and emotional volatility consistent with a personality disorder diagnosis. Sometimes she was angry and self-centered, verbally aggressive, and occasionally physically violent. At other times, she was depressed and self-critical, and would cut herself. Erica's most severe dysregulation occurred in interpersonal situations with romantic partners. Erica experienced identity diffusion. Her perception and construal of self and other were unstable rather than rigid, a pattern that can be described as splitting. She oscillated between states of narcissistic grandiosity and narcissistic vulnerability (Pincus, 2023; Pincus, Cain, & Wright, 2014), in which her interpersonal motives, perceptions, construals, affects, and behaviors were quite different. When grandiose, Erica had no awareness of her feelings of vulnerability and vice versa. This created chaotic and extreme shifts in self-, affect, and behavioral (field) dysregulation. Erica's split states can be represented by two common maladaptive interpersonal patterns in interpersonal situations.

Sometimes Erica experienced herself as entitled to "whatever I want whenever I want it," even if it meant taking advantage of or devaluing others. For example, Erica often engaged in casual sexual encounters even when living with a boyfriend in a committed relationship and felt quite comfortable lying about it. If discovered and accused of infidelity, Erica would perceive the other person as envious and whiny and construe their reactions as insignificant and annoying. Erica then experienced extreme self- and affect dysregulation, feeling angry (insecurity) and insulted (threat to self), which evoked self-protective motives. If yelling obscenities and insisting she did not care about their feelings failed to stifle their complaints, Erica would throw things, slam doors, and threaten physical violence. This maladaptive pattern is represented in Figure 13.6.

Erica's behavior led to repeated breakups, and soon after the relationships would end, her perception of self and others would shift sharply. Erica would feel alone, abandoned, ashamed, and regretful, and would seek to reconcile. However, bridges were often permanently burned and former boyfriends would not return. When Erica's apologies were spurned, she perceived and construed the other as entitled and withholding. Her self- and affect dysregulation was experienced as extreme self-hatred and hopelessness, which evoked self-protective motives. Erica would then express suicidal ideation and cut herself. Her former boyfriends were confused by this, unsure whether Erica wanted to die or was being manipulative. Erica was not sure about this, either. This maladaptive pattern is represented in Figure 13.7. A summary of both cases is presented in Table 13.2.

Description of Psychopathology: Interpersonal Case Conceptualization of Psychopathology

Categorical systems such as the DSM and dimensional systems such as the HiTOP describe psychopathology based on depictions of prominent symptoms grouped by expert committees or quantitative methods. The former provides familiar labels such as anxiety disorders, depressive disorders, eating disorders, etc., while the latter provides dimensional symptom profiles including internalizing, externalizing, thought disorder, etc. Whether conceptualized as categorical or dimensional, psychopathology emerges through interactions among interpenetrating biobehavioral systems and impacts interpersonal functioning even if the direct cause is situated outside the component systems of the interpersonal situation (e.g., amyloid plaques, formal thought disorder) (Wright et al., 2023). The interpersonal consequences

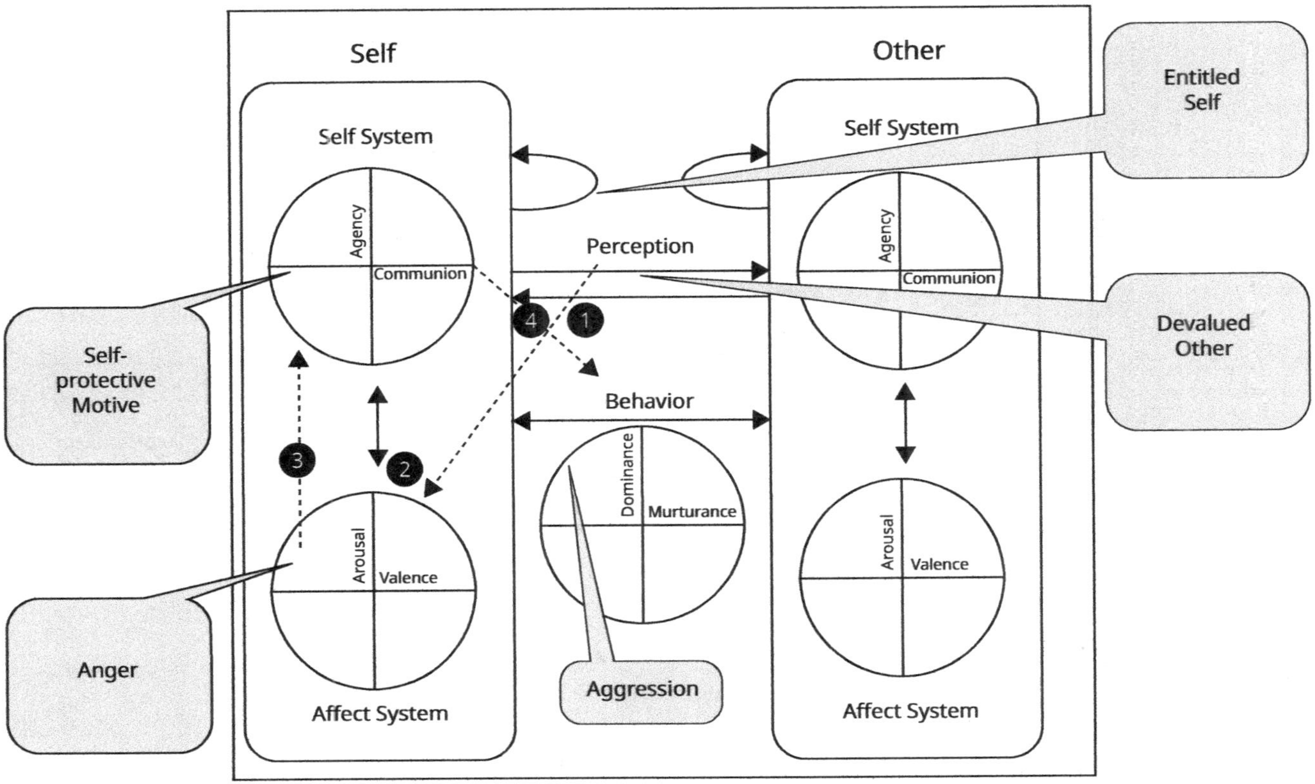

FIGURE 13.6 Erica's Grandiose Pattern of Distortion (1), Affect Dysregulation (2), Self-dysregulation (3), and Self-protection (4).

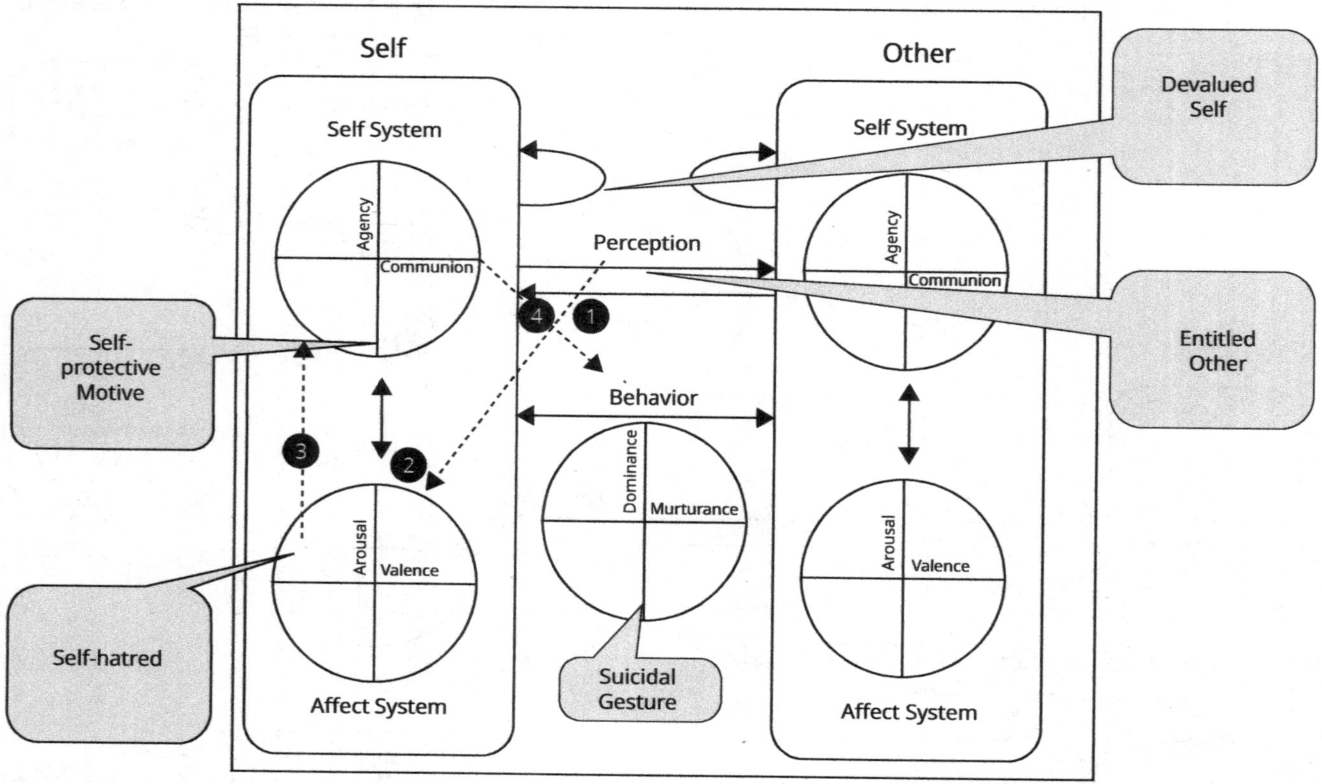

FIGURE 13.7 Erica's Vulnerable Pattern of Distortion (1), Affect Dysregulation (2), Self-dysregulation (3), and Self-protection (4).

TABLE 13.2 Maladaptive Interpersonal Patterns (Diego and Erica)

	System				Consequence
	Perception/ Construal	**Affect**	**Self**	**Behavior**	
Clinical Problem	Parataxic Distortion	Dysregulated Affect	Activation of Agentic and Communal Self-Protective Motives	Maladaptive Behavior	Vicious Circle/ Self-Fulfilling Prophecy
Diego's Suspicious Style	Perception of self as threatened and others as dangerous	Acute fear and shame	Motives to avoid threat via detachment	Self-isolating behavior	Perceived safety achieved through disconnection, and others' withdrawal confirms suspicion that they don't really care and cannot be trusted
Erica's Diffuse Identity (Splitting)	I am entitled and better than others / Others are entitled and better than me	Anger / Self-hatred	Motives to blame others for own indiscretion / Motives to harm self for own indiscretion and others' rejection	Unempathic and unkind acting out and blaming / Self-harming behavior	The repeated cycle of acting out, blaming others, getting rejected, and harming herself reinforces both grandiose and vulnerable beliefs, and the intensity of the pattern leaves little room for reflection and integration

Note. Parataxic Distortion and Dysregulation do not happen in clean sequences and are not always initiated by distortion as implied here. Instead, these are interpenetrating and mutually reinforcing phenomena that happen at various time scales and in various orders (often simultaneously). However, it is useful to represent them as a sequence in this standard order for case conceptualization.

of most symptoms and disorders can influence their maintenance and course. For example, Diego's interpersonal pattern of distortion, dysregulation, and detachment maintains his paranoia as he drifts away from consensus reality testing due to social isolation. Erica's unstable interpersonal patterns of entitlement and aggression, and self-hatred and self-harm, perpetuate her identity diffusion through chaotic, conflictual relationships and the long-term inability to form stable, mutual, supportive attachments.

The interpersonal approach to case conceptualization fundamentally differs from current categorical and dimensional systems. Rather than placing people into diagnostic categories based on descriptive characteristics or generating a profile of elevated symptom dimensions, the interpersonal approach centers on interpersonal dynamics articulated in the links between component systems of the interpersonal situation as a transdiagnostic and pantheoretical lens for conceptualizing adaptive and maladaptive human behavior. Interpersonal case conceptualization does not derive an inclusive taxonomy or etiological account for all possible presenting problems or symptoms, but rather provides an integrative nexus (Pincus et al., 2010) to describe and conceptualize how problems and symptoms emerge and impact relational functioning (Hopwood et al., 2015; Pincus & Hopwood, 2025; Pincus & Wright, 2011).

CIIT, along with the structures and processes of the interpersonal situation, can describe patients' distortions, dysregulation, and maladaptive behaviors in interpersonal transaction cycles. These temporally dynamic patterns of perception → construal → affect → motivation → behavior across contexts and situations include rigid or chaotic distortions of perception and construal of self and others, overvalued or extreme motivations or beliefs, deficits in basic interpersonal skills or repertoire, and exaggerated or suppressed links among perceptions, affect, and behavior. This lens can be used to describe a patient's interpersonal dysfunction and consequent socially reinforcing self-fulfilling prophecies and vicious circles, as well as identify salient targets for intervention. Combined with CIIT's developmental principles (Benjamin, 2003; Dawood et al., 2018; Horowitz, 2004; Pincus, 2005), interpersonal case conceptualization articulates patients' maladaptive interpersonal patterns, what triggers evoke and maintain them, and where they come from (Hopwood et al., 2019). Thus, the aim of interpersonal case conceptualization is to apply the interpersonal paradigm (theory and methodology) to understand how psychopathology manifests and is reciprocally reinforced via these interpersonal patterns of relational functioning (Leary, 1957; Sullivan, 1953b; Pincus & Wright, 2011). We view interpersonal case conceptualization as an informative explanatory and treatment system for any approach to describing and treating psychopathology and maladjustment (Pincus & Hopwood, 2025). Interpersonal case conceptualization represents a fundamentally different paradigm with different goals than most dimensional models of psychopathology.

CIIT and the interpersonal situation framework can be used to understand personality, psychopathology, and relational dynamics in an integrated way. Some clinical issues can be understood almost entirely in terms of interpersonal patterns (e.g., social anxiety, unassertiveness), whereas others (e.g., anorexia nervosa, schizotypy, Alzheimer's disease) clearly have central elements that are not directly interpersonal, but do have interpersonal antecedents, interpersonal consequences, or exhibit diverse manifestations in interpersonal situations. Finally, we view some clinical presentations as reflecting fundamental interpersonal disorders (Wright & Nielsen, 2025; Wright et al., 2022), including those conventionally associated with personality disorder diagnoses, as manifesting such ubiquitous and severe interpersonal distortion and dysregulation that it interferes with treatment, and the therapeutic relationship and treatment frame must be prioritized in psychotherapy. Thus, interpersonal case conceptualization can describe different forms of psychopathology through a clinically useful lens. This includes maladaptive interpersonal patterns reflecting interpersonal antecedents and interpersonal consequences of presenting problems and symptoms, how these may be differentially expressed in interpersonal situations depending on a patient's interpersonal style (i.e., interpersonal pathoplasticity), and the interpersonal disorders themselves.

Interpersonal Antecedents of Psychopathology

Social learning, often related to major developmental achievements and trauma (Benjamin, 1993; Dawood et al., 2018; Pincus & Ansell, 2013), along with certain dispositional tendencies, likely influence all forms of psychopathology. For example, early disruptions or traumas with caretakers lead to insecure forms of attachment, and this is often the wellspring for a variety of problems and symptoms (Horowitz, 2004; Mikulincer & Shaver, 2012). Further, as identity formation unfolds, the influence of interpersonal experience is both necessary and powerful (Dunlop et al., 2023; Sharp & Wall, 2021). CIIT and the interpersonal situation can operationalize a developmental understanding of client presentations by linking current interpersonal patterns to the social learning history of the client. This is referred to as interpersonal copying (Benjamin, 2003; Critchfield & Benjamin, 2008; Woehrle et al., 2023). For example, a non-binary patient who grew up in a family that was rejecting of this identity might (1) identify with their rejecting family and treat others as they were treated (e.g., dismissing others' authentic interest in them as phony), (2) recapitulate the socially learned pattern by persistently distorting perceptions and construals of others as signaling rejection and then withdrawing from them, and (3) introject the family rejection they received and reject themself as unlovable. Vicious circles reinforce this pattern over time, increasing its automaticity.

Interpersonal antecedents of psychopathology can also be relatively indirect regarding current symptom presentations. For example, the cognitive-interpersonal model of eating disorders (Treasure et al., 2020) asserts that early disruptions in social relationships predispose individuals to develop anorexia nervosa. If, across development, a person is constantly criticized or warned about their weight and eating habits, and/or is only appreciated by significant others for their appearance, this will impact their social cognition and interpersonal behavior, and disrupt identity development, stimulating perfectionistic strivings and narrowing self-worth to the achievement of an unrealistic body image. Here, the copy process of introjection is most relevant as the person with anorexia, having internalized valuing an unrealistic body image, now treats themselves as important others once did by being highly self-critical of their body, appearance, and eating habits, leading to continued food restriction.

As a final example, both cognitive-behavioral and psychodynamic theories of depression identify frustrated interpersonal motives as developmental antecedents of depression (Blatt, 2004). When deeply held agentic (introjective or autonomous) and communal (anaclitic or sociotropic) motives are chronically frustrated, risk for depression increases due to disruptions in self-concept (esteem) and interpersonal relatedness (security). Introjective/autonomous depression manifests in self-critical reactions to achievement failures, while anaclitic/sociotropic depression manifests in depressive and dependent reactions when needed others are unavailable (Kopala-Sibley et al., 2016).

Interpersonal Consequences of Psychopathology

Most symptoms of psychopathology, even those arising from dysfunction in systems outside the interpersonal situation, have consequences for interpersonal functioning that can contribute to the maintenance and exacerbation of problems and symptoms. CIIT and the interpersonal situation can operationalize the consequences of psychopathology by linking problems and symptoms to current interpersonal patterns to identify the vicious circles that reinforce and maintain psychopathology. For example, schizotypic symptoms clearly impact interpersonal functioning. Self-referential and persecutory thinking, social disinterest, unusual perceptions, flattened affect, avolition, and disorganization can all interfere with the mutual satisfaction of agentic and communal motivations in interpersonal situations (Asan et al., 2023). Although Diego's delusional disorder discussed earlier likely has fundamental origins in his neurophysiology, it profoundly impacts his interpersonal functioning. His interpersonal sensitivity and detachment contribute to symptom maintenance by reducing the presence and relevance of other people in his life such that Diego rarely has positive social experiences that could refute his persecutory beliefs and shameful self-concept. Over time, he drifts further away from consensus reality.

The cognitive-interpersonal model of eating disorders actually proposes both interpersonal antecedents and consequences of anorexia (Treasure et al., 2020). Early disruptions in interpersonal relations may lead to the internalization of unrealistic body image values that contribute to the development of anorexia. After its onset, acute starvation impacts social cognition and physical energy levels, both of which have numerous interpersonal consequences. Starvation can create deficits in nonverbal emotional expression, the ability to generate natural social narratives, and the recognition of others' interpersonal communications. It also can induce threat sensitivity and promote maladaptive social comparisons and conflict avoidance. Such consequences can lead to distortions and dysregulation in interpersonal situations and impair the ability to mutually satisfy agentic and communal motives of self and others (Ambwani et al., 2015; Cardi et al., 2018a, 2018b). Further, starvation-induced impairments in social responsiveness can evoke the vicious circle of complementary withdrawal and rejection from others, leading to further social exclusion. This can amplify the overvalued ideals of thinness and restricted eating for self-esteem.

Like anorexia, depression has both interpersonal antecedents and consequences. Individuals experiencing significant depression also experience impairments in self-focused social cognition, other-focused social cognition, and interpersonal behavior (Kupferberg & Hasler, 2023), which can be operationalized using the component systems of the interpersonal situation and their links. For example, depressive distortions in perception and construal of self include: (1) self-focused rumination on depressed mood, depression symptoms, and negative past and future events, as well as biased attention to negative social stimuli and inattention to positive social stimuli; (2) social-cognitive inflexibility, insufficient use of social-cognitive reappraisal of emotion-evoking situations, and an inability to revise initial impressions in interpersonal situations; and (3) severe social anhedonia including lack of interest and lack of pleasure in engaging in interpersonal interactions. Depressive distortions in perception and construal of others include: (1) impaired recognition of others' emotions; (2) impaired social trust, empathy, and forgiveness, (3) heightened sensitivity to social evaluation and rejection, and (4) frequent upward social comparisons. Consistent with CIIT, depressive social cognitive impairments are linked with maladaptive interpersonal behaviors, including: (1) difficulties with anger management (e.g., interpersonal irritability, inward-directed anger, passive aggressive acting out); (2) maladaptive reassurance seeking and social avoidance; and (3) inhibition of prosocial behaviors. These deficits directly impact interpersonal functioning, increasing interpersonal loneliness and stress, constraining the quality and diversity social networks, and limiting social support.

Interpersonal Pathoplasticity

Some symptoms and disorders may manifest similar patterns of interpersonal consequences in interpersonal situations for most individuals. However, this is not always the case. Pathoplasticity defines a non-causal but mutually influencing association between personality and psychopathology (Widiger & Smith, 2008). In simple terms, pathoplasticity refers to a moderation effect between the two. Pathoplasticity suggests that individual differences in personality can influence how symptoms manifest, as well as treatment course and outcome. This is also the case for interpersonal pathoplasticity (Pincus et al., 2010; Pincus & Wright, 2011), which occurs when similar symptoms or disorders exhibit diverse patterns of interpersonal consequences in interpersonal situations depending on an individual's prominent interpersonal motives and dispositions. Interpersonal pathoplasticity describes heterogeneity in presentation of psychopathology in terms of distinct patterns of distortion and dysregulation in interpersonal situations across individuals with the same symptom profile or diagnoses.

Research on interpersonal pathoplasticity has identified multiple interpersonal expressions across patients with the same categorical diagnoses or elevations on dimensionally assessed symptoms and clinical problems. Recognizing differences in patients' patterns of distortion and dysregulation provides clinically useful information above and beyond categorical diagnostic labels or dimensional profiles. Studies found support for interpersonal pathoplasticity in social phobia (e.g., Cain et al., 2010), generalized anxiety disorder (e.g., Przeworski et al., 2011), panic disorder (Zilcha-Mano et al., 2015), major depression (e.g., Cain et al., 2012), posttraumatic stress disorder (Thomas et al., 2014), eating pathology (Ambwani & Hopwood, 2009), substance use disorders (Boswell et al., 2017), maladaptive perfectionism (Slaney et al., 2006), and fear of failure (Wright et al., 2009).

Anxiety and depression are among the most common symptoms reported by patients seeking treatment. Whether considered categorical diagnoses or dimensions of psychopathology, both anxiety and depression include elements related to each of the component systems of the interpersonal situation: self, affect, perception, and behavior. But the interpersonal consequences of anxiety or depression (and internalizing symptoms more generally) are unlikely to manifest in similar interpersonal patterns of distortion and dysregulation for all patients. Figure 13.8 summarizes the findings of Przeworski et al. (2011) for generalized anxiety disorder (GAD) and Cain et al. (2012) for major depressive disorder (MDD). The interpersonal dispositions of patients diagnosed with GAD and patients diagnosed with MDD disperse around the IPC. All patients with GAD met threshold for the same diagnosis and thus reported uncontrollable worry. However, what worried them differed: Interpersonally cold

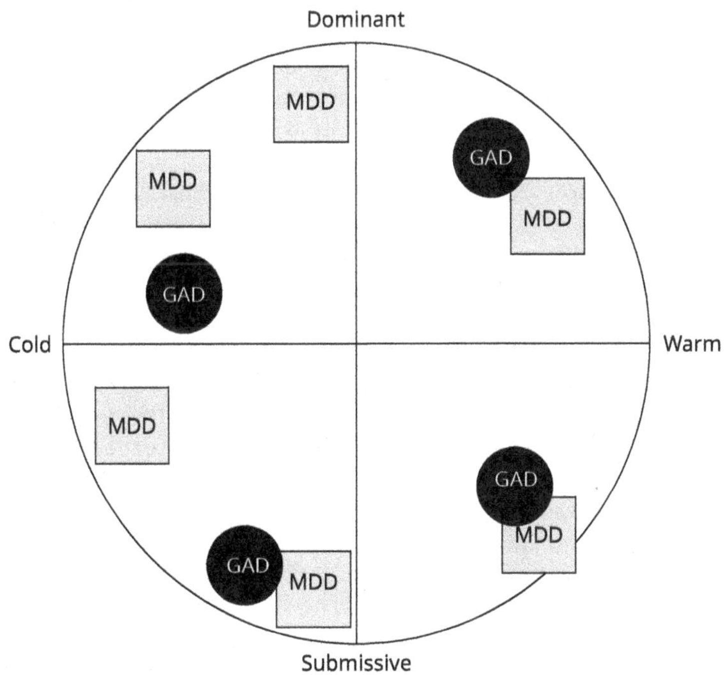

FIGURE 13.8 Interpersonal pathoplasticity for generalized anxiety disorder and major depression.

GAD patients worried that others would hurt them or take something from them, submissive GAD patients worried about their personal competency and the availability of help from others, warm-submissive GAD patients were most worried about whether others would like and approve of them, and warm-dominant GAD patients were most worried about punctuality. These interpersonally distinctive GAD patients also responded differently to cognitive behavioral therapy. The GAD patients with more submissive dispositions (bottom half of the IPC) exhibited greater improvement and post-treatment maintenance of gains than did the GAD patients with more dominant dispositions (upper half of the IPC). In CBT, therapists typically lead and patients follow. This type of therapeutic relationship may be more compatible with the interpersonal dispositions of submissive and warm-submissive GAD patients than with the cold and warm-dominant GAD patients.

Cain and colleagues (2012) found six interpersonal styles of patients who met threshold for MDD diagnosis, labeling them cold, submissive, unassuming, extraverted, dominant, and arrogant. The groups did not differ regarding baseline depression severity or comorbid diagnoses. However, over a 10-year period, the cold and submissive MDD patients experienced greater chronicity (i.e., months with significant depressive symptoms) than did the other groups, and the submissive MDD patients experienced the worst functioning (i.e., months with a Global Assessment of Functioning rating ≤ 70). CIIT's articulation of pathoplasticity of interpersonal consequences for many disorders, symptoms, and clinical problems provides important information beyond categorical diagnostic labels or dimensional symptom profiles to enhance case conceptualization and better tailor treatments.

Interpersonal Disorders

CIIT enhances understanding of psychopathology by accounting for diverse interpersonal antecedents and consequences of patients' disorders, symptoms, and clinical problems in terms of dispositional tendencies and interpersonal patterns of distortion and dysregulation operationalized by the interpersonal situation's component systems and their links. However, some clinical presentations, including those commonly diagnosed as personality disorders, are not interpersonal consequences of disorders or symptoms originating in other human systems. These reflect psychopathology we characterize as interpersonal disorders (Pincus, Cain, & Halberstadt, 2020; Wright & Nielsen, 2025; Wright et al., 2022). Interpersonal disorders reflect pervasive, deeply ensconced, socially learned, and extraordinarily rigid or highly unstable maladaptive interpersonal patterns of distortions and dysregulation that render individuals persistently unwilling and/or unable to form mutually satisfying and supportive relationships with others. Interpersonal disorders reflect pervasive dysfunction across most interpersonal situations such that individuals are chronically unable to accurately perceive and construe self or other (perceptual distortion), regulate emotions (affect dysregulation), behave in mutually satisfying and socially appropriate ways (behavior/field dysregulation), and achieve their interpersonal goals (self-dysregulation) (Pincus & Hopwood, 2012). Psychotherapy for patients with interpersonal disorders emphasizes management of the therapeutic relationship and the therapeutic frame as necessary requirements of treatment (Bateman et al., 2015; Clarkin et al., 2015; Critchfield & Benjamin, 2006).

In Table 13.3, the features of interpersonal disorders are grouped with reference to adaptive and maladaptive social processes and self-processes (the major distinguishing elements of personality disorder in the DSM-5 Alternative Model for Personality Disorders) and exemplified with DSM personality disorder symptoms. The pervasive characteristic distortions of interpersonal disorders lead individuals to experience diverse interpersonal situations as functionally equivalent threats to self-esteem and security, sparking extensive dysregulation. Examples

TABLE 13.3 Dysfunction in the Interpersonal Disorders and Ties with DSM Personality Disorders.

Process	Component System	Adaptive	Maladaptive	Example	DSM PD Symptom
Social processes	Perception/ Construal	Accurate encoding of others' intentions, affects, and behaviors	Chronic distortion of others' intentions, affects, and behaviors	Different interpersonal situations are experienced as functionally equivalent	Perceives all others as abandoning (borderline) or dangerous (paranoid)
				Distortions increase under stress	Perceives all situations as competitions to demonstrate self's superiority (narcissistic)
	Behavior	Selection of situationally and culturally appropriate interpersonal behavior that mutually satisfies self and other's agentic and communal motives and goals	Chronically unable or unwilling to enact situationally and culturally appropriate interpersonal behavior that mutually satisfies self and other's agentic and communal motives and goals	Behaviors are not contingent on other's interpersonal communications or typical expectations of the situation.	Chronic stubbornness (obsessive compulsive) or reassurance-seeking (dependent)
					Unstable push-pull dynamic of the need-fear dilemma (borderline)
Self-processes	Perception/ Construal	Accurate, coherent, stable sense of self	Inaccurate, incoherent, unstable sense of self.	Inflexible or rapidly shifting self-concept	Chronically views self as socially inept (avoidant) or superior to others (narcissistic)
				Chronically low or inflated self-esteem and felt security or volatile swings in self-esteem and felt security	Chronically unstable view of self (borderline)
	Motivation	Flexible selection and pursuit of agentic and communal goals consistent with situational demands	Inability to select or pursue agentic and communal goals consistent with situational demands	Overvalued, rigid, or unstable self-protective agentic and communal goals regardless of situational demands	Workaholism (obsessive-compulsive), disinterest in relating to others (schizoid), or urgent need for others (dependent)
	Affect	Emotional experience corresponds with situational and cultural norms	Emotional experience is inconsistent in kind and/or intensity with situational and cultural norms	Labile, incongruous, and/or inappropriate emotional experience relative to situational and cultural norms	Intolerance of being alone (dependent), discomfort when not center of attention (histrionic), exaggerated emotionality (histrionic), flat affect (schizoid)
		Stable sense of self across a variety of emotions	Unstable sense of self markedly varies across distinct emotional states		

include the chronic or unstable misperception of imminent abandonment associated with borderline personality disorder, the rigid misperception of harmful intent associated with paranoid personality disorder, or the construal of all interpersonal situations as competitions to win and opportunities to demonstrate superiority over others reflected in narcissistic personality disorder. These trigger maladaptive social behaviors that serve to protect the self (i.e., restore security and esteem) but are not contingent on others' behaviors or situational and cultural norms, and they impede mutual satisfaction of interpersonal motives. Examples of such rigid or unstable behaviors include the chronic stubbornness associated with obsessive-compulsive personality disorder, the constant reassurance-seeking associated with dependent personality disorder, or the unstable dynamic of the need-fear dilemma associated with borderline personality disorder.

Maladaptive self-processes include rigidly distorted or unstable self-concept and self-esteem; overvalued, rigid, or unstable agentic and communal motives/goals; and emotion dysregulation. Maladaptive self-processes lead to rigid, unstable, and/or confusing self-views and motives/goals, emotions that are incongruous in kind and/or intensity with situational demands and cultural norms, and self-protective motives that evoke maladaptive social behavior. Examples of distorted self-perceptions include chronically seeing oneself as socially inept (avoidant personality disorder) or superior to others (narcissistic personality disorder) or experiencing an erratic sense of self (borderline personality disorder). Examples of overvalued or rigid interpersonal motives include workaholism (obsessive compulsive personality disorder), profound disinterest in forming social bonds (schizoid personality disorder), and unrelenting desires to be close to and rely on supportive others (dependent personality disorder).

In contrast, some clients rapidly shift between keenly desiring closeness and anxiously avoiding it (borderline personality disorder). Finally, interpersonal disorders include chronic maladaptive labile and/or incongruous emotional experiences, such as discomfort being alone (dependent personality disorder), distress when not the center of attention and embellished emotions (histrionic personality disorder), flat affect (schizoid personality disorder), or abrupt emotional shifts such as narcissistic rage when entitled expectations are not met (narcissistic personality disorder) or suicidal depression in response to perceived abandonment (borderline personality disorder).

We suggest two additional advantages of conceptualizing personality pathology as interpersonal disorders. First, identifying core dysfunctions that are distinct from other forms of psychopathology (e.g., dissociative disorders, eating disorders, etc.) without labeling an individual's personality as disordered, reduces stigma regarding the diagnosis. Second, and perhaps most important, the interpersonal disorders indicate essential treatment implications, emphasizing that psychotherapy will need to concentrate on anticipated difficulties with alliance formation and treatment utilization. Notably, common factors found in validated treatments for interpersonal disorders include anticipating a longer length of treatment and committing more therapeutic time and attention to the therapeutic relationship and its boundaries, distorted perceptions and construals of self and others, and alliance ruptures (e.g., Bateman et al., 2015; Clarkin et al., 2015; Critchfield & Benjamin, 2006; Kramer et al., 2020; Pincus, Cain, & Halberstadt, 2020; Zhan Yuen Wong et al., 2023).

CIIT identifies maladaptive interpersonal patterns as antecedents of disorders, symptoms, and clinical problems; as consequences of disorders, symptoms, and clinical problems originating in other human systems (e.g., cognitive, arousal/regulatory, sensorimotor, endocrine); and as maladaptive interpersonal patterns that result from the pervasive core impairments of interpersonal disorders themselves, specifically, rigid or unstable distortions/construals of self and others and overvalued or inconsistent interpersonal motivations that evoke self-, affect, and behavioral (field) dysregulation, and severe impairments in forming and keeping close and supportive relationships. Importantly, maladaptive interpersonal patterns may be described similarly (e.g., social withdrawal and non-responsiveness), but this can be a consequence of other symptoms (e.g., starvation associated with anorexia nervosa) or a manifestation of deeply ingrained socially reinforced ways of organizing interpersonal experiences and motivations associated with important developmental experiences. Interpersonal consequences of psychopathology are driven by the individual's acute symptoms and problems, whereas interpersonal disorders represent such pervasive self and social impairments that may ultimately drive the individual's acute symptoms and problems.

Interpersonal Dynamics and Dimensional Models of Psychopathology

A useful taxonomy of psychopathology should describe variations in mental disorder, explain how they arise and are maintained, and inform treatment (Hopwood et al., 2023). This is more likely if a valid taxonomy is employed. It is clear that polythetic categorical diagnostic nosologies of psychopathology do not capture the covariation of disorders, symptoms, and problems across people in a valid manner, and in fact, introduce obfuscation by creating high rates of disorder comorbidity and highly heterogeneous presentations within diagnoses. This limits meaningful advancement in understanding the etiology and maintenance of discrete categories of psychopathology and development of effective disorder-specific treatments.

These failures have catalyzed new taxonomic approaches such as the Research Domain Criteria (RDoC; Cuthbert, 2014) and the HiTOP (Kotov et al., 2021). Both systems conceptualize symptoms and clinical problems as hierarchically arranged dimensions, with narrow symptoms relating to each other based on their mutual associations within broader dimensions. By conceptualizing psychopathology dimensionally, RDoC and HiTOP provide evidence-based taxonomies of how people differ from one another on average and facilitate more reliable estimates of psychopathological symptoms and problems in the population.

However, RDoC and HiTOP are missing two critical features that help to explain psychopathological symptoms and inform treatments. First, RDoC and HiTOP both account for psychopathology exclusively with reference to elevated levels of specific signs and symptoms within the person. This is a limited perspective, because psychopathology is expressed in dynamic patterns of person-environment transaction (Hopwood et al., 2022), commonly in the form of interpersonal situations (Pincus, Hopwood, & Wright, 2020). For example, individuals with anxiety symptoms misperceive benign situations as dangerous, individuals with psychotic symptoms misperceive information about the world around them, and individuals with antisocial features experience truly dangerous situations as exciting, increasing risks to self and others.

Second, neither RDoC nor HiTOP articulate temporally dynamic processes (e.g., interpersonal complementarity, interpersonal triggers) that can characterize how people move through their environments, and ultimately their lives, over time. Psychopathological symptoms and problems, and associated impairments, are generally not constant, but rather they more commonly emerge in particular situational contexts. The anxious person usually worries about certain kinds of concerns, the psychotic person misperceives certain kinds of things, and the antisocial person goes after certain kinds of thrills. HiTOP and RDoC can make predictions about which people are more or less likely to experience mental health problems in the abstract, but not when, where, and how those problems will manifest in the situations people encounter in their lives (Hopwood et al., 2023, p. 153).

CIIT conceptualizes psychopathology both in terms of how people differ from one another (what people are like) and how their transactions differ in various environmental contexts (what people do) (Pincus, 2005). Consistent with RDoC and HiTOP, CIIT offers a taxonomic model and set of well-validated methods to assess individual differences in personality and psychopathology (Pincus, Hopwood, & Wright, 2020). In contrast to RDoC and HiTOP, CIIT is concerned with how people function in the contexts in which they live. CIIT has two features that complement new dimensional approaches to diagnosis.

First, CIIT is relational. Transitioning from viewing individuals in a vacuum to understanding people in context has been an advancement across scholarly domains. Philosophy became intersubjective when Existentialists asserted that Descartes had to be thinking about something. The periodic table was based on the realization that electrons serve the function of connecting elements with one another. Nuclear power was facilitated by Einstein's understanding of the connection between energy and time. Major models of psychopathology still assume it can be understood as something that occurs in a vacuum, whereas CIIT's first assumption is that fundamentally important functional expressions of personality and psychopathology occur in interpersonal situations (Hopwood et al., 2021; Wright et al., 2023). In CIIT, the interpersonal situation is considered the basic unit of personality and psychopathology where self and other interact through the linkages of four interpenetrating component systems of perception/construal, self, affect, and behavior that identify the important features of socio-affective functioning. The links among these systems are key features of the dyadic processes that drive interpersonal situations as self and other dynamically cycle through continuous transactions.

Second, CIIT is temporally dynamic. It is assumed that the satisfaction of agentic and communal motives drives interpersonal behavior. This allows for probabilistic predictions about how people will relate to others via motivational, perceptual, affective, and behavioral processes, and how these can go awry. In CIIT, adaptive functioning is not defined by dispositional levels: rather, it is defined by the ability to harmonize and satisfy self and others' agentic and communal motives across different contexts of developmental, sociocultural, and situational demands consistently yet flexibly. Accordingly, psychopathology involves sustained breakdown in any of the processes that support and maintain consistent yet flexible and effective regulation of self, affect, and interpersonal behavior in relation to others.

CIIT also provides valid methods to assess interpersonal dispositions and temporally dynamic interpersonal processes that unfold in interpersonal situations. These include self- and informant-report questionnaires, experience sampling surveys via mobile devices, and computer-facilitated continuous observational assessment methods (Pincus, Sadler, et al., 2014). The dimensions of CIIT and the processes linking the interpersonal situation's component systems can be used to distinguish people from one another, on average, as do RDoC and HiTOP, but they can also be used to describe how people differ from themselves across time and situations. This allows for empirical tests of hypotheses about temporal dynamics in sample-based research and in individual clinical cases. Interpersonal dispositions and dynamic interpersonal processes have been empirically related to forms of psychopathology (e.g., Liu et al., 2025; Wright et al., 2017) and psychotherapeutic processes (e.g., Altenstein et al., 2013; Halberstadt et al., 2024; Luo et al., 2022).

CIIT advances dimensional models that describe how people differ from one another on average and how those differences pose risk for symptoms, by also providing a framework to operationalize how symptoms are expressed and the person-environment transactions that can aggravate or relieve them. CIIT integrates a structural model of individual differences with a functional model of temporally dynamic person-environment transactions to promote an integrated understanding of personality, psychopathology, assessment, and intervention that complements individual-based dimensional models of psychopathology like RDoC and HiTOP.

References

Allen, T. A., & DeYoung, C. G. (2017). Personality neuroscience and the Five Factor Model. In T. A. Widiger (Ed.), *The Oxford handbook of the Five Factor Model* (pp. 319–349). Oxford University Press.

Allen, T. A., Schreiber, A. M., Hall, N. T., & Hallquist, M. N. (2020). From description to explanation: Integrating across multiple levels of analysis to inform neuroscientific accounts of dimensional personality pathology. *Journal of Personality Disorders, 34*, 650–676.

Altenstein, D., Krieger, T., & Grosse Holtforth, M. (2013). Interpersonal microprocesses predict cognitive-emotional processing and the therapeutic alliance in psychotherapy for depression. *Journal of Counseling Psychology, 60*, 445–452.

Ambwani, S., & Hopwood, C. J. (2009). The utility of considering interpersonal problems in the assessment of bulimic features. *Eating Behaviors, 10*, 247–253.

Ambwani, S., Roche, M. J., Minnick, A. M., & Pincus, A. L. (2015). Negative affect, interpersonal perception, and binge eating behavior: An experience sampling study. *International Journal of Eating Disorders, 48*, 715–726.

Anchin, J. C., & Pincus, A. L. (2010). Evidence-based interpersonal psychotherapy with personality disorders: Theory, components, and strategies. In J. J. Magnavita (Ed.), *Evidence-based treatment of personality dysfunction: Principles, methods, and processes* (pp. 113–166). American Psychological Association.

Ansell, E. B., Kurtz, J. E., & Markey, P. M. (2008). Gender differences in interpersonal complementarity within roommate dyads. *Personality and Social Psychology Bulletin, 34*, 502–512.

Ansell, E. B., & Pincus, A. L. (2004). Interpersonal perceptions of the five-factor model of personality: An examination using the structural summary method for circumplex data. *Multivariate Behavioral Research, 39*(2), 167–201.

Asan, A. E., Pincus, A. L., & Ansell, E. B. (2024). A multi-method study of interpersonal complementarity and mentalization. *Journal of Research in Personality, 110*: 104478.

Asan, A. E., Pincus, A. L., & Hopwood, C. J. (2023). Interpersonal diagnosis of schizotypy. In S. Cheli & P. Lysaker (Eds.), *A dimensional approach to schizotypy: Conceptualization and treatment* (pp. 177–196). Springer.

Bakan, D. (1966). *The duality of human existence: Isolation and communion in Western man.* Beacon Press.

Bateman, A. W., Gunderson, J., & Mulder, R. (2015). Treatment of personality disorder. *Lancet, 385*, 735–743.

Baumeister, R. F., & Leary, M. R. (1995). The need to belong: Desire for interpersonal attachments as a fundamental human motivation. *Psychological Bulletin, 117*, 497–529.

Baumert, A., Schmitt, M., & Perugini, M. (2019). Towards an explanatory personality psychology: Integrating personality structure, personality process, and personality development. *Personality and Individual Differences, 147*, 18–27.

Benjamin, L. (1993). Every psychopathology is a gift of love. *Psychotherapy Research, 3*, 1–24.

Benjamin, L. S. (1974). Structural analysis of social behavior. *Psychological Review, 81*, 392–425.

Benjamin, L. S. (2003). *Interpersonal reconstructive therapy: Promoting change in nonresponders.* Guilford Press.

Blatt, S. J. (2004). *Experiences of depression: Theoretical, clinical, and research perspectives.* American Psychological Association.

Bornstein, R. F. (2019). From structure to process: On the integration of AMPD and HiTOP. *Journal of Personality Assessment, 101*, 360–366.

Boswell, J. F., Cain, N. M., Oswald, J. M., McAleavey, A. A., & Adelman, R. (2017). Interpersonal pathoplasticity and trajectories of change in routine adolescent and young adult residential substance abuse treatment. *Journal of Consulting and Clinical Psychology, 85*, 676–688.

Cain, N. M., Ansell, E. B., Wright, A. G. C., Hopwood, C. J., Thomas, K. M., Pinto, A., Markowitz, J. C., Sanislow, C. A., Zanarini, M. C., Shea, M. T., Morey, L. C., McGlashan, T. H., Skodol, A. E., & Grilo, C. M. (2012). Interpersonal pathoplasticity in the course of major depression. *Journal of Consulting and Clinical Psychology*, *80*, 78–86.

Cain, N. M., Hopwood, C. J., & Pincus, A. L. (2024). Psychotherapy through the lens of Contemporary Integrative Interpersonal Theory. In F. Leong (Ed.), *APA handbook of psychotherapy—Vol. 1: Theory-driven practice and disorder-driven practice* (pp. 141–156).American Psychological Association.

Cain, N. M., & Pincus, A. L. (2016). Treating maladaptive interpersonal signatures. In W. J. Livesley, G. Dimaggio, & J. F. Clarkin (Eds.), *Integrated treatment for personality disorder: A modular approach* (pp. 305–324). Guilford Press.

Cain, N. M., Pincus, A. L., & Grosse Holtforth, M. (2010). Interpersonal subtypes in social phobia: Diagnostic and treatment implications. *Journal of Personality Assessment*, *92*, 514–527.

Cardi, V., Mallorqui-Bague, N., Albano, G., Monteleone, A. M., Fernandez-Aranda, F., & Treasure, J. (2018). Social difficulties as risk and maintaining factors in anorexia nervosa: A mixed-method investigation. *Frontiers in Psychiatry*, *9*, 324997.

Cardi, V., Tchanturia, K., & Treasure, J. (2018). Premorbid and illness-related social difficulties in eating disorders: An overview of the literature and treatment developments. *Current Neuropharmacology*, *16*, 1122–1130.

Carson, R. C. (1969). *Interaction concepts of personality*. Aldine.

Carson, R. C. (1982). Self-fulfilling prophecy, maladaptive behavior, and psychotherapy. In J. C. Anchin & D. J. Kiesler (Eds.), *Handbook of interpersonal psychotherapy* (pp. 64–77). Pergamon Press.

Clarkin, J. F., Lenzenweger, M. F., & Meehan, K. B. (2015). Emerging approaches to the conceptualization and treatment of personality disorder. *Canadian Psychology*, *56*, 155–167.

Clegg, K. A., Moskowitz, D. S., Miners, C. T. H., Andrevski, G., Sadikaj, G., & Zuroff, D. C. (2021). Interpersonal perception and interpersonal spin. *Journal of Personality*, *89*, 483–499.

Côté, S., Moskowitz, D. S., & Zuroff, D. C. (2012). Social relationships and intraindividual variability in interpersonal behavior: Correlates of interpersonal spin. *Journal of Personality and Social Psychology*, *102*, 646–659.

Critchfield, K. L., & Benjamin, L. S. (2006). Principles for psychosocial treatment of personality disorder: Summary of the APA Division 12 Task Force/NASPR review. *Journal of Clinical Psychology*, *62*, 661–674.

Critchfield, K. L., & Benjamin, L. S. (2008). Internalized representations of early interpersonal experience and adult relationships: A test of copy process theory in clinical and non-clinical settings. *Psychiatry*, *71*, 71–92.

Cuthbert, B. N. (2014). The RDoC framework: Facilitating transition from ICD/DSM to dimensional approaches that integrate neuroscience and psychopathology. *World Psychiatry*, *13*, 28–35.

Dalgleish, T., Black, M., Johnston, D., & Bevan, A. (2020). Transdiagnostic approaches to mental health problems: Current status and future directions. *Journal of Consulting and Clinical Psychology*, *88*, 179–195.

Dawood, S., Dowgwillo, E. A., Wu, L. Z., & Pincus, A. L. (2018). Contemporary Integrative Interpersonal Theory of Personality. In V. Zeigler-Hill and T. Shackleford (Eds.), *The SAGE handbook of personality and individual differences—Vol. 1: The science of personality and individual differences* (pp. 171–202). Sage.

Depue, R. A. (2006). Interpersonal behavior and the structure of personality: Neurobehavioral foundation of agentic extraversion and affiliation. In T. Canli (Ed.), *Biology of personality and individual differences* (pp. 60–92). Guilford Press.

Dowgwillo, E. A., & Pincus, A. L. (2017). Differentiating dark triad traits within and across interpersonal circumplex surfaces. *Assessment*, *24*, 24–44.

Dowgwillo, E. A., Pincus, A. L., Newman, M. G., Wilson, S. J., Molenaar, P. C. M., & Levy, K. N. (2019). Two methods for operationalizing the interpersonal situation to investigate personality pathology and interpersonal perception in daily life. In L. I. Truslow & J. M. Rahmaan (Eds.), *Personality disorders: What we know and future directions for research* (pp. 31–106). Nova Science Publishers.

Du, T. V., Yardley, A. E., & Thomas, K. M. (2021). Mapping Big Five personality traits within and across domains of interpersonal functioning. *Assessment, 28*, 1358–1375.

Dunlop, W. L., Lind, M., & Hopwood, C. J. (2023). Synthesizing contemporary integrative interpersonal theory and the narrative identity approach to examine personality dynamics and regulatory processes. *Journal of Personality, 91*, 963–976.

Edershile, E. A., & Wright, A. G. C. (2025). Narcissism's effect on regulatory processes in interpersonal situations. *Personality Disorders: Theory, Research, and Treatment, 16*(3), 235–248.

Fournier, M. A., Moskowitz, D. S., & Zuroff, D. C. (2008). Integrating dispositions, signatures, and the interpersonal domain. *Journal of Personality and Social Psychology, 94*, 531–545.

Fournier, M. A., Moskowitz, D. S., & Zuroff, D. C. (2011). Origins and applications of the interpersonal circumplex. In L. M. Horowitz & S. Strack (Eds.), *Handbook of interpersonal psychology* (pp. 57–74). John Wiley & Sons.

Gibson, S., Slotter, E. B., & Markey, P. M. (2024). Fighting the good fight: Relating warmth and dominance across romantic conflict to resolution. *Journal of Social and Personal Relationships, 41*(9), 2716–2739.

Girard, J. M., Wright, A. G. C., Beeney, J. E., Lazarus, S. A., Scott, L. N., Stepp, S. D., & Pilkonis, P. A. (2017). Interpersonal problems across levels of the psychopathology hierarchy. *Comprehensive Psychiatry, 79*, 53–69.

Grosse-Holtforth, M., Thomas, A., & Caspar, F. (2011). Interpersonal motivation. In L. M. Horowitz & S. Strack (Eds.), *Handbook of interpersonal psychology* (pp. 107–122). John Wiley & Sons.

Gurtman, M. B., & Pincus, A. L. (2003). The circumplex model: Methods and research applications. In J. Schinka & W. Velicer (Eds.), *Handbook of psychology: Research methods in psychology* (2nd ed., pp. 407–428). John Wiley & Sons.

Halberstadt, A. L., Asan, A. E., & Pincus, A. L. (2024). Development and feasibility of a protocol to improve clinical trainees' awareness of interpersonal processes using Continuous Assessment of Interpersonal Dynamics. *Training and Education in Professional Psychology, 18*(4), 386–398.

Halberstadt, A. L., Pincus, A. L., Mogle, J., & Ansell, E. B. (2023). Interpersonal complementarity and affect in daily life. *Motivation and Emotion, 47*, 270–281.

Heck, S. A., & Pincus, A. L. (2001). Agency and communion in the structure of parental representations. *Journal of Personality Assessment, 76*, 180–184.

Helgeson, V. S. (1994). Relation of agency and communion to well-being: Evidence and potential explanations. *Psychological Bulletin, 116*, 412–428.

Hogan, R. J., & Roberts, B. W. (2000). A socioanalytic perspective on person-environment. In W. B. Walsh, K. H. Craik, & R. H. Price (Eds.), *Person-environment psychology: New directions and perspectives* (2nd ed.) (pp. 1–24). Lawrence Erlbaum.

Hopwood, C. J. (2018). Interpersonal dynamics in personality and personality disorders. *European Journal of Personality, 32*, 499–524.

Hopwood, C. J., Harrison, A. L., Amole, M., Girard, J. M., Wright, A. G., Thomas, K. M., Sadler, P., Ansell, E. G., Chaplin, T. M., Morey, L. C., Crowley, M. J., Durbin, C. E., & Kashy, D. A. (2020). Properties of the continuous assessment of interpersonal dynamics across sex, level of familiarity, and interpersonal conflict. *Assessment, 27*, 40–56.

Hopwood, C. J., Pincus, A. L., & Wright, A. G. C. (2019). The interpersonal situation: Integrating personality assessment, case formulation, and intervention. In D. B. Samuel & D. R. Lynam (Eds.), *Using basic personality research to inform personality pathology* (pp. 94–121). Oxford University Press.

Hopwood, C. J., Pincus, A. L., & Wright, A. G. C. (2021). Six assumptions of Contemporary Integrative Interpersonal Theory of personality and psychopathology. *Current Opinion in Psychology, 41*, 65–70.

Hopwood, C. J., Pincus, A. L., & Wright, A. G. C. (2023). A clinically useful model of psychopathology must account for interpersonal dynamics. *World Psychiatry, 22*, 152–154.

Hopwood, C. J., Wright, A. G. C., Ansell, E. B., & Pincus, A. L. (2013). The interpersonal core of personality pathology. *Journal of Personality Disorders, 27*, 270–295.

Hopwood, C. J., Wright, A. G. C., & Bleidorn, W. (2022). Person–environment transactions differentiate personality and psychopathology. *Nature Reviews Psychology, 1*, 55–63.

Hopwood, C. J., Zimmermann, J., Pincus, A. L., & Krueger, R. F. (2015). Connecting personality structure and dynamics: Towards a more evidence based and clinically useful diagnostic scheme. *Journal of Personality Disorders*, *29*, 431–448.

Horowitz, L. M. (2004). *Interpersonal foundations of psychopathology*. American Psychological Association.

Horowitz, L. M., Wilson, K. R., Turan, B., Zolotsev, P., Constantino, M. J., & Henderson, L. (2006). How interpersonal motives clarify the meaning of interpersonal behavior: A revised circumplex model. *Personality and Social Psychology Review*, *10*, 67–86.

Johnson, S. L., Leedom, L. J., & Muhtadie, L. (2012). The dominance behavioral system and psychopathology: Evidence from self-report, observational, and biological studies. *Psychological Bulletin*, *138*, 692–743.

Kaurin, A., Dombrovski, A. Y., Hallquist, M. N., & Wright, A. G. C. (2022). Momentary interpersonal processes of suicidal surges in borderline personality disorder. *Psychological Medicine*, *52*, 2702–2712.

Kaurin, A., Pilkonis, P. A., & Wright, A. G. (2022). Attachment manifestations in daily interpersonal interactions. *Affective Science*, *3*, 546–558.

Kiesler, D. J. (1983). The 1982 interpersonal circle: A taxonomy for complementarity in human interactions. *Psychological Review*, *90*, 185–214.

Kiesler, D. J. (1996). *Contemporary interpersonal theory and research: Personality, psychopathology, and psychotherapy*. John Wiley & Sons.

Kiesler, D. J., Schmidt, J. A., & Wagner, C. C. (1997). A circumplex inventory of impact messages: An operational bridge between emotion and interpersonal behavior. In R. Plutchik & H. R. Conte (Eds.), *Circumplex models of personality and emotions* (pp. 221–244). American Psychological Association.

Kopala-Sibley, D. C., Zuroff, D. C., Hermanto, N., & Joyal-Desmarais, K. (2016). The development of self-definition and relatedness in emerging adulthood and their role in the development of depressive symptoms. *International Journal of Behavioral Development*, *40*, 302–312.

Kotov, R., Krueger, R. F., Watson, D., Cicero, D. C., Conway, C. C., DeYoung, C. G., Eaton, N. R, Forbes, M. K, Hallquist, M. N., Latzman, R. D., Mullins-Sweatt, S. N., Ruggero, C. J., Simms, L. J., Waldman, I. D., Waszczuk, M. A., & Wright, A. G. (2021). The Hierarchical Taxonomy of Psychopathology (HiTOP): A quantitative nosology based on consensus of evidence. *Annual Review of Clinical Psychology*, *17*, 83–108.

Kramer, U., Beuchat, H., Grandjean, L., & Pascual-Leone, A. (2020). How personality disorders change in psychotherapy: A concise review of process. *Current Psychiatry Reports*, *22*(8), 41. https://doi.org/10.1007/s11920-020-01162-3

Kupferberg, A., & Hasler, G. (2023). The social cost of depression: Investigating the impact of impaired social emotion regulation, social cognition, and interpersonal behavior on social functioning. *Journal of Affective Disorders Reports*, *14*, 100631.

Kurzius, E., Borkenau, P., & Leising, D. (2022). Spontaneous interpersonal complementarity in the lab: A multilevel approach to modeling the antecedents and consequences of people's interpersonal behaviors and their dynamic interplay. *Journal of Personality and Social Psychology*, *122*, 244–264.

Leary, M. R., Tambor, E. S., Terdal, S. K., & Downs, D. L. (1995). Self-esteem as an interpersonal monitor: The sociometer hypothesis. *Journal of Personality and Social Psychology*, *68*, 518–530.

Leary, T. (1957). *Interpersonal diagnosis of personality*. Ronald Press.

Lewis, K. C., & Ridenour, J. M. (2020). The integration of EMA and single-occasion multimethod assessment data for a complex psychiatric patient. *Assessment*, *27*, 1532–1546.

Liu, Y., Hopwood, C. J., Pincus, A. L., Zhou, B., Yang, J., Bai, S., & Yang, B. (2025). Interpersonal problem profiles of personality and psychopathology constructs in Chinese undergraduates and offenders. *Assessment*, *32*(2), 253–268.

Lukowitsky, M. R., & Pincus, A. L. (2011). The pantheoretical nature of mental representations and their ability to predict interpersonal adjustment in a nonclinical sample. *Psychoanalytic Psychology*, *28*, 48–74.

Luo, X., Liu, S., Levendosky, A. A., Good, E. W., Turchan, J. E., & Hopwood, C. J. (2022). Idiographic and nomothetic relationships between momentary interpersonal behaviors, interpersonal

complementarity, and alliance ruptures in psychotherapy. *Journal of Counseling Psychology*, *69*, 642–655.
Mahadevan, N., Gregg, A. P., & Sedikides, C. (2019). Is self-regard a sociometer or a hierometer? Self-esteem tracks status and inclusion, narcissism tracks status. *Journal of Personality and Social Psychology*, *116*, 444–466.
Mahadevan, N., Gregg, A. P., & Sedikides, C. (2020). The ups and downs of social life: Within-person variations in daily status and inclusion differentially predict self-regard and interpersonal behavior. *Journal of Personality*, *88*, 1111–1128.
Meehan, K. B., Cain, N. M., Roche, M. J., Clarkin, J. F., & De Panfilis, C. (2018). Rejection sensitivity and interpersonal behavior in daily life. *Personality and Individual Differences*, *126*, 109–115.
Meehan, K. B., Cain, N. M., Roche, M. J., Clarkin, J. F., & De Panfilis, C. (2019). Rejection sensitivity and self-regulation of daily interpersonal events. *Journal of Contemporary Psychotherapy*, *49*, 223–233.
Meisel, S. N., Colder, C. R., & Hopwood, C. J. (2022). Assessing parent-adolescent substance use discussions using the Continuous Assessment of Interpersonal Dynamics. *Journal of Personality Assessment*, *104*, 800–812.
Mikulincer, M., & Shaver, P. R. (2012). An attachment perspective on psychopathology. *World Psychiatry*, *11*, 11–15.
Millon, T. (2011). *Disorders of personality: Introducing a DSM/ICD spectrum from normal to abnormal*. John Wiley & Sons.
Monteleone, A. M., Cascino, G., Salerno, L., Albano, G., Barone, E., Cardi, V., & Coco, G. L. (2023). The interplay between emotion regulation, interpersonal problems and eating symptoms in individuals with obesity: A network analysis study. *Journal of Affective Disorders*, *324*, 61–67.
Moskowitz, D. S. (2005). Unfolding interpersonal behavior. *Journal of Personality*, *73*, 1607–1632.
Moskowitz, D. S., Ho, M. H. R., & Turcotte-Tremblay, A. M. (2007). Contextual influences on interpersonal complementarity. *Personality and Social Psychology Bulletin*, *33*, 1051–1063.
Moskowitz, D. S., Zuroff, D. C., aan het Rot, M., & Young, S. N. (2011). Tryptophan and interpersonal spin. *Journal of Research in Personality*, *45*, 692–696.
Phalip, A., Netser, S., & Wagner, S. (2024). Understanding the neurobiology of social behavior through exploring brain-wide dynamics of neural activity. *Neuroscience & Biobehavioral Reviews*, *165*, 105856.
Pincus, A. L. (2005). A contemporary integrative interpersonal theory of personality disorders. In M. Lenzenweger & J. F. Clarkin (Eds.), *Major theories of personality disorder* (2nd Ed.) (pp. 282–331). Guilford Press.
Pincus, A. L. (2023). Narcissistic personality disorder and pathological narcissism. In R. F. Krueger & P. H. Blaney (Eds.), *Oxford textbook ofpsychopathology, 4th Ed.* (pp. 628–649). Oxford University Press.
Pincus, A. L., & Ansell, E. B. (2013). Interpersonal theory of personality. In J. Suls & H. Tennen (Eds.), *Handbook of psychology Vol. 5: Personality and social psychology* (2nd Ed.) (pp. 141–159). John Wiley & Sons.
Pincus, A. L., Cain, N. M., & Halberstadt, A. L. (2020). Importance of self and other in defining personality pathology. *Psychopathology*, *53*, 133–140.
Pincus, A. L., Cain, N. M., & Wright, A. G. C. (2014). Narcissistic grandiosity and narcissistic vulnerability in psychotherapy. *Personality Disorders: Theory, Research, and Treatment*, *5*, 439–443.
Pincus, A. L., & Hopwood, C. J. (2012). A contemporary interpersonal model of personality pathology and personality disorder. In T. A. Widiger (Ed.), *The Oxford handbook of personality disorders* (pp. 372–398). Oxford University Press.
Pincus, A. L., & Hopwood, C. J. (2025). *The interpersonal situation: Contemporary integrative interpersonal theory, assessment, and psychotherapy*. American Psychological Association.
Pincus, A. L., Hopwood, C. J., & Dawood, S. (2020). A contemporary interpersonal reassessment of Madeline G. In C. J. Hopwood & M. Waugh (Eds.), *Personality assessment paradigms and methods: A collaborative reassessment of Madeline G.* (pp. 112–131). Routledge.
Pincus, A. L., Hopwood, C. J., & Wright, A. G. C. (2020). The interpersonal situation: An integrative framework for the study of personality, psychopathology, and psychotherapy. In D. Funder, J. F. Rauthmann, & R. Sherman (Eds.), *Oxford handbook of psychological situations* (pp. 124–142). Oxford University Press.

Pincus, A. L., Lukowitsky, M. R., & Wright, A. G. C. (2010). The interpersonal nexus of personality and psychopathology. In T. Millon, R. F. Kreuger, & E. Simonsen (Eds.), *Contemporary directions in psychopathology: Scientific foundations for DSM-V and ICD-11* (pp. 523–552). Guilford Press.

Pincus, A. L., Lukowitsky, M. R., Wright, A. G. C., & Eichler, W. C. (2009). The interpersonal nexus of persons, situations, and psychopathology. *Journal of Research in Personality*, *43*, 264–265.

Pincus, A. L., Sadler, P., Woody, E., Roche, M. J., Thomas, K. M., & Wright, A. G. C. (2014). Multimethod assessment of interpersonal dynamics. In C. J. Hopwood & R. F. Bornstein (Eds.), *Multimethod clinical assessment* (pp. 51–91). Guilford Press.

Pincus, A. L. & Wright, A. G. C. (2011). Interpersonal diagnosis of psychopathology. In L. M. Horowitz and S. Strack (Eds.) *Handbook of interpersonal psychology* (pp. 359–381). John Wiley & Sons.

Posner, J., Russell, J. A., & Peterson, B. S. (2005). The circumplex model of affect: An integrative approach to affective neuroscience, cognitive development, and psychopathology. *Development and Psychopathology*, *17*, 715–734.

Przeworski, A., Newman, M. G., Pincus, A. L., Kasoff, M. B., Yamasaki, A. S., Castonguay, L. G., & Berlin, K. S. (2011). Interpersonal pathoplasticity in individuals with generalized anxiety disorder. *Journal of Abnormal Psychology*, *120*, 286–298.

Rappaport, L. M., Moskowitz, D. S., & D'Antono, B. (2014). Naturalistic interpersonal behavior patterns differentiate depression and anxiety symptoms in the community. *Journal of Counseling Psychology*, 61, 253–263.

Ringwald, W. R., Hallquist, M. N., Dombrovski, A. Y., & Wright, A. G. (2022). Transdiagnostic associations with interpersonal and affective variability in borderline personality pathology. *Journal of Personality Disorders*, *36*, 320–338.

Ringwald, W. R., Hopwood, C. J., Pilkonis, P. A., & Wright, A. G. (2021). Dynamic features of affect and interpersonal behavior in relation to general and specific personality pathology. *Personality Disorders: Theory, Research, and Treatment*, *12*, 365–376.

Roche, M. J. (2022). Tethering theory to timescale: Advances in measuring interpersonal complementarity and covariation. *Journal of Research in Personality*, *99*, 104264.

Roche, M. J., Pincus, A. L., Conroy, D. E., Hyde, A. L., & Ram, N. (2013). Pathological narcissism and interpersonal behavior in daily life. *Personality Disorders: Theory, Research, and Treatment*, *4*, 315–323.

Roche, M. J., Pincus, A. L., Hyde, A. L., Conroy, D. E., & Ram, N. (2013). Within-person co-variation of agentic and communal perceptions: Implications for interpersonal theory and assessment. *Journal of Research in Personality*, *47*, 445–552.

Roche, M. J., Pincus, A. L., Rebar, A. L., Conroy, D. E., & Ram, N. (2014). Enriching psychological assessment using a person-specific analysis of interpersonal processes in daily life. *Assessment*, *21*, 515–528.

Russell, J. J., Moskowitz, D. S., Zuroff, D. C., Sookman, D., & Paris, J. (2007). Stability and variability of affective experience and interpersonal behavior in borderline personality disorder. *Journal of Abnormal Psychology*, *116*, 578–588.

Sadikaj, G., Moskowitz, D. S., Russell, J. J., Zuroff, D. C., & Paris, J. (2013). Quarrelsome behavior in borderline personality disorder: Influence of behavioral and affective reactivity to perceptions of others. *Journal of Abnormal Psychology*, *122*, 195–207.

Sadikaj, G., Moskowitz, D. S., & Zuroff, D. C. (2011). Attachment-related affective dynamics: Differential reactivity to others' interpersonal behavior. *Journal of Personality and Social Psychology*, *100*, 905–917.

Sadikaj, G., Russell, J. J., Moskowitz, D. S., & Paris, J. (2010). Affect dysregulation in individuals with borderline personality disorder: Persistence and interpersonal triggers. *Journal of Personality Assessment*, *92*, 490–500.

Sadler, P., Ethier, N., Gunn, G. R., Duong, D., & Woody, E. (2009). Are we on the same wavelength? Interpersonal complementarity as shared cyclical patterns during interactions. *Journal of Personality and Social Psychology*, *97*, 1005–1020.

Sadler, P., Ethier, N., & Woody, E. (2011). Interpersonal complementarity. In L. M. Horowitz & S. Strack (Eds.), *Handbook of interpersonal psychology* (pp. 123–142). John Wiley & Sons.

Sanislow, C. A. (2016). Connecting psychopathology meta-structure and mechanisms. *Journal of Abnormal Psychology*, *125*, 1158–1165.

Sharp, C., & Wall, K. (2021). DSM-5 level of personality functioning: Refocusing personality disorder on what it means to be human. *Annual Review of Clinical Psychology*, *17*, 313–337.
Skowron, E. A., Kozlowski, J. M., & Pincus, A. L. (2010). Differentiation, self-other representations, and rupture-repair processes: Predicting child maltreatment-risk. *Journal of Counseling Psychology*, *57*, 304–316.
Slaney, R. B., Pincus, A. L., Uliaszek, A. A., & Wang, K. T. (2006). Conceptions of perfectionism and interpersonal problems: Evaluating groups using the structural summary method for circumplex data. *Assessment*, *13*, 138–153.
Slotter, E. B., Markey, P. M., Audigier, A., Dashineau, S. C., Finkel, E. J., & Luchies, L. B. (2023). Love's a dance you learn as you go: Evidence for interpersonal complementarity during romantic conflict and its association with relationship outcomes. *European Journal of Social Psychology*, *53*, 805–822.
Stadel, M., van Duijn, M. A. J., Wright, A. G. C., Bringmann, L. F., & Elmer, T. (2024). Considering the 'With Whom': Differences between event- and signal-contingent ESM data of person-specific social interactions. *Multivariate Behavioral Research*, 59(4), 841–858. https://doi.org/10.1080/00273171.2024.2335405.
Sullivan, H. S. (1953a). *Conceptions of modern psychiatry*. Norton.
Sullivan, H. S. (1953b). *The interpersonal theory of psychiatry*. Norton.
Sullivan, H. S. (1954). *The psychiatric interview*. Norton.
Sullivan, H. S. (1956). *Clinical studies in psychiatry*. Norton.
Sullivan, H. S. (1962). *Schizophrenia as a human process*. Norton.
Sullivan, H. S. (1964). *The fusion of psychiatry and social science*. Norton.
Thomas, K. M., Hopwood, C. J., Donnellan, M. B., Wright, A. G. C., Sanislow, C. A., McDevitt-Murphy, M. E., Ansell, E. B., Grilo, C. M., McGlashan, T. H., Shea, M. T., Markowitz, J. C., Skodol, A. E., Zanarini, M. C., & Morey, L. C. (2014). Personality heterogeneity in PTSD: Distinct temperament and interpersonal typologies. *Psychological Assessment*, *26*, 23–34.
Trapnell, P. D., & Paulhus, D. L. (2012). Agentic and communal values: Their scope and measurement. *Journal of Personality Assessment*, *94*, 39–52.
Treasure, J., Willmott, D., Ambwani, S., Cardi, V., Clark Bryan, D., Rowlands, K., & Schmidt, U. (2020). Cognitive interpersonal model for anorexia nervosa revisited: The perpetuating factors that contribute to the development of the severe and enduring illness. *Journal of Clinical Medicine*, *9*, 630.
Vize, C. E., Ringwald, W. R., Scott, L. N., Kamarck, T. W., Pilkonis, P. A., & Wright, A. G. C. (2024). Evidence for a vicious socioemotional cycle of negative emotions and interpersonal conflict. *Journal of Consulting and Clinical Psychology*, *92*, 479–492.
Wake, N., Frie, R., & Sauvayre, P. (2022). The roots of interpersonal psychoanalysis: Harry S. Sullivan, interdisciplinary inquiry, and subjectivity. In R. Frie & P. Sauvayre (Eds.), *Culture, politics, and race in the making of interpersonal psychoanalysis* (pp. 21–48). Routledge.
Waller, R., & Wagner, N. (2019). The Sensitivity to Threat and Affiliative Reward (STAR) model and the development of callous-unemotional traits. *Neuroscience & Biobehavioral Reviews*, *107*, 656–671.
Wang, S., Roche, M. J., Pincus, A. L., Conroy, D. E., Rebar, A. L., & Ram, N. (2014). Interpersonal dependency and emotion in everyday life. *Journal of Research in Personality*, *53*, 5–12.
Widiger, T. A., & Smith, G. T. (2008). Personality and psychopathology. In O. P. John, R. Robins, & L. A. Pervin (Eds.), *Handbook of personality: Theory and research* (3rd ed., pp. 743–769). Guilford Press.
Wiggins, J. S. (1979). A psychological taxonomy of trait descriptive terms: The interpersonal domain. *Journal of Personality and Social Psychology*, *37*, 395–412.
Wiggins, J. S. (1982). Circumplex models of interpersonal behavior in clinical psychology. In P. C. Kendall & J. N. Butcher (Eds.), *Handbook of research methods in clinical psychology* (pp. 183–221). John Wiley & Sons.
Wiggins, J. S. (1991). Agency and communion as conceptual coordinates for the understanding and measurement of interpersonal behavior. In D. Cicchetti & W. M. Grove (Eds.), *Thinking clearly about psychology: Essays in honor of Paul E. Meehl, Vol. 2: Personality and psychopathology* (pp. 89–113). University of Minnesota Press.
Wiggins, J. S. (1996). An informal history of the interpersonal circumplex tradition. *Journal of Personality Assessment*, *66*, 217–233.

Wiggins, J. S. (2003). *Paradigms of personality assessment*. Guilford Press.

Wiggins, J. S., & Trobst, K. K. (1999). The fields of interpersonal behavior. In L. Pervin and O. P. John (Eds.), *Handbook of personality: Theory and research* (2nd Ed.) (pp. 653–670). Guilford Press.

Wilson, S., Stroud, C. B., & Durbin, C. E. (2017). Interpersonal dysfunction in personality disorders: A meta-analytic review. *Psychological Bulletin, 143*, 677–734.

Woehrle, P. L., Critchfield, K. L., Anolik, S., Bobal, C., Pempek, T. A., & Skowron, E. A. (2023). Multigenerational patterns of parenting-at-risk: A test of interpersonal specificity using copy process theory. *Journal of Clinical Psychology, 79*, 186–200.

Woods, W. C., Edershile, E. A., Ringwald, W. R., Sharpe, B. M., Himmelstein, P. H., Newman, M. G., Wilson, S .J., Ellison, W. D., Levy, K. N., Pincus, A. L., Creswell, J. D., & Wright, A. G. C. (2023). Psychometric evaluation of a Visual Interpersonal Analog Scale. *Psychological Assessment, 35*, 311–324.

Wright, A. G. C., & Nielsen, S. R. (2025). A Contemporary Integrative Interpersonal Theory formulation of self and social pathology. In C. Banicki & P. Zachar (Eds.), *Conceptualizing personality disorder: Perspectives from philosophy, psychological science, and psychiatry* (pp. 108–129). Cambridge University Press.

Wright, A. G. C., Pincus, A. L., Conroy, D. E., & Elliot, A. J. (2009). The pathoplastic relationship between interpersonal problems and fear of failure. *Journal of Personality, 77*, 997–1024.

Wright, A. G. C., Pincus, A. L., & Hopwood, C. J. (2023). Contemporary Integrative Interpersonal Theory: Integrating structure, dynamics, temporal scale, and levels of analysis. *Journal of Psychopathology and Clinical Science, 132*, 263–276.

Wright, A. G. C., Pincus, A. L., Hopwood, C. J., Thomas, K. M., Markon, K. E., & Krueger, R. F. (2012). An interpersonal analysis of pathological personality traits in DSM-5. *Assessment, 19*, 263–275.

Wright, A. G. C., Ringwald, W. R., Hopwood, C. J., & Pincus, A. L. (2022). It's time to replace the personality disorders with the interpersonal disorders. *American Psychologist, 77*, 1085–1099.

Wright, A. G. C., Stepp, S. D., Scott, L. N., Hallquist, M. N., Beeney, J. E., Lazarus, S. A., & Pilkonis, P. A. (2017). The effect of pathological narcissism on interpersonal and affective processes in social interactions. *Journal of Abnormal Psychology, 126*, 898–910.

Zhan Yuen Wong, N., Barnett, P., Sheridan Rains, L., Johnson, S., & Billings, J. (2023). Evaluation of international guidance for the community treatment of personality disorders: A systematic review. *PLoS ONE, 18*, e0264239.

Zilcha-Mano, S., McCarthy, K. S., Dinger, U., Chambless, D. L., Milrod, B. L., Kunit, L., & Barber, J. P. (2015). Are there subtypes of panic disorder? An interpersonal perspective. *Journal of Consulting and Clinical Psychology, 83*, 938–950.

Zimmermann, J., & Wright, A. G. C. (2017). Beyond description in interpersonal construct validation: Methodological advances in the circumplex structural summary approach. *Assessment, 24*, 3–23.

CHAPTER 14

Psychodynamic Approaches

PATRICK LUYTEN AND PETER FONAGY

Introduction

THIS chapter builds on a number of recent exciting conceptual, methodological, and empirical developments in research concerning the nature and classification of personality and psychopathology, which have also led to a revival of interest in psychodynamic approaches to the conceptualization of psychopathology and its treatment (Luyten & Fonagy, 2022).

First, there is increasing evidence for the psychodynamic assumption that there is a fundamental continuity between normal and disrupted personality development, and between personality and psychopathology. The Hierarchical Taxonomy of Psychopathology (HiTOP) approach (Ruggero et al., 2019; Widiger et al., 2018), for instance, essentially proposes a unified multi-level approach to psychopathology and personality. The approach assumes that, at the highest level, there is a general psychopathology factor, beneath which groups of internalizing, externalizing, and thought disorders can be distinguished; and, at lower levels, five domains of personality functioning and psychopathology, namely, detachment, antagonistic externalizing, disinhibited externalizing, thought disorder, and internalizing (along with a provisional somatoform domain), can be differentiated. As in psychodynamic approaches, the HiTOP thus assumes that there is a fundamental continuity between personality and psychopathology, and proposes that different types of psychopathology reflect extreme variants of personality functioning.

From this description, it is also clear that the HiTOP shares a second fundamental assumption about the nature of personality and psychopathology with psychodynamic approaches, regarding the notion of severity of psychopathology and thus of disruptions in personality development. Research on a general psychopathology factor, or p factor, has been instrumental in this context, pointing to the existence of a higher-order factor explaining the associations between subordinate disorders and personality dimensions (Caspi et al., 2014; Caspi & Moffitt, 2018). Although they are not uncontested, substantive interpretations of the p factor suggest that it may represent a broad transdiagnostic vulnerability factor, which is highly associated with a history of adversity and compromised brain function in early life (Del Giudice, 2015; Laceulle et al., 2015; Lahey et al., 2015; Murray et al., 2016). These views are consistent with long-standing psychodynamic assumptions and research concerning the importance of distinguishing a severity factor in conceptualizing the nature of personality development and psychopathology. Consistent with these views, level of personality functioning is typically the most important predictor of the course of psychological disorders and response to treatment (Bach & Tracy, 2022; Cierpka et al., 2007; Kerber et al., 2024; Kernberg & Caligor, 2005; McWilliams, 2011; Sharp & Wall, 2021). Importantly, from a psychodynamic perspective, level of personality functioning is thought of as a factor that is orthogonal to the content of personality and types of psychopathology, meaning that different types of psychopathology can be expressed at different levels of functioning. As discussed in more detail in this chapter, the different types of personality and psychopathology are distinguished based on differences in internal working models of self and others that reflect strategies to try to adapt to a given environment (see Table 14.1).

These views and findings have been massively influential on recent versions of the major systems for classifying psychopathology. The emphasis in the DSM-5 (American Psychiatric Association, 2013) on severity as being characterized by various levels of disruption in the self (identity and self-direction) and interpersonal dysfunction (empathy and intimacy), in conceptualizing personality disorders, is to a large extent rooted in psychodynamic thinking and research (Bender et al., 2011; Blüml & Doering, 2021; Skodol et al., 2011). Similarly, the 11th revision of the International Classification of Diseases (ICD) (World Health Organization,

TABLE 14.1 Personality and Psychopathology Prototypes from a Psychodynamic Perspective

Prototypical Personality Types	Core conflict–defense constellation	Self-definition
Paranoid	Use of externalization to deal with issues related to autonomy, as expressed in high levels of distrust of others in particular	↑
Antisocial/psychopathic	Use of omnipotent control to deal with issues related to autonomy, and power issues in particular	
Narcissistic	Use of idealization of self and denigration of others to deal with issues related to autonomy, and (im)perfection in particular	
Schizoid/schizotypal	Use of withdrawal to deal with issues related to autonomy, particularly longings for intimacy in combination with high sensitivity to interpersonal stimulation and fear of others/intimacy	
Obsessive-compulsive	Use of reaction formation to deal with issues related to autonomy, and the need to control in particular	
Depressive-masochistic	Use of introjection and turning against the self to deal with issues related to autonomy, and achievement in particular	
Manic	Use of denial to deal with issues related to autonomy, and achievement in particular	
Anxious/avoidant	Avoidance of others to deal with fears of rejection and/or abandonment	
Dependent	Submissive clinging to others to deal with fears of rejection and/or abandonment	
Hysterical/histrionic	Sexualization to deal with fear of rejection and/or abandonment	
Dissociative	Use of dissociation to deal with a history of abuse and neglect	↓ Relatedness

2022) defines personality disorders in terms of problems in the functioning of aspects of the self (e.g., identity, self-worth, accuracy of self-view, self-direction) and/or interpersonal dysfunction (e.g., ability to develop and maintain close and mutually satisfying relationships, ability to understand others' perspectives and to manage conflict in relationships).

Yet, as explained in more detail later in this chapter, from a psychodynamic perspective, all types of psychopathology, and not only the group of disorders currently labeled as "personality disorders," are seen as reflecting, at different levels of functioning, either temporary or chronic problems with internal working models of self and others, and thus problems with the self and interpersonal relationships (Lingiardi & McWilliams, 2017; Luyten & Fonagy, 2022; McWilliams, 2011). This chapter will therefore first outline the basic assumptions of psychodynamic approaches to personality development and psychopathology, and relevant research in this area. This will also entail a reconsideration of the notion of personality based on recent social-communicative approaches to personality development that conceptualize personality and psychopathology as a problem of interaction with the (social) environment. These views also incorporate the influence of the environment as a much-neglected factor in considerations of the nature of personality and psychopathology (Fonagy et al., 2022). The chapter will also outline implications for the prevention of, and interventions for, psychopathology. Whereas more categorial models have led to a proliferation of treatments for specific disorders, a psychodynamic perspective on classification and diagnosis instead suggests a more transdiagnostic approach to treatment.

Assumptions of Psychodynamic Approaches to Psychopathology

All approaches to the nature of psychopathology and personality development are based on a number of assumptions. With regard to psychodynamic approaches, there is now considerable consensus concerning the following eight assumptions.

1. *The need for an empirically based approach.* Although this is perhaps self-evident, several dominant approaches toward the conceptualization and classification of psychopathology are based on professional consensus rather than research findings, and there is often only a loose coupling between research evidence and consensus views. In this regard, a central feature of clinical psychodynamic approaches toward psychopathology is that they involve the capacities to accept and tolerate uncertainty, complexity, and not-knowing. The same capacities should be embraced when considering various approaches to the understanding of psychopathology. Although research findings do not always confirm one's cherished theories, or may yield contradicting or unclear findings, it is imperative that clinicians and researchers embrace disconfirming evidence and uncertainty in the field of diagnosis and classification.
2. *The centrality of a developmental perspective.* There is now abundant research showing the multifactorial nature of the development of both normal and disrupted personality development throughout the lifespan (Caspi et al., 2016; Cicchetti, 2016). The principles of equifinality and multifinality, as formulated by Cicchetti and Rogosch (1996) nearly three decades ago, have shed light on the role of developmental factors in the emergence of psychopathology. Equifinality implies that different etiological factors are implicated in similar developmental outcomes, whereas, in multifinality, a specific etiological factor (e.g., temperament or trauma) can lead to different developmental outcomes depending on interactions with other factors. This means that the high prevalence of "comorbidity"

between psychological disorders, however they are conceptualized (e.g., in the DSM or in HiTOP), is largely artefactual (Beauchaine & Cicchetti, 2016; Forbes et al., 2016). The notion of comorbidity should therefore be reserved for etiologically distinct disorders, as was originally intended when the term was coined (Feinstein, 1970). Hence, a developmental perspective is fundamental for understanding the nature of psychopathology, and particularly for understanding the structure of psychopathology. Developmental research clearly suggests that there are spectra of disorders that share important etiological factors, and thus psychological disorders need to be distinguished on the basis of both developmental considerations and clinical utility as detailed in the next section.

3. *The function of psychopathology*. From a psychodynamic perspective, personality and psychopathology are considered to reflect an individual's attempts, however distorted, at adaptation in response to biological factors, a specific environment, and the interaction between the two. Different types of psychopathology thus represent different types of conflict–defense constellations that represent specific adaptation strategies. As with the assumptions listed above, there is good evidence for these views. For instance, empirical research increasingly suggests that attachment styles (and other personality dimensions) reflect adaptations to a particular environment (Ein-Dor et al., 2010; Ellis et al., 2011). Anxious attachment, for example, most probably reflects an adaptation to an environment characterized by inconsistently available attachment figures, with attachment hyperactivating strategies developing in an attempt to elicit care and support from these attachment figures. Research also suggests that personality and psychopathology represent conflict–defense constellations. Anxiously attached individuals, for example, typically report having positive models of others, but at the same time they experience feelings of jealousy and anger toward others, which they typically inhibit due to fear of abandonment and rejection (Mikulincer & Shaver, 2007). Similarly, avoidantly attached individuals often report experiencing the self as positive, but experimental and neurobiological findings suggest that this is a defensive strategy to defend against underlying feelings of vulnerability, anxiety, and inferiority (Mikulincer & Shaver, 2007).

   Similar findings have been reported in studies that focused more directly on the dynamics in psychological disorders. For instance, many individuals with features of narcissistic personality disorder often present with high self-esteem, but this serves to defend against and compensate for underlying feelings of inferiority and emptiness (Russ et al., 2008). As another example, individuals with obsessive-compulsive disorder are characterized by high levels of both conscientiousness and latent impulsive aggression that is experienced as ego-dystonic, leading to high levels of conscientiousness to defend against underlying impulses (Moritz et al., 2011).

   Hence, it is crucially important to consider contrasting and often highly conflicting thoughts and feelings—that is, simultaneously being very high and very low on the same "personality traits"—as a central feature of both normal and disrupted personality development. These findings also illustrate the idea that personality and psychopathology, conceived as an adaptation strategy, have both advantages and disadvantages, and may be more or less successful, referring to the severity dimension. For instance, an anxiously attached person might avoid being rejected by others or feeling unloved in the short term by constantly signaling their need for love, care, and support, but in the longer term this pattern of relating to others might lead others to become frustrated and resentful, and thus eventually to reject and abandon the person (Luyten & Fonagy, 2022).

4. *The interpersonal nature of psychopathology*. Research clearly suggests that human beings are fundamentally interpersonal. From an evolutionary perspective, human beings are

equipped with the capacities for attachment, mentalizing, and epistemic trust, which together facilitate complex relationships with others based on mutual understanding, intentionality, and collaboration (Luyten, Campbell, Allison et al., 2020; Tomasello, 2020). It is therefore very difficult to imagine any type of psychopathology in which interpersonal factors do not play a role in explaining either its origins or its course. From an evolutionary perspective, most types of psychopathology have important interpersonal functions, such as signalling distress (e.g., anxiety) or despair (e.g., depression), which communicate to others that the individual is in need of comfort or support, or wants to retreat from their social environment (Gilbert, 2016, 2024; Luyten & Fonagy, 2025). Likewise, interpersonal problems (e.g., rejection, abandonment, shaming) have been implicated in vulnerability for almost all types of psychopathology and the course of these disorders (Hopwood, 2024). Hence, consistent with contemporary interpersonal (Wright et al., 2023) and evolutionary (Gilbert, 2016, 2024) approaches, from a psychodynamic perspective, psychopathology is seen as fundamentally interpersonal.

5. *The primacy of a person-centered approach.* Psychodynamic approaches to psychopathology are also fundamentally person-centered. Their focus is on developmental pathways from infancy to adulthood—that is, how individuals are able to negotiate (more or less successfully) normative developmental tasks, and how failure to negotiate some of these tasks may give rise to maladaptation across the lifespan (Fonagy et al., 2024; Luyten et al., 2024). As a result, the focus has always been on developing a "taxonomy of people" rather than a "taxonomy of diseases" (Lingiardi & McWilliams, 2017, p. 17), and by extension a "taxonomy of brains" or a "taxonomy of genes." Psychodynamic approaches are centrally concerned with attempts to describe "what one is rather than what one has" (Lingiardi & McWilliams, 2017, p. 17).

These considerations are important in the current sociocultural climate, as scientific discussions concerning the nature and classification of psychopathology do not occur in a sociocultural vacuum. Despite increasing criticism of categorical approaches to psychopathology and personality, there is a clearly noticeable revival of biological reductionism with regard to the nature of psychopathology, which is to a considerable extent fueled by social media. The concept of neurodivergence is one example of this trend. This concept is often applied in discussions concerning the nature of autism spectrum problems and has more recently also been applied to other domains, such as attention-deficit/hyperactivity disorder (ADHD). The notion of neurodivergence exemplifies not only the biological reductionism that is often present in these discussions, as it is at odds with research findings concerning the biopsychosocial nature of psychopathology including autism spectrum disorders and ADHD. It also neglects decades of empirical research showing that personality dimensions are dimensionally distributed and that there is no such thing as a "neurotypical" brain or "normal" personality functioning (Russell, 2020). For example, in the case of individuals who are currently often considered to fall within the autism spectrum, decades of research have provided evidence for variations in personality development in terms of both the personality trait of introversion and schizoid (or in more extreme cases schizotypal) personality features. This body of research has also clearly documented both the individual and the societal values and advantages of such personality features, and also their potential disadvantages and intrapsychic and interpersonal "costs" (McWilliams, 2011), without reverting to an epistemologically problematic concept such as neurodiversity, nor to the problematic assumption of "normality" versus "abnormality." Reducing differences between people to differences in brain function not only implies a view of personality and psychopathology that is not supported by research, but also closes off consideration of the demonstrated developmental origins and functions of personality functioning; it has often also led to an unfortunate distinction between "us" and "them." Moreover, it has resulted in individuals not seeking treatment or refusing treatment altogether (Russell, 2020). Similarly, with regard to ADHD specifically, variations along the spectrum of extraversion and emotion-regulation problems have been described and investigated for many years (Ruggero et al., 2019). Hence, we need to be aware of the renewed growing influence of categorical and reductionist views on personality and psychopathology, which often seem to serve purposes other than scientific ones. These views are communicated on a very large scale through the internet and social media, and are hugely influential in the way individuals, particularly young people, are increasingly conceptualizing their psychological problems in unhelpful ways.

6. *The need for a focus on subjective experiences.* Psychopathology and personality are not merely static traits or endpoints. As Sharp and Wall (2021) noted, personality functions as a subjective intrapsychic system that is needed to fulfill adult life tasks, and thus there is a need to consider the contribution individuals make as agentic authors to the interpretation and management of the self and their interpersonal world. From this perspective, psychopathology arises when there is an (impending) failure of this intrapsychic system to adapt to ever-changing circumstances.
7. *A dimensional and categorical-prototypical view of psychopathology.* There is now abundant evidence that most types of psychopathology are dimensionally distributed and should be considered as reflecting extreme variants of normal personality functioning. In fact, these findings question whether there is such a thing as "healthy" or "normal" personality functioning, and whether there is a clear demarcation between "normal" and "disrupted" personality, and between "normality" and "pathology." A meta-analysis of 317 findings drawn from 183 papers found overwhelming support for a dimensional view of psychopathology (Haslam et al., 2020). Hence, although some psychological problems may be better represented by a categorical approach, most psychological problems seem to be dimensionally distributed. Moreover, research by Shedler, Westen, and colleagues has amply demonstrated the advantages of a combined dimensional and categorical approach where categories are defined not in terms of the presence or absence of specific features, but as personality prototypes (Shedler & Westen, 2010; Spitzer et al., 2008). Cognitive science has demonstrated that people prefer prototypical categorization, as this approach seems to reflect people's natural tendency to categorize objects. Prototypes are not only characterized by a good time/effort ratio (Spitzer et al., 2008); they also allow relatively fast and reliable recognition, and thus enhance clinical utility, which is a major issue for both descriptive and multivariate approaches to psychopathology, that is, approaches that primarily rely on multivariate statistical methods (e.g., factor analysis) to identify patterns among different personality dimensions (Shedler & Westen, 2010).

   The Shedler–Westen Assessment Procedure (SWAP), a tool in which clinicians follow a Q-sorting procedure of jargon-free descriptions of both descriptive phenomenology and psychological processes (including motives, defenses, and conflicts) typical of personality problems, has been used to identify distinct "naturally occurring" personality disorder prototypes in adolescents and adults that overlap to a large extent with the most common personality prototypes that have been identified by other methods (Westen, DeFife et al., 2014; Westen, Waller et al., 2014).

Interestingly, research also shows that "comorbidity" is greatly reduced when using a prototype approach, with most patients having elevated scores on only one prototype. There is also evidence that the prototypes are hierarchically organized into internalizing, externalizing, and borderline superordinate factors (Shedler & Westen, 2010; Westen, DeFife et al., 2014), suggesting that the concept of "borderline" reflects a level of personality functioning rather than a specific disorder or personality prototype, consistent with long-standing psychodynamic assumptions concerning the notion of borderline level of personality organization, discussed in more detail in the next section in this chapter. Finally, what is particularly interesting with regard to these prototypes is that they clearly point to the role of conflicting and opposing thoughts, feelings, and motives at the core of personality prototypes and personality disorders. For instance, high scores on the SWAP items "Has an exaggerated sense of self-importance (e.g., feels special superior, grand, or envied)" and "Tends to feel s/he is inadequate, inferior or a failure" are typical of the narcissistic prototype, and are indicative of the use of grandiosity to defend against underlying feelings of inferiority and unworthiness. Hence, as explained in more detail in the next section, a dimensional, developmental person-centered approach and a categorical prototype approach are not mutually exclusive.

8. *Clinical utility.* Clinical utility is of key importance from a psychodynamic perspective. It implies that there must be a close relationship between the conceptualization of personality prototypes and guidelines for assessment and intervention. Hence, the conceptualization that is adopted must allow clinicians to make the sophisticated distinctions and judgements that are needed in clinical practice. For instance, distinctions between personality prototypes or types of psychopathology are considered meaningful only if they are also related to differences in transference–countertransference dynamics when assessing the patient and their likely response to specific interventions in treatment (Betan et al., 2005; Bradley et al., 2005). In this context, given the centrality of dimensional considerations in psychodynamic approaches to psychopathology, any conceptual approach to psychopathology must also be able to explain the relationship between different types of psychopathology in terms of underlying vulnerability factors (e.g., the fact that different disorders may share trauma as a common etiological factor) and the role of conflicting and often opposing thoughts, feelings, and motives. Finally, a truly dimensional approach to psychopathology also implies that there is a fundamental continuity between "normality" and "pathology," and thus should assist clinicians in being attentive to both the advantages and disadvantages for the individual and their environment of a specific personality style that is implicated in their psychological problems (Luyten & Fonagy, 2022).

An Integrative Psychodynamic Approach to Psychopathology

Introduction

This section of the chapter will describe the integrative psychodynamic approach to the conceptualization of psychopathology that we have proposed and further developed over the years, informed by clinical practice and emerging research findings (Blatt & Luyten, 2009, 2010; Luyten & Blatt, 2007, 2011, 2013b; Luyten & Fonagy, 2022). This fundamentally dimensional approach situates different types of psychopathology within a hierarchical model that integrates theory-driven models that emphasize relatedness and self-definition as central developmental dimensions in normal and disrupted personality development with empirically derived models that focus on the role of temperament and multivariate personality factors. It also includes a more categorical approach, in that it distinguishes among prototypic conflict–defense constellations that can be delineated conceptually, clinically, and empirically, and reflect different adaptation strategies to an ever-changing environment.

Normal and Disrupted Personality Development: A Circumplex Approach

Although using somewhat different notions and being rooted in different conceptual frameworks, findings from various strands of research, ranging from Blatt's two-polarities model (Blatt, 2008; Luyten & Blatt, 2013a) to contemporary interpersonal approaches (Wright et al., 2023) and self-determination theory (Ryan et al., 2019), converge to suggest that different types of psychopathology can be arranged in a two-dimensional space defined by: (1) *relatedness*, ranging from high to low anxiety or warmth in relationships, and (2) *self-definition*, ranging from low to high avoidance of others (see Figure 14.1).

Over the course of psychological development, individuals are thought to develop internal working models of self and others, also referred to as "self and object representations" or "cognitive–affective schemas" of self and others, that underpin the capacity for relatedness and self-definition and that become increasingly complex, differentiated, and integrated, and enable individuals to negotiate different developmental tasks (Luyten et al., 2024). Across the lifespan, biological factors, in interaction with environmental influences, may lead to disruptions in the content and/or organizational or developmental level (also known as "structural level" or "level of personality organization") of these internal working models. Hence, this view implies that there is a fundamental continuity between "normal" personality features

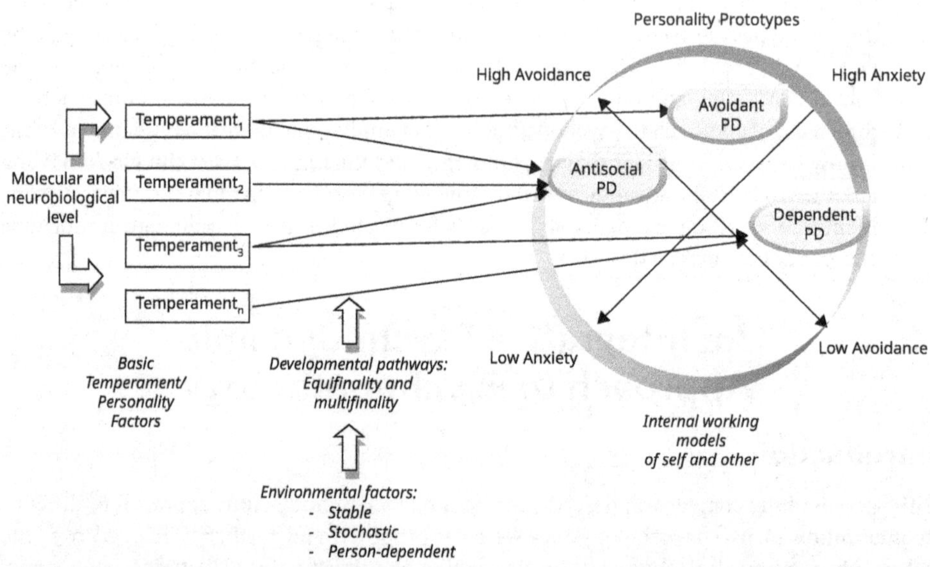

FIGURE 14.1 Personality prototypes as adaptation strategies in the context of a multilevel developmental psychopathology approach to personality development using the examples of antisocial, avoidant, and dependent personality prototypes.

and psychopathology, and fuzzy borders not only between "normality" and "pathology" but also between different personality prototypes.

As noted earlier in this chapter, both the DSM-5 and ICD-11 have incorporated the central assumptions of this approach, albeit only in their considerations concerning the conceptualization and classification of "personality" disorders. However, given the evidence for the dimensionality of psychopathology and the fundamental continuity between personality and psychopathology, we argue that all types of psychopathology should be conceptualized as reflecting temporary or more permanent disruptions in relatedness and self-definition. From this perspective, "symptom" disorders, such as depression, anxiety, or substance abuse, are the expression of the (impending) failure of the person's adaptation strategy and at the same time represent further attempts at (interpersonal) coping; for example, depression signals interpersonal distress and isolation while at the same time trying to reduce distress by entering into a state of "psychological hibernation" (Luyten & Fonagy, 2025). In this approach, the severity dimension, reflecting levels of functioning, distinguishes more temporary and potentially ego-dystonic psychological problems from more engrained and ego-syntonic psychological problems, which are currently typically understood as "personality disorders." Hence, from a psychodynamic perspective, different personality types can be expressed at different levels of functioning. As discussed in more detail in what follows, this view also necessitates changes in the way the notions of personality and personality disorder are defined and understood.

Before discussing these issues in more detail, it is important to point out that the approach outlined here also implies that co-occurrence and overlap between different disorders are expected to decrease as one moves around the circumplex (see Figure 14.1), which sheds an interesting light on the issue of "comorbidity" among disorders. Neither DSM-5 nor ICD-11 adopts this approach, despite its obvious psychometric and clinical advantages.

Yet, there is good evidence to suggest that personality prototypes follow a circular ordering, or circumplex, such that personality prototypes that fall close together are more related than variables that fall further apart on the circle. Decades of research have seen the development and validation of a range of measures of internal working models or cognitive–affective schemas around the circumplex, ranging from self-report questionnaires to interviews and observer-rated scales, that have often also demonstrated their clinical value for assessment, case formulation, and measurement of therapeutic change (Huprich & Greenberg, 2003; Locke, 2011; Mikulincer & Shaver, 2007; Ryan et al., 2019; Steele & Steele, 2008).

Severity and Levels of Personality Functioning

The severity of psychopathology has been conceptualized in various ways within psychodynamic approaches. One dominant approach, which has also influenced DSM-5 and ICD-11, originates in the work of Otto Kernberg and colleagues (Kernberg & Caligor, 2005) and in the writings of Nancy McWilliams (1994, 2011). Although both Kernberg and McWilliams conceive of the severity of psychopathology as being fundamentally dimensional, for both research and clinical purposes, they distinguish among three levels of personality functioning based on a number of criteria that refer to an individual's overall functioning. Kernberg, for instance, advanced the following features to distinguish among levels of personality functioning:

1. the level of identity integration
2. the predominant level of defenses (ranging from low-level defense mechanisms, such as splitting and projective identification, to higher-level and more mature defense mechanisms, such as repression and rationalization, to cope with external and internal stressors and conflicts)

3. the capacity for reality testing
4. the quality of object relations (and underlying representations of self and others)
5. moral functioning (ethical behavior, ideals, and values)
6. the nature of primary conflicts
7. the transference and countertransference potential of patients (i.e., the extent to which they tend to transfer interpersonal patterns in their relationships with others—including mental health professionals—and the extent to which they tend to evoke strong feelings in others as a result).

Based on combinations of these features, three levels of personality functioning or personality organization can be defined, from less severe to more severe, with fuzzy boundaries between each of these levels:

- Neurotic Personality Organization (NPO) is characterized by relatively high levels of identity integration, intact reality testing, and the predominant use of more mature (i.e., higher-level) defense or coping mechanisms
- Borderline Personality Organization (BPO) is characterized by identity diffusion and the use of lower-level defense mechanisms (e.g., splitting, projective identification), with relatively intact reality testing
- Psychotic Personality Organization (PPO) involves marked identity diffusion, impaired reality testing, and the often massive use of lower-level defense mechanisms (e.g., massive projection).

It should be noted that that the spectrum thus defined does not include "healthy personality organization," as it is a central assumption of psychodynamic approaches that the concept of "healthy functioning" and "normality" is intrinsically problematic (Van Haute, 2002), and thus that psychopathology is fundamentally dimensionally distributed. As a field, we also need to be aware that sociocultural factors tend to influence judgements about "normality" and "pathology," as we discussed in the context of the notion of neurodiversity (Stevanovic et al., 2017).

These views have led to various operationalizations of the concept of level of functioning, each with their respective assessment instruments, including the Structured Interview for Personality Organization and the Inventory of Personality Organization, which were developed based on Kernberg's views (Lenzenweger et al., 2001; Stern et al., 2010); the Operationalized Psychodynamic Diagnostics approach, which contains a strong emphasis on levels of personality functioning from a broad psychodynamic perspective (Doering et al., 2014; Ehrenthal & Benecke, 2019; Rosén & Hau, 2021); the Psychodynamic Diagnostic Manual (Lingiardi & McWilliams, 2017); the DSM-5 Level of Personality Functioning Scale (Morey, 2017) and the Semi-Structured Interview for Personality Functioning (STiP-5.1) (Balzen et al., 2025), which are based on the DSM-5; and the Standardized Assessment of Severity of Personality Disorder, which is based on the ICD-11 (Olajide et al., 2018).

Despite differences in the theoretical and methodological approaches of the above research traditions, substantial evidence is accruing for the importance of severity in considering psychopathology. This body of research has increasingly demonstrated that features referring to level of personality functioning can be reliably assessed and that they can be used to distinguish among patients with various diagnoses and levels of functional impairment, are associated with prognosis and treatment outcome, and have high levels of clinical utility (Ehrenthal & Benecke, 2019; Koelen et al., 2012; Morey et al., 2022). However, more research concerning this approach is needed. There is a particular need for large-scale population-representative longitudinal studies investigating the impact of level of personality functioning across a wide array of indices of functioning (Clark et al., 2024). A recent study in a large sample consisting of more than 27,000 community participants showed that indices of level of personality functioning largely accounted for the co-variance among dimensional personality traits in a hierarchical model of personality functioning, and for most of the variance in predicting well-being and psychosocial impairment over a two-year period over and above specific personality traits (Kerber et al., 2024). Similar studies are needed in the future, as well as studies that explore the relationships among the various measurement instruments that have been developed in this area. For instance, Kampe et al. (2018) found high correlations between overall scores of severity and domain scales of severity based on videotaped assessments of 30 psychotherapeutic inpatients and outpatients using the Structured Clinical Interview for the DSM-5 Alternative Model for Personality Disorders Module I (SCID-AMPD) and the Structured Interview of Personality Organization, providing evidence for convergent validity. Moreover, high correlations with criteria of clinical severity, an important index of predictive validity, were found.

If further validated, the view that each type of psychopathology can manifest at different levels of personality functioning (e.g., narcissistic personality can manifest at psychotic, borderline, and neurotic levels) (McWilliams, 2011) opens up important perspectives for a truly dimensional approach to psychopathology, with individuals being situated along a continuum of personality functioning. As we have seen, an important outstanding question in this respect is whether the notion of "borderline" is best conceived as referring to a level of functioning or to a specific personality disorder. Several studies (Sharp et al., 2015; Westen, DeFife et al., 2014) suggest that the term "borderline" can best be used to describe a hierarchically higher-order level of functioning under which several disorders (e.g., histrionic–impulsive personality disorder and emotionally dysregulated personality disorder) can be subsumed.

Research on a general psychopathology (p) factor may play an important role in this context, as it has further emphasized the importance of including a severity dimension in conceptualizing psychopathology. As noted, the p factor may not only represent a broad transdiagnostic vulnerability factor explaining the relationships among various types of psychopathology, but has also empirically shown a strong relationship with the onset, course, and persistence of psychopathology (Del Giudice, 2015; Laceulle et al., 2015; Lahey et al., 2015; Murray et al., 2016). For instance, Patalay et al. (2018) reported that the p factor explained future psychopathology and academic attainment, over and above internalizing and externalizing problems, in a large community-based sample of young adolescents ($n = 23477$). Similarly, Sallis et al. (2019) found the p factor to be more relevant in predicting long-term outcomes than specific symptoms in two independent birth cohort studies.

Figure 14.2 integrates Caspi and colleagues' (Caspi et al., 2023) theoretical framework concerning the p factor with psychodynamic approaches to level of personality functioning. The bottom of the pyramid in the figure depicts a large group of individuals who present with relatively mild psychological problems when faced with specific developmental tasks and other challenges. These problems are often relatively ubiquitous and transient, as shown by findings that only one in five people will *not* have a diagnosable mental health condition during their lifetime (Schaefer et al., 2017). Studies on resilience similarly point out that the normative response to most types of adversity is so-called "minimal impact resilience," implying that most individuals experience only temporary distress when faced with adversity, and then return to previous "normal" levels of functioning (Bonanno & Diminich, 2013; Southwick et al., 2014). Yet, there is also a substantial subgroup of individuals with neurotic levels of functioning who present with more persistent psychological problems, or high levels of relapse and recurrence (Luyten & Fonagy, 2022; Westen et al., 2002).

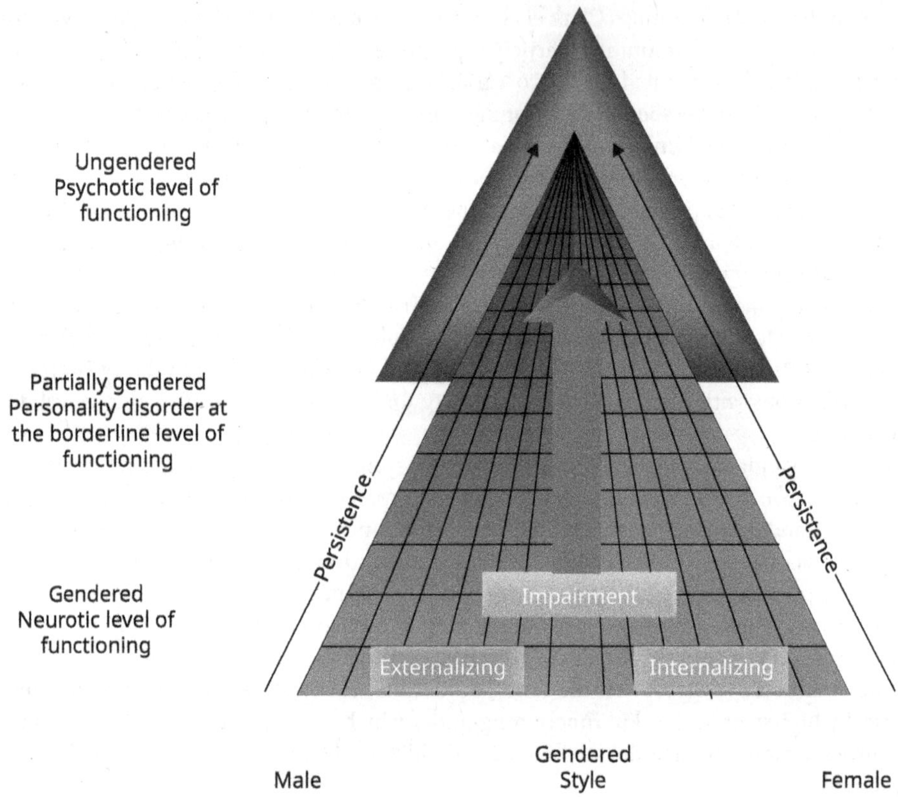

FIGURE 14.2 Levels of personality functioning, the general psychopathology factor and persistence of psychopathology (Adapted from Caspi et al., 2014.)

Moving higher up the pyramid (which represents increasing levels of the p factor), psychological problems tend to become more persistent and more ego-syntonic; that is, they become more ingrained in individuals' personalities. Moreover, as the level of p factor increases, it makes progressively less sense to distinguish among different psychological problems or disorders. For example, most people who are currently diagnosed with a personality disorder report feelings of depression and anxiety, meet criteria for substance abuse disorders and/or eating disorders, and engage in self-harm or in other impulsive behaviors. The distinction between internalizing and externalizing problems also begins to make less sense, as individuals at this level show a general dysregulation of emotional experience (Luyten, Campbell, & Fonagy, 2020; Sharp & Wall, 2021). At the psychotic level of functioning, the distinction between different disorders—and between the person and the disorder—is even more challenging, as problems with thought disorders are at the forefront (Luyten & Fonagy, 2022).

The persistence and rigidity of psychopathology associated with the p factor may well be associated with problems with two related key capacities in human functioning, namely, mentalizing and epistemic trust (Fonagy et al., 2022; Fonagy, Luyten, Allison et al., 2017). Epistemic trust refers to the capacity of humans to identify knowledge conveyed by others as personally relevant and generalizable to other contexts. Together with the capacity for shared intentionality and mentalizing (the human capacity to understand the self and others in terms of intentional mental states), epistemic trust enables complex forms of social learning involved in human communication and collaboration (Csibra & Gergely, 2009; Sperber et al., 2010; Tomasello, 2010; Tomasello & Vaish, 2013).

Developmental research shows that epistemic trust is a capacity that develops in the earliest years of life and involves the overcoming of epistemic vigilance, that is, a critical alertness to the believability, reliability, and validity of information provided by others (Mascaro & Sperber, 2009; Sperber et al., 2010; Wilson & Sperber, 2012). Relationships with attachment figures are crucial in this context, as they play a central role in the child developing the capacity to discern trustworthy knowledge (Csibra & Gergely, 2009). The broader family and the sociocultural climate are also important in this regard, which is most clearly evidenced by research involving children and young people who grow up in environments characterized by insecurity, abuse, neglect, violence, and mistrust (Luyten, Campbell, Allison et al., 2020; Luyten, Campbell, & Fonagy, 2020). These children and young people develop considerable epistemic vigilance toward others and the world around them. Traditionally, they are referred to as having considerable "rigidity" and many "maladaptive personality traits." In the extreme, they are typified as "hard to reach." However, we contend that epistemic vigilance, and the impairments in mentalizing associated with it, should be seen as an understandable adaptation strategy to a specific environment. For instance, for individuals growing up in a family environment marked by high expectations, the development of high levels of perfectionism and anxiety (characterized by both positive and negative models of the self and low levels of epistemic trust in others) is quite understandable. Similarly, the high levels of aggression (underpinned by negative models of self and others and high epistemic vigilance) typical of many young people and adults with "externalizing" problems represent a survival strategy for those growing up in an environment characterized by neglect, abuse, and violence. Moreover, current conceptualizations of this group of individuals fail to consider the fact that their aggression is not necessarily stable over time, as they can be caring and loving in some of their relationships. Hence, the stability that is typically observed in "personality" or "personality disorders" is observed only in contexts where the mechanisms that underpin their adaptation strategy are active. This does not imply a denial of the importance of genetic factors, and temperamental factors in particular, as discussed in the next section "A Prototype Approach to Personality and Psychopathology" (Fonagy & Luyten, 2018). However, the major influence of environmental factors such as social inequality on the prevalence, persistence, and course of personality and mental health problems (Rözer et al., 2016; Rözer & Volker, 2016) has been almost completely neglected in psychological models of personality and psychopathology.

There is emerging evidence that impairments in epistemic trust and associated impairments in mentalizing can be seen as another index, besides more "traditional" concepts such as defense mechanisms and reality testing, of the level of personality functioning (Byrne et al., 2019; Campbell et al., 2021; Zettl et al., 2020) and are associated with psychological problems across the internalizing (De Coninck et al., 2021; Kampling et al., 2022; Locati et al., 2023), externalizing (Malcorps et al., 2024), and thought disorder (Salaminios et al., 2024) spectrum. However, more longitudinal research is needed before firmer conclusions can be drawn with regard to the potential value of these views.

A Prototype Approach to Personality and Psychopathology

Within the epigenetic landscape of development, to use Waddington's (1957) famous metaphor to conceptualize the influence of developmental factors, there are probably only a small number of prototypical ways of negotiating developmental tasks and challenges, given existing biological and social constraints. This also means that it is highly likely that there are only a limited number of prototypical ways of dealing with life's challenges, which may explain the relatively small number of "naturally occurring" personality types. These represent prototypical conflict–defense constellations that reflect attempts, however maladaptive they may be for the individual and/or their environment, to establish and maintain a sense of relatedness and self-definition at different developmental levels of personality functioning (Blatt & Shichman, 1983; McWilliams, 1994). Table 14.1 depicts the prototypes that have received most empirical support in studies over the past decades and that may have the greatest clinical validity and utility, and the main conflict and defensive strategies employed by these individuals. Yet, it is important to realize that other defensive strategies are also typically used by individuals with these prototypical personality features, which also explains in part the fuzzy boundaries between these prototypes and differences in terms of severity (e.g., someone with obsessive-compulsive features at the borderline and particularly the psychotic level may use projection to defend against internal aggressive wishes, thus resembling the paranoid prototype). Moreover, as emphasized throughout this chapter, much remains uncertain in this field, and many important research and clinical questions have not yet been adequately addressed. There is therefore a need for large-scale longitudinal studies to trace the development of these prototypes over time. For instance, it is not yet clear whether the schizoid-schizotypal personality disorder prototype should be considered to be two separate personality prototypes or if the schizotypal prototype may reflect a more severe expression of the schizoid prototype. Similarly, it is not yet clear whether a dissociative personality prototype can be distinguished, or whether it is better to conceptualize dissociation as a defensive strategy that may be present across different personality prototypes.

Despite these limitations, a prototype approach has substantial clinical utility, as it is not subject to the major limitations of traditional categorical approaches that rely on arbitrary consensus-based cut-off criteria, or on empirically determined cut-off scores in multivariate dimensional approaches to psychopathology. As noted earlier, the advantages in terms of clinical utility and validity are the following:

1. Human beings prefer prototypes, which reflect their natural tendency when they are asked to categorize objects. Clinicians can easily compare similarities (and differences) between a given patient and a prototypical description (Spitzer et al., 2008; Westen et al., 2006). Prototypes go beyond a list of manifest descriptors and conditional statements (e.g., "someone with high levels of both neuroticism and extroversion is likely to become depressed when he is alone"). Prototypes are abstractions; yet, as there are only a relatively limited number of prototypical ways of dealing with the challenges humans are typically confronted with, they are relatively easy for clinicians to recognize.
2. A prototype approach facilitates identifying fundamental similarities as well as differences among different types of personality and psychopathology, such as the preoccupation with the sense of self in paranoid, obsessive-compulsive, and narcissistic personality, or the preoccupation with issues of attachment and relatedness in dependent, anxious-avoidant, and histrionic personality (Blatt & Shichman, 1983). For instance, conflicts around separation and abandonment, depending on their interaction with other factors (e.g., child temperament, identification with attachment figures, and sociocultural pressures), may be dealt with in different ways as expressed in dependent, avoidant, or histrionic personality prototypes (see Table 14.1).
3. It also helps in understanding the "natural" co-occurrence of various personality types and features, such as antisocial and narcissistic features, or depressive and anxious features, as similar defense and coping strategies are involved in the development of these personality features (see Table 14.1), and they often also share similar developmental factors.

The Need for a Developmental Psychopathology Perspective

The findings reviewed in this chapter lead to developmental considerations and issues related to equifinality and multifinality in the development of personality and psychopathology. It is here that the temperamental features identified by empirically driven, multivariate models of personality might provide a powerful approach to understanding the emergence of personality prototypes.

It is often forgotten in this context that psychodynamic approaches to personality and psychopathology have historically placed a strong emphasis on the role of biological factors, in particular, temperament. From these early formulations onward, Kernberg and Caligor (2005), for instance, proposed introversion and extraversion as a second dimension (besides the level of personality organization or severity dimension) underpinning personality development. Consistent with these views, basic temperament and personality factors studied by multivariate personality models have been shown to have an important influence on developmental trajectories. In this context, a combination of person-centered and variable-centered approaches is needed in order to more fully understand the development of personality and psychopathology at various levels of analysis, ranging from the molecular, neurobiological, and neural, which are central in the Research Domain Criteria (RDoC) approach (Cuthbert & Insel, 2013), to the level of temperament and basic personality factors, and, finally, environmental factors, such as life stress and broader sociocultural factors, as personality development does not occur in a social vacuum (see Figure 14.1).

For example, research findings suggest that the dependent personality prototype is located in the low avoidance–high anxiety quadrant, and thus reflects strong desires for attachment and love, in combination with strong fears of abandonment, rejection, and loss of love (Luyten & Blatt, 2011). The avoidant personality prototype is located in the high anxiety–high avoidance quadrant, reflecting an approach/avoidance conflict. Although these individuals want to be accepted and admired, they are at the same time also afraid of being criticized and rejected by others. Hence, these two personality prototypes represent two prototypical ways of finding a balance between relatedness and self-definition. Note that these represent continuous personality prototypes, ranging from normal-neurotic variations to more extreme variants that can be expressed at more borderline and psychotic levels of functioning. Moreover, these prototypes can give rise to similar "symptom" disorders (e.g., depression, anxiety, substance abuse, externalizing problems) when their dominant adaptation strategy fails, suggesting that symptom disorders are not an appropriate basis for the conceptualization and classification of psychopathology.

Importantly, basic temperament/personality factors that have been identified by multivariate studies may play an important role in determining the phenotypic expression of the above described prototypes along the internalizing, externalizing, and thought disorder spectra (see Figure 14.2). For example, research findings suggest that individuals with high levels of effortful control (i.e., the opposite of disinhibition) are more prone to express their psychological issues in terms of internalizing problems (Leadbeater et al., 1999). Those with low levels of effortful control tend to express their problems in terms of both internalizing and externalizing problems (Leadbeater et al., 1999; Luyten & Blatt, 2011). Similarly, sociocultural factors are likely to influence the expression of personality issues and psychopathology, as demonstrated by cross-cultural research. For instance, dependency is very differently valued across different cultures, and thus may not only be expressed differently depending on sociocultural factors, but may also be differentially related to indices of psychopathology across cultures (Bornstein,

2012; Luyten & Blatt, 2013a). Temperamental factors are similarly differentially valued across cultures (Campagna et al., 2023). This leads us to a consideration of the value, but also the limitations, of considering spectra in the conceptualization of psychopathology.

There Is More than One Spectrum in the Domain of Psychopathology

Current dimensional approaches to psychopathology often argue that psychopathology is organized along internalizing, externalizing, and thought disorder spectra. There is indeed considerable research evidence from multivariate studies supporting this assumption (Caspi et al., 2023; Widiger et al., 2018). Yet, as we have discussed, high comorbidity among disorders within and across the different spectra is the rule rather than the exception, as evidenced by research on a general p factor. For example, depression, anxiety, and substance abuse disorder are highly "comorbid" and thus the distinction among these "disorders," although important from a descriptive and phenomenological perspective, provides little guidance for prevention and intervention. Moreover, these different "disorders" share many etiological features (e.g., trauma, chronic stress) while they are at the same time very heterogeneous in terms of etiological factors, again providing little guidance for prevention and intervention strategies. It may thus be helpful to remind ourselves that a number of other spectra in the domain of psychopathology can be distinguished, namely, those based on underlying etiological factors, ranging from genetic to neural and psychosocial factors. For instance, there is good evidence for a spectrum of stress-related disorders, which includes depression, anxiety disorders, PTSD, and functional somatic disorders (Lowe et al., 2024; McEwen, 2007). Similarly, there is good evidence that early adversity provides an ecophenotype that cuts across many different diagnoses and the internalizing, externalizing, and thought disorder spectra (Teicher & Samson, 2013).

From a psychodynamic perspective, personality prototypes are therefore seen as a better basis for conceptualizing the nature and structure of psychopathology from a dimensional perspective because of their greater clinical utility, as

a. these prototypes are relatively limited in number, thus providing a parsimonious explanation for individual differences,
b. they can be readily translated to assessment, prevention, and intervention strategies, as each of the prototypes is associated with relatively unique intrapersonal and interpersonal dynamics,
c. different descriptive disorders (e.g., depression and anxiety) are seen as responses that aim to regain one's equilibrium (hence why they are so highly "comorbid" as individuals typically make various attempts to restore their equilibrium), and
d. they also provide a clear heuristic framework to investigate equifinality and multifinality implicated in both the various prototypes (including temperamental dimensions identified by multivariate research in personality science) as well as the severity dimension that is central in psychodynamic considerations concerning psychopathology.

Implications for Assessment, Prevention, and Intervention

The views expressed in this chapter stress the value in assessment, prevention, and intervention on the content of personality and psychopathology on the one hand, and severity of psychopathology on the other. For instance, research findings increasingly suggest that patient features, conceptualized in terms of the underlying dynamics, explain a sizeable portion of the outcome of psychological intervention across different therapeutic orientations. For example, there is a sizeable research literature that suggests that individuals who are primarily preoccupied with issues of relatedness, consistent with their focus on relationships, are primarily responsive to relational factors in psychotherapy across descriptive diagnoses (Blatt et al., 2010; Luyten & Fonagy, 2025). Similarly, level of personality functioning (i.e., the severity dimension) is another important predictor of the course and outcome of psychological disorders, as discussed. These findings have led the various therapeutic schools to adapt their treatment approach to the level of functioning of patients. For instance, in research on BPD, various evidence-based treatments focus on the lack of structure and coherence of individuals with these features, to the point that all treatments for individuals with BPD currently probably share more similarities than differences in terms of treatment interventions; length of treatment; and emphasis on the consistency, coherence, and continuity of treatment (Fonagy, Luyten, & Bateman, 2017). Similarly, in the treatment of individuals with chronic depression, all evidence-based treatments share a focus on the recovery and development of metacognition or mentalizing, an important severity dimension (Luyten et al., 2013; Luyten & Fonagy, 2025), rather than a focus on the content of the dynamics, particularly in the first stages of treatment. Besides severity, all therapeutic schools increasingly emphasize the need to identify the relatively unique dynamics associated with personality prototypes described above, and address their core dynamics. For instance, schema therapy stresses the need to identify the core schemas and schema modes (Arntz et al., 2022). Similarly, psychodynamic therapies have a long history of adapting treatment to address the specific needs and dynamics associated with personality prototypes (McWilliams, 2011).

These trends may exemplify the growing realization of a fundamental parallel between developmental processes involved in personality development and mechanisms of therapeutic change (Blatt & Behrends, 1987; Luyten et al., 2012). All effective treatment approaches appear to facilitate the experiencing of thoughts and feelings in the context of an attachment relationship with a therapist, engendering an experience of feeling understood, validated, and appreciated by another. This process entails a change in the internal working models or cognitive–affective schemas of self and others. This experience also seems to enable individuals to begin to better understand and appreciate their own thoughts and feelings and those of others, thus fostering the capacity for mentalizing or metacognition, which enables them, much as in normal development, to establish reciprocal, mutually facilitating, intersubjective interpersonal relationships and to benefit from their environment through a salutogenic process (Fonagy et al., 2015; Luyten, Campbell, Allison et al., 2020).

Conclusions and Future Directions

Psychodynamic approaches to personality and psychopathology are fundamentally dimensional, as they assume continuity between "normal" and "disrupted" personality functioning. These views are increasingly incorporated in new approaches to classification and diagnosis, given the increasing consensus that both personality and psychopathology are largely dimensionally distributed. Yet, a number of key assumptions of psychodynamic approaches to personality and psychopathology, despite growing empirical support, remain unintegrated in contemporary approaches to diagnosis and classification. Tables 14.2 and 14.3 summarize these assumptions and their advantages for clinical practice and research.

However, although there is growing empirical evidence for psychodynamic assumptions concerning psychopathology, much work remains to be done. Throughout this chapter, we

TABLE 14.2 Key Points of Psychodynamic Approaches to Diagnosis and Classification

Key points
- Psychodynamic approaches to psychopathology are fundamentally dimensional; they assume the existence of a continuity between normal personality development and disrupted personality development along a dimension of severity.
- These approaches also incorporate a categorical-prototype approach based on findings concerning naturally emerging prototypical personality organizations; these personality prototypes are conceived as dynamic conflict–defense constellations that have developed as adaptation strategies to a given environment and biological predisposition.
- Each of these personality prototypes may occur at different levels of personality functioning, reflecting a severity dimension that is orthogonal to the content dimension of personality functioning (i.e., the different personality prototypes).
- Symptom disorders (e.g., depression and anxiety) are seen from this perspective as o the expression of the failure, or impending failure, of prototypical adaptation strategies (e.g., feelings of depression and anxiety reflect the failure to establish an essentially positive sense of self across the various prototypes, which explains the high "comorbidity" of symptomatic disorders); and o evolutionarily determined secondary adaptation strategies that are activated when the primary adaptation strategy (the conflict–defense constellation) fails, or is about to fail, from both an intrapersonal and an interpersonal perspective (e.g., depression can be seen as an attempt at psychological "hibernation" to protect the individual from further distress, but it also signals to others the need for help).

TABLE 14.3 Main Advantages of a Psychodynamic Combined Dimensional-Prototype Approach

- Clinical utility: personality prototypes provide a parsimonious explanation for individual differences, can be relatively easily identified in clinical practice, and can be readily translated to specific strategies for assessment, prevention, and intervention.
- Provides a comprehensive and empirically supported conceptual framework to investigate the equifinality and multifinality implicated in these various prototypes, including temperamental dimensions identified by multivariate research in personality science and the role of environmental and sociocultural factors as a much-neglected aspect in consideration of the nature of personality and psychopathology.
- Includes an emphasis on a severity dimension that has been identified in empirical research, as these adaptation strategies might be more or less "successful" in terms of their consequences for the self and others.
- Is able to explain the high "comorbidity" among "symptom disorders," as there are only a limited number of ways in which individuals can express the psychological consequences of distress associated with failure to adapt to their environment and their attempts to cope with this distress; it is also able to explain the high "comorbidity" among "personality disorders," as different personality prototypes share core conflicts (i.e., conflicts regarding self-definition versus relatedness) and involve the use of related defense strategies to deal with these conflicts.

have emphasized the need for large-scale, interdisciplinary studies tracing the development of prototypic ways of dealing with life's inevitable changes and challenges, and how these give rise to relatively stable "personality" prototypes. Yet, the stability of the intrapersonal and interpersonal features associated with these "personality" prototypes may be to a large extent in the eye of the beholder, as environmental factors may play an important role in explaining the apparent stability of the adaptation strategies that we have historically termed "personality." As discussed, this does not imply a naive environmental position, and temperament dimensions may play an important role in explaining part of the stability in personality features besides the environment.

Finally, we have stressed the need for a user- and clinician friendly approach to psychopathology, with immediate implications for assessment, prevention, and intervention. The combined dimensional and prototype approach advanced in this chapter provides such a transtheoretical and transdiagnostic approach (see also Table 14.3). It is hoped that this chapter gives rise to collaborative research efforts to further investigate the views expressed here.

References

American Psychiatric Association. (2013). *Diagnostic and statistical manual of mental disorders (5th ed., DSM-5)*. American Psychiatric Press.

Arntz, A., Jacob, G. A., Lee, C. W., Brand-de Wilde, O. M., Fassbinder, E., Harper, R. P., Lavender, A., Lockwood, G., Malogiannis, I. A., Ruths, F. A., Schweiger, U., Shaw, I. A., Zarbock, G., & Farrell, J. M. (2022). Effectiveness of predominantly group schema therapy and combined individual and group schema therapy for borderline personality disorder: A randomized clinical trial. *JAMA Psychiatry, 79*(4), 287–299. https://doi.org/10.1001/jamapsychiatry.2022.0010

Bach, B., & Tracy, M. (2022). Clinical utility of the alternative model of personality disorders: A 10th year anniversary review. *Personality Disorders: Theory, Research, and Treatment, 13*(4), 369–379. https://doi.org/10.1037/per0000527

Balzen, K. M., Kerr, S., Gecha, T., Hutsebaut, J., Berghuis, H., & Sharp, C. (2025). First psychometric evaluation of the English version of the Semi-Structured Interview for Personality Functioning (STiP-5.1). *Journal of Personality Assessment, 107*(1), 1–11. https://doi.org/10.1080/00223891.2024.2365325

Beauchaine, T. P., & Cicchetti, D. (2016). A new generation of comorbidity research in the era of neuroscience and Research Domain Criteria. *Development and Psychopathology, 28*(4pt1), 891–894. https://doi.org/10.1017/S0954579416000602

Bender, D. S., Morey, L. C., & Skodol, A. E. (2011). Toward a model for assessing level of personality functioning in DSM-5, Part I: A review of theory and methods. *Journal of Personality Assessment, 93*(4), 332–346. https://doi.org/10.1080/00223891.2011.583808

Betan, E., Heim, A. K., Zittel Conklin, C., & Westen, D. (2005). Countertransference phenomena and personality pathology in clinical practice: An empirical investigation. *American Journal of Psychiatry, 162*(5), 890–898. https://doi.org/10.1176/appi.ajp.162.5.890

Blatt, S. J. (2008). *Polarities of experience: Relatedness and self-definition in personality development, psychopathology, and the therapeutic process*. American Psychological Association.

Blatt, S. J., & Behrends, R. S. (1987). Internalization, separation-individuation, and the nature of therapeutic action. *International Journal of Psychoanalysis, 68*(Pt 2), 279–297.

Blatt, S. J., & Luyten, P. (2009). A structural-developmental psychodynamic approach to psychopathology: Two polarities of experience across the life span. *Development and Psychopathology, 21*(3), 793–814. https://doi.org/10.1017/S0954579409000431

Blatt, S. J., & Luyten, P. (2010). Reactivating the psychodynamic approach to classify psychopathology. In T. Millon, R. F. Krueger, & E. Simonsen (Eds.), *Contemporary directions in psychopathology. Scientific foundations of the DSM-V and ICD-11* (pp. 483–514). Guilford Press.

Blatt, S. J., & Shichman, S. (1983). Two primary configurations of psychopathology. *Psychoanalysis and Contemporary Thought, 6*, 187–254.

Blatt, S. J., Zuroff, D. C., Hawley, L. L., & Auerbach, J. S. (2010). Predictors of sustained therapeutic change. *Psychotherapy Research*, *20*, 37–54. https://doi.org/10.1080/10503300903121080

Blüml, V., & Doering, S. (2021). ICD-11 personality disorders: A psychodynamic perspective on personality functioning. *Frontiers in Psychiatry*, *12*, 654026. https://doi.org/10.3389/fpsyt.2021.654026

Bonanno, G. A., & Diminich, E. D. (2013). Annual research review: Positive adjustment to adversity—trajectories of minimal-impact resilience and emergent resilience. *Journal of Child Psychology and Psychiatry*, *54*(4), 378–401. https://doi.org/10.1111/jcpp.12021

Bornstein, R. F. (2012). From dysfunction to adaptation: An interactionist model of dependency. *Annual Review of Clinical Psychology*, *8*(1), 291–316. https://doi.org/10.1146/annurev-clinpsy-032511-143058

Bradley, R., Heim, A. K., & Westen, D. (2005). Transference patterns in the psychotherapy of personality disorders: Empirical investigation. *British Journal of Psychiatry*, *186*(4), 342–349. https://doi.org/10.1192/bjp.186.4.342

Byrne, G., Sleed, M., Midgley, N., Fearon, P., Mein, C., Bateman, A., & Fonagy, P. (2019). Lighthouse Parenting Programme: Description and pilot evaluation of mentalization-based treatment to address child maltreatment. *Clinical Child Psychology and Psychiatry*, *24*(4), 680–693. https://doi.org/10.1177/1359104518807741

Campagna, A. X., Desmarais, E. D., French, B., Underwood, J. J., Majdandžić, M., Beijers, R., de Weerth, C., Lee, E. G., Huitron, B., Ahmetoglu, E., Benga, O., Raikkonen, K., Heinonen, K., Gonzalez-Salinas, C., Slobodskaya, H., Kozlova, E., Linhares, M. B. M., Lecannelier, F., Casalin, S., Acar, I., Tuovinen, S., Wang, Z., Montirosso, R., Giusti, L., Park, S. Y., Han, S. Y., Putnam, S., & Gartstein, M. A. (2023). Temperament and behaviour problems in children: A multilevel analysis of cross-cultural differences. *Infant and Child Development*, *32*(5), e2443. https://doi.org/10.1002/icd.2443

Campbell, C., Tanzer, M., Saunders, R., Booker, T., Allison, E., Li, E., O'Dowda, C., Luyten, P., & Fonagy, P. (2021). Development and validation of a self-report measure of epistemic trust. *PLoS One*, *16*(4), e0250264. https://doi.org/10.1371/journal.pone.0250264

Caspi, A., Houts, R. M., Belsky, D. W., Goldman-Mellor, S. J., Harrington, H., Israel, S., Meier, M. H., Ramrakha, S., Shalev, I., Poulton, R., & Moffitt, T. E. (2014). The p factor: One general psychopathology factor in the structure of psychiatric disorders? *Clinical Psychological Science*, *2*(2), 119–137. https://doi.org/10.1177/2167702613497473

Caspi, A., Houts, R. M., Belsky, D. W., Harrington, H., Hogan, S., Ramrakha, S., Poulton, R., & Moffitt, T. E. (2016). Childhood forecasting of a small segment of the population with large economic burden. *Nature Human Behaviour*, *1*, 0005. https://doi.org/10.1038/s41562-016-0005

Caspi, A., Houts, R. M., Fisher, H. L., Danese, A., & Moffitt, T. E. (2023). The general factor of psychopathology (p): Choosing among competing models and interpreting p. *Clinical Psychological Science*, *12*(1), 53–82. https://doi.org/10.1177/21677026221147872

Caspi, A., & Moffitt, T. E. (2018). All for one and one for all: Mental disorders in one dimension. *American Journal of Psychiatry*, *175*(9), 831–844. https://doi.org/10.1176/appi.ajp.2018.17121383

Cicchetti, D. (2016). *Developmental psychopathology. Vol. 3: Maladaptation and psychopathology*. John Wiley & Sons.

Cicchetti, D., & Rogosch, F. A. (1996). Equifinality and multifinality in developmental psychopathology. *Development and Psychopathology*, *8*(4), 597–600. https://doi.org/10.1017/s0954579400007318

Cierpka, M., Grande, T., Rudolf, G., von der Tann, M., & Staschf, M. (2007). The operationalized psychodynamic diagnostics system: Clinical relevance, reliability and validity. *Psychopathology*, *40*(4), 209–220. https://doi.org/10.1159/000101363

Clark, L. A., Ro, E., Vittengl, J. R., & Jarrett, R. B. (2024). Longitudinal prediction of psychosocial functioning outcomes: Diagnostic and Statistical Manual of Mental Disorders, Fifth Edition, Section-II personality disorders versus alternative model personality dysfunction and traits. *Personality Disorders: Theory, Research, and Treatment*, *15*(5), 341–351. https://doi.org/10.1037/per0000673

Csibra, G., & Gergely, G. (2009). Natural pedagogy. *Trends in Cognitive Sciences*, *13*(4), 148–153. https://doi.org/10.1016/j.tics.2009.01.005

Cuthbert, B. N., & Insel, T. R. (2013). Toward the future of psychiatric diagnosis: The seven pillars of RDoC. *BMC Medicine, 11*(1), 126. https://doi.org/10.1186/1741-7015-11-126

De Coninck, D., Matthijs, K., & Luyten, P. (2021). Depression in Belgian first-year university students: A longitudinal study of self-definition, interpersonal relatedness, mentalizing, and integration. *Journal of Clinical Psychology, 77*(7), 1715–1731. https://doi.org/10.1002/jclp.23149

Del Giudice, M. (2015). The life history model of psychopathology explains the structure of psychiatric disorders and the emergence of the p factor. *Clinical Psychological Science, 4*(2), 299–311. https://doi.org/10.1177/2167702615583628

Doering, S., Burgmer, M., Heuft, G., Menke, D., Bäumer, B., Lübking, M., Feldmann, M., & Schneider, G. (2014). Assessment of personality functioning: Validity of the Operationalized Psychodynamic Diagnosis axis IV (structure). *Psychopathology, 47*(3), 185–193. https://doi.org/10.1159/000355062

Ehrenthal, J. C., & Benecke, C. (2019). Tailored treatment planning for individuals with personality disorders. In U. Kramer (Ed.), *Case formulation for personality disorders* (pp. 291–314). Academic Press. https://doi.org/10.1016/b978-0-12-813521-1.00015-1

Ein-Dor, T., Mikulincer, M., Doron, G., & Shaver, P. R. (2010). The attachment paradox: How can so many of us (the insecure ones) have no adaptive advantages? *Perspectives on Psychological Science, 5*(2), 123–141. https://doi.org/10.1177/1745691610362349

Ellis, B. J., Boyce, W. T., Belsky, J., Bakermans-Kranenburg, M. J., & van Ijzendoorn, M. H. (2011). Differential susceptibility to the environment: An evolutionary–neurodevelopmental theory. *Development and Psychopathology, 23*(1), 7–28. https://doi.org/10.1017/S0954579410000611

Feinstein, A. R. (1970). The pre-therapeutic classification of co-morbidity in chronic disease. *Journal of Chronic Diseases, 23*(7), 455–468.

Fonagy, P., Campbell, C., Constantinou, M., Higgitt, A., Allison, E., & Luyten, P. (2022). Culture and psychopathology: An attempt at reconsidering the role of social learning. *Development and Psychopathology, 34*(4), 1205–1220. https://doi.org/10.1017/S0954579421000092

Fonagy, P., & Luyten, P. (2018). Conduct problems in youth and the RDoC approach: A developmental, evolutionary-based view. *Clinical Psychology Review, 64*, 57–76. https://doi.org/10.1016/j.cpr.2017.08.010

Fonagy, P., Luyten, P., & Allison, E. (2015). Epistemic petrification and the restoration of epistemic trust: A new conceptualization of borderline personality disorder and its psychosocial treatment. *Journal of Personality Disorders, 29*(5), 575–609. https://doi.org/10.1521/pedi.2015.29.5.575

Fonagy, P., Luyten, P., Allison, E., & Campbell, C. (2017). What we have changed our minds about: Part 1. Borderline personality disorder as a limitation of resilience. *Borderline Personality Disorder and Emotion Dysregulation, 4*, 11. https://doi.org/10.1186/s40479-017-0061-9

Fonagy, P., Luyten, P., Allison, E., & Campbell, C. (2024). Taking stock to move forward: Where the field of developmental psychopathology might be heading. *Development and Psychopathology, 36*(5), 2056–2065. https://doi.org/10.1017/S0954579424000312

Fonagy, P., Luyten, P., & Bateman, A. (2017). Treating borderline personality disorder with psychotherapy: Where do we go from here? *JAMA Psychiatry, 74*(4), 316–317. https://doi.org/10.1001/jamapsychiatry.2016.4302

Forbes, M. K., Tackett, J. L., Markon, K. E., & Krueger, R. F. (2016). Beyond comorbidity: Toward a dimensional and hierarchical approach to understanding psychopathology across the life span. *Development and Psychopathology, 28*(4pt1), 971–986. https://doi.org/10.1017/S0954579416000651

Gilbert, P. (2016). *Depression: The evolution of powerlessness*. Routledge.

Gilbert, P. (2024). Caring and the evolution of guilt: A biopsychosocial approach to a pro-social emotion. In L. Al-Shawaf & T. K. Shackelford (Eds.), *The Oxford handbook of evolution and the emotions* (pp. 282–296). Oxford University Press. https://doi.org/10.1093/oxfordhb/9780197544754.013.18

Haslam, N., McGrath, M. J., Viechtbauer, W., & Kuppens, P. (2020). Dimensions over categories: A meta-analysis of taxometric research. *Psychological Medicine, 50*(9), 1418–1432. https://doi.org/10.1017/S003329172000183X

Hopwood, C. J. (2024). If personality disorder is just maladaptive traits, there is no such thing as personality disorder. *Journal of Psychopathology and Clinical Science, 133*(6), 427–428. https://doi.org/10.1037/abn0000922

Huprich, S. K., & Greenberg, R. P. (2003). Advances in the assessment of object relations in the 1990s. *Clinical Psychology Review*, *23*(5), 665–698. https://doi.org/10.1016/s0272-7358(03)00072-2

Kampe, L., Zimmermann, J., Bender, D., Caligor, E., Borowski, A. L., Ehrenthal, J. C., Benecke, C., & Hörz-Sagstetter, S. (2018). Comparison of the Structured DSM-5 Clinical Interview for the Level of Personality Functioning Scale with the Structured Interview of Personality Organization. *Journal of Personality Assessment*, *100*(6), 642–649. https://doi.org/10.1080/00223891.2018.1489257

Kampling, H., Kruse, J., Lampe, A., Nolte, T., Hettich, N., Brähler, E., Sachser, C., Fegert, J. M., Gingelmaier, S., Fonagy, P., Krakau, L., Zara, S., & Riedl, D. (2022). Epistemic trust and personality functioning mediate the association between adverse childhood experiences and posttraumatic stress disorder and complex posttraumatic stress disorder in adulthood. *Frontiers in Psychiatry*, *13*, 919191. https://doi.org/10.3389/fpsyt.2022.919191

Kerber, A., Ehrenthal, J. C., Zimmermann, J., Remmers, C., Nolte, T., Wendt, L. P., Heim, P., Müller, S., Beintner, I., & Knaevelsrud, C. (2024). Examining the role of personality functioning in a hierarchical taxonomy of psychopathology using two years of ambulatory assessed data. *Translational Psychiatry*, *14*(1), 340. https://doi.org/10.1038/s41398-024-03046-z

Kernberg, O. F., & Caligor, E. (2005). A psychoanalytic theory of personality disorders. In M. F. Lenzenweger & J. F. Clarkin (Eds.), *Major theories of personality disorder* (2nd ed., pp. 114–156). Guilford Press.

Koelen, J. A., Luyten, P., Eurelings-Bontekoe, L. H., Diguer, L., Vermote, R., Lowyck, B., & Buhring, M. E. (2012). The impact of level of personality organization on treatment response: A systematic review. *Psychiatry*, *75*(4), 355–374. https://doi.org/10.1521/psyc.2012.75.4.355

Laceulle, O. M., Vollebergh, W. A. M., & Ormel, J. (2015). The structure of psychopathology in adolescence: Replication of a general psychopathology factor in the TRAILS study. *Clinical Psychological Science*, *3*(6), 850–860. https://doi.org/10.1177/2167702614560750

Lahey, B. B., Rathouz, P. J., Keenan, K., Stepp, S. D., Loeber, R., & Hipwell, A. E. (2015). Criterion validity of the general factor of psychopathology in a prospective study of girls. *Journal of Child Psychology and Psychiatry*, *56*(4), 415–422. https://doi.org/10.1111/jcpp.12300

Leadbeater, B. J., Kuperminc, G. P., Blatt, S. J., & Hertzog, C. (1999). A multivariate model of gender differences in adolescents' internalizing and externalizing problems. *Developmental Psychology*, *35*(5), 1268–1282. https://doi.org/10.1037/0012-1649.35.5.1268

Lenzenweger, M. F., Clarkin, J. F., Kernberg, O. F., & Foelsch, P. A. (2001). The Inventory of Personality Organization: Psychometric properties, factorial composition, and criterion relations with affect, aggressive dyscontrol, psychosis proneness, and self-domains in a nonclinical sample. *Psychological Assessment*, *13*(4), 577–591. https://doi.org/10.1037/1040-3590.13.4.577

Lingiardi, V., & McWilliams, N. (2017). *Psychodynamic diagnostic manual: PDM-2*. Guilford Press.

Locati, F., Milesi, A., Conte, F., Campbell, C., Fonagy, P., Ensink, K., & Parolin, L. (2023). Adolescence in lockdown: The protective role of mentalizing and epistemic trust. *Journal of Clinical Psychology*, *79*(4), 969–984. https://doi.org/10.1002/jclp.23453

Locke, D. (2011). Circumplex measures of interpersonal constructs. In L. M. Horowitz & S. Strack (Eds.), *Handbook of interpersonal psychology: Theory, research, assessment, and therapeutic intervention* (pp. 313–324). John Wiley & Sons.

Lowe, B., Toussaint, A., Rosmalen, J. G. M., Huang, W. L., Burton, C., Weigel, A., Levenson, J. L., & Henningsen, P. (2024). Persistent physical symptoms: Definition, genesis, and management. *Lancet*, *403*(10444), 2649–2662. https://doi.org/10.1016/S0140-6736(24)00623-8

Luyten, P., & Blatt, S. J. (2007). Looking back towards the future: Is it time to change the DSM approach to psychiatric disorders? The case of depression. *Psychiatry: Interpersonal and Biological Processes*, *70*(2), 85–99.

Luyten, P., & Blatt, S. J. (2011). Integrating theory-driven and empirically-derived models of personality development and psychopathology: A proposal for DSM V. *Clinical Psychology Review*, *31*(1), 52–68. https://doi.org/10.1016/j.cpr.2010.09.003

Luyten, P., & Blatt, S. J. (2013a). Interpersonal relatedness and self-definition in normal and disrupted personality development: Retrospect and prospect. *American Psychologist*, *68*(3), 172–183. https://doi.org/10.1037/a0032243

Luyten, P., & Blatt, S. J. (2013b). Relatedness and self-definition in normal and disrupted personality development: Retrospect and prospect. *American Psychologist*, *68*(3), 172–183.

Luyten, P., Blatt, S. J., & Fonagy, P. (2013). Impairments in self structures in depression and suicide in psychodynamic and cognitive behavioral approaches: Implications for clinical practice and research. *International Journal of Cognitive Therapy*, *6*(3), 265–279. https://doi.org/10.1521/ijct.2013.6.3.265

Luyten, P., Blatt, S. J., & Mayes, L. C. (2012). Process and outcome in psychoanalytic psychotherapy research: The need for a (relatively) new paradigm. In R. A. Levy, J. S. Ablon, & H. Kächele (Eds.), *Psychodynamic psychotherapy research: Evidence-based practice and practice-based evidence* (pp. 345–359). Humana Press/Springer.

Luyten, P., Campbell, C., Allison, E., & Fonagy, P. (2020). The mentalizing approach to psychopathology: State of the art and future directions. *Annual Review of Clinical Psychology*, *16*, 297–325. https://doi.org/10.1146/annurev-clinpsy-071919-015355

Luyten, P., Campbell, C., & Fonagy, P. (2020). Borderline personality disorder, complex trauma, and problems with self and identity: A social-communicative approach. *Journal of Personality*, *88*(1), 88–105. https://doi.org/10.1111/jopy.12483

Luyten, P., & Fonagy, P. (2022). Integrating and differentiating personality and psychopathology: A psychodynamic perspective. *Journal of Personality*, *90*(1), 75–88. https://doi.org/10.1111/jopy.12656

Luyten, P., & Fonagy, P. (2025). Psychodynamic treatments of depression. In J. W. Pettit, T. M. Olino, R. C. Boyd, B. C. Chu, P. E. Hayden, & D. A. Pizzagalli (Eds.), *APA handbook of depression. Vol. 2: Minoritized populations, lifespan development, assessment, and treatment* (pp. 579–602). American Psychological Association Publishing.

Luyten, P., Malcorps, S., Mayes, L. C., Target, M., & Fonagy, P. (2024). Developmental research. In G. O. Gabbard, B. Litowitz, & P. Williams (Eds.), *Textbook of psychoanalysis* (3rd ed., pp. 403–418). American Psychiatric Press.

Malcorps, S., Vliegen, N., & Luyten, P. (2024). Childhood adversity and adolescent acting-out behaviors: The mediating role of mentalizing difficulties and epistemic vigilance. *European Child & Adolescent Psychiatry*, *33*(7), 2153–2162. https://doi.org/10.1007/s00787-023-02302-9

Mascaro, O., & Sperber, D. (2009). The moral, epistemic, and mindreading components of children's vigilance towards deception. *Cognition*, *112*(3), 367–380. https://doi.org/10.1016/j.cognition.2009.05.012

McEwen, B. S. (2007). Physiology and neurobiology of stress and adaptation: Central role of the brain. *Physiological Reviews*, *87*(3), 873–904. https://doi.org/10.1152/physrev.00041.2006

McWilliams, N. (1994). *Psychoanalytic diagnosis*. Guilford Press.

McWilliams, N. (2011). *Psychoanalytic diagnosis: Understanding personality structure in the clinical process* (2nd ed.). Guilford Press.

Mikulincer, M., & Shaver, P. R. (2007). *Attachment in adulthood: Structure, dynamics and change*. Guilford Press.

Morey, L. C. (2017). Development and initial evaluation of a self-report form of the DSM–5 Level of Personality Functioning Scale. *Psychological Assessment*, *29*(10), 1302–1308. https://doi.org/10.1037/pas0000450

Morey, L. C., McCredie, M. N., Bender, D. S., & Skodol, A. E. (2022). Criterion A: Level of personality functioning in the alternative DSM-5 model for personality disorders. *Personality Disorders: Theory, Research, and Treatment*, *13*(4), 305–315. https://doi.org/10.1037/per0000551

Moritz, S., Kempke, S., Luyten, P., Randjbar, S., & Jelinek, L. (2011). Was Freud partly right on obsessive-compulsive disorder (OCD)? Investigation of latent aggression in OCD. *Psychiatry Research*, *187*(1–2), 180–184. https://doi.org/10.1016/j.psychres.2010.09.007

Murray, A. L., Eisner, M., & Ribeaud, D. (2016). The development of the general factor of psychopathology 'p factor' through childhood and adolescence. *Journal of Abnormal Child Psychology*, *44*(8), 1573–1586. https://doi.org/10.1007/s10802-016-0132-1

Olajide, K., Munjiza, J., Moran, P., O'Connell, L., Newton-Howes, G., Bassett, P., Akintomide, G., Ng, N., Tyrer, P., Mulder, R., & Crawford, M. J. (2018). Development and psychometric properties of the Standardized Assessment of Severity of Personality Disorder (SASPD). *Journal of Personality Disorders*, *32*(1), 44–56. https://doi.org/10.1521/pedi_2017_31_285

Patalay, P., Fonagy, P., Deighton, J., Belsky, J., Vostanis, P., & Wolpert, M. (2018). A general psychopathology factor in early adolescence. *British Journal of Psychiatry*, *207*(1), 15–22. https://doi.org/10.1192/bjp.bp.114.149591

Rosén, T., & Hau, S. (2021). Operationalized psychodynamic diagnosis in childhood and adolescence (OPD-CA-2)—A useful tool for improving diagnoses of psychological illnesses. *Nordic Psychology*, *73*(4), 291–299. https://doi.org/10.1080/19012276.2021.2001677

Rözer, J., Kraaykamp, G., & Huijts, T. (2016). National income inequality and self-rated health: The differing impact of individual social trust across 89 countries. *European Societies*, *18*(3), 245–263. https://doi.org/10.1080/14616696.2016.1153697

Rözer, J. J., & Volker, B. (2016). Does income inequality have lasting effects on health and trust? *Social Science & Medicine*, *149*, 37–45. https://doi.org/10.1016/j.socscimed.2015.11.047

Ruggero, C. J., Kotov, R., Hopwood, C. J., First, M., Clark, L. A., Skodol, A. E., Mullins-Sweatt, S. N., Patrick, C. J., Bach, B., Cicero, D. C., Docherty, A., Simms, L. J., Bagby, R. M., Krueger, R. F., Callahan, J. L., Chmielewski, M., Conway, C. C., De Clercq, B., Dornbach-Bender, A., Eaton, N. R., Forbes, M. K., Forbush, K. T., Haltigan, J. D., Miller, J. D., Morey, L. C., Patalay, P., Regier, D. A., Reininghaus, U., Shackman, A. J., Waszczuk, M. A., Watson, D., Wright, A. G. C., & Zimmermann, J. (2019). Integrating the Hierarchical Taxonomy of Psychopathology (HiTOP) into clinical practice. *Journal of Consulting and Clinical Psychology*, *87*(12), 1069–1084. https://doi.org/10.1037/ccp0000452

Russ, E., Shedler, J., Bradley, R., & Westen, D. (2008). Refining the construct of narcissistic personality disorder: Diagnostic criteria and subtypes. *American Journal of Psychiatry*, *165*(11), 1473–1481. https://doi.org/10.1176/appi.ajp.2008.07030376

Russell, G. (2020). Critiques of the neurodiversity movement. In S. K. Kapp (Ed.), *Autistic community and the neurodiversity movement: Stories from the frontline* (pp. 287–303). Springer Singapore. https://doi.org/10.1007/978-981-13-8437-0_21

Ryan, R. M., Soenens, B., & Vansteenkiste, M. (2019). Reflections on self-determination theory as an organizing framework for personality psychology: Interfaces, integrations, issues, and unfinished business. *Journal of Personality*, *87*(1), 115–145. https://doi.org/10.1111/jopy.12440

Salaminios, G., Barrantes-Vidal, N., Luyten, P., & Debbane, M. (2024). Editorial: Mentalization in the psychosis continuum: Current knowledge and new directions for research and clinical practice. *Frontiers in Psychiatry*, *15*, 1447937. https://doi.org/10.3389/fpsyt.2024.1447937

Sallis, H., Szekely, E., Neumann, A., Jolicoeur-Martineau, A., van IJzendoorn, M., Hillegers, M., Greenwood, C. M. T., Meaney, M. J., Steiner, M., Tiemeier, H., Wazana, A., Pearson, R. M., & Evans, J. (2019). General psychopathology, internalising and externalising in children and functional outcomes in late adolescence. *Journal of Child Psychology and Psychiatry*, *60*(11), 1183–1190. https://doi.org/10.1111/jcpp.13067

Schaefer, J. D., Caspi, A., Belsky, D. W., Harrington, H., Houts, R., Horwood, L. J., Hussong, A., Ramrakha, S., Poulton, R., & Moffitt, T. E. (2017). Enduring mental health: Prevalence and prediction. *Journal of Abnormal Psychology*, *126*(2), 212–224. https://doi.org/10.1037/abn0000232

Sharp, C., & Wall, K. (2021). DSM-5 level of personality functioning: Refocusing personality disorder on what it means to be human. *Annual Review of Clinical Psychology*, *17*(1), 313–337. https://doi.org/10.1146/annurev-clinpsy-081219-105402

Sharp, C., Wright, A. G., Fowler, J. C., Frueh, B. C., Allen, J. G., Oldham, J., & Clark, L. A. (2015). The structure of personality pathology: Both general ('g') and specific ('s') factors? *Journal of Abnormal Psychology*, *124*(2), 387–398. https://doi.org/10.1037/abn0000033

Shedler, J., & Westen, D. (2010). The Shedler-Westen Assessment Procedure: Making personality diagnosis clinically meaningful. In J. F. Clarkin, P. Fonagy, & G. O. Gabbard (Eds.), *Psychodynamic psychotherapy for personality disorders. A clinical handbook* (pp. 125–161). American Psychiatric Publishing.

Skodol, A. E., Bender, D. S., Morey, L. C., Clark, L. A., Oldham, J. M., Alarcon, R. D., Krueger, R. F., Verheul, R., Bell, C. C., & Siever, L. J. (2011). Personality disorder types proposed for DSM-5. *Journal of Personality Disorders*, *25*(2), 136–169. https://doi.org/10.1521/pedi.2011.25.2.136

Southwick, S. M., Bonanno, G. A., Masten, A. S., Panter-Brick, C., & Yehuda, R. (2014). Resilience definitions, theory, and challenges: Interdisciplinary perspectives. *European Journal of Psychotraumatology*, *5*(1), 25338. https://doi.org/10.3402/ejpt.v5.25338

Sperber, D., Clement, F., Heintz, C., Mascaro, O., Mercier, H., Origgi, G., & Wilson, D. (2010). Epistemic vigilance. *Mind & Language*, *25*(4), 359–393. https://doi.org/10.1111/j.1468-0017.2010.01394.x

Spitzer, R. L., First, M. B., Shedler, J. P., Westen, D. P., & Skodol, A. E. (2008). Clinical utility of five dimensional systems for personality diagnosis: A "consumer preference" study. *Journal of Nervous and Mental Disease*, *196*(5), 356–374. https://doi.org/10.1097/NMD.0b013e3181710950

Steele, H., & Steele, M. (2008). *Clinical applications of the Adult Attachment Interview*. Guilford Press.

Stern, B. L., Caligor, E., Clarkin, J. F., Critchfield, K. L., Horz, S., MacCornack, V., Lenzenweger, M. F., & Kernberg, O. F. (2010). Structured Interview of Personality Organization (STIPO): Preliminary psychometrics in a clinical sample. *Journal of Personality Assessment*, *92*(1), 35–44. https://doi.org/10.1080/00223890903379308

Stevanovic, D., Jafari, P., Knez, R., Franic, T., Atilola, O., Davidovic, N., Bagheri, Z., & Lakic, A. (2017). Can we really use available scales for child and adolescent psychopathology across cultures? A systematic review of cross-cultural measurement invariance data. *Transcultural Psychiatry*, *54*(1), 125–152. https://doi.org/10.1177/1363461516689215

Teicher, M. H., & Samson, J. A. (2013). Childhood maltreatment and psychopathology: A case for ecophenotypic variants as clinically and neurobiologically distinct subtypes. *American Journal of Psychiatry*, *170*(10), 1114–1133. https://doi.org/10.1176/appi.ajp.2013.12070957

Tomasello, M. (2010). *Origins of human communication*. MIT Press.

Tomasello, M. (2020). The adaptive origins of uniquely human sociality. *Philosophical Transactions of the Royal Society of London. Series B, Biological Sciences*, *375*(1803), 20190493. https://doi.org/10.1098/rstb.2019.0493

Tomasello, M., & Vaish, A. (2013). Origins of human cooperation and morality. *Annual Review of Psychology*, *64*, 231–255. https://doi.org/10.1146/annurev-psych-113011-143812

Van Haute, P. (2002). *Against adaptation*. Other Press.

Waddington, C. H. (1957). *The strategy of the genes*. Allen & Unwin.

Westen, D., DeFife, J. A., Malone, J. C., & DiLallo, J. (2014). An empirically derived classification of adolescent personality disorders. *Journal of the American Academy of Child and Adolescent Psychiatry*, *53*(5), 528–549. https://doi.org/10.1016/j.jaac.2013.12.030

Westen, D., Heim, A., Morrison, K., Patterson, M., & Campbell, L. (2002). Simplifying diagnosis using a prototype-matching approach: Implications for the next edition of the DSM. In L. E. Beutler & M. L. Malik (Eds.), *Rethinking the DSM: A psychological perspective* (pp. 221–250). American Psychological Association.

Westen, D., Shedler, J., & Bradley, R. (2006). A prototype approach to personality disorder diagnosis. *American Journal of Psychiatry*, *163*(5), 846–856. https://doi.org/10.1176/ajp.2006.163.5.846

Westen, D., Waller, N. G., Shedler, J., & Blagov, P. S. (2014). Dimensions of personality and personality pathology: Factor structure of the Shedler-Westen Assessment Procedure-II (SWAP-II). *Journal of Personality Disorders*, *28*(2), 281–318. https://doi.org/10.1521/pedi_2012_26_059

Widiger, T. A., Sellbom, M., Chmielewski, M., Clark, L. A., DeYoung, C. G., Kotov, R., Krueger, R. F., Lynam, D. R., Miller, J. D., Mullins-Sweatt, S., Samuel, D. B., South, S. C., Tackett, J. L., Thomas, K. M., Watson, D., & Wright, A. G. C. (2018). Personality in a hierarchical model of psychopathology. *Clinical Psychological Science*, *7*(1), 77–92. https://doi.org/10.1177/2167702618797105

Wilson, D., & Sperber, D. (2012). *Meaning and relevance*. Cambridge University Press.

World Health Organization. (2022). *ICD-11: International classification of diseases (11th revision)*. WHO.

Wright, A. G. C., Pincus, A. L., & Hopwood, C. J. (2023). Contemporary integrative interpersonal theory: Integrating structure, dynamics, temporal scale, and levels of analysis. *Journal of Psychopathology and Clinical Science*, *132*(3), 263–276. https://doi.org/10.1037/abn0000741

Zettl, M., Volkert, J., Vögele, C., Herpertz, S. C., Kubera, K. M., & Taubner, S. (2020). Mentalization and criterion a of the alternative model for personality disorders: Results from a clinical and nonclinical sample. *Personality Disorders: Theory, Research, and Treatment*, *11*(3), 191–201. https://doi.org/10.1037/per0000356

PART III

Methodologies for Creating and Evaluating Dimensional Models

CHAPTER 15

Factor Analysis in Psychopathology Research

ASHLEY L. WATTS AND ZHEYUE PENG

Introduction

FACTOR analysis is a statistical method designed to reduce a given set of variables into a smaller set of factors, a process known as dimension reduction (Mulaik, 1987; Spearman, 1927). Its central purpose is to explain the correlations or covariances among observable variables in terms of fewer unobservable, latent variables. Factor analysis is particularly useful when researchers suspect that a smaller set of underlying dimensions might influence complex, multidimensional data. In studies of psychopathology, factor analysis can help reveal hidden patterns within symptom clusters, which in turn may represent different dimensions of psychopathology, from narrow (e.g., anhedonia) to broad (e.g., externalizing, internalizing; Forbes, Baillie et al., 2025; Forbes, Neo et al., 2023).

The use of factor analysis has arguably defined the zeitgeist of alternative classification movements that propose reorganizing the structure of psychopathology (Kotov et al., 2017, 2021). These movements have leveraged factor analytic techniques to challenge the categorical diagnostic framework of the *Diagnostic and Statistical Manual of Mental Disorders* (DSM; American Psychiatric Association, 2013) and propose more dimensional, data-driven approaches to describing mental health conditions and how they interface with one another (Rief et al., 2023). By articulating the latent factor structure underlying symptom patterns, these alternative classification systems aim to better capture the heterogeneity and comorbidity observed in clinical practice, moving away from the discrete, mutually exclusive diagnostic categories of the DSM (e.g., Kotov et al., 2021). Factor analysis has been instrumental in driving calls for a paradigm shift in the conceptualization and classification of mental disorders.

Historical Applications of Factor Analysis

The roots of factor analysis trace back to the early 20th century, largely credited to psychologists Charles Spearman and Louis Leon Thurstone. Spearman (1904) first introduced the concept of factor analysis in his research on human intelligence, where he developed a "two-factor theory" of intelligence. This theory proposed that individual performance on cognitive tasks could be explained by a general intelligence factor, known as "g." This theory laid the groundwork for what would become the single factor model, or common factor analysis, marking a pivotal moment for fields that investigate complex, interconnected variables (Spearman, 1927).

Thurstone (1934), a contemporary of Spearman, made significant contributions to the development of factor analysis. He expanded upon Spearman's work by introducing the concept of "simple structure," which emphasized the idea that each observed variable (indicators) should load highly on only one factor, with minimal "cross-loadings" on secondary factors. Thurstone also developed methods for factor rotation, such as the "multiple-factor analysis" technique, which allowed for the identification of more meaningful and interpretable factors.

During the mid-20th century, factor analysis gained further traction as computational capabilities expanded, allowing researchers to analyze larger datasets with greater precision. Achenbach (1966) pioneered the application of factor analysis to study empirically derived dimensions of psychopathology, specifically in the context of youth mental health (reviewed by Copeland, this volume). These efforts explored whether certain psychiatric symptoms tended to co-vary with one another, providing empirical support for existing diagnostic categories or suggesting new groupings altogether.

Achenbach's innovative use of factor analysis revealed dimensions of psychopathology that stood in relatively stark contrast with the DSM-defined conditions that were (and remain) dominant at that time. Indeed, Achenbach's efforts paved the way for a more empirically driven, data-based understanding of the structure of psychopathology, which generated the now-canonical differentiation between internalizing (such as anxiety and depression) and externalizing (such as antisocial behavior and substance use) psychopathology. Factor analysis continued to gain traction in psychopathology research, such as in scale validation efforts, but it was not for another 40 or so years that others applied factor analysis to study the structure of mental disorder in adults. Externalizing and internalizing now take center stage in alternative classification systems, such as the Hierarchical Taxonomy of Psychopathology (HiTOP; Kotov et al., 2021; Krueger et al., 2021; Watson et al., 2022).

Factor Analysis in Modern Nosology

Factor analysis has become essential in psychopathology research that aims to evaluate and revise existing diagnostic frameworks. The field increasingly recognizes that existing classification systems, such as the DSM, inadequately characterize and organize mental disorders (Cuthbert, 2014; Kotov et al., 2017; Rief et al., 2023; Whooley, 2014). First and foremost, many mental disorders are probably best described as dimensionally graded as opposed to categorical (Haslam et al., 2020). There is probably no qualitative difference between mild and moderate depression, for instance, beyond what is accounted for by differential severity. Dimensional nosologies posit that mental disorders can be better understood as varying along dimensions of functioning, where symptoms and features exhibit gradual differences across individuals rather than sharp distinctions. Factor analysis is compatible with this conceptualization, because it assumes that there are underlying continua or dimensions that describe variation in psychopathology. Thus, factor analysis allows for the representation of symptom severity and diversity along a spectrum.

Second, traditional diagnostic frameworks such as the DSM tend to categorize disorders discretely, often neglecting the significant overlap across symptoms and diagnoses. Factor analysis reduces this complexity by identifying a smaller number of latent factors that can account for the correlations observed among a wide range of symptoms or behaviors, thus providing a more parsimonious understanding of mental disorders. In particular, factor analysis' role in identifying broad, transdiagnostic dimensions has been pivotal in understanding and reconceptualizing comorbidity, a common challenge in psychopathology in which individuals experience multiple overlapping disorders. By modeling their overlap, factor analysis has led to widespread acceptance of transdiagnostic dimensions of psychopathology (e.g., externalizing) whose components (e.g., conduct disorder, attention-deficit/hyperactivity disorder) are potentially undergirded by shared causal mechanisms (e.g., low effortful control).

Factor analysis' ability to describe and organize psychopathology as a hierarchically arranged set of phenomena offers unique advantages over other quantitative methods. It explicitly accommodates the increasing reality that psychopathology is best characterized by broad and narrow features, some of which are shared across many mental disorders, and many of which are unique to a given mental disorder (Conway et al., 2022; Williams et al., 2025). Thus, factor analysis can represent psychopathology at various levels of specificity, with differing degrees of specificity serving different functions depending on the research question.

Fundamentals of Factor Analysis

The theoretical foundations of factor analysis are closely tied to the development of psychometric theory and the conceptualization of psychological constructs as latent variables. Factor analysis is based on the premise that there are underlying, unobserved constructs or factors that account for the relationships observed among a set of measured variables. These latent factors are hypothesized to influence the co-variation among the observed variables. Observed variables are, ostensibly, manifestations or indicators of the underlying latent factors.

Factor analysis aims to identify these latent factors and determine the strength of their relationships with the observed variables. Mathematically, factor analysis models the observed variables as linear combinations of the latent factors, with factor loadings representing the strength of the relationships between the factors and the observed variables (for a tutorial on the mathematical mechanics of factor analysis using Excel spreadsheets, see Brusco et al., 2025). The goal of factor analysis is to find the smallest number of factors that can adequately explain the observed correlations or covariances among the observed variables. This parsimonious representation of the data helps researchers better understand the underlying structure of the constructs being measured.

With this broad overview completed, we can now explore the two main types of factor analysis: exploratory factor analysis (EFA) and confirmatory factor analysis (CFA).

Exploratory Factor Analysis. Exploratory factor analysis was developed by Spearman (1904) to examine the interrelatedness of intelligence tasks. The goal of EFA is to describe the number of latent dimensions and to maximize the amount of variance explained in the data. EFA is referred to as "exploratory," because it does not require a priori hypotheses or specification surrounding the patterning of variables' loadings (or strength of association with the factor) onto factors, and all variables are allowed to load onto all factors (Mulaik, 1987). The researcher is not even required to have a hypothesis about the number of factors that best describe the data, though they may and often do. EFA takes an inductive approach, allowing the data to guide the identification of the underlying factor structure (Haig, 2005). This approach makes EFA a useful tool for uncovering the dimensional organization of a set of variables, particularly when there is limited prior knowledge about the measured constructs.

EFA begins with the analysis of the correlation or covariance matrix of the observed variables. From there, EFA uses an extraction method to identify the latent factors by accounting for the shared variance among the observed variables (or indicators). Common factor extraction methods include principal axis factoring and maximum likelihood. The choice of extraction method often depends on the characteristics of the data and the researcher's objectives, but any choice should be well-justified, or the researcher should demonstrate that their results are robust across factor extraction methods.

After extraction, EFA applies a rotation technique to enhance the interpretability of the factor structure by achieving a simpler and more meaningful pattern of factor loadings. Factor loadings indicate the degree to which each observed variable is associated with or "loads onto" the underlying latent factors. Just as regression coefficients quantify the change in the dependent variable associated with a one-unit change in the independent variable, factor loadings quantify the expected change in the observed variable associated with a one-unit change in the latent factor.

Factor rotation minimizes the complexity of factor loading matrices to get better differentiation among the factors and to achieve a simpler structure for ease of interpretation. There are dozens of rotation techniques, with two major classes of them: orthogonal and oblique. Orthogonal rotations (e.g., varimax, quartimax) constrain the factors to be uncorrelated with one another, whereas oblique rotations (e.g., oblimin, geomin, promax) allow the factors to be correlated with one another. Some have argued that orthogonal rotations offer a simpler, more interpretable factor structure, because each observed variable tends to load highly on one factor and has low loadings on the other factors, but they are most useful when the underlying factors are believed to be independent. In contrast, oblique rotations can result in more complex factor structures. Variables may load moderately on multiple factors, and the factor intercorrelation(s) complicate the interpretation of each factor as purely independent of the others. Still, oblique rotations are most appropriate when the underlying factors are hypothesized to be related.

Ultimately, the goal of rotation is to achieve a clear and interpretable factor structure that aligns with the researcher's theoretical understanding of the latent constructs. Careful consideration and justification of the rotation technique are critical, and researchers ought to consider whether their chosen factor solution is robust across rotation methods.

Confirmatory Factor Analysis. More than 60 years after EFA was developed, Jöreskog (1969) developed confirmatory factor analysis (CFA) to test more specific hypotheses regarding the hierarchical arrangement of performance on intelligence tasks. In contrast with EFA, CFA requires researchers to make more explicit a priori decisions about the model specification, including the number of factors, whether those factors are correlated (oblique) or uncorrelated (orthogonal), and which observed variables load onto which factors (Figure 15.1).

In some ways, CFA is considered a more rigorous test of the hypothesized factor structure. The "confirmatory" nature of CFA means that model testing begins by assuming a proposed factor structure is correct, and then uses the data to examine whether that model provides an accurate summary of the observed relationships. This hypothesis-driven approach stands in contrast to the more exploratory nature of EFA, where the factor structure emerges from the data without requiring strong a priori assumptions.

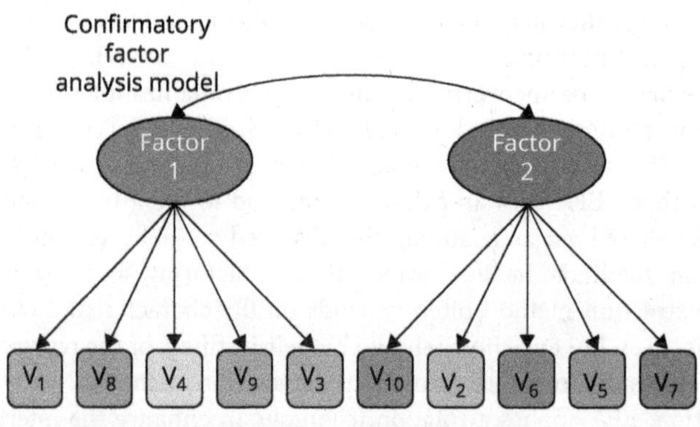

NOTE. THIS CONFIRMATORY FACTOR ANALYSIS MODEL ASSUMES SIMPLE STRUCTURE, WITH ITEMS LOADING ONTO ONLY ONE FACTOR. V = VARIABLE.

FIGURE 15.1 Confirmatory factor analysis model

Over time, the use of CFA has eclipsed EFA, as the field has increasingly prioritized theory testing about what latent variables are captured in the data over exploration of how many variables might be captured. The increased focus on CFA over time reflects the field's growing emphasis on theory testing and validation rather than purely exploratory investigations of the dimensional structure of psychological constructs. Nevertheless, the need for strong theoretical justification of the proposed factor structure remains an important consideration when implementing CFA. Further, a major and often untenable assumption in CFA is the notion of simple structure, where each observed variable is expected to load onto only one factor with no cross-loadings (Marsh et al., 2010). This strict requirement can be limiting, as real-world psychological constructs are often more complex, with variables relating to multiple latent factors.

Exploratory Structural Equation Modeling. Exploratory structural equation modeling (ESEM) was developed to address issues with overly restrictive CFA models, namely, that simple structure is rarely observed in practice (Marsh et al., 2010, 2014; Figure 15.2).

Although specific variables may be intended to represent one factor, such as externalizing, certain variables might represent that factor as well as another, such as internalizing. In factor analysis, when a variable indicates multiple factors, that phenomenon is referred to as a "cross-loading," whereby the variable indexes both the intended construct as well as another (or multiple others; Morin et al., 2016).

The psychopathology field has numerous examples of potential cross-loadings. Consider a model with internalizing and externalizing dimensions. Borderline personality disorder, for instance, tends to cross-load onto both factors (for a review, see Krueger et al., 2021). Anger and irritability, although technically viewed as forms of negative affect that should hence load onto internalizing, also load onto externalizing (Krueger et al., 2021). Similarly, were one to model the latent structure of anxiety disorders, "excessive worry" might load primarily onto a factor representing generalized anxiety disorder but may also cross-load onto a factor representing obsessive-compulsive disorder.

If we take the case of borderline personality disorder in a model with correlated externalizing and internalizing factors, failing to account for the disorder's cross-loading onto the internalizing factor would be problematic. It would imply that the aspects of borderline personality disorder that overlap with internalizing are the same aspects of externalizing that overlap with internalizing. Such an assumption would overlook the unique relationship that

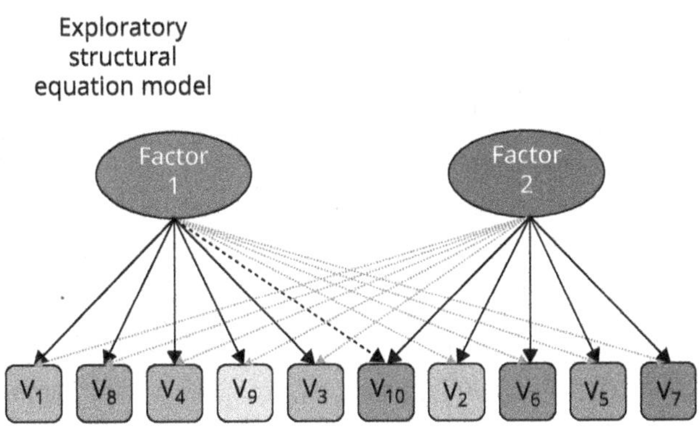

Note. Cross-loadings are depicted as dotted lines, with a substantial loading for V10 (variable 10) onto Factor 1 in addition to its primary loading on Factor 2.

FIGURE 15.2 Exploratory structural equation model

borderline personality disorder has with internalizing and could lead to an oversimplified understanding of the overlap between externalizing and internalizing. As an example, if we assume that the overlap between externalizing and internalizing reflects something akin to irritability, we assume in the case of borderline personality disorder that its overlap with internalizing is due solely to the irritability features of borderline personality disorder. In contrast, borderline personality disorder may have additional features that overlap with internalizing that do not overlap with externalizing. Nevertheless, borderline personality disorder contains other features, such as affective instability (frequent, intense emotional shifts), that overlap with conditions of internalizing (e.g., depression) but are not characteristic of externalizing.

As a result, CFA factor correlations are often inflated and the models can fit relatively poorly. Regarding factor correlations, this inflation occurs in CFA without cross-loadings, because the variance that borderline personality disorder shares with internalizing can be modeled only through the correlation between externalizing and internalizing—borderline personality disorder has no direct path to internalizing. When borderline personality disorder's cross-loading is modeled, the correlation between externalizing and internalizing may drop (at least to some extent), because the features of borderline that are better accounted for by internalizing are directly linked to it.

Regarding model fit, which quantifies the extent to which the model represents the data, CFA models without necessary cross-loadings can be associated with poorer fit. The estimated model does not reflect the true patterns in the data (i.e., borderline personality disorder's overlap with internalizing), and the model explains less variance in borderline personality disorder than is ideal, resulting in lower fit. The more variance a model explains in its variables, the better the model fit. Thus, if some of the residual variance in borderline personality disorder ought to be accounted for by internalizing, a model without a cross-loading accounts for less variance in borderline personality disorder, and model fit statistics will penalize the model for that issue. All told, even if the data generally resemble the hypothesized structure modeled in a CFA, a researcher might conclude that their overarching, conceptual model is refuted based on the poor fit of the CFA that could be improved by allowing cross-loadings.

ESEM allows for cross-loadings, but a hypothesized factor structure is still defined using "target rotation." In contrast with EFA, where the patterning of loadings is not specified, ESEM allows the researcher to specify the number of factors and marker variables for one or more of them. A marker variable is one that "most defines" a latent factor, so the researcher selects variables that are thought to reflect relatively "pure" indicators of the factor (Simmering et al., 2015). Then, the factor model is rotated with that specification in mind, meaning that the analysis attempts to find a rotation that maximizes loadings from a predefined set of indicators and minimizes cross-loadings for those items onto other factors. In this way, ESEM is thought to reflect a balance between EFA and CFA, because it allows tests of a hypothesized CFA structure that allows for cross-loadings (Marsh et al., 2014).

Bass-ackward Modeling. Goldberg's (2006) bass-ackward method can facilitate exploration of multiple levels of a hierarchy, which is useful, given that psychopathology is widely regarded as hierarchically organized (Kotov et al., 2017; Figure 15.3).

Although CFA can model higher-order factor structures, the typical CFA application typically addresses two levels of a hierarchical structure: the observed variables and a set of latent factors (Gignac, 2016; Molenaar, 2016). In contrast, the bass-ackwards method can model numerous levels of a hierarchy.

To do so, the bass-ackward method uses either principal components analysis or EFA with orthogonal or oblique rotation to extract a single component or factor at the highest level of

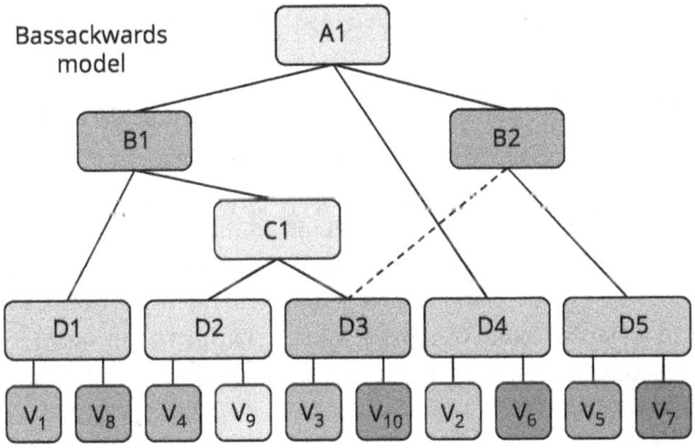

Note. Variables are organized from the top down into a series of hierarchically-organized dimensions. Dotted lines reflect cross-loadings.

FIGURE 15.3 Bass-ackwards model

the hierarchy, adding one more component or factor at each subsequent level (i.e., two on the second level and three on the third). Correlations between sequential levels of the structure characterize the hierarchical relationships among the components or factors. Forbes (2024) proposed several modifications to the bass-ackward method to provide a simpler yet more complete picture of the hierarchical structure by examining the correlations among all levels of the structure, rather than only sequential levels.

Related Statistical Techniques

Principal Component Analysis. Principal component analysis (PCA) is a dimension-reduction technique that is closely related to EFA (Greenacre et al., 2022). EFA is based on the common factor model, which assumes that the observed variables arise as a function of latent factors plus unique variance. In contrast, PCA does not make any assumptions about the underlying factor structure. EFA accounts for the shared variance among the observed variables, whereas PCA extracts both the shared and unique variance of the observed variables. PCA is not a model per se, and its components should be interpreted based on the linear combinations of the original variables. PCA is simply concerned with explaining the total variance in the data through linear combinations of the original variables.

Hierarchical Clustering. Hierarchical clustering is a multivariate statistical technique that can be used to uncover the underlying structure in data (Murtagh & Contreras, 2012). It nevertheless differs fundamentally from factor analysis in that it does not assume a latent variable model but instead creates a dendrogram (tree-like structure) that illustrates the iterative process of grouping variables based on their similarity. Hierarchical clustering operates on the notion of proximity or distance, such as Euclidean distance or Pearson correlation, grouping entities that are close to one another in a multidimensional space. Whereas factor analysis typically assumes a linear relationship among variables, hierarchical clustering does not make such an assumption and is simply a descriptive summary of the data. In psychopathology, these techniques might serve complementary roles (for joint implementations of factor analysis and hierarchical clustering, see Forbes, Baillie et al., 2025; Watts et al., 2021).

Key Assumptions in Factor Analysis

Common Cause Model

The most foundational principle of factor analysis is that latent factors are responsible for the correlations observed among various manifest variables. Factor analysis presupposes that each underlying component, or common cause, accounts for the shared variance of its observables. Invoking historical context, Spearman's theory of a general intelligence factor (g) exemplifies this logic by attributing the correlations among different intelligence tests to a single cognitive capability (Bollen, 1989; Bollen & Diamantopoulos, 2017; Spearman, 1904).

Nevertheless, a well-fitting factor model does not confirm a common cause hypothesis (DeYoung & Krueger, 2020; Watts, Lane et al., 2020). Latent variables primarily serve to encapsulate the co-variation among manifest variables without explicating the underlying processes responsible for their co-variation. For instance, simulation studies have demonstrated that the data congruent with a one-factor model could be generated by a diversity of structures, including a singular common cause, a mixture of independent or interrelated latent variables, and even complex causal loops among variables (Fried, 2020; Hayduk, 2014; van Bork et al., 2017, 2021).

Although factor analysis can reveal patterns of co-variation that suggest a common cause, the construction of latent variables within the analysis is, fundamentally, a method of summarizing co-variation without asserting causal mechanisms. Factor models do not inherently explain why items co-vary—they provide a parsimonious way to represent the covariance structure as an inductive summary rather than a deductive confirmation of a common cause (cf., Haig, 2005). Although the common cause assumption is a convenient explanatory tool, it should not be the only one considered. Rather than solely ascribing the shared variance among a set of variables to a single common mechanism, it is plausible that numerous influences are at play.

Linearity

Factor analysis assumes that the relationships among observed variables and underlying latent factors are linear. If the linearity assumption is not upheld, factor analysis might fail to capture the actual structure of the underlying data. When conducting factor analysis, the goal is to make inferences about the population based on the sample data. The estimated factor loadings from the sample are viewed as approximations of the true population loadings. These estimates should be close to the true population values when the sample is representative, sufficiently large, and the factor analysis assumptions (including linearity) are met.

Beyond random variability, systematic influences on factor loadings can suggest violations of the linearity assumption. The technique of measurement invariance, which explores whether a factor model is consistent across different groups, over time, or in relation to other variables, deals with potential linearity assumption violations (Millsap, 2012). For example, if the factor loading for substance use disorder on an externalizing latent factor differs between men and women, it would indicate a non-linear association between substance use disorder and externalizing, with gender acting as a moderator. Thus, the population-level factor loading is not a fixed value and instead varies as a function of individual or contextual factors.

The field has often focused on time and sociodemographic variables that may cause factor loadings to vary across subpopulations. Nevertheless, the potential for non-linearity, including interactions between factors, has not been as thoroughly examined. For instance, the correlation between externalizing and internalizing might change depending on one's level of externalizing. This underexplored possibility may pose significant challenges to the prevailing notion of a unified, population-wide psychopathology meta-structure. Perhaps there is no single way to organize psychopathology.

Local Independence

Local independence pertains to the assumption that all items are related to one another by way of the latent variable, meaning that items should be uncorrelated after accounting for the latent factor (Bauer, 2017; Christensen et al., 2023). This assumption goes hand in hand with the common cause assumption: What is responsible for the interrelatedness of the items is that latent factor and the latent factor only. Unfortunately, this assumption is often unmet.

In the case of a multidimensional model that is forced to be unidimensional, items will likely correlate with one another above and beyond what is shared by the single latent variable extracted. For instance, if a measure is composed of 10 items, eight of which are positively keyed and two of which are negatively keyed, the negatively keyed items may correlate with one another above and beyond what they share with the positively keyed items (e.g., Lindwall et al., 2012; Seng Kam & Meyer, 2015). In this case, when there is local dependence among items, the meaning of the latent variable will be biased toward the source of the local dependence.

As another example, if a subset of items is especially prone to drawing out response bias (e.g., attractive, popular), such as social desirability, they will correlate with one another more strongly than they will with all other items (e.g., tidy, curious). Thus, in both of these cases, the latent variable's meaning shifts away from the intended substantive construct and toward method bias. A solution to this issue is to—within each sample—examine the dimensionality of one's measure before assuming it is unidimensional. This step includes extracting a single dimension and examining its factor loadings (or item response theory-based severities), and also includes examining alternative, multidimensional factor solutions (Watts et al., 2021). In the most general sense, failing to meet the basic assumption of the use of scale scores results in (1) a non-trivial bias in individual scale score estimates compared to their "true" score and (2) the estimation of scores that are *less* reliable than they otherwise would have been had they been estimated from the correct psychometric model (McNeish, 2018).

Indicator Interchangeability

Indicator interchangeability, or what Spearman (1927) referred to as the principle of "indifference of indicators" (p. 197), is a fundamental assumption in factor analysis that has implications for the construction and interpretation of latent factors. That is, the observed variables that indicate a latent factor should be interchangeable, meaning that the interpretation of the latent variable should not change as a function of the exact combination of relevant indicators that is used to model it. This principle is predicated on the understanding that latent factors are inferred from observed variables, and there are numerous possible indicators of any given construct. For instance, there are hundreds of ways we could describe the personality trait of extraversion, and a given extraversion measure contains only a subset of those possible adjectives. Consequently, latent variables are not considered fixed, because they are not defined by a definitive list of indicators that perfectly represent the construct. Latent variables are instead random, because they are necessarily composed of a random sample of indicators drawn from the larger pool (Steyer, 1989).

Researchers use dozens of different measures to model psychopathology using factor analysis, most of which contain unique idiosyncrasies. But we also assume that "externalizing" in one study is identical to "externalizing" in another, hence the shared name. In many instances, the meaning of externalizing factors probably varies across studies, and varies in systematic ways that are not attributable to sampling variation. As an example, externalizing in young children is defined by behavioral problems, but it is not routinely defined by constructs that are central to accounts of externalizing in adolescents and adults, such as truancy, fire setting, and substance use, because these behaviors are exceedingly rare among very young children. Still, we assume that externalizing as assessed in four-year-olds is perfectly equivalent to externalizing assessed in 16- and 50-year-olds. Researchers are implicitly, if not explicitly, adopting the interchangeability assumption by asserting that the meaning of externalizing is consistent even when assessed with different sets of indicators.

The literature on general factors of psychopathology has highlighted instances in which different general factors across studies do not replicate well, with low congruence across patterns of factor loadings (i.e., an intraclass correlation of. 23) across 15 published general factors of psychopathology (Watts, Lane et al., 2020). This lack of consistency suggests that general factors of psychopathology may be sensitive to the particular indicators chosen, challenging the principle of indicator interchangeability. Two other studies further tested this possibility by modeling general factors of psychopathology within the same sample, dropping only one variable from the latent factor. General factors of psychopathology, in particular, were highly sensitive to their contents, with the varied versions of general factors producing dramatically different loading patterns (Waldman et al., 2023; Watts et al., 2019). Externalizing and internalizing factors were prone to violations of the interchangeability assumption, too, but to a far lesser extent (Waldman et al., 2023). If the inclusion or exclusion of certain indicators alters the fundamental nature of the latent variable, then the latent variable may not reflect a true latent construct.

Common Types of Factor Models

There are four major types of models used in factor analyses of psychopathology. First, the unidimensional model posits that a single factor is responsible for the shared variance among a variable set (e.g., a one-factor model of alcohol use disorder symptoms; Figure 15.4).

Second, in contrast, the correlated factors model contains two or more distinct but related factors that summarize the shared variance among their variables (Figure 15.5).

Typically, these factors are allowed to correlate with one another, but that is not a requirement of the model.

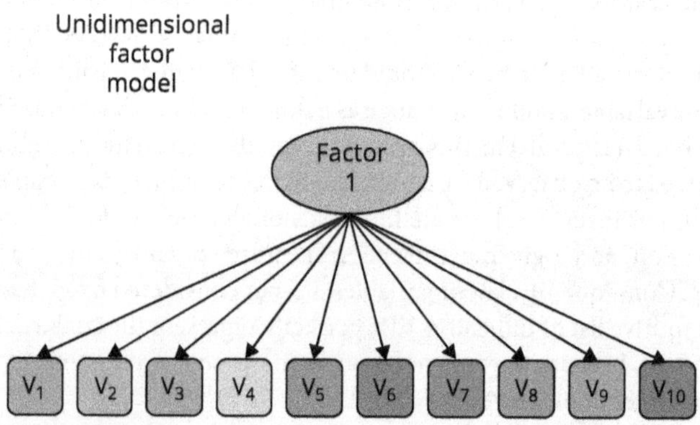

NOTE. V = VARIABLE.

FIGURE 15.4 Unidimensional factor model

Correlated factors model

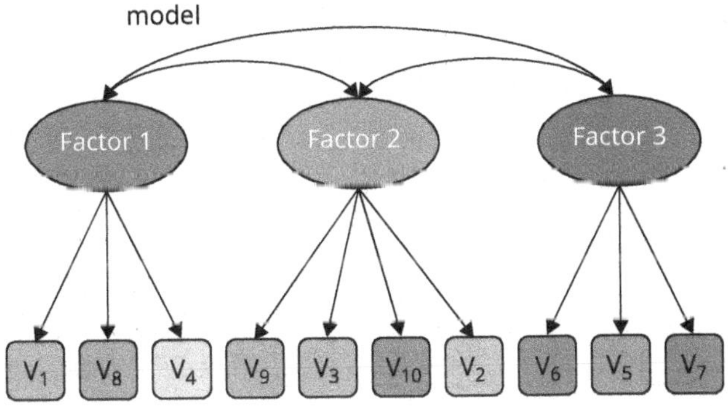

Note. V = VARIABLE.

FIGURE 15.5 Correlated factors model

Bifactor model

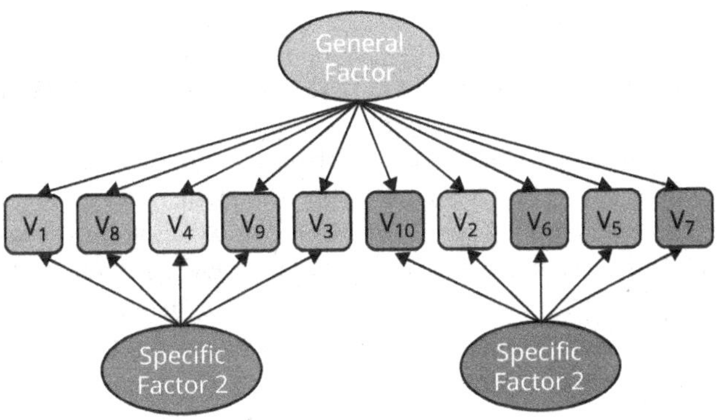

Note. V = VARIABLE.

FIGURE 15.6 Bifactor model

Third, a hierarchical structure could be modeled with a bifactor model, which includes a general factor that influences all variables in the model, and specific factors that influence specific subsets of indicators (Figure 15.6).

General factors reflect a single source of co-variation among all variables included in the model. Any remaining co-variation among subsets of variables is captured with specific factors. To properly identify the model, the general factor is constrained to be uncorrelated with the specific factors. Traditionally, specific factors are constrained to be uncorrelated with one another, under the assumption that the general factor is the sole source of covariance among variables that load on different specific factors, but this constraint is not necessary to identify the model and is often conceptually untenable. As an example, specific factors might influence subsets of indicators that reflect externalizing and internalizing, respectively.

Fourth, a higher-order model could also model psychopathology in a hierarchical manner, this time with lower-order externalizing and internalizing dimensions that are further explained by a higher-order factor (Figure 15.7).

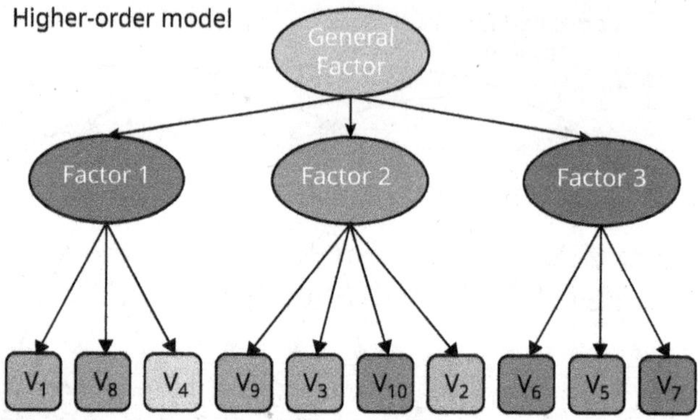

NOTE. V = VARIABLE.

FIGURE 15.7 Higher-order model

Similar to specific factors in a bifactor model, first-order factors represent residuals such that their contents reflect the shared variance of their constituent items net of the variance captured by the second-order factor(s).

The Exploratory-Confirmatory Continuum

In factor analysis, it is common for researchers to have in mind an exploratory-confirmatory continuum, with EFA, CFA, and ESEM ostensibly occupying different regions of it. It is also common, although misguided, for people to evoke a rigid dichotomy between EFA and CFA (Jacobucci, 2022). Conventionally speaking, EFA and CFA are thought to occupy opposite poles of the continuum, with ESEM falling somewhere in between them (Jacobucci, 2022; Sass & Schmitt, 2010; Wright, 2017). Nevertheless, the extent to which EFA is sufficiently exploratory and CFA sufficiently confirmatory depends on how they are implemented. Others have critiqued the labels "exploratory" and "confirmatory" altogether, suggesting that they are oversimplified and problematic (Jacobucci, 2022)—the generic use of the terms "exploratory" and "confirmatory" is misleading, in that the labels can mask the myriad local decisions and varied degrees of theoretical justification during the analytic process.

For instance, the implementation of EFA can take many forms, some of which are far more exploratory than others. The use of a single factor extraction method and a single factor rotation method (e.g., geomin with maximum likelihood) is technically exploratory, although it is advisable to ensure that one's factor solution is robust to the factor extraction and rotation methods, lest the factor solution reflect an artifact of the peculiarities of a given method (see also Greene et al., 2023).

Similarly, researchers could use multiple random starts to ensure that their factor solution replicates. Factor analysis is an iterative process that aims to find the optimal factor loadings and structure that best explain the correlations among observed variables. It is not guaranteed that factor analysis will produce the best solution, which means that a given factor solution may not be the one that most closely describes the data or is most interpretable. This issue occurs because, due to computational constraints, the estimation process (algorithm) starts with an initial set of factor loadings as "starting values," and then iteratively updates these loadings to improve model fit. Sometimes the estimation process can get stuck in what is called a "local optimum," which is a solution that fits best but only within a confined region of the multivariate space, and it may not be the ideal or truest model, the "global optimum." When initial starting values are poorly chosen, the estimation procedure often produces a locally optimal solution as opposed to the globally optimal one. Using multiple random starts means that you ask the algorithm to re-estimate the model a given number of times with different starting values. To ensure the robustness of a factor solution, researchers should inspect the factor loadings for all available optima (often fewer than 10 solutions) to examine agreement across them. When there is strong agreement, the researcher can feel more confident about their solution (see Nguyen & Waller, 2023, for a more detailed discussion).

Although examining EFAs under multiple different analytic conditions is arguably even more exploratory than conducting an EFA using one set of model specifications, this practice is also arguably far more likely to yield a robust and generalizable solution as opposed to an artefactual one. In this way, the label "exploratory" can take many different forms, and some approaches are far more exploratory than others, so "exploratory" may not be sufficiently descriptive of the researcher's decision-making process.

Similarly, the implementation of CFA is often far less "confirmatory" than is implied by its name. Of course, researchers specify the number of factors in the model, whether factors are correlated, and which variables indicate which factors. But it is rare for researchers to specify characteristics such as the degree of factor loadings and factor inter-correlations in a CFA framework (Bonifay et al., 2024), rendering the typical CFA model fairly agnostic with respect to a priori hypotheses regarding the observed model, particularly aspects of the model that have the potential to adjudicate between competing factor explanations and theories. In these sorts of implementations of CFA, the CFA is hardly confirmatory (Greene, Watts et al., 2022; Watts, Greene, Ringwald et al., 2023; Watts, Lane et al., 2020).

Further, the use of model modification indices, which provide the improvement in the chi-squared fit statistic if the parameter were to be modeled, is often used to improve model fit. Post hoc model modifications (e.g., dropping items with low factor loadings) that improve fit render the model specification less and less confirmatory as a function of the number of model modifications. In many circumstances, chasing model fit in CFA is arguably akin to p-hacking or making methodological decisions to achieve statistically "significant" results (Jacobucci, 2022; Watts, Greene, Ringwald et al., 2023). Within the context of CFA and the use of conventional fit benchmarks to "prove" one's hypothesized structure is valid, attaining "good" fit is analogous to a hypothesis test (McNeish & Wolf, 2023).

Of course, sources of model misfit can indicate serious problems with model specification, so they should not be ignored completely. Likewise, some degree of data-driven decision-making is appropriate, particularly when unexpected features of the data (e.g., non-normality and influential cases) render a hypothesized model inappropriate. The same is true for using EFA as a guide for future CFA specifications or as a tool for probing problematic CFA results (Watts, Smith et al., 2020). In either case, EFA results should be presented to prevent the questionable research practice of framing CFA specifications as though they were hypothesis-driven when they were actually guided by EFA results (i.e., the factor analytic analog to hypothesizing after results are known or HARKing; Crede & Harms, 2019). Regardless of the specific choices made, the decision-making behind every factor model should be transparent, clearly described, and defended (Jacobucci, 2022).

Model Selection and Evaluation

We open this section with a complicated question: "How do we select the right model, and how do we know if we have selected the right model?" The answer to complicated questions such as this one is almost always that "it's complicated." Model evaluation and selection is a topic that is constantly evolving with the advent of novel methods to adjudicate statistical models.

To further complicate the issue, when conducting factor analysis, the process of selecting the "right" or "best" model depends on the type of factor analysis being performed, either exploratory or confirmatory. Regardless of the type of factor analysis, however, modern practices entail the consideration of numerous factors as opposed to any one factor in isolation. Here, we focus on features of factor models that should be vetted before adopting a specific model according to contemporary best practices (e.g., Waldman et al., 2023).

EFA-specific Criteria

Perhaps the most crucial decision in conducting EFA surrounds how many factors one should extract. In EFA, one can extract as many factors as there are indicators, but that approach generally undermines the goal of reducing the data into a more parsimonious set of dimensions. Because researchers can conduct an EFA with few expectations about its results, EFA requires the use of additional statistical criteria to determine which model best describes the data.

Generally, modern practice involves considering a number of criteria that guide selection of the optimal EFA model (Howard, 2016). Historically, researchers visually inspected the scree plot, which displays the eigenvalues (corresponding to the amount of variance explained in the variable set) for each factor, and selected the number of factors that appear prior to the elbow in the plot. The elbow indicates that extracting additional factors does not explain a substantially greater amount of variance in the observed variables. Others promoted the Kaiser criterion, arguing that one should extract the number of factors with an eigenvalue greater than one. Both practices are considered outdated (Preacher & MacCallum, 2003).

Modern methods include parallel analysis (Garrido et al., 2013; Horn, 1965), Velicer's minimum average partial test (MAP; Velicer, 1976), and the test of very simple structure (VSS; Revelle & Rocklin, 1979). Parallel analysis compares the eigenvalues of the observed correlation matrix to the eigenvalues generated from random datasets of the same size. It is common for researchers to generate 500 or more random datasets. Parallel analysis then selects the number of factors for which the observed eigenvalues are larger than the randomly generated eigenvalues, which ensures that the extracted latent factors account for more variance in the observed variables than would be expected by chance.

The MAP test calculates the average of the squared partial correlations among the variables after removing the effects of the extracted factors. The number of factors is determined by the point at which the average partial correlation is minimized, as this indicates the appropriate number of factors to account for the common variance in the data. Finally, the VSS test evaluates the degree to which the factor structure conforms to a "very simple structure," where each variable loads highly on only one factor. It does this by comparing the obtained factor structure to an ideal simple structure and calculating an index that reflects how close the actual structure is to this ideal. The number of factors is determined by the point at which the VSS index is maximized, yielding a parsimonious and interpretable factor solution.

It is common for these methods (parallel analysis, MAP test, VSS test) to disagree. In those instances, each factor structure that these methods suggest is optimal should be studied and scrutinized. In hierarchically organized constructs, such as psychopathology, it is typical for these methods to converge on solutions that reflect different rungs of the hierarchy. For instance, VSS might support a two-factor solution, with internalizing and externalizing factors. MAP might support a three-factor solution, with an internalizing factor and two moderately to highly correlated externalizing factors, one for disinhibited externalizing and another for antagonistic externalizing. From there, the researcher might inspect the factor loadings and factor correlations. Is each of the factors well-defined? Are the two externalizing factors in the three-factor solution so highly correlated (e.g., $r > .85$) that they are unlikely to have different correlates? Would this study benefit from parsing subforms of externalizing? Still other aspects of the factor model may benefit from further scrutiny before selection.

Before we move on to other topics relevant to model selection, we want to make a case for fully exploiting the "exploratory" nature of EFA. Sometimes researchers will conduct an EFA but will specify the number of factors they would like to extract on an a priori basis. If there is a strong theoretical rationale for extracting a certain number of factors, such a practice is generally defensible, particularly if researchers expect that there are a fair amount of cross-loadings that would render a CFA that forces simple structure untenable. That said, there is little harm in using various EFA-specific model selection techniques to explore alternative solutions, and there is no harm in studying all possible EFA solutions to become intimately familiar with the data and how the variables interface with one another. To become most familiar with their data, researchers could extract all possible factor solutions and study how the differing factor structures unfold. To be sure, many solutions will be over-extracted, uninterpretable, and weak. Studying patterns in the data can lead to a stronger understanding of the covariance patterns in the data, potentially generating novel insights into the interrelatedness of one's constructs of interest. Such insights are not gained if one simply focuses on one or two potential EFA solutions.

Similarly, EFA can be used after CFA to ensure that the pre-specified, a priori structure holds using modeling techniques that do not necessarily force such a structure. In this way, EFA can be used as a diagnostic tool or robustness check (Watts, Smith et al., 2020). That is, to be sure that one's CFA is the optimal structure to represent the data, the EFA should generally support that same structure (although it may reveal weak cross-loadings, and so on). Of course, all EFAs and CFAs should be reported as such, especially to guard against the practice of reporting CFA models only when they were first tested using EFA.

Factor Interpretability

First and foremost, a factor model must be interpretable to be useful. That is, researchers should aim for the most parsimonious factor solution that adequately explains the data, avoiding overly complex models. Ideally, one would ensure that the interpretation of the extracted factors is meaningful and aligns with the theoretical framework. Researchers should not be so enamored by quantitative metrics that their common sense—and substantive expertise in their phenomena of interest—falls to the wayside.

Although multiple competing EFA factor solutions may be interpretable and ultimately compatible with one another, there are other instances in which model selection criteria can mislead us. The most obvious example is when factor selection criteria, such as parallel analysis, suggest an unrealistic number of factors to extract. When sample sizes are large ($N > 500$), parallel analysis will tend to suggest an over-extracted solution, meaning it will recommend too many factors that are not well represented by the observed variables. For instance, parallel analysis could indicate that a five-factor solution is best, but inspection of the factor loadings on that factor might reveal that no observed variables with standardized loadings above .2 onto the fifth factor. Similarly, parallel analysis might prefer a five-factor solution whereby the fourth and fifth factors are correlated above .90. Although extracting a fifth factor may explain more variance in the observed variables, there is likely little utility in extracting the fifth factor, particularly if the four-factor solution includes a factor that reflects a blend of the fourth and fifth factors in the five-factor solution.

Additionally, there are many construct-irrelevant sources of variance that may reveal themselves in various factor structures. Method variance, in particular, can cause challenges in factor analysis (Campbell & Fiske, 1959). For instance, Watts, Smith, and colleagues (2020) conducted an EFA of the UPPS-P Impulsivity scales, presupposing that a five-factor solution would best describe the data. Parallel analysis nevertheless supported a seven-factor solution. Inspection of that solution revealed that there were five substantive factors in the solution that corresponded to the five impulsivity domains in the UPPS-P. The remaining two factors reflected two method factors. The UPPS-P Lack of Premeditation items formed two factors, one for positively worded items and another for negatively worded items. Hence, the seven-factor solution was not only over-extracted, meaning that not all of the seven factors were well represented by their indicators, but also the method factors are of little interest compared with the substantive factors in the five-factor solution. In the event that method variance is so prominent in the observed covariance matrix, there are several classes of CFA models that can directly model method variance by removing it from the substantive factors of interest (for thorough treatments, see: Eid, 2000; Pohl & Steyer, 2010).

Factor Reliability

As a general rule of thumb, a robust factor should generally have loadings greater than .40 from three or more observed variables. The "three or more" rule—that at least three variables should load strongly onto the latent factor—is particularly useful for translating factor solutions between EFA and CFA, with the latter requiring three or more variables to statistically identify the factor.

Robust factor loadings are non-negotiable—the potency of a factor is in direct proportion to its loadings. When factor loadings are low, it suggests that a substantial portion of the variance in the observed variables is not explained by the common factor but rather by other sources—one of which is measurement error. For instance, a standardized loading of. 40 indicates that a latent variable explains only 16% of the variance in the observed variable, a rather paltry amount of variance explained by a presumably robust latent variable. In contrast, if a variable loads at 1.0 on the latent factor, the latent factor explains 100% of that variable's variance and the latent factor is essentially defined by that variable. Ultimately, latent factors that explain little variance in their variables are underwhelming in their interpretability and explanatory power.

Loading strength feeds directly into a well-known psychometric issue: reliability. As is the case with a desirable measure, a desirable factor model will yield reliable factors that are well defined by their indicators. A variety of modern indices quantify model-based reliability, and there are several helpful primers on these indices (Brunner et al., 2012; Rodriguez et al., 2016b, 2016a). Most commonly used in factor analysis today are the omega family of indices (e.g., omega hierarchical, omega total), which estimate the proportion of variance in the indicators accounted for by each latent factor (omega hierarchical) or by all latent factors combined (omega total; McNeish, 2018). Omegas quantify the proportion of variance in observed scores that is attributable to all true score variance for a given latent factor. True score variance includes both the common variance the factor shares with other variables/factors, as well as the unique reliable variance that is specific to that factor. A high omega suggests that the items consistently measure the same construct and are not influenced by random error or unrelated dimensions.

A related index is explained common variance, which is a measure of the proportion of common variance in the indicators—that is, variance that is shared among a set of observed variables due to their relationship with one or more factors—explained by each factor or the entire factor solution. Omega considers the reliability of scale scores relative to the latent factor, accounting for both common and unique reliable sources of indicator variances, whereas explained common variance focuses exclusively on the proportion of common variance explained by each factor. A high explained common variance indicates that the factor(s) identified in the model account for a substantial portion of the variance that is shared among observed variables, implying that the factor solution effectively summarizes the data.

Calculating and interpreting reliability indices offers a range of benefits that collectively serve to evaluate the suitability of a model. To begin, these indices enable researchers to communicate the robustness of factors in accessible terms, such as by quantifying the variance a factor accounts for within its indicators—a mere 10%, for instance, might signal a weak and noisy factor. Furthermore, such indices provide context to the overarching fit of the model. A model with weak factors may fit well, due to being heavily parameterized. Specifying greater numbers of factors with small factor loadings can inflate some model fit indices but provide a solution that is unique to the observed data and hence less replicable (Montoya & Edwards, 2021), but low factor reliability indicates that weak factors do not explain much variance in the indicator(s). When small-to-moderate loadings are also unreliable (e.g., with large standard errors), we are likely overfitting our data, leaving us with little useful information from our estimated model (Forbes et al., 2021; Watts et al., 2019).

Model Fit

Model fit refers to the ability of a model to reproduce the data, typically the variance–covariance matrix associated with the data. That is, model fit statistics quantify the degree to which the proposed factor model's implied covariance matrix reproduces the observed covariances in the data. The observed covariance matrix refers to the matrix of the actual, empirically observed covariances or correlations among the measured variables in the dataset, whereas the model-implied covariance matrix is the covariance matrix that is implied or predicted by the tested factor model. The better the model fits according to some fit index, the more closely it approximates the data. The general goal of factor analysis is to find the model that best reproduces the observed data as closely as possible.

Imagine a two-factor CFA model where variables x1, x2, and x3 load on one factor, and variables x4, x5, and x6 load on another factor (Figure 15.8).

Let's say the standardized factor loadings for x-x3 on f1 are all 0.6, and the standardized loadings for x4-x6 on f2 are all 0.7. The correlation between the two factors, f1 and f2, is 0.3. In this hypothetical model, the observed correlation between x1 and x4 might be 0.25. But the model-implied correlation between y1 and y4 would be calculated based on the factor loadings and the factor correlation. Specifically, the model-implied correlation would be: (0.6 * 0.7 * 0.3) = 0.126. So, the observed correlation of 0.25 between x1 and x4 differs from the model-implied correlation of 0.126. Model fit statistics quantify the degree to which the

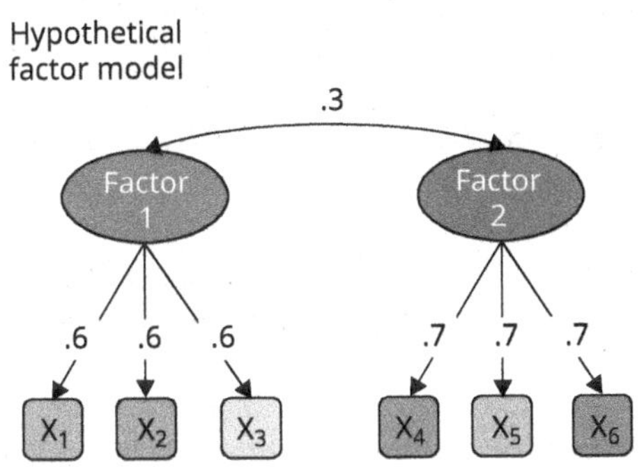

FIGURE 15.8 Hypothetical factor model

model-implied covariance matrix, calculated from the factor loadings and factor correlations, reproduces the observed covariance matrix in the data. The greater the discrepancies between the two, the poorer the fit.

For reasons we will describe later, model fit is most commonly evaluated within the context of CFA (as opposed to EFA), with the focus being evaluating how well a theoretically driven factor structure fits the observed data. Hence, whether or not a model fits well is interpreted as support for a hypothesized factor model based on prior theory or empirical evidence. There are numerous classic fit indices available to researchers to serve this goal, and they fall into three major categories: absolute fit indices, relative (or incremental) fit indices, and information-theoretic indices.

Absolute Fit Indices. Absolute fit indices evaluate the overall model fit by comparing the observed covariance matrix to the model-implied covariance matrix. Common examples of absolute fit indices include the chi-squared fit statistic, the Root Mean Square Error of Approximation (RMSEA), and the Standardized Root Mean Square Residual (SRMR). Each of these fit indices assesses the degree to which the proposed factor model is able to reproduce the observed data, without comparing it to any baseline or alternative model. For absolute fit indices, perfect fit is equivalent to 0, and the bigger the index, the worse the model fits. As an example, RMSEA estimates the amount of unexplained variance in the model, adjusting for model complexity, with low values indicating that the model explains much of the (co)variance in the variables.

The chi-squared test of model fit was once regarded as the preferred model fit index, but it has fallen out of favor in modern practice because it is highly sensitive to sample size. Specifically, the chi-squared statistic is directly proportional to sample size, so as sample size increases, chi-squared will increase even if the proportional fit of the model remains the same. The p-value associated with the chi-squared statistic is often interpreted, with non-significant values indicating "good" fit. But with large sample sizes (e.g., $N > 300$), even small differences between the observed and model-implied covariance matrices can lead to a significant p value for the chi-squared test, indicating poor model fit, even when the model is actually a good fit to the data. Further, with small sample sizes, the chi-square test may not be sensitive enough to detect meaningful lack of fit. The chi-squared fit statistic is generally appropriate when the sample size falls between 75 and 200 and is almost always significant when the sample size exceeds 400 (Kline, 2016). With the psychopathology literature increasingly acknowledging the need to rely on larger samples due to concerns regarding statistical power, the chi-squared fit statistic has limited utility in informing model fit. Indeed, its fallible nature highlights the need to rely on multiple fit indices to determine global model fit.

Relative Fit Indices. Relative fit indices, in contrast to absolute fit indices, evaluate the fit of a proposed factor model by comparing it against a baseline or "null" model. Typically, this null model is one in which all observed variables are assumed to be uncorrelated, suggesting the absence of common factors influencing the data. Two commonly used relative fit indices are the Comparative Fit Index (CFI) and the Tucker-Lewis Index (TLI). Both indices gauge the improvement of the target model's fit over that of the null model. Values closer to 1 reflect better fit, with 1 itself indicating a perfect fit. Lower values, approaching 0, indicate progressively poorer fit. CFI and TLI are particularly informative, because they assess fit improvement in a way that accounts for varying model complexities. This offers a relative measure of fit that helps determine whether the added complexity of the proposed model leads to a substantially better representation of the underlying data structure compared to a model with no latent variables at all.

Information-theoretic Indices. Information-theoretic fit indices, such as the Akaike Information Criterion (AIC) and Bayesian Information Criterion (BIC), provide a different approach to evaluating the fit of factor analysis models compared with some of the more traditional absolute and relative fit indices. A key benefit to information-theoretic fit indices is that they penalize for a model's parametric complexity, or its number of estimated parameters. This penalty best facilitates the comparison of models that vary in their number of parameters. BIC, compared with AIC, can further penalize for sample size (see the sample-size-adjusted BIC), which can facilitate the comparison of models whose sample sizes vary.

Given that they penalize the estimated number of parameters in the model, AIC and BIC are often promoted as the indices that balance model fit with model complexity, presumably prioritizing the most parsimonious model (e.g., Lahey et al., 2012), but such a statement is misguided for at least two reasons. First, some relative fit indices also penalize for the number of estimated parameters, including CFI and RMSEA, so AIC and BIC are not inherently better at detecting parsimonious models than certain other fit indices and hence should not be prioritized as such. Second, AIC and BIC penalize for one component of model complexity, parametric complexity, but do not penalize for another important form of model complexity, configural complexity. Parametric complexity refers to the number of estimated parameters in the model, whereas configural complexity refers to the specific arrangement or structure of the factor model (e.g., the number of factors, the pattern of factor loadings; see Bonifay & Cai, 2017; Preacher, 2006, for longer discussions). As such, information-theoretic fit indices, at this time, do not fully account for model complexity.

Limitations of Model Fit. Fit indices, though prioritized in CFA, are not without their controversies. There are literally hundreds of fit indices available to researchers today, many of which have been criticized for various reasons. Here, we highlight some of the contemporary issues around model fit statistics.

Limited Applicability to EFA. Recommended cutoff values for commonly used fit indices are not apt for EFA because they are overly sensitive to correlated residuals and nonspecific model misspecification (Montoya & Edwards, 2021). Fit indices in the context of EFA will generally support overfactored solutions. Hence, reliance on model fit indices in EFA can lead to incorrect conclusions about the number of factors, resulting in the endorsement of complex models that may not be replicable in new datasets.

Model fit evaluation in the context of ESEM shares the same concerns when it comes to determining the number of factors to retain. When both EFA and ESEM extract the same numbers of factors, they are fit-equivalent, meaning that their model fit to any given dataset is identical (Marsh et al., 2010, 2014). Relying on conventional fit indices to support an ESEM is not consistent with best practice, as ESEM models that allow for all possible cross-loadings (even when very small) benefit from modeling sample-specific noise and containing a relatively large number of parameters. Uncritical application of such fit indices may detract from the intended balance of exploratory and confirmatory elements of factor analysis.

Sensitivity to Variable Distribution. Conventional model fit statistics such as RMSEA and CFI are prone to misrepresenting model fit with categorical data, particularly binary data that are common in psychopathology studies (e.g., models of symptom or diagnosis presence versus absence). More specifically, traditional fit indices often overestimate the extent to which factor models actually fit such data, potentially leading researchers to accept models that, in reality, fail to capture the underlying structure accurately (Savalei, 2021). One clear implication from this common practice is that conventional fit indices could mislead us into concluding that many phenomena are unidimensional when they are, in fact, not (Watts et al., 2021). Savalei (2021) proposed the use of robust fit indices that modify the calculation of these indices to correctly reflect the fit when data are categorical, which generate more valid estimates of model fit for categorical data (see also Brosseau-Liard et al., 2012; Brosseau-Liard & Savalei,

2014; Xia & Yang, 2019). Although these fit indices are not widely adopted in the field at the time of this writing, wider adoption of them would benefit the field.

Arbitrary and Inappropriate Benchmark Guidelines. It is common practice to rely on static (benchmark) cutoffs for model fit (e.g., good fit is indicated by Comparative Fit Index > .95 and Root Mean Square Error of Approximation <.05; Hu & Bentler, 1999; cf., Groskurth et al., 2023). These cutoffs, however, were established under certain conditions and for specific types of models, and they do not consistently extend to all modeling contexts, such as one-factor CFA or hierarchical factor models. In turn, certain cutoffs may be inappropriate for a given model, leading to false conclusions about the appropriateness of a given factor model. McNeish and Wolf (2023) created dynamic fit indices, which derive fit index cutoffs that are tailored to the unique specifications of one's factor model (see also McNeish & Manapat, 2024; McNeish & Wolf, 2022).

This bespoke approach to evaluating model fit considers variations in model characteristics—model size, sample size, number of indicators, and strength of loadings—that influence the sensitivity of fit indices, thereby providing a more reliable and nuanced assessment of model fit. Numerous simulation studies have shown that dynamic fit indices outperform traditional cutoffs in terms of classification accuracy. Dynamic fit indices can recalibrate the sensitivity of fit indices like RMSEA and CFI to address issues such as the "reliability paradox" noted by Hancock and Mueller (2011), where stronger loadings can result in worse fit according to static cutoffs. These dynamic cutoffs prevent spurious conclusions about model performance, ensuring that the assessment of fit accurately reflects the data's theoretical constructs.

Overfitting the Data. An ideal model is sufficiently complex to capture the essential structures and relationships among variables but not so complex as to include superfluous parameters. Overfitting occurs when a model is too closely tailored to the peculiarities of a specific dataset, capturing noise—or random fluctuations—in addition to the true underlying patterns. To put it simply, overfitting compromises the model's generalizability and predictive power. Although an overfitted model might produce an excellent fit to one's data, it may fail to replicate when applied to new data sets. That is, certain parameters (e.g., residual covariances, loadings, factor correlations) are unlikely to replicate in other samples. One such explanation of such lack of replication is because extra parameters that seemed necessary to describe the data were, in fact, modeling variance that is specific to the sample as opposed to generalizable to the population.

The dangers of overfitting are amplified by the traditional reliance on fixed cutoff values for fit indices—standards set to determine the adequacy of model fit, often regardless of the model's specific features or the data's nature. Benchmark cutoffs may inadvertently encourage overfitting data by leading researchers to add parameters until the fit improves. Researchers, motivated to achieve good fit by these arbitrary benchmarks, might modify their models by incrementally adding parameters until the fit improves, thus straying into the realm of overfitting. To mitigate the risk of overfitting, it is essential to approach model fitting with a judicious balance between complexity and parsimony, prioritizing a simpler model if it fits the data nearly as well as a more complex one.

Unfortunately, well-fitting models are not inherently replicable. Focusing primarily, or exclusively, on model fit can fail to capture significant variations between original and replication studies, leading to flawed conclusions about the replicability of models. A two-factor model of psychopathology with externalizing and internalizing factors may fit well in two studies but have dramatically different factor loadings and factor correlations. Bonifay and colleagues (2024) proposed the use of Bayesian prior predictive similarity checking to appraise how closely the data patterns and parameter estimates of a replication study align with those from the original study. Applying their method to the National Comorbidity Survey and its replication, they found that despite the excellent fit of their tested model to both datasets, the similarity checks often indicated significant disparities in data patterns and parameters. This finding led to the realization that achieving high goodness-of-fit does not guarantee that the relationship among variables is consistent across datasets. Fit statistics mask meaningful differences between datasets.

Alternative, Equally Well-fitting Models. One can use a variety of classes of models to model their constructs: factor models, network models, and class-based models, to name a few. Factor models assume the underlying structure is composed of one or more normally distributed dimensions, network models assume the modeled structure arises from complex interactions among the indicators, and class-based models assume that there are discrete groupings (i.e., classes) of individuals in the population that do not vary on the construct of interest. Even though various models often make dramatically different assumptions about the nature of the constructs being modeled, they are often statistically equivalent.

The problem of statistical equivalence can occur both within a type of modeling (e.g., factor analysis) as well as across types (e.g., factor and network analysis). Consider two factor models of psychopathology, one with correlated externalizing and internalizing factors, and a bifactor model with a broad ("general") psychopathology factor and narrower externalizing and internalizing dimensions (Figure 15.6). The former model posits that two correlated dimensions describe the structure of psychopathology across people, and the latter posits that there is a general liability to experience psychopathology in addition to liabilities to experience externalizing and internalizing beyond general liability. These models reflect distinct hypothetical structures with different interpretations, but they are often equivalent in terms of model fit (e.g., Greene et al., 2019).

Even more distinct in terms of hypothesized causal structure are factor and network models. Under many conditions, factor and network structures are also statistically equivalent (van Bork et al., 2021). Taking our depression example, the data may be generated from a common cause process such that underlying depression vulnerability causes an array of symptoms, but they may also be generated by a series of interactions among the symptoms included in the model, such that sadness causes sleeplessness, which causes fatigue, which causes trouble concentrating and irritability, and so on (see Slipetz & Henry, this volume).

In each of these cases, different models with divergent substantive interpretations or structural pathways can and do yield identical fit statistics, a phenomenon known as model equivalence. In turn, a model that fits the data perfectly may not necessarily be the "true" model (Tomarken & Waller, 2003). Even when a model demonstrates a minimal discrepancy between the observed covariance matrix and the covariance matrix implied by the model, this does not prove the model is uniquely correct. Indeed, many different models can produce the same covariance matrix, leading to the same fit statistics.

As an extreme example, there are exactly identified models, also known as just-identified models, that have zero degrees of freedom. These models will always perfectly fit the data, because they have enough parameters to exactly reproduce the observed covariances, but they provide no information about the true nature of the data-generating process.

Imagine you have three observed variables, x1, x2, and x3. You want to use these three variables to estimate a single latent factor. In this case, the number of free parameters you need to estimate is equal to the number of unique (i.e., non-redundant) variances and covariances in the 3x3 observed covariance matrix. Specifically, the model would estimate three factor loadings and three unique (residual) variances (one for each observed variable), meaning that we are estimating six parameters. The 3x3 observed covariance matrix also contains only six unique elements—three variances (one for each observed variable) and three covariances

(N covariances = (k*(k-1))/2, or (3(3-1))/2, or 6). In this example, the number of estimated parameters is equal to the number of elements in the observed covariance matrix, meaning that the model is just identified. Degrees of freedom correspond to the number of unique elements in the covariance matrix minus the number of estimated parameters, with zero degrees of freedom meaning that there are no remaining "extra" pieces of information to test the model fit. In turn, a just-identified model will always fit the data perfectly because the number of parameters matches the number of unique statistics in the observed data. But this perfect fit does not prove the model is the "true" underlying structure—it simply means the model is able to reproduce the observed covariances without any remaining degrees of freedom to test the model.

Apart from exact equivalence, near-equivalent models that are not mathematically identical still produce model fit statistics that are so similar they lie within their margins of error. Equivalent models can severely limit the inferences that can be drawn about the validity of any given model based solely on fit indices, because two models with markedly different theoretical foundations can appear virtually identical in terms of statistical fit.

Ultimately, good fit tells us little about the processes that generated the observed data. Two equivalent (or nearly equivalent) models can neither confirm nor disconfirm a theory unless an equivalent model can be ruled out with stronger tests, and any well-fitting model should not be confused with one that reflects nature simply because a researcher extracted it (Bonifay et al., 2017; Fried, 2020; Watts, Greene, Bonifay et al., 2024; Yarkoni, 2020).

Model Complexity. Many fit indices, particularly those that are information-theoretic, are praised for their ability to penalize model complexity. Fit indices will, generally speaking, favor more complex models. But again, existing fit indices (e.g., CFI, RMSEA, AIC, BIC) penalize for parametric complexity (the number of parameters) and not configural complexity (the particular arrangement of those parameters, e.g., how many factors, factor loadings, and residual covariances are estimated), meaning that these fit statistics fail to appropriately penalize for all components of model complexity (Bonifay & Cai, 2017; Falk & Muthukrishna, 2023; Preacher, 2006).

Models that differ in their configural complexity can yield different fits to the data even when they are equivalent in terms of their parametric complexity. Holding constant the number of parameters in a series of competing models, Bonifay and Cai (2017) showed that certain types of models—in this case, a bifactor CFA model—achieved good fit for almost as many data patterns as alternative models, including an EFA model. Furthermore, the confirmatory bifactor model achieved better fit than the exploratory factor model for a small proportion of the data patterns. These data were randomly generated, with no specified data-generating mechanism that would indicate that the bifactor model was "truer" than others. The increased configural complexity of the bifactor CFA model was the likely cause of its better fit relative to other models. Ironically, although confirmatory models are supposed to impose more constraints on the data, the bifactor model's configuration allowed it to fit the data quite well, so well that it bordered on atheoretical (Greene, Eaton et al., 2022; Greene et al., 2019; Greene, Watts et al., 2022).

Models that tend to fit well, even to randomly generated datasets, have what other researchers have termed a high degree of "fitting propensity," or an inherent tendency to accommodate a wide range of possible data patterns. As such, model fit cannot be treated as the single most important indicator of model validity, given its tendency to favor models that are not necessarily strongly aligned with the data-generating mechanisms. Models with a high fitting propensity may be selected not because they best capture the true data-generating mechanisms, but simply because they are otherwise adept at reproducing the observed covariance patterns, including noise or error. In short, configurally complex models can find creative ways to overfit the data. In turn, the field may have proliferated certain types of models (i.e., the bifactor model) due to their ability to achieve good model fit rather than their validity.

The problems of model complexity and fitting propensity make it especially challenging to choose among competing factor models, which is the name of the game in modern quantitative psychopathology studies (Reise et al., 2016, referred to this practice as "fit contests"). Fit indices will place models with differing numbers of parameters on a more even playing field, but they cannot help us adjudicate among models with differing configurations, rendering most "fit contests" virtually impossible to interpret. Recent simulation studies show, for instance, that certain fit indices will unduly favor certain factor models (i.e., the bifactor model) even when the true data generating model conforms to a correlated factors structure. That is, model fit statistics encourage selection of the model that is, by definition, wrong because it is more complex. What's more, these same simulation studies have shown that fit indices that penalize for parametric complexity (such as BIC) are consistently biased toward more complex models, which contradicts the common assumption that they discourage complexity.

Global Fit Can Mask Local Misfit. Some authors have argued that reliance on model fit indices is often overprioritized, and omnibus fit can obscure construct heterogeneity and lead to model misspecification (Stanton et al., 2021). In short, factor analysis can oversimplify complex phenomena, pointing to relative unidimensionality for complex disorders (e.g., alcohol use disorders) or psychopathology in general (cf., Watts et al., 2021; Watts, Greene, Bonifay et al., 2024). To demonstrate this problem, Stanton and colleagues (2021) showed that although one-factor models for interpersonal dysfunction and internalizing each fit well, EFAs showed that each construct could be parsed into multiple dimensions that had unique correlates. Watts and colleagues (2021) demonstrated how model fit intersects with measurement, with model fit indices favoring one-factor models when there are relatively few indicators of complex constructs, such as alcohol use disorder. With more thorough assessment of alcohol use disorder, a multidimensional, three-factor structure that was highly consistent with theoretical models was supported. The authors argue for a balanced use of exploratory and confirmatory methods that reflect both broad and narrow dimensions, aligning with hierarchical frameworks such as HiTOP. They suggest incorporating exploratory analyses to ensure that emerging structures align with theoretical expectations, and they advocate for supplementing fit indices with a critical evaluation of other model features and alternative structures. Model fit indices are but one source of information and should not be the sole determinant of model selection.

The Necessity for Holistic Model Evaluation

Some researchers have argued that fit indices add no value to factor analysis (Barrett, 2007). Others have argued that fit indices are challenging to interpret, with simulation studies offering benchmarks for good fit that are fallible, because they are inherently model-specific and context dependent. That is, although quantitative researchers have provided cutoffs for good fit, they rightly point out that the ability of any benchmark to actually inform good fit will depend on the sample size, magnitude of factor loadings, number of factors, extent of cross-loadings, distributions of the indicators, and so on (Hu & Bentler, 1999; Marsh et al., 2004). Hence, numerous researchers have concluded that conventional benchmarks for model fit are subject to abuse, if not virtually meaningless (Hayduk et al., 2007). Today, most researchers acknowledge that model fit statistics have some value, but that conventional benchmarks should be avoided, and model fit should be evaluated holistically, prioritizing convergence across varied fit indices and not cherry-picking a single fit index.

Given the fallibility of model fit indices, researchers should incorporate several other methodological considerations beyond fit when validating their factor models. In addition to the considerations we raised (e.g., factor interpretability, factor reliability), researchers should prioritize theoretical robustness. Factor models should align with existing theoretical frameworks, and a good factor model should reflect established knowledge and theories about the constructs being measured. Before even considering factor analysis, researchers must have a clear understanding of why factor analysis is an appropriate method given their data, constructs, and theory. They should also have a clear understanding of how the latent variables are conceptually defined and are expected to relate to one another and to observed variables. Fit indices are just one piece of a larger puzzle of model adequacy.

Conclusion

Factor analysis is a powerful tool for describing the structure of psychopathology, but it is a technique that is as easily misused as it is used. Here, we described current issues in factor analysis and advise against exclusive reliance on singular model performance metrics to assess a model's suitability. The implications of poorly conducted factor analyses extend well beyond academic discourse, affecting classification systems, shaping clinical practice, and influencing policymaking. We advocate for a more integrated and cautious approach to factoring in model performance that includes theoretical coherence and factor interpretability. To this end, before applying factor analysis, researchers should critically assess whether the method is warranted given their data, their constructs, and, critically, theory. This holistic framework strikes at the heart of what we aspire toward in the development of rigorous, reliable, and clinically meaningful models.

References

Achenbach, T. M. (1966). The classification of children's psychiatric symptoms: A factor-analytic study. *Psychological Monographs: General and Applied*, 80(7), 1–37. https://doi.org/10.1037/h0093906

American Psychiatric Association & American Psychiatric Association (Eds.). (2013). *Diagnostic and statistical manual of mental disorders: DSM-5* (5th ed.). American Psychiatric Association.

Bauer, D. J. (2017). A more general model for testing measurement invariance and differential item functioning. *Psychological Methods*, 22(3), 507–526. https://doi.org/10.1037/met0000077

Bollen, K. A. (1989). *Structural equations with latent variables*. Wiley.

Bollen, K. A., & Diamantopoulos, A. (2017). In defense of causal-formative indicators: A minority report. *Psychological Methods*, 22(3), 581–596. https://doi.org/10.1037/met0000056

Bonifay, W., & Cai, L. (2017). On the complexity of item response theory models. *Multivariate Behavioral Research*, 52(4), 465–484. https://doi.org/10.1080/00273171.2017.1309262

Bonifay, W., Lane, S. P., & Reise, S. P. (2017). Three concerns with applying a bifactor model as a structure of psychopathology. *Clinical Psychological Science*, 5(1), 184–186. https://doi.org/10.1177/2167702616657069

Bonifay, W., Winter, S. D., Skoblow, H. F., & Watts, A. L. (2024). Good fit is weak evidence of replication: Increasing rigor through prior predictive similarity checking. *Assessment*, 32(2), 10731911241234118. https://doi.org/10.1177/10731911241234118

Brosseau-Liard, P. E., & Savalei, V. (2014). Adjusting incremental fit indices for nonnormality. *Multivariate Behavioral Research*, 49(5), 460–470. https://doi.org/10.1080/00273171.2014.933697

Brosseau-Liard, P. E., Savalei, V., & Li, L. (2012). An investigation of the sample performance of two nonnormality corrections for RMSEA. *Multivariate Behavioral Research*, 47(6), 904–930. https://doi.org/10.1080/00273171.2012.715252

Brunner, M., Nagy, G., & Wilhelm, O. (2012). A tutorial on hierarchically structured constructs: Hierarchically structured constructs. *Journal of Personality*, 80(4), 796–846. https://doi.org/10.1111/j.1467-6494.2011.00749.x

Brusco, M., Steinley, D., & Watts, A. L. (2025). Teaching the mechanics of factor analysis using excel spreadsheets. *Structural Equation Modeling: A Multidisciplinary Journal*, *32*(4), 730–751. https://doi.org/10.1080/10705511.2024.2424815

Campbell, D. T., & Fiske, D. W. (1959). Convergent and discriminant validation by the multitrait-multimethod matrix. *Psychological Bulletin*, *56*(2), 81–105. https://doi.org/10.1037/h0046016

Christensen, A. P., Garrido, L. E., & Golino, H. (2023). Unique variable analysis: A network psychometrics method to detect local dependence. *Multivariate Behavioral Research*, *58*(6), 1165–1182. https://doi.org/10.1080/00273171.2023.2194606

Conway, C. C., Forbes, M. K., & South, S. C. (2022). A Hierarchical Taxonomy of Psychopathology (HiTOP) primer for mental health researchers. *Clinical Psychological Science*, *10*(2), 236–258. https://doi.org/10.1177/21677026211017834

Crede, M., & Harms, P. (2019). Questionable research practices when using confirmatory factor analysis. *Journal of Managerial Psychology*, *34*(1), 18–30. https://doi.org/10.1108/JMP-06-2018-0272

Cuthbert, B. N. (2014). The RDoC framework: Facilitating transition from ICD/DSM to dimensional approaches that integrate neuroscience and psychopathology: Forum—The Research Domain Criteria Project. *World Psychiatry*, *13*(1), 28–35. https://doi.org/10.1002/wps.20087

DeYoung, C. G., & Krueger, R. F. (2020). To wish impossible things: On the ontological status of latent variables and the prospects for theory in psychology. *Psychological Inquiry*, *31*(4), 289–296. https://doi.org/10.1080/1047840X.2020.1853462

Eid, M. (2000). A multitrait-multimethod model with minimal assumptions. *Psychometrika*, *65*(2), 241–261. https://doi.org/10.1007/BF02294377

Falk, C. F., & Muthukrishna, M. (2023). Parsimony in model selection: Tools for assessing fit propensity. *Psychological Methods*, *28*(1), 123–136. https://doi.org/10.1037/met0000422

Forbes, M. K. (2024). Improving hierarchical models of individual differences: An extension of Goldberg's bass-ackward method. *Psychological Methods*, *29*(6), 1062–1073. https://doi.org/10.1037/met0000546

Forbes, M. K., Baillie, A., Batterham, P. J., Calear, A., Kotov, R., Krueger, R. F., Markon, K. E., Mewton, L., Pellicano, E., Roberts, M., Rodriguez-Seijas, C., Sunderland, M., Watson, D., Watts, A. L., Wright, A. G. C., & Clark, L. A. (2025). *Reconstructing psychopathology: A data-driven reorganization of the symptoms in the Diagnostic and Statistical Manual of Mental Disorders. Clinical Psychological Science*, *13*(3), 462–488. https://doi.org/10.31234/osf.io/7um9a

Forbes, M. K., Greene, A. L., Levin-Aspenson, H. F., Watts, A. L., Hallquist, M., Lahey, B. B., Markon, K. E., Patrick, C. J., Tackett, J. L., Waldman, I. D., Wright, A. G. C., Caspi, A., Ivanova, M., Kotov, R., Samuel, D. B., Eaton, N. R., & Krueger, R. F. (2021). Three recommendations based on a comparison of the reliability and validity of the predominant models used in research on the empirical structure of psychopathology. *Journal of Abnormal Psychology*, *130*(3), 297–317. https://doi.org/10.1037/abn0000533

Forbes, M. K., Neo, B., Nezami, O. M., Fried, E. I., Faure, K., Michelsen, B., Twose, M., & Dras, M. (2023). *Elemental psychopathology: Distilling constituent symptoms and patterns of repetition in the diagnostic criteria of the DSM-5* [Preprint]. PsyArXiv. https://doi.org/10.31234/osf.io/u56p2

Fried, E. I. (2020). Lack of theory building and testing impedes progress in the factor and network literature. *Psychological Inquiry*, *31*(4), 271–288. https://doi.org/10.1080/1047840X.2020.1853461

Garrido, L. E., Abad, F. J., & Ponsoda, V. (2013). A new look at Horn's parallel analysis with ordinal variables. *Psychological Methods*, *18*(4), 454–474. https://doi.org/10.1037/a0030005

Gignac, G. E. (2016). The higher-order model imposes a proportionality constraint: That is why the bifactor model tends to fit better. *Intelligence*, *55*, 57–68. https://doi.org/10.1016/j.intell.2016.01.006

Greenacre, M., Groenen, P. J. F., Hastie, T., D'Enza, A. I., Markos, A., & Tuzhilina, E. (2022). Principal component analysis. *Nature Reviews Methods Primers*, *2*(1), 100. https://doi.org/10.1038/s43586-022-00184-w

Greene, A. L., Eaton, N. R., Forbes, M. K., Fried, E. I., Watts, A. L., Kotov, R., & Krueger, R. F. (2022). Model fit is a fallible indicator of model quality in quantitative psychopathology research: A reply to Bader and Moshagen. *Journal of Psychopathology and Clinical Science*, *131*(6), 696–703. https://doi.org/10.1037/abn0000770

Greene, A. L., Eaton, N. R., Li, K., Forbes, M. K., Krueger, R. F., Markon, K. E., Waldman, I. D., Cicero, D. C., Conway, C. C., Docherty, A. R., Fried, E. I., Ivanova, M. Y., Jonas, K. G., Latzman, R. D., Patrick, C. J., Reininghaus, U., Tackett, J. L., Wright, A. G. C., & Kotov, R. (2019). Are fit indices used to test psychopathology structure biased? A simulation study. *Journal of Abnormal Psychology*, *128*(7), 740–764. https://doi.org/10.1037/abn0000434

Greene, A. L., Watts, A. L., Forbes, M. K., Kotov, R., Krueger, R. F., & Eaton, N. R. (2023). Misbegotten methodologies and forgotten lessons from Tom Swift's electric factor analysis machine: A demonstration with competing structural models of psychopathology. *Psychological Methods*, *28*(6), 1374–1403. https://doi.org/10.1037/met0000465

Groskurth, K., Bluemke, M., & Lechner, C. M. (2023). Why we need to abandon fixed cutoffs for goodness-of-fit indices: An extensive simulation and possible solutions. *Behavior Research Methods*, *56*(4), 3891–3914. https://doi.org/10.3758/s13428-023-02193-3

Haig, B. D. (2005). Exploratory factor analysis, theory generation, and scientific method. *Multivariate Behavioral Research*, *40*(3), 303–329. https://doi.org/10.1207/s15327906mbr4003_2

Hancock, G. R., & Mueller, R. O. (2011). The reliability paradox in assessing structural relations within covariance structure models. *Educational and Psychological Measurement*, *71*(2), 306–324. https://doi.org/10.1177/0013164410384856

Haslam, N., McGrath, M. J., Viechtbauer, W., & Kuppens, P. (2020). Dimensions over categories: A meta-analysis of taxometric research. *Psychological Medicine*, *50*(9), 1418–1432. https://doi.org/10.1017/S003329172000183X

Hayduk, L. (2014). Seeing perfectly fitting factor models that are causally misspecified: Understanding that close-fitting models can be worse. *Educational and Psychological Measurement*, *74*(6), 905–926. https://doi.org/10.1177/0013164414527449

Hayduk, L., Cummings, G., Boadu, K., Pazderka-Robinson, H., & Boulianne, S. (2007). Testing! Testing! One, two, three—Testing the theory in structural equation models! *Personality and Individual Differences*, *42*(5), 841–850. https://doi.org/10.1016/j.paid.2006.10.001

Horn, J. L. (1965). A rationale and test for the number of factors in factor analysis. *Psychometrika*, *30*(2), 179–185. https://doi.org/10.1007/BF02289447

Howard, M. C. (2016). A review of exploratory factor analysis decisions and overview of current practices: What we are doing and how can we improve? *International Journal of Human-Computer Interaction*, *32*(1), 51–62. https://doi.org/10.1080/10447318.2015.1087664

Hu, L., & Bentler, P. M. (1999). Cutoff criteria for fit indexes in covariance structure analysis: Conventional criteria versus new alternatives. *Structural Equation Modeling: A Multidisciplinary Journal*, *6*(1), 1–55. https://doi.org/10.1080/10705519909540118

Jacobucci, R. (2022). A critique of using the labels confirmatory and exploratory in modern psychological research. *Frontiers in Psychology*, *13*, 1020770. https://doi.org/10.3389/fpsyg.2022.1020770

Jöreskog, K. G. (1969). A general approach to confirmatory maximum likelihood factor analysis. *Psychometrika*, *34*(2), 183–202. https://doi.org/10.1007/BF02289343

Kline, R. B. (2016). *Principles and practice of structural equation modeling* (4th edition). The Guilford Press.

Kotov, R., Krueger, R. F., Watson, D., Achenbach, T. M., Althoff, R. R., Bagby, R. M., Brown, T. A., Carpenter, W. T., Caspi, A., Clark, L. A., Eaton, N. R., Forbes, M. K., Forbush, K. T., Goldberg, D., Hasin, D., Hyman, S. E., Ivanova, M. Y., Lynam, D. R., Markon, K., . . . Zimmerman, M. (2017). The Hierarchical Taxonomy of Psychopathology (HiTOP): A dimensional alternative to traditional nosologies. *Journal of Abnormal Psychology*, *126*(4), 454–477. https://doi.org/10.1037/abn0000258

Kotov, R., Krueger, R. F., Watson, D., Cicero, D. C., Conway, C. C., DeYoung, C. G., Eaton, N. R., Forbes, M. K., Hallquist, M. N., Latzman, R. D., Mullins-Sweatt, S. N., Ruggero, C. J., Simms, L. J., Waldman, I. D., Waszczuk, M. A., & Wright, A. G. C. (2021). The Hierarchical Taxonomy of Psychopathology (HiTOP): A quantitative nosology based on consensus of evidence. *Annual Review of Clinical Psychology*, *17*(1), 83–108. https://doi.org/10.1146/annurev-clinpsy-081219-093304

Krueger, R. F., Hobbs, K. A., Conway, C. C., Dick, D. M., Dretsch, M. N., Eaton, N. R., Forbes, M. K., Forbush, K. T., Keyes, K. M., Latzman, R. D., Michelini, G., Patrick, C. J., Sellbom, M., Slade, T., South, S. C., Sunderland, M., Tackett, J., Waldman, I., Waszczuk, M. A., . . . HiTOP Utility

Workgroup. (2021). Validity and utility of Hierarchical Taxonomy of Psychopathology (HiTOP): II. Externalizing superspectrum. *World Psychiatry*, *20*(2), 171–193. https://doi.org/10.1002/wps.20844
Lahey, B. B., Applegate, B., Hakes, J. K., Zald, D. H., Hariri, A. R., & Rathouz, P. J. (2012). Is there a general factor of prevalent psychopathology during adulthood? *Journal of Abnormal Psychology*, *121*(4), 971–977. https://doi.org/10.1037/a0028355
Lindwall, M., Barkoukis, V., Grano, C., Lucidi, F., Raudsepp, L., Liukkonen, J., & Thøgersen-Ntoumani, C. (2012). Method effects: The problem with negatively versus positively keyed items. *Journal of Personality Assessment*, *94*(2), 196–204. https://doi.org/10.1080/00223891.2011.645936
Marsh, H. W., Hau, K.-T., & Wen, Z. (2004). In search of golden rules: Comment on hypothesis-testing approaches to setting cutoff values for fit indexes and dangers in overgeneralizing Hu and Bentler's (1999) findings. *Structural Equation Modeling: A Multidisciplinary Journal*, *11*(3), 320–341. https://doi.org/10.1207/s15328007sem1103_2
Marsh, H. W., Lüdtke, O., Muthén, B., Asparouhov, T., Morin, A. J. S., Trautwein, U., & Nagengast, B. (2010). A new look at the big five factor structure through exploratory structural equation modeling. *Psychological Assessment*, *22*(3), 471–491. https://doi.org/10.1037/a0019227
Marsh, H. W., Morin, A. J. S., Parker, P. D., & Kaur, G. (2014). Exploratory structural equation modeling: An integration of the best features of exploratory and confirmatory factor analysis. *Annual Review of Clinical Psychology*, *10*(1), 85–110. https://doi.org/10.1146/annurev-clinpsy-032813-153700
McNeish, D. (2018). Thanks coefficient alpha, we'll take it from here. *Psychological Methods*, *23*(3), 412–433. https://doi.org/10.1037/met0000144
McNeish, D., & Manapat, P. D. (2024). Dynamic fit index cutoffs for hierarchical and second-order factor models. *Structural Equation Modeling: A Multidisciplinary Journal*, *31*(1), 27–47. https://doi.org/10.1080/10705511.2023.2225132
McNeish, D., & Wolf, M. G. (2022). Dynamic fit index cutoffs for one-factor models. *Behavior Research Methods*, *55*(3), 1157–1174. https://doi.org/10.3758/s13428-022-01847-y
McNeish, D., & Wolf, M. G. (2023). Dynamic fit index cutoffs for confirmatory factor analysis models. *Psychological Methods*, *28*(1), 61–88. https://doi.org/10.1037/met0000425
Millsap, R. E. (2012). *Statistical approaches to measurement invariance*. Routledge.
Molenaar, D. (2016). On the distortion of model fit in comparing the bifactor model and the higher-order factor model. *Intelligence*, *57*, 60–63. https://doi.org/10.1016/j.intell.2016.03.007
Montoya, A. K., & Edwards, M. C. (2021). The poor fit of model fit for selecting number of factors in exploratory factor analysis for scale evaluation. *Educational and Psychological Measurement*, *81*(3), 413–440. https://doi.org/10.1177/0013164420942899
Morin, A. J. S., Arens, A. K., Tran, A., & Caci, H. (2016). Exploring sources of construct-relevant multidimensionality in psychiatric measurement: A tutorial and illustration using the Composite Scale of Morningness: Construct-Relevant Multidimensionality. *International Journal of Methods in Psychiatric Research*, *25*(4), 277–288. https://doi.org/10.1002/mpr.1485
Mulaik, S. A. (1987). A brief history of the philosophical foundations of exploratory factor analysis. *Multivariate Behavioral Research*, *22*(3), 267–305. https://doi.org/10.1207/s15327906mbr2203_3
Murtagh, F., & Contreras, P. (2012). Algorithms for hierarchical clustering: An overview. *WIREs Data Mining and Knowledge Discovery*, *2*(1), 86–97. https://doi.org/10.1002/widm.53
Nguyen, H. V., & Waller, N. G. (2023). Local minima and factor rotations in exploratory factor analysis. *Psychological Methods*, *28*(5), 1122–1141. https://doi.org/10.1037/met0000467
Pohl, S., & Steyer, R. (2010). Modeling common traits and method effects in multitrait-multimethod analysis. *Multivariate Behavioral Research*, *45*(1), 45–72. https://doi.org/10.1080/00273170903504729
Preacher, K. J. (2006). Quantifying parsimony in structural equation modeling. *Multivariate Behavioral Research*, *41*(3), 227–259. https://doi.org/10.1207/s15327906mbr4103_1
Preacher, K. J., & MacCallum, R. C. (2003). Repairing Tom Swift's electric factor analysis machine. *Understanding Statistics*, *2*(1), 13–43. https://doi.org/10.1207/S15328031US0201_02
Reise, S. P., Kim, D. S., Mansolf, M., & Widaman, K. F. (2016). Is the bifactor model a better model or is it just better at modeling implausible responses? Application of iteratively reweighted least squares to the Rosenberg Self-Esteem Scale. *Multivariate Behavioral Research*, *51*(6), 818–838. https://doi.org/10.1080/00273171.2016.1243461

Revelle, W., & Rocklin, T. (1979). Very simple structure: An alternative procedure for estimating the optimal number of interpretable factors. *Multivariate Behavioral Research, 14*(4), 403–414. https://doi.org/10.1207/s15327906mbr1404_2

Rief, W., Hofmann, S. G., Berg, M., Forbes, M. K., Pizzagalli, D. A., Zimmermann, J., Fried, E., & Reed, G. M. (2023). Do we need a novel framework for classifying psychopathology? A discussion paper. *Clinical Psychology in Europe, 5*(4), e11699. https://doi.org/10.32872/cpe.11699

Rodriguez, A., Reise, S. P., & Haviland, M. G. (2016a). Applying bifactor statistical indices in the evaluation of psychological measures. *Journal of Personality Assessment, 98*(3), 223–237. https://doi.org/10.1080/00223891.2015.1089249

Rodriguez, A., Reise, S. P., & Haviland, M. G. (2016b). Evaluating bifactor models: Calculating and interpreting statistical indices. *Psychological Methods, 21*(2), 137–150. https://doi.org/10.1037/met0000045

Sass, D. A., & Schmitt, T. A. (2010). A comparative investigation of rotation criteria within exploratory factor analysis. *Multivariate Behavioral Research, 45*(1), 73–103. https://doi.org/10.1080/00273170903504810

Savalei, V. (2021). Improving fit indices in structural equation modeling with categorical data. *Multivariate Behavioral Research, 56*(3), 390–407. https://doi.org/10.1080/00273171.2020.1717922

Seng Kam, C. C., & Meyer, J. P. (2015). Implications of item keying and item valence for the investigation of construct dimensionality. *Multivariate Behavioral Research, 50*(4), 457–469. https://doi.org/10.1080/00273171.2015.1022640

Simmering, M. J., Fuller, C. M., Richardson, H. A., Ocal, Y., & Atinc, G. M. (2015). Marker variable choice, reporting, and interpretation in the detection of common method variance: A review and demonstration. *Organizational Research Methods, 18*(3), 473–511. https://doi.org/10.1177/1094428114560023

Spearman, C. (1904). "General Intelligence," objectively determined and measured. *The American Journal of Psychology, 15*(2), 201. https://doi.org/10.2307/1412107

Spearman, C. (with Osmania University & Digital Library of India). (1927). *The abilities of man*. Macmillan and Company, Limited. http://archive.org/details/abilitiesofman031969mbp

Stanton, K., Watts, A. L., Levin-Aspenson, H. F., Carpenter, R., & Emery, N. N. (2021). *Focusing narrowly on model fit in factor analysis can mask construct heterogeneity and model misspecification: Applied demonstrations across sample and assessment types* [Preprint]. Open Science Framework. https://doi.org/10.31219/osf.io/6te2b

Steyer, R. (1989). Models of classical psychometric test theory as stochastic measurement models: Representation, uniqueness, meaningfulness, identifiability, and testability. *Methodika, 3*, 25–60.

Thurstone, L. L. (1934). The vectors of mind. *Psychological Review, 41*(1), 1–32. https://doi.org/10.1037/h0075959

Tomarken, A. J., & Waller, N. G. (2003). Potential problems with "well fitting" models. *Journal of Abnormal Psychology, 112*(4), 578–598. https://doi.org/10.1037/0021-843X.112.4.578

van Bork, R., Epskamp, S., Rhemtulla, M., Borsboom, D., & van der Maas, H. L. J. (2017). What is the *p*-factor of psychopathology? Some risks of general factor modeling. *Theory & Psychology, 27*(6), 759–773. https://doi.org/10.1177/0959354317737185

van Bork, R., Rhemtulla, M., Waldorp, L. J., Kruis, J., Rezvanifar, S., & Borsboom, D. (2021). Latent variable models and networks: Statistical equivalence and testability. *Multivariate Behavioral Research, 56*(2), 175–198. https://doi.org/10.1080/00273171.2019.1672515

Velicer, W. F. (1976). Determining the number of components from the matrix of partial correlations. *Psychometrika, 41*(3), 321–327. https://doi.org/10.1007/BF02293557

Waldman, I. D., King, C. D., Poore, H. E., Luningham, J. M., Zinbarg, R. M., Krueger, R. F., Markon, K. E., Bornovalova, M., Chmielewski, M., Conway, C., Dretsch, M., Eaton, N. R., Forbes, M. K., Forbush, K., Naragon-Gainey, K., Greene, A. L., Haltigan, J. D., Ivanova, M., Joyner, K., . . . Zald, D. (2023). Recommendations for adjudicating among alternative structural models of psychopathology. *Clinical Psychological Science, 11*(4), 616–640. https://doi.org/10.1177/21677026221144256

Watson, D., Levin-Aspenson, H. F., Waszczuk, M. A., Conway, C. C., Dalgleish, T., Dretsch, M. N., Eaton, N. R., Forbes, M. K., Forbush, K. T., Hobbs, K. A., Michelini, G., Nelson, B. D., Sellbom, M.,

Slade, T., South, S. C., Sunderland, M., Waldman, I., Witthöft, M., Wright, A. G. C., ... Zinbarg, R. E. (2022). Validity and utility of Hierarchical Taxonomy of Psychopathology (HiTOP): III. Emotional dysfunction superspectrum. *World Psychiatry*, *21*(1), 26–54. https://doi.org/10.1002/wps.20943

Watts, A. L., Boness, C. L., Loeffelman, J. E., Steinley, D., & Sher, K. J. (2021). Does crude measurement contribute to observed unidimensionality of psychological constructs? A demonstration with DSM–5 alcohol use disorder. *Journal of Abnormal Psychology*, *130*(5), 512–524. https://doi.org/10.1037/abn0000678

Watts, A. L., Greene, A. L., Bonifay, W., & Fried, E. I. (2024). A critical evaluation of the p-factor literature. *Nature Reviews Psychology*, 3, 108–122. https://doi.org/10.1038/s44159-023-00260-2

Watts, A. L., Greene, A. L., Ringwald, W., Forbes, M. K., Brandes, C. M., Levin-Aspenson, H. F., & Delawalla, C. (2023). Factor analysis in personality disorders research: Modern issues and illustrations of practical recommendations. *Personality Disorders: Theory, Research, and Treatment*, *14*(1), 105–117. https://doi.org/10.1037/per0000581

Watts, A. L., Lane, S. P., Bonifay, W., Steinley, D., & Meyer, F. A. C. (2020). Building theories on top of, and not independent of, statistical models: The case of the p-factor. *Psychological Inquiry*, *31*(4), 310–320. https://doi.org/10.1080/1047840X.2020.1853476

Watts, A. L., Poore, H. E., & Waldman, I. D. (2019). Riskier tests of the validity of the bifactor model of psychopathology. *Clinical Psychological Science*, *7*(6), 1285–1303. https://doi.org/10.1177/2167702619855035

Watts, A. L., Smith, G. T., Barch, D. M., & Sher, K. J. (2020). Factor structure, measurement and structural invariance, and external validity of an abbreviated youth version of the UPPS-P Impulsive Behavior Scale. *Psychological Assessment*, 32(4), 336–347. https://doi.org/10.1037/pas0000791

Whooley, O. (2014). Nosological reflections: The failure of *DSM* -5, the emergence of RDoC, and the decontextualization of mental distress. *Society and Mental Health*, *4*(2), 92–110. https://doi.org/10.1177/2156869313519114

Williams, A. L., Conway, C. C., Olino, T. M., Revelle, W., & Zinbarg, R. E. (2025). Testing criterion validity in hierarchical models of psychopathology: Comparison of latent-variable and factor-score approaches. *Clinical Psychological Science*, 13(1), 128–145. https://doi.org/10.1177/21677026231225414

Wright, A. G. C. (2017). The current state and future of factor analysis in personality disorder research. *Personality Disorders: Theory, Research, and Treatment*, *8*(1), 14–25. https://doi.org/10.1037/per0000216

Xia, Y., & Yang, Y. (2019). RMSEA, CFI, and TLI in structural equation modeling with ordered categorical data: The story they tell depends on the estimation methods. *Behavior Research Methods*, *51*(1), 409–428. https://doi.org/10.3758/s13428-018-1055-2

Yarkoni, T. (2020). Implicit realism impedes progress in psychology: Comment on Fried (2020). *Psychological Inquiry*, *31*(4), 326–333. https://doi.org/10.1080/1047840X.2020.1853478

CHAPTER 16

Taxometrics and Dimensional Models of Psychopathology

NICK HASLAM

Introduction

ON receiving a major career award in 1994, Paul Meehl, the doyen of American clinical psychology, made an audacious claim: "taxometrics," an approach to numerical taxonomy that he pioneered, could solve the classification problem in psychopathology. "Solve" is a strong word. Meehl could have hedged his bets with "advance" or "improve," but he chose an expression that implied a once-and-for-all rectification. "Revision of diagnostic systems," he wrote pointedly (Meehl, 1995, p. 266), the DSM franchise very much in his sights, "should be based on taxometric analysis rather than on committee decisions based on clinical impressions and nontaxometric research."

Meehl's views on the nature of the classification problem in psychopathology informed his confidence that taxometrics should provide the solution. The problem was one of applied mathematics, he said, requiring us to clarify the structure underlying variation in symptoms, signs, and other aspects of mental illness. In particular, it asks: "Is the latent structure of these phenotypic indicator correlations taxonic (categories) or nontaxonic (dimensions, factors)?" (p. 266). Psychopathology could be underpinned by "taxons"—discrete natural categories—or by continuous dimensions, and taxometric analysis was the preferred method for adjudicating between these options.

Meehl held a firm conviction in the existence of psychopathological taxons and believed that detecting and characterizing them was the fundamental task of classification. A mature nosology would be one that collected and systematized these taxons, winnowing out those clinical variations that were simply matters of degree. Meehl had no time for "dogmatic antinosologists" who believed that no such latent categories could exist, or for constructionists, nominalists, or pragmatists who believed that the classification of mental illness was a matter of social convention, mere labeling, or practical utility. Taxometrics could cut through to the reality behind the messy confusion of clinical phenomena and set classification on a firmer footing.

Looking back three decades after Meehl's bold pronouncement, it is fair to say that taxometrics did not solve the classification problem in psychopathology. However, the taxometric research program he initiated has played a major role in the radical developments in classification that are the focus of this volume. Ironically, the primary conclusion from hundreds of taxometric research studies is that few if any forms of psychopathology are taxonic. The legacy of Meehl's taxometrics has not been a classification system populated by proven taxons, but one that dispenses with latent categories altogether. Taxometrics has shown that the realm of psychopathology is primarily dimensional and that classifications must reflect that reality.

This chapter provides an overview of taxometric analysis, and the findings it has generated. First, I describe the historical and conceptual background of taxometrics and what it aspires to do. I then briefly describe the main taxometric procedures that have been employed by researchers. Following this, I provide an overview of the main foci of taxometric research on psychopathology, before summarizing the findings of a major quantitative review of the taxometric literature published in 2020. The chapter concludes with an extended discussion of the implications of that review for dimensional models of psychopathology.

Historical and Conceptual Context

Meehl (1992) comprehensively lays out the historical and theoretical background for his interest in latent structure. The distinction between types and continuous dimensions has endured in psychology and psychiatry over the past century and beyond, he argues, and commitments to particular positions on the issue have often been strong. In psychology, especially, researchers in personality and individual differences have typically adopted an anti-typological position: psychological variation is a matter of degree, it should be measured quantitatively rather than as a collection of types, and factor analysis should be used to determine its dimensional structure. Thinkers who proposed personality types, such as Carl Jung, were criticized as misrepresenting dimensions as categories. Similarly, many psychologists have also challenged the existence of psychopathological types, seeing these as embodying a biomedical view of mental illnesses as discrete disease entities. More generally, dimensional thinking was seen as intrinsically more advanced and scientific than "essentialist" categorical thinking.

Meehl agreed that personality is likely to be underpinned by continuous dimensions and that mental illnesses cannot be presumed to be discrete categories. However, he argued that these default assumptions should not be held dogmatically, because the issue of latent structure should be evaluated on a case-by-case basis and informed by scientific evidence.

> Whether or not the entities, properties, and processes of a particular domain (such as psychopathology, or vocational interest patterns) are purely dimensional, or are instead a mix of dimensional and taxonic relations, *is an empirical question*, not to be settled by a methodological dogma about "how science works." Among psychologists, particularly those who have a trade union animus against psychiatrists, and sometimes an extremely dogmatic treatment of the so called "medical model" . . . one hears remarks such as, "Of course there are no entities, comparable to mumps or measles, in psychopathology." The *of course* is unwarranted. (Meehl, 1992, p. 119)

In addition to making the case for empirical investigations of latent structure, Meehl defended the plausibility of discrete categories in psychology. Such categories are commonplace in other sciences, he noted, listing as examples "chemical elements, biological species, organic diseases, geological strata, kinds of stars, elementary particles, races, cultures, Mendelizing mental deficiencies, major psychoses, vocations, ideologies, religions" (Meehl, 1992, p. 117). Meehl proposed the "taxon" concept to capture categories of these kinds. Although he did not define the concept explicitly, he used it to refer to naturally existing, objectively discoverable categories—a kind of thing that "is in some sense really out there, whether human scientists identify it or not" (p. 122)—to be contrasted with categories that were simply matters of convention or arbitrarily imposed on a continuum. Taxon is sometimes translated as "natural kind," but that idea carries unwanted philosophical baggage and overlooks the fact that Meehl allowed taxons to be socially shaped and generated rather than restricting it to human-independent facts of nature. Among the "environment mold" taxons that he recognized were Trotskyist and bridge player.

If taxons might exist in the psychological domain, as Meehl proposed, their identification might have significant implications. Taxons call for different approaches to psychological assessment than dimensions do (category assignment versus quantification). They are likely to require different causal models (i.e., explanations capable of generating discontinuous outcomes, such as major gene effects in the case of Huntington's disease; or identity formation processes, such as self-labeling, joining clubs, and engaging in years of practice in the case of "bridge player"). In a clinical context, knowing a patient's taxon membership may afford more far-reaching inferences about their history, etiology, treatment, and course than would a diagnosis based on a dimensional spectrum. More basically, any realist science worth its salt should strive to develop an accurate picture of the phenomena it studies. In this spirit, Meehl proposed taxometric methods as a rigorous means of detecting taxons from fallible, psychological data.

Taxometric Procedures

Taxometrics is an approach to multivariate data analysis that was unusual when it first appeared and has remained distinctive ever since among methods with related aims (Borsboom et al., 2016). Approaches to clarifying the latent structure of multivariate data typically have three features that taxometric analysis initially did not. Most quantitative methods employ a single primary procedure and are couched in the paradigm of inferential statistics, producing significance tests for the fit of their structural models and simple, numerical evidence to support their conclusions. In contrast, taxometric methodology involves seeking consistent evidence regarding latent structure from multiple, mathematically independent procedures. It does not involve null hypothesis significance testing and originally did not provide simple output such as fit statistics. Instead, classical taxometric methods involved visual inspection of data plots to find evidence favoring categorical or dimensional conclusions.

Another point of distinction from many forms of structural analysis such as factor analysis or cluster analysis is that taxometrics is not primarily an inductive method for finding and characterizing patterns in observed variables. Taxometric analyses typically proceed from a known or hypothesized latent variable and determine whether or not it is taxonic. The research question is not what co-varies with what, but whether the co-variation known to exist is more compatible with a categorical or a dimensional latent structure. In this respect, taxometrics is also idiosyncratic. Whereas more familiar statistical approaches for characterizing the latent structure of differences among people assume that they can be modeled dimensionally (e.g., traditional factor analysis) or categorically (e.g., latent class analysis), taxometrics evaluates the more fundamental question of which structure occurs in particular cases.

The four most popular taxometric procedures are briefly described below, followed by a discussion of an important general innovation in taxometric methodology that emerged in the middle of the first decade of the 21st century. Readers interested in a more detailed discussion of taxometric analysis should consult Ruscio, Haslam, and Ruscio (2006), and those wanting a state-of-the-art overview of how to implement it using the RTaxometrics package are directed to Ruscio and Wang (2022).

MAXCOV

MAXCOV, for "maximum co-variance," was the original taxometric procedure. It was first presented in Meehl's classic text *Psychodiagnosis* (Meehl, 1973), where it was described as "a taxonomic search method for loose genetic syndromes." The procedure requires at least three "indicators": variables, preferably continuous, that are strongly associated with the latent variable of interest, such as a quantitative measure of a specific symptom of a mental illness whose latent structure is in question. Meehl recommended that MAXCOV and other taxometric procedures be used with samples of at least 300 and also provided guidelines on the required validity level for indicator variables.

To conduct MAXCOV, one indicator is defined as the input indicator and the remaining two as output indicators. The co-variance of the output indicators is calculated within successive intervals of the input indicator and plotted. The analysis can be repeated for every pair of output indicators, and overlapping ("sliding") regions on the input indicator can be used to produce a smoother plot. The multiple plots that are produced can be inspected separately as a panel or averaged. When the latent variable is dimensional, MAXCOV plots tend to be flat: the co-variation of indicators is constant along the range of the latent variable. In the taxonic case, MAXCOV plots rise to a peak, representing the region on the input indicator where taxon members and non-members (i.e., the complement) co-occur. When a taxon is present, the output indicators co-vary, because they differentiate it from its complement, and therefore they do not tend to co-vary among the taxon or the complement (i.e., at each end of the input indicator). If a taxonic peak is observed, its prevalence or "base rate" can be estimated from properties of the plot.

MAXEIG

The MAXEIG, or "maximum eigenvalue" procedure, is a later elaboration of MAXCOV that has the same basic rationale. Instead of examining the co-variance of output indicators as a function of an input indicator, like MAXCOV, MAXEIG examines their eigenvalues: the proportion of variance of a set of observed variables that is accounted for by factors extracted by factor analysis. MAXEIG plots the maximum eigenvalue for a set of output indicators as a function of sliding regions of an input indicator, repeating the process so that every indicator serves as the input indicator. As with MAXCOV, a peaked plot implies a taxon and a flat plot implies a latent dimension.

MAMBAC

Unlike MAXCOV and MAXEIG, the MAMBAC ("means above minus below a cut") requires only two indicators, although it is typically conducted with many more in order to capture the key elements of the phenomenon of interest and to obtain consistent and robust findings. In the simplest case, one indicator is defined as input and the other as output, and the analysis is then repeated with the roles reversed. A moving cut-point is placed on the input indicator, and the difference between the mean score on the output indicator for cases scoring above and those scoring below the cut is calculated. This difference is then plotted along the length of the input indicator as a function of the cut-point location. When the latent structure is dimensional the MAMBAC plot tends to be U-shaped, and when it is taxonic the plot tends to have a convex hump. As with MAXCOV/MAXEIG, the shape of the taxonic plot allows the taxon base rate to be estimated.

L-Mode

Like MAXCOV, the L-Mode ("latent mode") procedure requires at least three indicators. These are factor-analyzed and the density distribution of scores on the first factor is examined. When the latent structure is dimensional, that distribution should be unimodal, but in the taxonic case, a bimodal distribution representing the admixed taxon and complement members is expected.

Data Simulations and Fit Indices

It should be clear that traditional taxometric analysis relied heavily on visual inspection of plots rather than on clear-cut statistical decision criteria. This reliance was problematic for several reasons. Some plots or panels of plots were ambiguous or inconsistent. Inferences could be affected by arbitrary choices about indicator selection and data plotting in ways that increased researcher degrees of freedom. Some plot shapes, such as upward linear trends in MAXCOV, were commonly obtained in research studies but were neither prototypically taxonic (peaked) nor dimensional (flat). Evidence emerged that it could be challenging to differentiate taxometric plots derived from low base-rate taxons from those derived from positively skewed dimensions, a significant problem given the prevalence of positive skew in psychopathology data.

John Ruscio and colleagues (Ruscio, Ruscio, & Meron, 2007) developed a promising solution to these challenges. Their method involves generating thousands of simulated datasets that match key properties of the observed research data, such as its sample size and indicator inter-correlations, but that are based either on a taxonic structure or on a dimensional structure. The same taxometric analyses that are run on the research data are repeated on these taxonic and dimensional simulated datasets, providing an easily visualized comparison of how findings derived from the research data, with all its idiosyncrasies, would look under the two structural alternatives.

To further aid interpretation and inference, Ruscio and colleagues developed the Comparison Curve Fit Index (CCFI), which quantifies the degree to which the observed taxometric findings fit those derived from one set of simulated data better than the other. A CCFI value of 0.5 represents an equally good or bad fit to both sets of simulated data, implying an ambiguous structural finding, whereas values below 0.5 support dimensional structure and values above 0.5 support taxonic structure. Typically, separate CCFI values are generated for each taxometric procedure that is employed. Extensive Monte Carlo research (e.g., Ruscio & Kaczetow, 2009) has supported the validity, sensitivity, and lack of bias of this approach to taxometric inference, even under adverse psychometric conditions, and it quickly became popular among researchers for offering a rigorous and unambiguous approach to taxometric inference.

Domains of Taxometric Research on Psychopathology

Research using taxometric procedures has a four-decade history at the time of writing. Its center of attention has been the domain of psychopathology, although numerous studies have been carried out on personality variables and smaller numbers on such diverse phenomena as relationship types, sexual orientations, physical illnesses, and social attitudes. For the purposes of the present chapter, I focus on the main lines of psychopathology research to give a flavor of that work, citing key early articles as appropriate.

Although Meehl unveiled MAXCOV in 1973, the first published taxometric research article appeared six years later (Golden & Meehl, 1979). It explored the possibility of the "schizoid taxon" proposed in Meehl's theory of schizophrenia, which postulated a categorical vulnerability grounded in a dominant schizogene (Meehl, 1990). The article found support for a taxon and has been followed by over 20 studies. These articles generally replicated the taxonic finding with different indicators, populations, and conceptualizations or facets of schizotypy (e.g., schizotypal personality disorder symptoms, measures of physical and social anhedonia, measures of perceptual aberration), although in more recent years many have challenged the taxonic conclusion (e.g., Rawlings et al., 2008). Nevertheless, the latent structure of schizotypy and associated constructs has been one of the most popular ongoing foci of taxometric research (e.g., Morton et al., 2016; Linscott et al., 2018).

The psychopathology domain that has received the greatest taxometric attention has been that of the anxiety disorders. Beginning in 2005, a flurry of work addressed the latent structure of anxiety sensitivity (Bernstein et al., 2005), a vulnerability factor for anxiety disorders, and generally found evidence of a taxon. Other phenomena to receive significant attention from taxometric researchers included PTSD (e.g., A. Ruscio, 2001), OCD subtypes (e.g., Haslam et al., 2005), and social anxiety disorder (e.g., Kollman et al., 2006), although small quantities of work investigated GAD, health anxiety or hypochondriasis, and pathological worry, among others. Although some evidence for taxons emerged from this research, dimensional findings were more typical, a pattern that is noteworthy in view of later evidence, reviewed in the next section, that taxometric research conducted prior to about 2010 had a pro-taxonic bias.

Mood disorders also received substantial attention from taxometric researchers, with much of the focus falling on subtypes such as melancholic, endogenous, or "nuclear" depression (e.g., Grove et al., 1987). Some evidence for the taxonic status of this subtype emerged but other proposed subtypes tended to yield dimensional results, as did multiple studies of general depression or dysthymia (e.g., Ruscio & Ruscio, 2000), vulnerability for depression (e.g., Gibb et al., 2004), and mania (Prisciandaro & Roberts, 2011).

After mood and anxiety disorders and schizotypy, the next most popular field of taxometric research on psychopathology has been (non-schizotypal) personality pathology. The greatest concentration of this work by far has been antisocial personality disorder and the closely related construct of psychopathy. The first study in this line of work (Harris, Rice & Quinsey, 1994) found surprising evidence of a psychopathic taxon, although a large volume of subsequent research (e.g., Marcus et al., 2006) has provided evidence of dimensionality for psychopathy, antisocial personality and behavior, and assorted criminal tendencies (e.g., Walters, 2007). Seven other DSM personality disorders have received at least some taxometric attention, with borderline and paranoid personalities, in particular, the target of a handful of studies. Early evidence suggested the presence of a borderline taxon (Trull et al., 1990), but as with antisocial personality and psychopathy, later studies have tended to challenge that conclusion.

Smaller bodies of work have examined the latent structure of eating disorders and substance use problems. The findings of studies of eating disorders, which include some investigations of related phenomena such as dietary restraint, drive for thinness, and body dissatisfaction, are difficult to summarize, because these studies have commonly carried out complex analyses of differences between proposed subtypes of anorexia and bulimia nervosa rather than examining whether these conditions themselves differ taxonically from normal variations in eating behavior. Some early work found evidence for some taxons (Gleaves et al., 2000; Williamson et al., 2002), but these findings have not been consistently replicated since. In the substance use field, there have been a surprising number of taxonic findings in relation to alcohol use disorders (e.g., Walters, 2009). Few studies have examined the use of other substances although evidence tentatively points to marijuana use being dimensional (e.g., Denson & Earleywine, 2006) and nicotine dependence being taxonic (Goedeker & Tiffany, 2008).

Most taxometric research on psychopathology has addressed adult disorders, but disorders of and in childhood have not been entirely neglected. Among these are multiple studies of ADHD (e.g., Haslam et al., 2006), autism and its proposed subtypes (e.g., Ingram et al., 2008), and specific language impairment (e.g., Dollaghan, 2004). This work has tended to support the taxonic status of some aspects of autism but has consistently backed a dimensional view of ADHD and language impairments.

The taxometric literature on psychopathology has been expansive in its coverage but often thinly spread, and this overview can offer only a sketch of the most popular topics. Additional phenomena that have been the subject of at least one study include dementia (Gavett & Stern, 2012), pathological dissociation (Waelde et al., 2005), psychotic symptoms (Ahmed et al., 2012), suicidal ideation (Witte et al., 2017), and somatization (Jasper et al., 2012). Many "normal" personality factors that may be of interest to psychopathologists have also been investigated. Readers interested in a comprehensive listing of taxometric publications should consult the meta-analysis to which this chapter now turns.

Meta-analytic Evidence

In an effort to synthesize the rapidly growing evidence base outlined in the preceding section, Haslam, McGrath, Viechtbauer, and Kuppens (2020) carried out the first meta-analysis of the taxometric literature. Their analysis examined an exhaustive set of 279 peer-reviewed articles, published or in press by the end of 2019, that employed one or more taxometric procedures to investigate the latent structure of one or more observed variables. The analysis aimed to evaluate the prevalence of taxonic findings across a diverse array of construct domains, and to determine any methodological and substantive factors that moderate that prevalence. Secondarily it aimed to identify latent variables that were especially plausible candidates for taxonic status.

The primary level of analysis for the meta-analysis was the study "finding," namely, the conclusion drawn by the researchers about the taxonic versus dimensional status of a variable based on their analysis. The 279 articles yielded 502 findings, as many reported multiple studies or analyzed multiple variables. Findings were classified into 17 content domains, of which 11 were psychopathology-related (mood, anxiety, eating, substance use, other externalizing, schizotypy, other personality, childhood, psychotic and somatoform disorders, plus an "other psychopathology" grouping [e.g., dissociation, dementia]), five related to additional psychological variables (personality, sexuality, gender, response styles and biases, and other individual differences [e.g., attitudes, interests]), and one "miscellaneous" domain containing findings about non-psychological variables such as biological sex and handedness.

An assortment of methodological variables was also evaluated for each finding. These included the size and nature of the study sample (e.g., community, clinical, college student, child or adolescent), the type of data employed (e.g., self-ratings, interviews), and properties of the indicators used in the analyses (e.g., whether they were dichotomous, based on single items versus multi-item scales, and whether they had undergone a validation process). Finally, the taxometric methods themselves were evaluated, including the specific procedures (e.g., MAXCOV, MAMBAC), the number of procedures carried out, and whether Ruscio's simulation method was used to generate values of the comparative curve fit index (CCFI).

Arguably the most striking result to emerge from the meta-analysis arose from the comparison of studies that employed the CCFI and those that did not. Taxonic findings were rare in the former (53 of 317: 16.7%) but common in the latter (107 of 185: 57.8%). Analyses confirmed that this gaping discrepancy was not due to the respective studies examining different variables. Given extensive Monte Carlo research evidence that the simulation/CCFI method is unbiased with respect to judgments of taxonicity (Ruscio & Kaczetow, 2009; Ruscio, Walters, Marcus & Kaczetow, 2010), the discrepancy points to a serious pro-taxonic bias in taxometric research that does not use the simulation method. A previous quantitative review of taxometric research up to 2011 (Haslam, Holland & Kuppens, 2012) further showed that several additional aspects of study methodology that were common in early taxometric studies—the use of small samples, fewer taxometric procedures, and dichotomous and unvalidated indicator variables—also generated such a pro-taxonic bias. In that review, a broad index of overall methodological quality was associated with a lower likelihood of taxonic findings.

Studies that did not employ the simulation method began in 1979, whereas those that did first appeared in 2004, after which it became standard. The methodological quality of studies (independent of the use of the simulation method) also tended to improve over time. As a result, the historical trend in taxometric research has led steadily away from the enthusiasm for taxa that marked the early years. Figure 16.1 plots the cumulative proportion of taxonic findings in taxometric studies of psychopathology variables (solid line) and the cumulative proportion of taxometric findings that employed the simulation method (dotted line). Taxonic findings predominated well into the 2000s, but with the rapid and widespread adoption of the simulation method, their cumulative proportion fell to 34% by 2019. This figure substantially overestimates the true rate at which taxa exist, because it includes a substantial proportion of presumptively biased studies that did not use the simulation method.

The main component of the Haslam et al. (2020) meta-analytic study was restricted to the 317 taxometric findings, drawn from 183 articles, that were based on the simulation method, where the CCFI could be used as a quantitative index akin to an effect size. The overall mean CCFI of 0.40 indicated that latent dimensionality was the rule across all construct domains. Taxonic findings were in the minority in all 17 of these except the (non-psychological) miscellaneous domain. Overall evidence for the presence of taxa was not significantly greater in the psychopathology domains (mean CCFI = 0.42) than in the "normal" psychological domains (mean CCFI = 0.36). Internalizing and externalizing domains did not differ in this regard. The personality disorder domain was significantly less taxonic than other domains of psychopathology, but despite the decades-long interest in the possible taxonic status of schizotypy, it was no more taxonic than other personality disorders. In short, a comprehensive review of the taxometric research literature as of 2020 indicated that taxa were rare, that early taxometric studies greatly inflated their prevalence, and that psychopathology was no different from

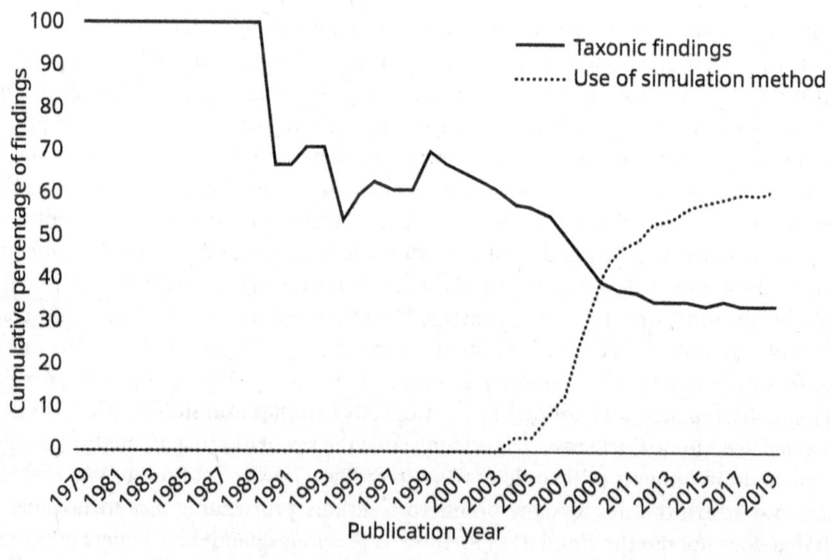

FIGURE 16.1 Cumulative proportion of taxonic findings over the history of taxometric research on psychopathology, and cumulative rate of use of Ruscio's comparative data simulation procedure.

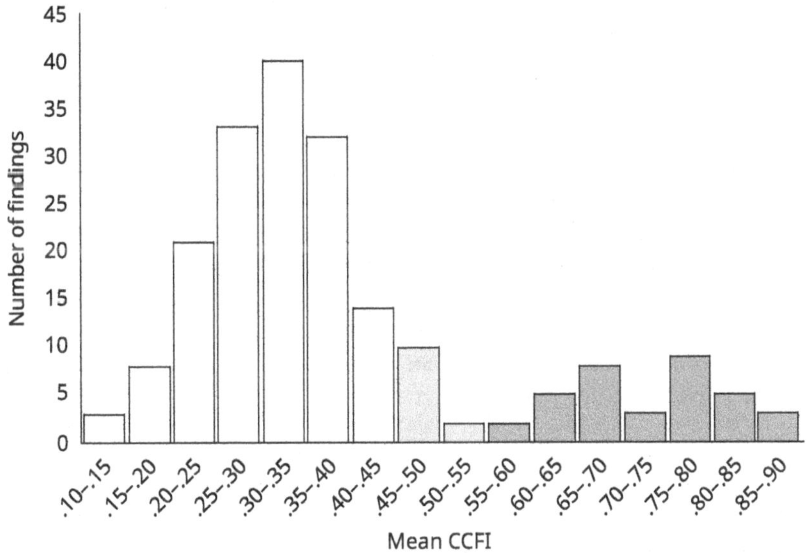

FIGURE 16.2 Distribution of CCFI values for taxometric studies of psychopathology (no shading = dimensional findings, light shading = ambiguous findings, dark shading = taxonic findings)

normal variation in personality and other psychological phenomena in being predominantly dimensional.

One last finding of the Haslam et al. (2020) meta-analysis deserves mention. The analysis revealed that CCFI values were distributed bimodally, with a majority of findings concentrated symmetrically at low CCFI values and a small minority concentrated at high values. Figure 16.2 plots this distribution for the 198 CCFI values from analyses of psychopathology variables. Two key implications can be drawn from this striking pattern. First, there is a modest proportion (18%) of taxonic findings in the psychopathology domain, despite it being primarily dimensional. Second, the bimodality is consistent with taxonic and dimensional latent structures being genuinely distinct alternatives. If there was a spectrum of structural variants from fully dimensional and fully taxonic, a unimodal and perhaps skewed distribution might be expected. We should conclude that taxonicity is itself taxonic and that taxonic latent structure is real but rare in the field of psychopathology.

Implications

Although taxometric research studies continue to be published, the rate at which they appear has declined significantly in recent years. Given the very extensive range of phenomena that has been studied and the consistent support for dimensional conclusions in the vast majority of cases, it is unlikely that the overall complexion of taxometric findings will change in future. It is, therefore, appropriate to take stock of the lessons taxometric research teaches us about dimensional models in the domain of psychopathology.

Dimensional Models and Dimensional Diagnoses

The most obvious lesson from the body of taxometric research is that phenotypic variation in this domain is overwhelmingly dimensional. That conclusion holds for specific mental disorders, for an assortment of proposed subtypes of these disorders, and for a wide assortment of personality diatheses. If, as Meehl supposed, a true psychiatric nosology must contain categories, then either no such nosology is possible or it is possible but very sparsely populated, omitting most of the phenomena that have typically been considered fundamental forms of mental illness.

The more defensible approach is to propose that a systematic nosology is possible, but it must be primarily dimensional in nature. The findings of five decades of taxometric research therefore support the ontological assumptions of new dimensional models of psychopathology. HiTOP, for example (Kotov et al., 2007), proposes that differences among people in the psychopathology domain are chiefly matters of degree, and taxometric research is one of several lines of positive support for that assumption. Relatedly, that research also supports the adoption of continuum beliefs about mental illness among laypeople, which appear to have positive implications for reducing stigma toward people experiencing mental illness (Schomerus, Matschinger, & Angermeyer, 2013).

Whether these findings also support the complete abandonment of categorical classifications such as the DSM is less obvious. While retaining categorical diagnosis, recent editions of the DSM have disavowed any implication that its diagnoses correspond to discrete latent categories. It is entirely legitimate to believe that the latent structure of psychopathology is continuous but believe it is beneficial to make discontinuous diagnoses for pragmatic reasons such as easing clinical communication and determining need for treatment. This belief is increasingly challenged by research showing the pragmatic benefits of dimensional diagnosis (Bornstein & Natoli, 2019), but it remains a defensible way to retain some aspects of categorical diagnosis while recognizing its structural inadequacy. On this view, DSM disorders could be understood as categorical distinctions that are imposed on dimensional realities for the purposes of pragmatic simplification rather than reflecting a deep commitment to a categorical view of psychopathology.

The distinction between the pragmatics of clinical diagnosis and the ontology of mental illness—whether it is latently dimensional or categorical—was not appreciated sufficiently by the taxometric pioneers. There is no necessary connection between the latent structure of psychopathology and the most useful way of identifying cases. Evidence that a form of psychopathology is taxonic does not entail that all taxon members warrant a diagnosis: perhaps only more severe expressions of the taxon reach clinical significance. A pragmatic decision about where the diagnostic threshold should be located on the severity spectrum would then be required. Evidence for a taxon does not even strongly entail the use of categorical diagnosis, as it is conceivable that quantifying the severity of its manifestations is more clinically meaningful than making a binary clinical judgment. The same weak link between ontology and pragmatics—between the true nature of a difference and the most useful way to represent it—justifies why DSM-style categorical diagnosis applied to dimensional psychopathology is not intrinsically inappropriate. It is only inappropriate if the diagnostic cutoff is poorly located (i.e., too stringent so that significantly affected people fail to meet criteria or too liberal so that over-diagnosis occurs) or if the benefits of graded, severity-based diagnosis relative to categorical diagnosis outweigh the possible costs in added complexity. Nevertheless, it is highly likely that many DSM cutoffs are inappropriate by this pragmatic criterion as well as by misrepresenting a dimension as a category.

That said, the strong taxometric evidence for the dimensionality of psychopathology represents a strike against categorical classification and diagnosis. Even if there is no necessary parallel between latent structure and practical diagnosis on the issue of categories versus dimensions, there should surely be some general alignment. If the reality a classification attempts to capture is categorical, for example, it would make little sense to represent it dimensionally, and there should be a presumption that accurately identifying category members may be clinically informative. Similarly, if the underlying reality is dimensional, the presumption should be that diagnoses that recognize degrees of severity will be more valid than dichotomous ones. In addition, because categorical diagnosis systems such as DSM tend to proliferate diagnostic entities that overlap and emphasize the local distinctiveness of disorders rather than their broad similarities, they are ill-suited to identifying a parsimonious structure for psychopathology. Evidence for the dimensionality of psychopathology, therefore, tends to undermine categorical models in practice even if it does not rule out the use of categorical diagnosis in principle.

In essence, my point is simple. The strong general support that taxometric research offers to dimensional models of psychopathology does not represent the fatal blow to categorical diagnosis in general or DSM in particular that it is sometimes taken to be. Even in a dimensional universe, it may be useful to make categorical distinctions. For example, it might be clinically beneficial to set multiple cut points on a severity continuum to define levels of disturbance for targeted interventions, as is done in staging models (McGorry & Mei, 2021). Once we abandon the idea that these distinctions or cut points carve nature at its non-existent joints, we need to ensure that we make them wisely.

Inappropriate Quantitative Methods

In addition to its implications for systems of classification and diagnosis, the taxometric evidence that psychopathology is generally dimensional also has implications for research. If mental illness, its variants, and its vulnerability factors are latently dimensional, then they should be measured and modeled as continua. Continuous, quantitative measurement is standard in psychopathology research, with well-known benefits for statistical power relative to dichotomous assessment. However, when it comes to multivariate modelling of variation, psychopathology researchers routinely employ multivariate methods that presume the existence of latent categories such as latent class analysis, latent profile analysis, cluster analysis or, for longitudinal data, latent growth curve modelling. If latent structure in the psychopathology domain is usually dimensional, then methods that represent variation as dimensions, such as factor analysis, are more suitable.

To illustrate, a search of the "Psychiatry" field in the Web of Science database located more than one thousand articles matching the search term "latent class analy*" published in the five-year period from 2018 to 2022. Inspection of the most recent 100 items found that they identified a median of four latent classes. No article in this sample obtained a one-class solution, which would correspond to the dimensional model supported by the overwhelming majority of taxometric studies. There is strong evidence that taxometric research using the data simulation approach is not biased for or against dimensional conclusions (Ruscio & Kaczetow, 2009; Ruscio, Walters, Marcus, & Kaczetow, 2010), so these findings point to a severe categorical bias in research using latent class analysis. In brief, such research almost always misrepresents the latent structure of psychopathology. If latent class methods that pre-ordain the existence of classes are to be used, they should ideally be explicitly compared to other latent variable methods that do not share their assumptions (e.g., Eaton et al., 2013).

This criticism may sound harsh, but if most psychopathology is latently dimensional, then category-presuming methods are unlikely to be fit for purpose in the field. Latent class analysis and related methods assume that datasets can be represented as a set of latent classes and will therefore tend to mistakenly identify classes when none exist. Just as it would be wrong to use factor analysis to uncover the latent structure of a sample of household pets—cats, dogs, turtles, goldfish—because biological species are taxonic, it is wrong to model the spectral reality of mental illness with analyses that invariably find categories.

Two caveats should be considered on this point. First, it is possible that some researchers employing latent class analyses understand the classes they generate to be pragmatic simplifications rather than objectively real taxons. Sophisticated researchers might acknowledge that their classes are based on arbitrary but potentially helpful cut-offs imposed on a dimensional reality, like considering people over 1.83 meters to be tall, or those with a body mass index over 30 to be obese. In this case, researchers would not be misrepresenting the latent structure of psychopathology after all. Although this defense could be credible, latent classes are typically reified as real, discovered entities without any ontological qualification or backpedaling. Second, the critique of class-favoring methods may apply less to those that examine temporal patterns, given that taxometric studies have exclusively examined cross-sectional variation. Latent growth curve modelling analyses that find evidence of distinct temporal trajectories of psychopathology variables might be more plausible than analyses finding distinct cross-sectional "types." Nevertheless, the striking empirical support for dimensionality in taxometric research on psychopathology surely reduces the likelihood that categorically distinct temporal trajectories exist. That support implies that category-presuming quantitative methods should be employed very sparingly and cautiously in psychopathology research. Current data-analytic practice in psychiatry, at least, runs contrary to this advice.

Some Taxons May Still Exist

Although taxometric research has generally offered powerful support for dimensional models of psychopathology, it is important not to forget that it has also obtained many taxonic findings. In the Haslam et al. (2020) meta-analysis, for example, studies employing the simulation method obtained taxonic CCFI values on 53 occasions, compared to 240 nontaxonic values (a further 24 intermediate values were ambiguous values). If 18% of decisive taxometric findings point to the existence of latent categories, then dimensional models of psychopathology should be open to the possibility that some latent categories exist.

Identifying these potential taxa is challenging. Haslam et al. (2020) considered plausible candidates to be variables for which a taxonic finding had been replicated by independent research groups, and for which the majority of all taxometric findings favored the taxonic conclusion. Of the 53 taxonic findings from simulation-based studies, six psychopathological variables passed this test, most of them barely: alcohol dependence, intermittent explosive disorder, problem gambling, autism, suicide risk, and pedophilia. Taxometric studies published since the meta-analysis' 2019 cut-off have strengthened the case for the taxonic status of autism (Frazier et al., 2023) and pedophilia (Brankley, Knight, & Hanson, 2022) and weakened the case for suicidal thinking (Siddaway, Holm-Denoma, Witte, & Ruscio, 2021).

Evidence for the existence of replicable taxa is clearly modest, but it suggests that some are likely to exist. Many additional taxonic findings have been obtained but have yet to be replicated, given the often thin and patchy coverage of taxometric research, implying that latent categories may be found beyond the six potential candidates described in the previous paragraph.

In view of this possibility, it is important for proponents of dimensional models of psychopathology to be open to some non-dimensional exceptions. Some degree of pluralism regarding latent structure may be needed (Haslam, 2002). Although the tide has turned in favor of dimensional classification, we should heed Paul Meehl's sage advice that the issue should be resolved empirically, rather than by theoretical preference, convention, or committee. Even if psychopathological taxons are rare, we should not become "dogmatic antinosologists."

Conclusion

Taxometrics has played an important role in the unfolding recent history of how we classify mental ill health. It has sharpened the conceptual distinction between categorical and dimensional models of psychopathology and helped to clarify what is at stake theoretically. It was the first rigorous method for testing between these models. It has generated a large and still-growing body of research evidence that supports the general validity of dimensional models of psychopathology and illuminates the latent structure of specific phenomena. Although Meehl and his followers set out to revolutionize the classification of psychopathology by populating it with verified taxons, the scarcity of those taxons revealed by their scientific work has ended up helping to revolutionize it in a very different way.

References

Ahmed, A. O., Buckley, P. F., & Mabe, P. A. (2012). Latent structure of psychotic experiences in the general population. *Acta Psychiatrica Scandinavica, 125*, 54–65.

Bernstein, A., Zvolensky, M. J., Weems, C., Stickle, T., & Leen-Feldner, E. W. (2005). Taxonicity of anxiety sensitivity: An empirical test among youth. *Behaviour Research and Therapy, 43*, 1131–1155.

Bornstein, R. F., & Natoli, A. P. (2019). Clinical utility of categorical and dimensional perspectives on personality pathology: A meta-analytic review. *Personality Disorders: Theory, Research, and Treatment, 10*(6), 479–490.

Borsboom, D., Rhemtulla, M., Cramer, A. O. J., van der Maas, H. L., Scheffer, M., & Dolan, C. V. (2016). Kinds versus continua: A review of psychometric approaches to uncover the structure of psychiatric constructs. *Psychological Medicine, 46*, 1567–1579.

Brankley, A. E., Knight, R. A., & Hanson, R. K. (2022). Pedophilia is a taxon among 706 adult males assessed at a civil commitment center. *Journal of psychopathology and clinical science, 131*(2), 209–220.

Denson, T. F., & Earleywine, M. (2006). Pothead or pot smoker? A taxometric investigation of cannabis dependence. *Substance Abuse Treatment, Prevention, and Policy, 1*, 22.

Dollaghan, C. A. (2004). Taxometric analyses of specific language impairment in 3- and 4-year-old children. *Journal of Speech, Language and Hearing, 47*, 464–475.

Eaton, N. R., Krueger, R. F., Markon, K. E., Keyes, K. M., Skodol, A. E., Wall, M., Hasin, D. S., & Grant, B. F. (2013). The structure and predictive validity of the internalizing disorders. *Journal of Abnormal Psychology, 122*(1), 86–92.

Frazier, T., Chetcuti, L., Al-Shaban, F., Haslam, N., Ghazal, I., Klingemier, E. W., Aldosari, M., Whitehouse, A. J. O., Youngstrom, E. A., Hardan, A. Y., & Uljarevic, M. (2023). Categorical versus dimensional structure of autism spectrum disorder: A multi-method investigation. *JCCP Advances*, 3(2), e14142.

Gavett, B. E., & Stern, R. A. (2012). Dementia has a categorical, not dimensional, latent structure. *Psychology and Aging, 27*, 791–797.

Gibb, B. E., Alloy, L. B., Abramson, L. Y., Beevers, C. G., Miller, I. W. (2004). Cognitive vulnerability to depression: A taxometric analysis. *Journal of Abnormal Psychology, 113*, 81–89.

Gleaves, D. H., Lowe, M. R., Snow, A. C., Green, B. A., & Murphy-Eberenz, K.P. (2000). Continuity and discontinuity models of bulimia nervosa: A taxometric investigation. *Journal of Abnormal Psychology, 109*, 56–68.

Goedeker, K. C., & Tiffany, S. T. (2008). On the nature of nicotine addiction: A taxometric analysis. *Journal of Abnormal Psychology, 117*, 896–909.

Golden, R. R., & Meehl, P. E. (1979). Detection of the schizoid taxon with MMPI indicators. *Journal of Abnormal Psychology, 88*, 217–233.

Grove, W. M., Andreasen, N. C., Young, M., Endicott, J., Keller, M. B., Hirschfeld, R. M. A., & Reich, T. (1987). Isolation and characterization of a nuclear depressive syndrome. *Psychological Medicine, 17*, 471–484.

Harris, G. T., Rice, M. E., & Quinsey, V. L. (1994). Psychopathy as a taxon: Evidence that psychopaths are a discrete class. *Journal of Consulting and Clinical Psychology*, *62*, 387–397.

Haslam, N. (2002). Kinds of kinds: A conceptual taxonomy of psychiatric categories. *Philosophy, Psychiatry, & Psychology*, *9*, 203–217.

Haslam, N., Holland, E., & Kuppens, P. (2012). Categories versus dimensions in personality and psychopathology: A quantitative review of taxometric research. *Psychological Medicine*, *42*, 903–920.

Haslam, N., McGrath, M. J., Viechtbauer, W., & Kuppens, P. (2020). Dimensions over categories: A meta-analysis of taxometric research. *Psychological Medicine*, *50*(9), 1418–1432.

Haslam, N., Williams, B. J., Kyrios, M., McKay, D., & Taylor, S. (2005). Subtyping obsessive-compulsive disorder: A taxometric analysis. *Behavior Therapy*, *36*, 381–391.

Haslam, N., Williams, B., Prior, M., Haslam, R., Graetz, B., & Sawyer, M. (2006). Testing the latent structure of ADHD: A taxometric analysis. *Australian and New Zealand Journal of Psychiatry*, *40*, 639–647.

Ingram, D. G., Takahashi, T. N., & Miles, J. H. (2008). Defining autism subgroups: A taxometric solution. *Journal of Autism and Developmental Disorders*, *38*, 950–960.

Jasper, F., Hiller, W., Rist, F., Bailer, J., & Witthöft, M. (2012). Somatic symptom reporting has a dimensional latent structure: Results from taxometric analyses. *Journal of Abnormal Psychology*, *121*, 725–738.

Kollman, D. M., Brown, T. A., Liverant, G. I., & Hofmann. S. G. (2006). A taxometric investigation of the latent structure of social anxiety disorder in outpatients with anxiety and mood disorders. *Depression and Anxiety*, *23*, 190–199.

Kotov, R., Krueger, R. F., Watson, D., Achenbach, T. M., Althoff, R. R., Bagby, R. M., Brown, T. A., Carpenter, W. T., Caspi, A., Clark, L. A., & Eaton, N. R. (2017). The Hierarchical Taxonomy of Psychopathology (HiTOP): A dimensional alternative to traditional nosologies. *Journal of Abnormal Psychology*, *126*, 454–477.

Linscott, R. J., & Morton, S. E. (2018). The latent taxonicity of schizotypy in biological siblings of probands with schizophrenia. *Schizophrenia Bulletin*, *44*, 922–932.

Marcus, D. K., Lilienfeld, S. O., Edens, J. F., & Poythress, N. G. (2006). Is antisocial personality disorder continuous or categorical? A taxometric analysis. *Psychological Medicine*, *36*, 1571–1581.

McGorry, P. D., & Mei, C. (2021). Clinical staging for youth mental disorders: Progress in reforming diagnosis and clinical care. *Annual Review of Developmental Psychology*, *3*, 15–39.

Meehl, P. E. (1973). *Psychodiagnosis: Selected papers*. University of Minnesota Press.

Meehl, P. E. (1990). Toward an integrated theory of schizotaxia, schizotypy, and schizophrenia. *Journal of Personality Disorders*, *4*(1), 1–99.

Meehl, P. E. (1992). Factors and taxa, traits and types, difference of degree and differences in kind. *Journal of Personality*, *60*, 117–174.

Meehl, P. E. (1995). Bootstraps taxometrics: Solving the classification problem in psychopathology. *American Psychologist*, *50*, 266–275.

Morton, S. E., O'Hare, K. J., Maha, J. L., Nicolson, M. P., Machado, L., Topless, R., Merriman, T. R., & Linscott, R. J. (2017). Testing the validity of taxonic schizotypy using genetic and environmental risk variables. *Schizophrenia Bulletin*, *43*, 633–643.

Prisciandaro, J. J., & Roberts, J. E. (2011). Evidence for the continuous latent structure of mania in the Epidemiological Catchment Area from multiple latent structure and construct validation methodologies. *Psychological Medicine*, *41*, 575–588.

Rawlings, D., Williams, B., Haslam, N., & Claridge, G. (2008). Taxometric analysis supports a dimensional latent structure for schizotypy. *Personality and Individual Differences*, *44*, 1640–1651.

Ruscio, A.M., Ruscio, J., & Keane, T. M. (2002). The latent structure of post-traumatic stress disorder: A taxometric investigation of reactions to extreme stress. *Journal of Abnormal Psychology*, *111*, 290–301.

Ruscio, J., Haslam, N., & Ruscio, A. M. (2006). *Introduction to the taxometric method: A practical guide*. Lawrence Erlbaum Associates.

Ruscio, J., & Kaczetow, W. (2009). Differentiating categories and dimensions: Evaluating the robustness of taxometric analyses. *Multivariate Behavioral Research*, *44*, 259–280.

Ruscio, J., & Ruscio A. M. (2000). Informing the continuity controversy: A taxometric analysis of depression. *Journal of Abnormal Psychology*, *109*, 473–487.

Ruscio, J., Ruscio, A. M., & Meron, M. (2007). Applying the bootstrap to taxometric analysis: Generating empirical sampling distributions to help interpret results. *Multivariate Behavioral Research*, *42*, 349–386.

Ruscio, J., Walters, G. D., Marcus, D. K., & Kaczetow, W. (2010). Comparing the relative fit of categorical and dimensional latent variable models using consistency tests. *Psychological Assessment*, *22*, 5–21.

Ruscio, J., & Wang, S. B. (2022). Taxometric analysis. In G. J. G. Asmundson (Ed.), *Comprehensive clinical psychology* (2nd ed., pp. 148–175). Elsevier.

Schomerus, G., Matschinger, H., & Angermeyer, M. C. (2013). Continuum beliefs and stigmatizing attitudes towards persons with schizophrenia, depression, and alcohol dependence. *Psychiatry Research*, *209*, 665–669.

Siddaway, A. P., Holm-Denoma, J., Witte, T. K., & Ruscio, J. (2021). Reexamining the latent structure of suicidal thoughts using taxometric analysis: Implications for testing ideation to action theoretical models of suicidal thoughts and behavior. *Psychological Assessment*, *33*(3), 243–254.

Trull, T. J., Widiger, T. A., & Guthrie, P. (1990). Categorical versus dimensional status of borderline personality disorder. *Journal of Abnormal Psychology*, *99*, 40–48.

Waelde, L. C., Silvern, L., & Fairbank, J. A. (2005). A taxometric investigation of dissociation in Vietnam veterans. *Journal of Traumatic Stress*, *18*, 359–369.

Walters, G. D. (2007). The latent structure of the criminal lifestyle: a taxometric analysis of the lifestyle criminality screening form and psychological inventory of criminal thinking styles. *Criminal Justice and Behavior*, *34*, 1623–1637.

Walters, G. D. (2009). Taxometric analysis of alcohol dependence in male prisoners: Measuring latent structure with indicators from DSM-IV. *Addiction Research and Theory*, *17*, 372–380.

Williamson, D. A., Womble, L. G., Smeets, M. A. M., Netemeyer. R. G., Thaw, J., Kutlesic, V., & Gleaves, D. H. (2002). The latent structure of eating disorder symptoms: A factor analytic and taxometric investigation. *American Journal of Psychiatry*, *159*, 412–418.

Witte, T. K., Holm-Denoma, J. M., Zuromski, K. L., Gauthier, J. M., & Ruscio, J. (2017). Individuals at high risk for suicide are categorically distinct from those at low risk. *Psychological Assessment*, *29*, 382–393.

CHAPTER 17

What Can Twin and Molecular Research Tell Us about Dimensionality of Psychopathology?

MARINA BORNOVALOVA, MICHAEL NEALE, ASIF ZAARUR, HAYA FATIMAH, AND EUN-SUN LEE

Introduction

THE question of whether psychopathological constructs are continuously or discontinuously distributed can be approached from multiple methodological perspectives, many of which are covered in this book. The overarching purpose of this chapter is to explain how one can leverage univariate and multivariate twin and molecular genetic methods to answer the continuous versus discontinuous question. We begin with a brief primer on common methods in psychiatric genetics. We then outline how the data might look under either condition—continuous or discontinuous—and provide examples from existing literature. We finish with future directions and opportunities in this area.

Brief Overview of Statistical and Molecular Genetics Methods Relevant to Current Discussion

Molecular Genetics. The early years of psychiatric molecular genetics focused on candidate gene research—theory-based selection of single genes and association of said genes or their interactions with some environmental event with psychiatric disorders (Caspi et al., 2003), frequently in (what are now considered) very small samples (Aguilera et al., 2009; Åslund et al., 2010). After the first few years of enthusiasm, more and more studies reported replication failures (Culverhouse et al., 2018), except for a few potentially intriguing but rare cases (Arioka et al., 2021; Lee et al., 2018; Sanchez-Roige et al., 2019). These failures are hardly surprising; as is discussed below, even the most influential single genes each have small to miniscule effects on psychiatric disorders. Other factors adding to replication difficulties include but are not limited to: lack of statistical power, differences in sampling, incomplete coverage of genetic variation within the candidate genes, and publication bias (L. E. Duncan & Keller, 2011; Ioannidis et al., 2001; Johnson et al., 2017). As such, candidate gene research has mostly fallen into disuse. Instead, the field has moved to genome-wide association studies (GWASs), which compare individuals with to those without a disorder on variants in single nucleotide polymorphisms (SNPs) at multiple locations throughout the genome. Because one is essentially doing hundreds of thousands of t-tests, the significance level has to be adjusted downward to avoid widespread Type I errors. Results of a GWAS are typically presented as a Manhattan plot, in which the y-axis is in negative base-10 logarithm units. Loci (usually SNPs) with p-values less than $.5x10^{-8}$, reach up above this value on the y-axis, so significant "hits" look like the taller buildings on the New York skyline.

Most genome-wide association studies (GWAS) are designed for identifying common genetic variants with small to medium effect sizes. These studies primarily focus on common alleles, which are genetic variants that occur frequently in the population. The frequency of these variants is measured by the minor allele frequency (MAF), which indicates how often the less common allele appears in a given population. Common alleles are arbitrarily classified as those for which the MAF is greater than 1%. This limit is in part due to the use of a SNP array technology, which directly assesses a subset of some 200,000–1,000,000 SNPs from the 3.1 billion on the human genome. Relatively common SNPs are usually selected to be on the array, as these are more informative. Often, additional sites are assayed by proxy, using imputation to derive probably genotypes at SNPs between those directly assayed. More recently, technological advances have afforded whole-exome sequencing (WES) and even whole-genome sequencing (WGS), both of which provide much denser sampling of the genome and may identify rare variants, whose MAF is less than 1%. These rare variants include single-nucleotide variants (SNVs) and copy number variants (CNVs), which can have substantial biological effects despite their lower frequency in the population. Single-nucleotide variants (SNVs) are changes in a single nucleotide, appearing at low frequencies in the population. Copy number variants (CNVs) involve segments of DNA that are deleted or duplicated, with duplications and especially deletions potentially disrupting gene function and downstream functioning. Some CNVs can have significant effects on biological processes, although, like single nucleotide polymorphisms (SNPs), many CNVs typically have smaller individual effects. However, different CNVs can contribute to the same psychopathological condition, such as schizophrenia, in different individuals (Kato et al., 2023). This variability suggests that there is genetic heterogeneity, such that there isn't a single genetic pathway leading to the disorder; rather, various genetic disruptions can result in similar clinical outcomes, indicating a complex genetic landscape.

With the realization that (a) most psychiatric phenotypes will be influenced by multiple SNPs, CNVs, and SNVs across multiple genes, and (b) much of the variance will be accounted for by common SNPs with very small to miniscule effect sizes (Trubetskoy et al., 2022), the sample size requirements for GWAS have become enormous. In short, for gene discovery efforts, the bigger, the better, and this partly explains the popularity of the U.K. Biobank, comprising 1.5 million participants (Bycroft et al., 2018). The advantage of large sample sizes has in turn led to the development of consortia such as the Psychiatrics Genetics Consortium, which enables researchers across the globe to pool multiple modestly sized datasets. Notably, this sort of pooling necessarily leads to a tradeoff of precision versus power: the data are generally harmonized at the level of the disorder rather than symptom, and often using a categorical system (e.g., a binary, DSM-based diagnosis of schizophrenia). These gene-detection methods have led to the emergence of several valuable by-products, including the estimation of SNP-based heritability and of polygenic risk scores (PRSs). SNP heritability is the proportion of the total phenotypic variance that can be attributed to the additive effects of all SNPs on a genotyping array (Yang et al., 2010), now expanded to refer to the variance explained by any set of SNPs (e.g., all genetic variants from in-depth WGS, (Yang et al., 2015)). One primary method for estimating SNP heritability is to use Genomic-Relatedness-Based Restricted Maximum Likelihood (GREML; Benjamin et al., 2012; Yang et al., 2011). This approach partitions the phenotypic variance into genetic and environmental components based on the genetic similarity among unrelated (in reality, distantly related) individuals. PRSs are calculated by summing the effects of many genetic variants across the genome, weighted by their effect sizes derived from a large GWAS. Essentially, a beta regression coefficient is estimated for the regression of the trait on every available SNP. The PRS for an individual is then calculated as the sum of these SNP beta coefficients. An individual's PRS can be used to estimate an individual's genetic predisposition to a particular trait or disorder (e.g., schizophrenia) in any other genotyped sample. A major advantage of a PRS is that it combines information across many SNPs, even those with very small individual effects, to create a composite score that can predict the trait or disorder in new samples. Since PRS are individual-based scores, one can do the same thing to them as they would to any column representing some variable (e.g., neuroticism), such as calculate (genetic) correlations. While there are many other GWAS-based methods (Mendelian randomization, genomic structural equation modeling) but those are not as directly relevant to the continuous vs. discontinuous liability distribution question that is the focus of this chapter.

Family and Twin Studies. Family, sibling, cousin, adoptive, classical twin, and children of twins studies all fall under the umbrella of family-based data structures. Historically, family studies compared rates or levels of disease or risk in families of affected probands and unaffected controls. However, this method does not disambiguate between genetic and family environmental influences. Thus, many have moved to methods that allow one to associate phenotypic variance with genetic and environmental sources. Most popular of those is the classical twin design (CTD), which capitalizes on similarities and differences between monozygotic (MZ) twin pairs (who share 100% of their genes) and dizygotic (DZ) twins (who share on average 50% of their genes). The resulting differences in twin similarities on a phenotype (e.g., depression symptoms) then are modeled as latent variables of additive genetic (A), shared environment (C), and non-shared environment factors (E). Additive genetic influences are the cumulative effects of genes summed across loci and are inferred if the phenotypic correlation between MZ twins is greater than that between DZ twins. Shared environmental influences refer to environmental influences that contribute to similarity among relatives (e.g., parenting style, neighborhood, school). Non-shared environmental influences include anything that contributes to difference between MZ twins (difference in perception of same parenting, different circle of friends) and are inferred if the MZ twin correlations are less than 1. The non-shared environment parameter also contains measurement error. Other variance components are possible as well, such as the effects of allelic dominance (D). Dominance genetic influences refer to the interaction between alleles at the same locus, where the mean of heterozygote individuals (Aa) is not halfway between the means of the two homozygotic genotypes AA and aa. These dominance effects can be manifested as an MZ twin correlation that is significantly greater than twice the DZ twin correlation. In the classical twin design, C and D are confounded, and absent additional data, estimates of C should be regarded as the sum total of C, D, and other sources including epistasis (interactions between different loci on the genome) or assortative mating (the tendency for like to marry like). Notably, the A, C (or D), and E estimates may be moderated by many things—SES, environmental risk, sex, age, and even level of severity of psychopathology (Bergen et al., 2007; Kendler, Gardner et al., 2011; Purcell & Sham, 2002; Rathouz et al., 2008). The simple ACE (or ADE) model can be extended to a bivariate case, where the A, C, and E exert influences on two phenotypes simultaneously (e.g., major depressive disorder and alcohol use disorder, or major depressive disorder diagnosis and neuroticism). Moreover, this bivariate ACE model allows one to estimate the genetic, shared environmental, and non-shared environmental correlations between two phenotypes. This can, in turn, give a sense of shared versus unique genetic and environmental risk to the two disorders or phenotypes (see Figure 17.1). Multivariate versions of this model are possible, such that genetic and environmental overlap can be estimated on multiple disorders simultaneously (Kendler, Aggen et al., 2011; Martin & Eaves, 1977; Neale & Cardon, 1992).

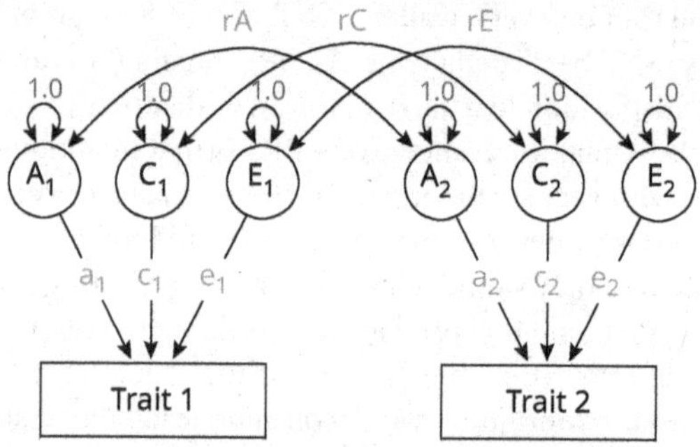

FIGURE 17.1 Path diagram of model for one twin bivariate analysis of major depressive disorder (MDD) and minor depressive disorder (MiDD). Each observed variable (in rectangles) is influenced by additive genetic (A), shared environmental (C) and nonshared environmental (E) sources of variation (in circles). Co-variation between these sources is shown by correlational paths rA, rC, and rE, that is, genetic, shared environmental, and non-shared environmental correlations.

Other models that compare twins (multiple threshold models) are also possible and are discussed below.

Sources of Evidence

In this section, we set up the logic of what the data would look like if the underlying liability is dimensional or discontinuous; we then follow up with examples when available. When not available, we outline potential studies that could address the question. Drawing on a recent commentary (Hopwood et al., 2023), we define a dimensional (continuous) model as one in which the sum of genetic (or environmental) influences forms a continuous distribution without gaps, where individuals can vary in degree of liability for a disorder. Thus, the genetic factors can be summed to reflect a continuum of severity. The definition of discontinuity is much more complex, and nailing it down (perhaps in a series of simulations) is beyond the goals of the current chapter. Many of the tests of continuity covered below primarily focus on deviations from continuity in one way or another; that is, they test for mixtures in the data. They also test whether the liability dimension is the same or different across various levels of a disorder (i.e., if different genetic influences for different severity levels, potentially indicating separate etiological pathways for those above and below the threshold). Under this framework, individuals classified as "affected" or "unaffected" do not share the same (or at least, not completely the same) underlying genetic liability, implying the presence of qualitatively distinct genetic risks. However, the tests we provide don't always test if the two (or however many) liability dimensions themselves are binary (constants), whether they are dimensional themselves, and how much the dimensions overlap.

Molecular Studies

Check for Multiple, Small Effects. A strong source of support for the liability to psychopathology being continuous is the polygenic nature of most psychiatric disorders. Polygenic effects are what they sound like—that many genes can (and typically do) influence psychiatric phenotypes. We argue that for a phenotype to show evidence for continuity, we should see many SNPs contributing to the phenotype, all with small effect sizes. This cumulative effect of multiple variants with small effect sizes is consistent with what has been postulated about complex traits more than a century ago. Fisher's seminal work demonstrated that quantitative traits could result from the combined effect of multiple susceptibility alleles, each with a small effect size, across various loci, leading to a normally distributed liability in genetically heterogeneous populations under varied environments (Fisher, 1918; Norton & Pearson, 1976; Visscher & Goddard, 2019). The tendency toward a normal distribution is largely due to the central limit theorem; that is, when independent and identically distributed random variables are added, their sum tends toward a normal distribution, regardless of the original distribution of the variables. Extensions of Fisher's model introduced the idea of a threshold, positing that individuals express a trait when their genetic liability exceeds a specific burden of risk (Carter, 1967; Carter, 1961). In this liability-threshold model, individuals exhibiting the trait might be referred to as "affected" and those not exhibiting as "unaffected" (Figure 17.2).

A biologically categorical phenotype, in contrast, would be influenced by one or two SNPs or other variants with disproportionately large effect sizes. Paul Meehl, the brilliant schizophrenia theorist, for example, thought that both the liability to schizophrenia and schizophrenia itself were categorically distributed, based on taxometric evidence (Meehl, 1989, 1990). Meehl expected to see a dominant gene, which accounts for a large proportion of the variance in liability to schizophrenia, as well as interactions with the environment and other polygenic potentiators (e.g., anxiety, anhedonia) (Meehl, 1962). To date, that hypothesis has not been supported by genomic studies, which reveal loci accounting for less than 1% of phenotypic variance in almost all psychiatric disorders studied to date. In contrast, as is discussed in more detail below, alcohol use disorder presents a much more interesting case. In European

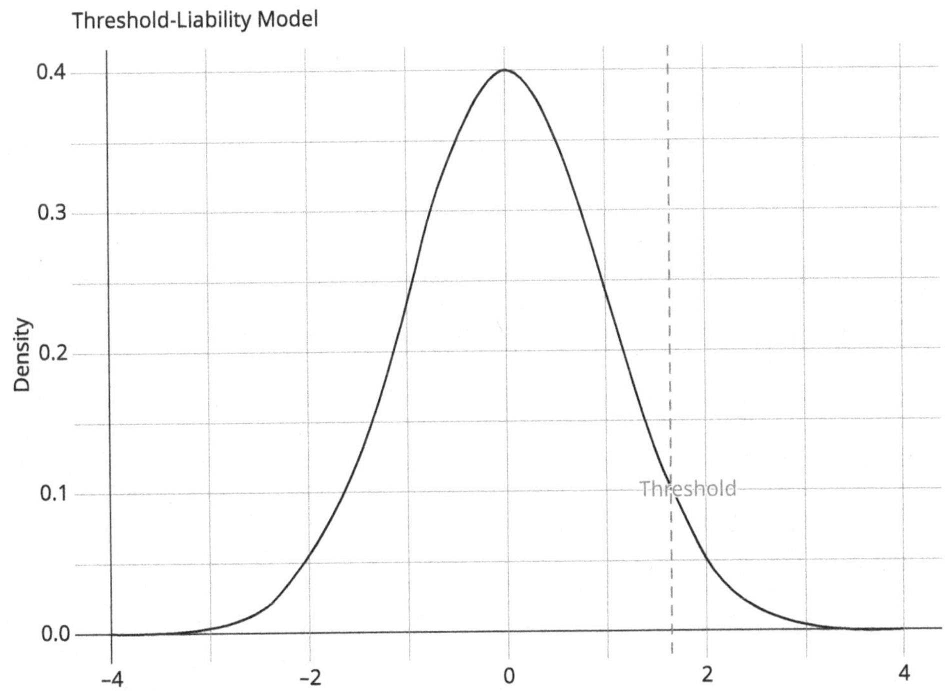

FIGURE 17.2 Population trait variation, where the extreme end of a continuous distribution of a trait is associated with a continuous underlying genetic liability, that is, the sum of the genetic factors contributing to it (A1+A2+A3+A4 . . . +A10).

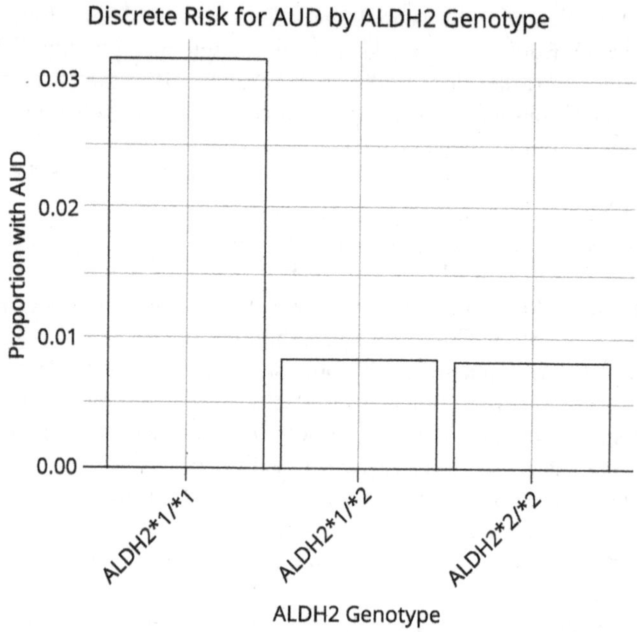

FIGURE 17.3 Illustration of discrete risk based on patterns of the relationship between ALDH2 alleles and alcohol use disorder (AUD). Note: A dominant effect is shown such that homozygous (ALDH2*2/ALDH2*2) and heterozygous (ALDH2*1/ ALDH2*2) individuals have nearly equal risk for AUD (Edenberg, 2007).

ancestry populations, AUD appears to be more dimensionally distributed; however, in Asian populations (among some others), genes involved in alcohol metabolism (e.g., ADH1B, ALDH2) account for a (relatively) large (~1-2%) proportion of the variance (Zaso et al., 2019) in alcohol use disorder, possibly presenting a discontinuous, even a categorical risk (Figure 17.3), or more likely, a mixture distribution, such that a proportion of the population has a dimensionally distributed risk, whereas for a portion of the population, that risk is steeply reduced (Figure 17.4).

Current evidence suggests that most complex traits (most forms of psychopathology, personality) that are downstream of genetics, depend on *many* genes (>250 distinct genetic loci for schizophrenia, >80 depression, 29 for alcohol use disorder) (Howard et al., 2019; Legge et al., 2021; Levey et al., 2021; Ripke et al., 2014; Trubetskoy et al., 2022; Welter et al., 2014; Zhou et al., 2020). For example, ~71% of 1 megabase (1,000,000 base pairs) genomic regions have at least one variant influencing liability to schizophrenia, but no one region explains more than .1% of schizophrenia liability (Loh et al., 2015).

Moreover, the individual SNP effect sizes tend to be extraordinarily small. To give the reader the scope of the effect sizes involved, consider the non-psychiatric phenotype of height, which is highly heritable (Yang et al., 2010). Park and colleagues, for example (Park et al., 2010; Visscher et al., 2017), conducted a power calculation for GWAS based on the known distribution of the effect sizes for height (.04–1.13% of genetic variance accounted for by each SNP). At N of 10,000, the expected cumulative (i.e., aggregate, across SNPs) genetic variance explained was ~7% (~27 discoveries); at 20,000, 10.3% (74 discoveries); at 30,000, 13.2% (125 discoveries); at 40,000, 14.9% (161 discoveries), and at 50,000, 15.7% (182 discoveries). Note that there is a diminishing marginal returns–type effect to genetic variance accounted for, such that with

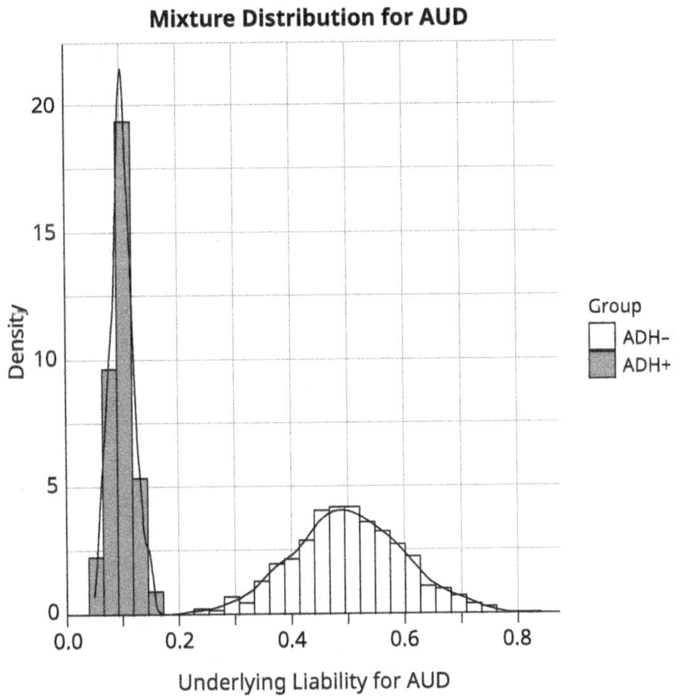

FIGURE 17.4 Illustration of mixture distribution as applied to AUD; ADH+, individuals with *2 versions of the alcohol dehydrogenase genes and subsequent aversive effects; ADH-, individuals with no *2 versions of the genes.

subsequent increases of sample size, less and less of the additional (total) genetic variance is explained. This occurs because the effect sizes of the SNPs that can be discovered at such large sample sizes will become smaller and smaller. Rare variants (e.g., single-nucleotide variants and copy number variants) can have larger (sometimes quite a bit larger) effect sizes. However, the sample size requirements to detect them (given low population frequency, < 1% in population) are very large indeed, and they still explain a relatively small proportion of variance (Kato et al., 2023; Visscher et al., 2017).

For complex phenotypes such as schizophrenia or depression, most individual SNPs will have miniscule, near-zero effect sizes, requiring very large sample sizes to be detected (Howard et al., 2019; Legge et al., 2021; Ripke et al., 2014; Schizophrenia Working Group of the Psychiatric Genomics Consortium et al., 2020; Zhou et al., 2020). To contextualize, at 30% MAF in the population, and 1% population base rate of schizophrenia, an odds ratio of 1.3 (r = ~.05, .3% variance accounted for) is considered a fairly large effect (Shi et al., 2009); common variants will generally have odds ratios < 1.2 (Kato et al., 2023; Legge et al., 2021; Welter et al., 2014). Even combined to form polygenic risk scores (PRS), they explain a very limited proportion of the variance in psychiatric disorders. The most recent schizophrenia PRS tends to explain only ~8%[1] of the variance in schizophrenia (Lee et al., 2012; Legge et al., 2021; Ripke et al., 2013, 2014). Many other phenotypes follow the same polygenic pattern. Very

[1] Caution must be taken when interpreting genetic variance accounted for, as it can refer to either multiple r-squared in the disorder, or estimates derived from GCTA, which has similar principles but is calculated somewhat differently (and using all available SNPs); GCTA estimates tend to be higher.

large GWASs of depression [N = ~1,000,000, for example, (Howard et al., 2019)] reported associations with 102 variants, 87 of which replicated in an independent and also very large sample. Each individual SNP had extremely small effect sizes; in aggregate, they explained around 2–3% of the variance in the liability to depression (Howard et al., 2019; Wray et al., 2018). The largest GWAS of alcohol dependence and problem drinking to date (Zhou et al., 2020) identified 29 risk variants; the aggregate PRS predicted < 2% of the variance in alcohol-related phenotypes. Notably, the relatively underpowered datasets (e.g., largest GWAS for schizophrenia contains ~300,000 individuals) also mean that many of the variants with smaller effect sizes remain unidentified. In other words, given large enough sample sizes, we are likely to find many more SNPs with extremely small effect sizes contributing to the phenotype. Indeed, variance explained in schizophrenia and bipolar disorder increases (with a diminishing returns–type shape) as the p-value requirement for SNPs included in a polygenic risk score becomes less stringent; at larger sample sizes, these effects would become significant at the genome-wide level (Visscher et al., 2017).

One might expect that if there were substantial support for the categorical hypothesis, it would likely be found in prominent genetic regions associated with major hypotheses about the underlying biology of disorders—such as the serotonin theory of depression or the dopamine theory of schizophrenia—since these theories are partly derived from the observed effects of pharmacological treatments. These treatments often target specific neurotransmitter systems, suggesting that if a disorder were driven by large, distinct genetic effects, they might be linked to the biological pathways influenced by these drugs. Of course, treatment mechanisms don't have to match etiology to work; highly heritable disorders are subject to effects of environmental intervention (e.g., Phenylketonuria, myopia, (Li & Zhang, 2017)). Nevertheless, these regions were a reasonable place to start looking for causal variants. However, a large meta-analysis (Culverhouse et al., 2018) reported that the association of depression with the serotonin transporter gene (which many expected to be the main genetic cause of depression) does not significantly differ from zero. Likewise, variants from the theoretically derived candidate genes "for" schizophrenia have very small effect sizes [ORs < 1.1; GWAS database, (Welter et al., 2014)], and are no more related to schizophrenia than variants from genes associated with Type II diabetes (Johnson et al., 2017). One exception in schizophrenia (discussed further below) is that rare copy number variants tend to have much larger effect sizes. However, these variants appear in only about 2–8% of patients with schizophrenia (Kato et al., 2023; Kushima et al., 2018; Rees et al., 2014); thus, they cannot be necessary for the development of schizophrenia.

It is also worthwhile to consider some potential exceptions to this pattern of small, additive effects of genes contributing to psychiatric phenotypes. One such notable exception is the association between genes involved in alcohol metabolism and alcohol use disorder (e.g., ADH1B, ALDH2). This relationship is one of the largest and frequently replicated effects in psychiatric genetics. However, "largest" effect is still relative; a GWAS meta-analysis of alcohol use disorder (Sanchez-Roige et al., 2019) found that the top "hit" was a SNP belonging to the alcohol dehydrogenase gene family, explaining .25–.45% of variance in the alcohol use disorder identification test score. A meta-analysis suggested that the ALDH2, ADH1B, and ADH1C genes account for a whopping 1–2% in AUD among East Asian populations (Zaso et al., 2019). Interestingly, some studies find that the effect is dominant, such that neither homozygous (two ALDH*2 variants) or heterozygous (i.e., one each of ALDH2*1 and ALDH2*2 alleles) individuals have no ALDH2 activity in the liver—that is, both show the increased aversive reactions to alcohol (Edenberg, 2007, but see Chen et al., 1999; Muramatsu et al., 1995). In smoking research, the SNP rs16969968 (located in nicotinic receptor gene cluster) accounts for a behemoth 1–2% of the variance (OR = 1.33) in number of cigarettes smoked (Lee et al.,

2018; Saccone et al., 2010). Note that in both cases the genes are related to the direct processing of the drug itself, and the "large" effect sizes are still very modest.

In schizophrenia, rare copy number variants have disproportionate effect sizes. One of the largest and most replicated effects seems to be in a glia function related gene RTN4R, located in the 22q11.2 region, which includes ~40 genes expressed in the brain (1:3000-1:6000 live births; odds ratio with schizophrenia > 50) (Kato et al., 2023; Maynard et al., 2003; McDonald-McGinn et al., 2015); it is related to protein processing in the endoplasmic reticulum in dopaminergic neurons (Arioka et al., 2021). An animal model in which the 22q11.2 deletion was reproduced showed behavioral features strongly reminiscent of the endophenotypes in schizophrenia: auditory prepulse inhibition, attenuated cue-dependent fear memory, impaired early visual processing, and hypoactivity (Saito et al., 2020). As interesting as these effects are, it's worth remembering that these CNVs, even collectively, account for a small proportion of individuals with schizophrenia (Kato et al., 2023; Kushima et al., 2018; Rees et al., 2014). They are also pleiotropic, predicting not only schizophrenia but also autism, intellectual disability, and Parkinson's (Kushima et al., 2018). Thus, such CNVs partially explain a generalized neuronal development and function vulnerability among a limited proportion of schizophrenics. In a way, this is along the lines of Meehl's prediction of a genetic mutation producing an integrative neural defect, which, under the right conditions, can convert to schizophrenia (Meehl, 1962). Yet, these CNVs are neither necessary nor sufficient to explain schizophrenia. Of course, given the potential for the etiology of schizophrenia to be heterogeneous and our imperfect measurement and classification systems, it is possible that there are subclasses of patients with differing etiologies. For example, one could propose that there is a mixture distribution underlying the population, some with underlying dimensional risk, and others with a discontinuous risk. That, in turn, would imply that schizophrenia is (at least) two different disorders with differing etiologies.

Use a Psychometric Approach. A second method for testing dimensionality would be to take a psychometric approach, and use a pre-selected set of SNPs and, if available, CNVs and SNVs, as survey items. The pre-selection process would be much like the one used in the creation of a PRS at the initial stages (i.e., use summary statistics in, e.g., PGC to generate SNP associations at different levels of significance). Subsequently, as with survey items, it would be possible to subject the variants to a series of model fitting of dimensional models (factor analysis), categorical models (latent class), and mixture distributions (both, as in the case of, e.g., schizophrenia) in an independent sample. This modeling sequence can be done with variants for a single phenotype (e.g., schizophrenia), or, given massive genetic overlap and pleiotropy among psychiatric disorders (Kato et al., 2023; Kendler, Aggen et al., 2011; Lee et al., 2021; Visscher et al., 2017), for multiple phenotypes simultaneously. Although the idea of treating variants as items is not new, to our knowledge, no one has actually tried fitting mixture models to individual variants directly. There are a few reasons for this: (1) the "items" (SNPs, CNVs, etc.) are not independent, and their non-independence depends largely on their proximity in the genome; (2) population stratification and assortative mating can affect co-variance among variants; and (3) most common variants are identified under an additive model with tiny effects, implying a normally distributed genomic liability. The first two points would require imaginative modeling, such as including these factors into the model itself. As to the latter point, including variants with larger effects (e.g., CNVs) may help with clarifying if there are indeed deviations from the underlying normality.

Look at Consistency of Genetic Influences across Disorder Severity. A third test for dimensionality involves examining how the genetic contribution varies across levels of severity in a phenotype. To do so, one might examine SNP-based heritability across the continuum of severity. Under a continuous model, heritability would remain similar across levels of severity (e.g., SNP-based heritability same at extremes or in the middle of the liability distribution). A discontinuous model would predict that the genetic influences would change across levels of severity (e.g., SNP-based heritability may be different on the extremes of the liability distribution than it is closer to the middle). It should be noted that examining contributions across the continuum of liability can test if the liability for, for example, severe MDD is different from the liability to subclinical or moderate MDD, but it doesn't necessarily inform if either liability is continuous (both, or neither could be). Follow-up tests would be needed, such as finding a major locus with a large effect size for that level of severity. For instance, for a non-psychiatric phenotype of advanced macular degeneration, heritability was greater at the extremes than at the normal range (Seddon, 2005); subsequently, a major locus was found (The AMD Gene Consortium, 2013). In psychiatric genetics, Nguyen and colleagues (Nguyen et al., 2022) examined SNP-based heritability and LD regression-based genetic correlations among many subtypes of MDD, including moderate versus severe symptoms, and mild, medium, and high levels of impairment. The severe MDD subtype had similar heritability to the moderate MDD subtype. However, when examining mild, moderate, and severe impairment, moderate and severe impairment had significantly higher heritability than mild impairment. Similarly, Direk and colleagues (Direk et al., 2017) reported that SNP-based heritability differed significantly between depressive symptoms and MDD (.04% versus 20% heritability). While it's tempting to interpret these results as evidence of discontinuity, methodological artifacts can strongly contribute to differences in heritability. A clean interpretation of the results requires equating the discovery power, measurement modalities, and precision across levels of severity (e.g., using structured clinical interviewing for both moderate and severe MDD; see below).

Similarly, it might be useful to examine the overlap in SNPs (and CNV, etc.) across the continuum of disorder severity. We might, for example, conduct two GWAS: one for moderate MDD, and one for severe MDD. Next, we would examine the overlap of the SNPs. A continuous model predicts that only the number but not the combination of specific SNPs matters; thus, we should identify the same SNPs in both GWAS (provided, of course, sufficient power). On average, individuals with moderate MDD should have a lower burden of risk (fewer SNPs) than those with severe MDD. A discontinuous model would predict that, for example, severe MDD has at least a somewhat separate etiology. Thus, for example, we might find that there are 10 SNPs contributing to moderate MDD, whereas the same 10 plus an additional 5 contribute to severe MDD. This pattern would also suggest that (1) the 10 SNPs are necessary for severe depression, and (2) there is an interaction effect between these 10 and the additional 5. Cai and colleagues, for example (Cai et al., 2020), compared the genetic contributions to "minimal phenotyping" of MDD (help-seeking, cardinal symptoms of depression, self-reported diagnosis) with the same on clinical records and formal, clinician-ascertained diagnosis. Minimal phenotypes had lower SNP-based heritability than did the stricter versions (~14% v 26%); the genetic correlations were significantly different from unity as well. Before drawing conclusions, however, it should be noted that the minimal phenotypes were not equivalent to just lowering the threshold for disease liability; they were also prone to misclassifying controls as cases, and had low discriminant validity (high genetic overlap with other forms of psychopathology, e.g., anxiety). Moreover, a series of simulations within the same study illustrated how dropping the threshold to include milder cases (on the same instrument) would not decrease SNP-based heritability. This study is notable not just for highlighting an approach in a very cool way, but also in the way it brings up the importance of method differences and measurement error.

A rougher version of the same idea is to examine if the PRS developed for lower levels of severity (e.g., broadband or moderate depression) will predict severe depression in an independent sample as well as a PRS developed for higher levels of severity (provided equal power across both GWAS), and vice versa. Several studies used a PRS that was developed using clinical case-control status to predict milder versions of psychiatric disorders in the population (Martin et al., 2018). For example, some schizophrenia studies find no association between the schizophrenia PRS and lower-grade psychotic experiences (Sieradzka et al., 2014). Conversely, other studies have reported positive associations of schizophrenia PRS with childhood thought problems (Jansen et al., 2018), and a dose-response relationship between PRS burden and severity (Bigdeli et al., 2014; Legge et al., 2019). In the very large U.K. Biobank (Jermy et al., 2022), the MDD PRS is associated with various lower-grade depression symptoms. Similarly, the MDD PRS, along with PRSs for broad depression, anxiety, and neuroticism, predicted depressive symptoms in a longitudinal community cohort of adolescents, with the strength of prediction increasing over time (Kwong et al., 2021). Most impressively, Taylor and colleagues (Taylor et al., 2019) estimated PRSs for autism spectrum disorder, ADHD, bipolar disorder, obsessive-compulsive disorder, anxiety, MDD, and schizophrenia, along with PRSs for subclinical, dimensionally measured ADHD symptoms, and depressive symptoms. The PRSs for the psychiatric disorders were associated with the relevant traits for everything except bipolar disorder. Moreover, the PRS for quantitatively measured MDD symptoms predicted a diagnosis of MDD (but the same was not true for ADHD).

Look at the Pattern of Risk in Families. Examining the genetic liability in affected and unaffected family members of probands with a disorder provides yet another test of continuity. Under a continuity model, relatives of individuals with, for example, severe MDD would have the highest genetic risk (as measured by a PRS score); relatives of individuals with moderate MDD would have an intermediate PRS score; and relatives of individuals with no MDD would have the lowest score. Under a discontinuity model, two PRS scores would be needed to describe risk to relatives completely: the moderate and the severe. To our knowledge, no studies have set up the question this way in the past, although some have looked at PRS within families. For example, one study (Bigdeli et al., 2014) reported that the schizophrenia PRS is elevated among family members of probands with schizophrenia. Moreover, the PRS score increased monotonically with severity of schizophrenia-spectrum disorders in the family members. Similar results have been reported for bipolar disorder (Fullerton et al., 2015), along with elevated PRS scores in at-risk affected and unaffected young.

Examine Genetic Correlations between Different Levels of Severity of the Disorder. One can also examine genetic correlations between milder and more severe versions of a disorder (e.g., moderate and severe MDD) using linkage disequilibrium (LD) score regression. Essentially, LD regression takes two datasets containing correlations of each commonly tested SNP with a phenotype (e.g., schizophrenia) and correlates these with a different dataset of the same SNPs with another phenotype (e.g., nicotine dependence), thus obtaining a genetic correlation between the two. When correlating two forms of a disorder, any genetic correlation with a confidence interval not including one would suggest differences in genetic etiology and provide evidence against continuity.

Recently, Na Cai's group (Huang et al., 2024) compared the genetic architecture of the Patient Health Questionnaire-9 (PHQ-9, current symptoms) and the Composite International Diagnostic Interview (CIDI, worst episode). The two instruments had moderate genetic correlations (rg = 0.43 - 0.87). Moreover, PHQ-9 polygenic scores (PGS) exhibited more pleiotropy relative to CIDI and were associated with traits reflective of general negative emotionality. Nguyen and colleagues (Nguyen et al., 2022) reported that both the genetic correlations between severe and moderate MDD subtypes and the cross-correlations among mild, moderate, and severe impairment were significantly less than one (but see Direk et al. (2017) for conflicting results). This study is notable not only for providing evidence of discontinuity but also for distinguishing between severity (often symptom count) and impairment. Although a binary psychiatric diagnosis conflates the two, they are unlikely to be interchangeable.

Family Studies

Look at Consistency of Genetic Influences across Disorder Severity. There are at least two approaches for the underlying continuity of a phenotype using family (in particular, twin) studies. The first is to examine whether the etiological influences—the genetic and environmental contributions—change across the range of disorder severity. In essence, this approach tests whether extreme groups on a phenotype—for example, severe MDD—show equivalent genetic and environmental influences (A, C, and E) as milder versions (moderate MDD). The logic for continuous versus discontinuous liability here is similar to that in molecular studies: similar etiological structure across the range of severity is consistent with a dimensional model. On the other hand, changes in heritability or shared environment provide evidence of distinct etiological processes for different levels of severity. As with the equivalent molecular approach above, the test by itself does not inform about the distributional shape of the distinct etiological processes, if present. This approach has been used to examine etiological processes across the continuum in multiple psychiatric phenotypes, including but not limited to autism spectrum (Frazier et al., 2014; Robinson et al., 2011), schizophrenia (Zavos et al., 2014), ADHD (Larsson et al., 2012), nicotine use (Rende et al., 2005), and MDD (Corfield et al., 2017; Eley, 1997; Rende et al., 2006). For the most part, these studies show similar etiological influences across the severity dimension, although MDD and autism spectrum show mixed results.

Look at the Pattern of Risk in Families. The second approach (termed "multiple threshold model") involves comparing risk in families of probands. Under a continuity model, relatives of individuals with, for example, severe MDD would have the highest risk for severe MDD; relatives of individuals with moderate MDD would have intermediate risk; and relatives of individuals with no MDD would have the lowest risk (Reich et al., 1972, 1975, 1979). Under a discontinuity model, with entirely different causes of moderate versus severe disorder, relatives of individuals with moderate MDD are not at any higher risk of severe MDD than relatives of individuals with no MDD. Similarly (but perhaps more surprisingly), relatives of those with severe MDD would not have higher risks of moderate MDD. Such modeling makes predictions about risks to relatives, which can be quantified and assessed for rejecting the simple model of a continuous single underlying dimension of liability. Practically, this test is accomplished by setting up a 3 X 3 contingency table between one family member's levels of disorder (no symptoms, moderate MDD, severe MDD) and the second. Next, observed frequencies are compared with the frequencies expected under the bivariate normal distribution of the underlying liability with two thresholds to delineate among no, moderate, and severe disorder categories. If there are deviations from normality, then the place in the distribution where they deviate likely comes from a different class rather than from a homogenous group. In essence, this is a test for mixtures using twins or relatives.

Notably, the multiple threshold test, like in all null hypothesis theory testing, does not let you accept the null (the data come from a different group), but only to reject the null (the data are generated under a bivariate normal underlying liability). A few papers have applied the principle in MDD (Corfield et al., 2017); ADHD and conduct disorder (Thapar et al., 2001); panic, fears, and phobias (Kendler et al., 2001; Kendler et al., 2001); pathological gambling (Blanco et al., 2012; Slutske et al., 2000); nicotine withdrawal (Pergadia et al., 2006); personality disorders (Kendler et al., 2006; Reichborn-Kjennerud et al., 2010; Torgersen et al., 2008); schizophrenia (Kendler et al., 1995); and bipolar disorder (McGuffin et al., 2003). In most of these cases, the hypothesis that the underlying liability is normally distributed could not be rejected. For instance, although minor (subclinical/moderate) and major MDD come from the same underlying distribution (Corfield et al., 2017), unipolar MDD and bipolar affective disorder do not (McGuffin et al., 2003). One should, however, model the influence of third variables as needed (e.g., sex, age, socioeconomic status), as failure to do so could artificially induce something that looks like discontinuity. Consider an example of a disorder with three levels of severity (mild, moderate, and severe), where the onset of the severe form does not occur until age 40. Prior to age 40, mild and moderate forms are possible. One might analyze data from a sample of relatives that has an age range of 18 to 60. At younger ages, the relative of an affected person with the moderate form of the disorder might have the moderate or mild form of the disorder, consistent with a continuous risk. At older ages, however, the co-twin of the twin affected with the severe form of the disorder is unlikely to have mild or moderate versions of the disorder.

Examine Genetic Correlations among Different Levels of Severity of the Disorder. In the third approach, one may use the bivariate ACE (twin) model to directly estimate the genetic and environmental correlations between, for example, clinical diagnosis of MDD and a quantitative scale derived from symptoms of depression. Notably, a key requirement is that the same individual has data on both phenotypes simultaneously (which is impossible with, e.g., mild and moderate MDD levels). As with molecular approaches, any correlation that is significantly different from one would be evidence against continuity, as it would suggest differences in genetic etiology (Neale & Kendler, 1995). For example, in a large Swedish twin sample, Taylor and colleagues (Taylor et al., 2019) examined genetic and environmental correlations among clinical diagnoses of autism-spectrum disorder, ADHD, anxiety, and MDD with corresponding quantitively measured traits (Taylor et al., 2019); both genetic and environmental correlations between the binary diagnoses and corresponding dimensional traits were significant, but their confidence intervals failed to reach a correlation of unity. Thus, only a proportion of genetic risk was indicated to be shared across disorders and quantitively measured traits. The big concern here is method variance and amount of error; if, for example, a quantitative scale is more prone to misclassifying controls as cases and picking up generalized psychopathology (low sensitivity, low specificity, such as asking one if they've ever sought treatment for depression), the correlations with, for example, MDD clinical diagnosis would drop. Thus, the two phenotypes on which the twins are measured must be equated on measurement properties (method of administration, item difficulty, variance).

Methodological Considerations

Several methodological considerations should be discussed concerning distinguishing between continuous and discontinuous models. The first is the issue of measurement. Many of the tests of continuity discussed above compare more versus less severe versions of the disorder on etiological influences or rates in families. As noted above, to make correct inferences, it is critical to equate the measurement modality (and preferably even the measure itself) across levels of severity; otherwise, methodological artifacts may affect empirical conclusions. Similarly, there should be equivalent measurement precision at all levels. For example, Kendler et al. (Kendler et al., 2019) used a twin model to examine joint and unique genetic and environmental effects on two self-report measures and one clinically ascertained measure of MDD. The clinically ascertained measure showed unique genetic influences not shared with the self-report measures of depression, and this was interpreted to suggest that MDD is at least somewhat on a different continuum. However, the results may have been purely a function of a measurement artifact, as clinically ascertained depression will have more difficult depression items and is obtained via a different method (interactive interview with probe questions vs.

self-report questionnaire items). Similarly, many GWAS studies will either compare heritability, compare SNP discovery rates, or examine a genetic correlation between GWAS of clinically ascertained disorder and GWAS of self-reported and less severe symptoms (Direk et al., 2017; Taylor et al., 2019). The differences in content across scales, their psychometric difficulty levels, and method variance frequently make it messy to determine whether the differences in severity versus the differences in scales is driving, for example, differences in heritability. Ideally, as we mention above, researchers would develop dimensional scales that equally well measure the full range of subclinical variation to clinical severity for use in GWAS, and such efforts are underway (Simms et al., 2022). In reality, however, it's a big ask. Clinical measures differ from self-report measures by more than just psychometric difficulty. Semi-structured interviews, for example, ask follow-up questions to each symptom regarding duration, severity, impairment, and pervasiveness (structured interviews are more scripted). Moreover, the assessment method (clinician ascertainment) may be indelibly intertwined with assessment itself, as follow-up questions (at least in semi-structured interviews) can be idiosyncratic to obtain detail. And, of course, there is the difficult-to-define rapport between the interviewer and interviewee, which, compared to answering questions on a sheet of paper, can make a difference in how someone responds to a probe. It would be very difficult to write a questionnaire capturing nuances of this type. There are currently two suggestions for imperfect ways around this issue. First, one might computerize a structured clinical interview as a computer adaptive test, thereby partially handling variance due to clinician. Second, one might use a combination of self-report and clinically ascertained measures, and take the shared variance (i.e., a common factor) between the two. For example, Torgersen and colleagues (Torgersen et al., 2012) fit a psychometric or common factor model to each personality disorder as measured by self-report, dimensional measures, and an interview. The heritability of the latent personality disorder factor was considerably higher than was the heritability of either the dimensional measures or the personal interview alone. Moreover, self-report measures showed unique, significant genetic influences. This uniqueness can be interpreted as distinct genetic influence, or, more likely, method variance. As such, this last approach doesn't actually solve the problem but does allow for better dimension coverage and stronger genetic signal.

A broader issue is that the trait, the measure of said trait, and the underlying liability are often conflated, but they are not quite the same thing, and may not mirror one another's distributional patterns. For example, Paul Meehl would have said that the liability for schizophrenia is a dominant gene, which results in schizotypy, a class in which nevertheless individuals vary in levels of severity due to other genetic and environmental factors. Thus, even though the underlying genetic risk is binary, the actual vulnerability expressed, if Meehl was right, would have been at least semi-continuous, or at least would vary in severity. Similarly, a seemingly dimensional trait might actually contain two etiological "mixtures" (e.g., a mix of individuals with MDD due to genetic versus environmental factors). As long as the means of the two mixtures on MDD are close, they may remain undetected, leading to the assumption of the same underlying etiology. This same principle is seen in the traits of intelligence and height. Intelligence is thought to be normally distributed in the population, but there are genetic disorders such as trisomy 21 that result in intellectual disability. The trait of height is likewise dimensionally distributed in the population, but there are genetic conditions such as mutations of the FGFR3 gene leading to achondroplasia. Fitting mixture distributions may recover such patterns; so can the use of relatives, as is seen below. Finally, as alluded to above, the distribution of a measure of psychopathology should not be conflated with the distribution of the trait itself. The measures of trait can be quite different in terms of psychometric properties such as content and item difficulty; some are more appropriate for population samples (but are not very good at measuring clinical-range pathology), and some are more appropriate for clinical samples (which would be too "difficult" for most population samples and would produce a pile of zeros for item endorsement). These different measures might, in turn, produce different answers on any phenotypic, twin, or molecular study. Consider, as an illustration, three measures of depression: the self-reported Center for Epidemiological Studies Depression (CESD) scale; the self-reported Beck Depression Inventory (BDI); and the clinician-ascertained, semi-structured clinical interview that involves multiple follow-up questions as to the severity, impairment, and pervasiveness of each symptom. Each of these will have their own distribution. The CESD has psychometrically "easy" items, the BDI has more difficult and less frequently endorsed items, and the clinical interview has items more difficult still, producing less and less normal-looking distributions. Yet it's quite likely that the three approaches simply measure different locations within the same underlying dimensional latent trait, which progressive model fitting in an item response theory framework would likely reveal. Moreover, even if the latent trait is normal, it is still possible that different genetic or environmental liabilities might be operating at different locations of the trait (e.g., genetic influences for one location and environmental for another). All in all, caution should be taken from drawing inferences about the underlying risk by simply looking at a distribution of a particular measure of a phenotype.

Finally, it is important to equate the power in GWAS discovery samples across levels of severity; because the mean differences between moderate depression and controls is smaller than the mean differences between, for example, severe depression and controls, the moderate category will have less power to detect GWAS hits. Thus, differences in heritability and/or GWAS "hits" across levels of severity may also reflect differences in power. Finally, it is important to pay attention to how individuals in GWAS (or family) studies were sampled, as non-epidemiological (e.g., enriched) sampling can lead to odd effects in the underlying distribution. For example, compared to population-based sampling, the ability of PRS to explain schizophrenia case-control status is reduced (Zheutlin et al., 2019)

Future Directions

Level of Analysis for Genetically Informed Studies. A major consideration is whether the targets of our investigation should be measured at the level of symptom, individual disorder, higher-order common factor, or mechanism. Disorder-level approaches (e.g., GWAS of MDD, examining underlying continuum of MDD) are flawed for several reasons, primarily stemming from discriminant validity. Our current classification system for psychiatric disorders suffers from high symptom overlap, comorbidity, and heterogeneity. Fried (Fried & Nesse, 2015a), for instance, made a point that the overall MDD disorder category masks the massive heterogeneity in depression by counting over a thousand different depression profiles in his sample. There is also substantial pleiotropy across disorders, as indicated by shared risk SNP and CNV variants, high genetic and environmental correlations, and the cross-correlations of various PRSs (Kato et al., 2023; Kendler, Aggen et al., 2011; Lee et al., 2021; Leppert et al., 2020; Visscher et al., 2017). Moreover, there appears to be a "core" that is shared across disorders that is related to negative emotionality (Brandes et al., 2019; Tackett et al., 2013), and might be driving much of the pleiotropy. Given that our disorders are "open constructs" (Meehl, 1977), and are not conditional upon finding specific etiology, it is hard to tell whether this is the true state of affairs or a methodological artifact (e.g., stemming from symptom overlap). Several alternative targets for genetic studies have been proposed, including individual symptoms, mechanisms, and shared common variance across disorders. For example, some theorists (Fried & Nesse, 2015b) see individual symptoms as the fundamental building blocks that interact to form psychopathology and suggest that GWAS should be done at the level of the individual symptomatology (Fried et al., 2014). Other perspectives, such as the research domain criteria (Cuthbert & Insel, 2013), might suggest that transdiagnostic systems such as circadian or sleep systems should be the primary targets for gene discovery and search for discontinuity. For example, the hierarchical taxonomy of psychopathology (Kotov et al., 2017) would suggest approaching gene discovery and out-of-sample prediction using a multivariate framework rather than a case-control one. Under this framework, one can simultaneously conduct a GWAS for what is common across disorders (i.e., broad, upstream, possibly causal factors of internalizing, externalizing or general psychopathology factors) and what is unique to each disorder. To select among these different diagnostic frameworks, one might compare the success (with success roughly defined as number of significant genetic "hits") of the current disorder-level diagnostic model to these alternative models. Likewise, one might examine whether, after accounting for mechanism-related or common factor-related PRS, the DSM-based PRS (e.g., for MDD) continues to uniquely predict MDD.

Moving to Dimensional Measurement. Typically, large consortium data sufficiently powered for GWAS use binary measurement (case-control) of psychopathology. In a recent paper, Waszczuk (Waszczuk et al., 2023) reviewed the benefits of a dimensional approach to phenotype measurement in GWAS and other genetic studies. We briefly reiterate some of the main points here. On this note, it's worthwhile to consider the benefits conferred by measuring psychopathology dimensionally more broadly. First, relative to categorical case-control method, dimensional approaches have more power (and thus, may be somewhat gentler on the sample size requirements). Second, dimensional measures are generally not set up for skip-out logic, which is a key feature of DSM-based clinician-administered diagnostic instruments. This dimensional measurement in turn would complete datasets where either gene discovery, PGS-type work/genomic SEM, or twin/family studies can be done at the level of symptoms or syndromes. Moreover, overlap among constructs (i.e., double-dipping of the items across multiple disorders) could be detected and removed.

Third, dimensional measures could be pre-processed prior to GWAS analysis to test—at the phenotypic level—whether the constructs are categorical, dimensional, or a mixture distribution (combination of both). This could be done at the level of individual studies, or, with combined consortium data. Taking the step to pre-process the data at the phenotypic level may give better GWAS targets and enhance signal. Fourth, dimensional measures of psychopathology allow researchers to compare etiological contributions across levels of severity using the same instrument and measurement modality (provided equal measurement precision at low, moderate, and high levels of the scale). For example, severe versus moderate MDD could be derived using the same instrument (e.g., ranges on a self-report measure of depression), which would rule out method effects. Fifth, dimensional measurement allows one to get more precise estimates about someone's location on the latent psychopathology variable of interest (and how much measurement error may contribute to their score), compared to binary (or even absent/subclinical/present) measures. Sixth, dimensional measurement can start distinguishing between the severity of a disorder (e.g., via symptom count or a scale score across a dimension) and impairment. One, for instance, could argue that impairment is separate from overall symptom count and might reflect something like the impact of each symptom on academic, social, educational, or family functioning. Unfortunately, few genetically informed studies have investigated the different genetic contributions to symptom count versus impairment, because binary, DSM-based assessment collapses the two into a single diagnosis. Yet, it's not clear that they can be treated interchangeably, at least with respect to genetic risk. For example, Nguyen and colleagues (Nguyen et al., 2022) investigated the genetic correlations between various types and features of depression, and reported that the correlation between MDD with severe, moderate, and mild impairment was significantly different from one.

Finally, dimensional scales are paradoxically both more temporally stable and more sensitive to situational and clinical change, compared to categorical diagnoses. As genetic models incorporate more and more of the ebb and flow of the dynamics of pathology over short and longer time periods (e.g., GWAS of stability and change of, e.g., psychosis), this property of dimensional measures will become increasingly important. Consider, for instance, that one might want to look at the genetic influences on the persistence of anhedonia in depression, with anhedonia measured repeatedly multiple times per day over a week. We might index persistence as the autocorrelation of anhedonia over time. Measuring anhedonia via a 10-point scale or even a sum of three items would allow examination of finer changes in average levels, and may have higher autocorrelations, than a comparable binary (diagnosed with anhedonia or not) approach.

Using Longitudinal Studies to Understand the Underlying Risk Distribution. An important but oft-overlooked area in genetics concerns the longitudinal patterning, trajectories, and dynamics of psychiatric disorders. Indeed, there is an increasing recognition that disorders, and disorder features, show temporal dynamics, even in the short term. The focus on temporal dynamics is useful in many ways. It can add to power (if each column is a time point, the data frame essentially acquires more columns; if conducting intensive longitudinal designs, exponentially more columns). However, temporal dynamics may also be able to tell us something about continuous or discontinuous processes. Combined with twin studies this can be a powerful tool to tell us something about the distribution of the underlying risks.

Developmental family and twin studies can, for example, examine the genetic contributions to temporally stable versus time-varying elements of a disorder (or a higher-order factor such as internalizing) over time. If data are available, the same can be done in molecular studies. That is, incorporating a longitudinal design and breaking a phenotype down to stable and time-varying components may result in a better signal in GWAS discovery studies, or at least provide complimentary evidence. Moreover, longitudinal data can account for temporal non-invariance of expression and change in expression in psychiatric disorders over development (Bornovalova et al., 2010). It can also detect non-linear change, which could signal non-linear shifts in risk. Likewise, the parameters obtained from such developmental models can be subjected to much the same logic as we describe above (e.g., patterns in families, comparison of genetic effects at multiple thresholds).

Moreover, in recent years, there has been an increased focus on measuring short-term dynamics using intensive longitudinal data and fitting dynamical systems models such as the damped oscillator model (Hu et al., 2014; McKee et al., 2020) to data on psychiatric disorders. Such models can provide person-level parameters including, but not limited to, equilibrium or attractor position (a state to which a person tends to return), number of attractors, spring (movement away from equilibrium), and damping reduction in spring over time. Such models can in principle detect qualitative differences across people in their types of trajectory over time. Combined with a genetically informative approach, dynamical systems can be a powerful tool to understand the distribution of the underlying genetic risk (McKee, 2020, 2021). Indeed, as with developmental longitudinal models, the parameters derived from dynamical systems models can be used in family studies or as GWAS targets. Instead of conducting a GWAS for a trait at different levels of severity, a GWAS would be conducted on parameters of the dynamical system model (e.g., depressive symptoms patterned over time in terms of attractor position, number of attractors, spring, damping, overall shape). Similarly, these parameters can also be subjected to the logic outlined in this chapter for understanding the underlying distribution of risk (e.g., examine risk in families, compare genetic influences across the full range of parameter). Complimentary phenotypic work might examine whether the parameters and overall shape of change can be equated between clinical and non-clinical populations. Failure to achieve equivalence suggests different processes across clinical and subclinical levels and would be expected if the underlying liability is discrete.

Subjecting Environmental Risk to Continuous/Discontinuous Logic. The study of behavioral and molecular genetics is also the study of the environment, although that can get less attention. It would be informative to subject the environmental factors to the same sort of analyses as outlined above to understand whether the environmental risk for some phenotype(s) is continuous or discontinuous. Indeed, given a large enough dataset and with enough environmental measures, one could conduct every test outlined above with environmental variables (including LD score regression). Thus, one might conduct an "EWAS" to detect associations of individual environmental events with psychopathology, and then ask questions such as: does the liability on the environmental front also follow a threshold-liability type model? What is the distribution of effect sizes of environmental events on psychopathology, and how specific are the factors? Does psychopathology come from some big stressors (as we hypothesize in PTSD or depression), or is it produced by the add-up of daily hassles? Are there non-linear effects? Are the environmental risk factors the same (number over type) across levels of psychopathology severity, or are there some specific environmental "variants" that push one over the edge into the severe category on, for example, MDD? Would a PeRS (poly-environmental risk score) keyed to moderate MDD predict severe MDD in an independent sample as well as the one keyed to severe MDD? A limited set of studies has started examining the "environmentome" in large, longitudinal datasets such as the Adolescent Brain and Cognitive Development, which has ~12,000 kids and ~900+ environmental variables (Moore et al., 2021). Using longitudinal datasets for work like this also allows one to take care with direction of causation issues (i.e., environmental variables preceding versus following disorder onset). Let us hope that the sample size requirements won't turn out to be as astronomical as they are for genetic effects.

Improving the Generalizability of Our Studies. The final consideration is the sampling that restricts generalizability and cross-cultural comparisons of the underlying genetic risk. Indeed, it is a well-known limitation of most twin, family, and especially molecular genetic studies that the participants are primarily of European ancestry. There are several reasons for this, many of them due to the greater frequency of European ancestry in many of the nations conducting genetic research in its early years. Modeling ancestry explicitly in a multi-ancestry approach may lead to more accurate inferences for a greater proportion of people (Kim et al., 2024). However, because relatively few discovery studies have been conducted on individuals of non-European ancestry, PRSs derived on European ancestry samples have limited prediction in non-European populations (Bigdeli et al., 2020; Duncan et al., 2019; Lam et al., 2019; Martin et al., 2019). The ideal solution would be to build a U.K. Biobank–type repository in every participating country and ask the same questions of the data across countries. In turn, a cross-cultural approach to the genetics of psychiatric disorders can tell us whether psychopathology is built using the same genetic building blocks across the world, and whether the distribution of risk is equivalent. Non-trivially, before delving into GWAS of, for example, depression or schizophrenia or putative mechanisms of these disorders around the world, cross-cultural measurement invariance of the constructs should be established.

Conclusions

To summarize, the goal here is not to definitively claim that all liabilities to psychiatric disorders are continuous, although many appear to be based on current evidence. Instead, we aim to demonstrate the methods and logic for assessing whether a given disorder follows a continuous or discontinuous model. Indeed, there is an accumulating body of evidence for most common disorders that can be systematically reviewed or meta-analyzed using the framework presented in this chapter. Moreover, the field would greatly benefit from standardized measurement across studies, integrating longitudinal and environmental perspectives, and conducting analyses at multiple levels. This comprehensive approach will enhance our understanding of underlying mechanisms, ultimately informing targeted prevention and intervention efforts. Moving forward, it is crucial to build on the existing research while adopting innovative methodologies to refine our understanding of psychiatric disorders.

References

Aguilera, M., Arias, B., Wichers, M., Barrantes-Vidal, N., Moya, J., Villa, H., Os, J. van, Ibáñez, M. I., Ruipérez, M. A., Ortet, G., & Fañanás, L. (2009). Early adversity and 5-HTT/BDNF genes: New evidence of gene–environment interactions on depressive symptoms in a general population. *Psychological* Medicine, 39(9), 1425–1432. https://doi.org/10.1017/S0033291709005248

Arioka, Y., Shishido, E., Kushima, I., Suzuki, T., Saito, R., Aiba, A., Mori, D., & Ozaki, N. (2021). Chromosome 22q11.2 deletion causes PERK-dependent vulnerability in dopaminergic neurons. *eBioMedicine*, *63*, 103138. https://doi.org/10.1016/j.ebiom.2020.103138

Åslund, C., Nordquist, N., Comasco, E., Leppert, J., Oreland, L., & Nilsson, K. W. (2010). Maltreatment, MAOA, and delinquency: Sex differences in gene–environment interaction in a large population-based cohort of adolescents. *Behavior Genetics*, *41*(2), 262–272. https://doi.org/10.1007/s10519-010-9356-y

Benjamin, D. J., Cesarini, D., Van Der Loos, M. J., Dawes, C. T., Koellinger, P. D., Magnusson, P. K., Chabris, C. F., Conley, D., Laibson, D., & Johannesson, M. (2012). The genetic architecture of economic and political preferences. *Proceedings of the National Academy of Sciences*, *109*(21), 8026–8031.

Bergen, S. E., Gardner, C. O., & Kendler, K. S. (2007). Age-related changes in heritability of behavioral phenotypes over adolescence and young adulthood: A meta-analysis | twin research and human genetics. *Twin Research and Human Genetics*, *10*(3), 423–433. https://doi.org/10.1375/twin.10.3.423

Bigdeli, T. B., Bacanu, S.-A., Webb, B. T., Walsh, D., O'Neill, F. A., Fanous, A. H., Riley, B. P., & Kendler, K. S. (2014). Molecular validation of the schizophrenia spectrum. *Schizophrenia Bulletin*, *40*(1), 60–65. https://doi.org/10.1093/schbul/sbt122

Bigdeli, T. B., Genovese, G., Georgakopoulos, P., Meyers, J. L., Peterson, R. E., Iyegbe, C. O., Medeiros, H., Valderrama, J., Achtyes, E. D., Kotov, R., Stahl, E. A., Abbott, C., Azevedo, M. H., Belliveau, R. A., Bevilacqua, E., Bromet, E. J., Byerley, W., Carvalho, C. B., Chapman, S. B., . . . Pato, C. N. (2020). Contributions of common genetic variants to risk of schizophrenia among individuals of African and Latino ancestry. *Molecular Psychiatry*, *25*(10), 2455–2467. https://doi.org/10.1038/s41380-019-0517-y

Blanco, C., Myers, J., & Kendler, K. S. (2012). Gambling, disordered gambling and their association with major depression and substance use: A web-based cohort and twin-sibling study. *Psychological Medicine*, *42*(3), 497–508. https://doi.org/10.1017/S0033291711001401

Bornovalova, M. A., Hicks, B. M., Iacono, W. G., & McGue, M. (2010). Familial transmission and heritability of childhood disruptive disorders. *American Journal of Psychiatry*, *167*(9), 1066–1074. https://doi.org/10.1176/appi.ajp.2010.09091272

Brandes, C. M., Herzhoff, K., Smack, A. J., & Tackett, J. L. (2019). The p factor and the n factor: Associations between the general factors of psychopathology and neuroticism in children. *Clinical Psychological Science*, *7*(6), 1266–1284. https://doi.org/10.1177/2167702619859332

Bycroft, C., Freeman, C., Petkova, D., Band, G., Elliott, L. T., Sharp, K., Motyer, A., Vukcevic, D., Delaneau, O., O'Connell, J., Cortes, A., Welsh, S., Young, A., Effingham, M., McVean, G., Leslie, S., Allen, N., Donnelly, P., & Marchini, J. (2018). The UK Biobank resource with deep phenotyping and genomic data. *Nature*, *562*(7726), 203–209. https://doi.org/10.1038/s41586-018-0579-z

Cai, N., Revez, J. A., Adams, M. J., Andlauer, T. F. M., Breen, G., Byrne, E. M., Clarke, T.-K., Forstner, A. J., Grabe, H. J., Hamilton, S. P., Levinson, D. F., Lewis, C. M., Lewis, G., Martin, N. G., Milaneschi, Y., Mors, O., Müller-Myhsok, B., Penninx, B. W. J. H., Perlis, R. H., . . . Flint, J. (2020). Minimal phenotyping yields genome-wide association signals of low specificity for major depression. *Nature Genetics*, *52*(4), 437–447. https://doi.org/10.1038/s41588-020-0594-5

Carter, C. (1967). Clinical aspects of genetics, the genetics of common malformations and diseases. *Transactions of the Medical Society of London*, *83*, 84–91. https://pubmed.ncbi.nlm.nih.gov/4228764/

Carter, C. O. (1961). The inheritance of congenital pyloric stenosis. *British Medical Bulletin*, *17*(3), 251–253. https://doi.org/10.1093/oxfordjournals.bmb.a069918

Caspi, A., Sugden, K., Moffitt, T. E., Taylor, A., Craig, I. W., Harrington, H., McClay, J., Mill, J., Martin, J., Braithwaite, A., & Poulton, R. (2003). Influence of life stress on depression: Moderation by a polymorphism in the 5-HTT gene. *Science*, *301*(5631), 386–389. https://doi.org/10.1126/science.1083968

Chen, C.-C., Lu, R.-B., Chen, Y.-C., Wang, M.-F., Chang, Y.-C., Li, T.-K., & Yin, S.-J. (1999). Interaction between the functional polymorphisms of the alcohol-metabolism genes in protection against alcoholism. *The American Journal of Human Genetics*, *65*(3), 795–807. https://doi.org/10.1086/302540

Corfield, E. C., Yang, Y., Martin, N. G., & Nyholt, D. R. (2017). A continuum of genetic liability for minor and major depression. *Translational Psychiatry*, *7*(5), e1131–e1131. https://doi.org/10.1038/tp.2017.99

Culverhouse, R. C., Saccone, N. L., Horton, A. C., Ma, Y., Anstey, K. J., Banaschewski, T., Burmeister, M., Cohen-Woods, S., Etain, B., Fisher, H. L., Goldman, N., Guillaume, S., Horwood, J., Juhasz, G., Lester, K. J., Mandelli, L., Middeldorp, C. M., Olié, E., Villafuerte, S., . . . Bierut, L. J. (2018). Collaborative meta-analysis finds no evidence of a strong interaction between stress and 5-HTTLPR genotype contributing to the development of depression. *Molecular Psychiatry*, *23*(1), 133–142. https://doi.org/10.1038/mp.2017.44

Cuthbert, B. N., & Insel, T. R. (2013). Toward the future of psychiatric diagnosis: The seven pillars of RDoC. *BMC Medicine*, *11*(1), 126. https://doi.org/10.1186/1741-7015-11-126

Direk, N., Williams, S., Smith, J. A., Ripke, S., Air, T., Amare, A. T., Amin, N., Baune, B. T., Bennett, D. A., Blackwood, D. H. R., Boomsma, D., Breen, G., Buttenschøn, H. N., Byrne, E. M., Børglum, A. D., Castelao, E., Cichon, S., Clarke, T.-K., Cornelis, M. C., . . . Sullivan, P. F. (2017). An analysis of two genome-wide association meta-analyses identifies a new locus for broad depression phenotype. *Biological Psychiatry*, *82*(5), 322–329. https://doi.org/10.1016/j.biopsych.2016.11.013

Duncan, L. E., & Keller, M. C. (2011). A critical review of the first 10 years of candidate gene-by-environment interaction research in psychiatry. *American Journal of Psychiatry*, *168*(10), 1041–1049. https://doi.org/10.1176/appi.ajp.2011.11020191

Duncan, L., Shen, H., Gelaye, B., Meijsen, J., Ressler, K., Feldman, M., Peterson, R., & Domingue, B. (2019). Analysis of polygenic risk score usage and performance in diverse human populations. *Nature Communications*, *10*(1), 3328. https://doi.org/10.1038/s41467-019-11112-0

Edenberg, H. J. (2007). The genetics of alcohol metabolism: Role of alcohol dehydrogenase and aldehyde dehydrogenase variants. *Alcohol Research & Health*, *30*(1), 5.

Eley, T. C. (1997). Depressive symptoms in children and adolescents: Etiological links between normality and abnormality: A research note. *Journal of Child Psychology and Psychiatry*, *38*(7), 861–865. https://doi.org/10.1111/j.1469-7610.1997.tb01604.x

Fisher, R. A. (1918). The correlation between relatives on the supposition of Mendelian inheritance. *Earth and Environmental Science Transactions of The Royal Society of Edinburgh*, *52*(2), 399–433. https://doi.org/10.1017/S0080456800012163

Frazier, T. W., Thompson, L., Youngstrom, E. A., Law, P., Hardan, A. Y., Eng, C., & Morris, N. (2014). A twin study of heritable and shared environmental contributions to autism. *Journal of Autism and Developmental Disorders*, *44*(8), 2013–2025. https://doi.org/10.1007/s10803-014-2081-2

Fried, E. I., & Nesse, R. M. (2015a). Depression is not a consistent syndrome: An investigation of unique symptom patterns in the STAR*D study. *Journal of Affective Disorders*, *172*, 96–102. https://doi.org/10.1016/j.jad.2014.10.010

Fried, E. I., & Nesse, R. M. (2015b). Depression sum-scores don't add up: Why analyzing specific depression symptoms is essential. *BMC Medicine*, *13*(1), 72.

Fried, E. I., Nesse, R. M., Zivin, K., Guille, C., & Sen, S. (2014). Depression is more than the sum score of its parts: Individual DSM symptoms have different risk factors. *Psychological Medicine*, *44*(10), 2067–2076. *Cambridge Core*. https://doi.org/10.1017/S0033291713002900

Fullerton, J. M., Koller, D. L., Edenberg, H. J., Foroud, T., Liu, H., Glowinski, A. L., McInnis, M. G., Wilcox, H. C., Frankland, A., Roberts, G., Schofield, P. R., Mitchell, P. B., Nurnberger, J. I., & Bipolar High Risk Study Group, B. C. (2015). Assessment of first and second degree relatives of individuals with bipolar disorder shows increased genetic risk scores in both affected relatives and young At-Risk Individuals. *American Journal of Medical Genetics Part B: Neuropsychiatric Genetics*, *168*(7), 617–629. https://doi.org/10.1002/ajmg.b.32344

Hopwood, C. J., Morey, L. C., & Markon, K. E. (2023). What is a psychopathology dimension? *Clinical Psychology Review*, *106*, 102356. https://doi.org/10.1016/j.cpr.2023.102356

Howard, D. M., Adams, M. J., Clarke, T.-K., Hafferty, J. D., Gibson, J., Shirali, M., Coleman, J. R. I., Hagenaars, S. P., Ward, J., Wigmore, E. M., Alloza, C., Shen, X., Barbu, M. C., Xu, E. Y., Whalley, H. C., Marioni, R. E., Porteous, D. J., Davies, G., Deary, I. J., . . . McIntosh, A. M. (2019). Genome-wide meta-analysis of depression identifies 102 independent variants and highlights the importance of the prefrontal brain regions. *Nature Neuroscience*, *22*(3), 343–352. https://doi.org/10.1038/s41593-018-0326-7

Hu, Y., Boker, S., Neale, M., & Klump, K. L. (2014). Latent differential equation with moderators: Simulation and application. *Psychological Methods*, *19*(1), 56–71. https://doi.org/10.1037/a0032476

Huang, L., Tang, S., Rietkerk, J., Appadurai, V., Krebs, M. D., Schork, A. J., Werge, T., Zuber, V., Kendler, K., & Cai, N. (2024). Polygenic analyses show important differences between major depressive disorder symptoms measured using various instruments. *Biological Psychiatry*, *95*(12), 1110–1121. https://doi.org/10.1016/j.biopsych.2023.11.021

Ioannidis, J. P. A., Ntzani, E. E., Trikalinos, T. A., & Contopoulos-Ioannidis, D. G. (2001). Replication validity of genetic association studies. *Nature Genetics*, *29*(3), 306–309. https://doi.org/10.1038/ng749

Jansen, P. R., Polderman, T. J. C., Bolhuis, K., van der Ende, J., Jaddoe, V. W. V., Verhulst, F. C., White, T., Posthuma, D., & Tiemeier, H. (2018). Polygenic scores for schizophrenia and educational attainment are associated with behavioural problems in early childhood in the general population. *Journal of Child Psychology and Psychiatry*, *59*(1), 39–47. https://doi.org/10.1111/jcpp.12759

Jermy, B. S., Hagenaars, S. P., Glanville, K. P., Coleman, J. R. I., Howard, D. M., Breen, G., Vassos, E., & Lewis, C. M. (2022). Using major depression polygenic risk scores to explore the depressive symptom continuum. *Psychological Medicine*, *52*(1), 149–158. https://doi.org/10.1017/S0033291720001828

Johnson, E. C., Border, R., Melroy-Greif, W. E., de Leeuw, C. A., Ehringer, M. A., & Keller, M. C. (2017). No evidence that schizophrenia candidate genes are more associated with schizophrenia than noncandidate genes. *Biological Psychiatry*, *82*(10), 702–708. https://doi.org/10.1016/j.biopsych.2017.06.033

Kato, H., Kimura, H., Kushima, I., Takahashi, N., Aleksic, B., & Ozaki, N. (2023). The genetic architecture of schizophrenia: Review of large-scale genetic studies. *Journal of Human Genetics*, *68*(3), 175–182. https://doi.org/10.1038/s10038-022-01059-4

Kendler, K., Myers, J., Prescott, C., & Neale, M. (2001). The genetic epidemiology of irrational fears and phobias in men. *Archives of General Psychiatry*, *58*, 257–265. https://doi.org/10.1001/archpsyc.58.3.257

Kendler, K. S., Aggen, S. H., Knudsen, G. P., Røysamb, E., Neale, M. C., & Reichborn-Kjennerud, T. (2011). The structure of genetic and environmental risk factors for syndromal and subsyndromal common DSM-IV Axis I and all Axis II disorders. *American Journal of Psychiatry*, *168*(1), 29–39. https://doi.org/10.1176/appi.ajp.2010.10030340

Kendler, K. S., Czajkowski, N., Tambs, K., Torgersen, S., Aggen, S. H., C. Neale, M., & Reichborn-Kjennerud, T. (2006). Dimensional representations of DSM-IV Cluster A personality disorders in a population-based sample of Norwegian twins: A multivariate study. *Psychological Medicine*, *36*(11), 1583–1591. https://doi.org/10.1017/S0033291706008609

Kendler, K. S., Gardner, C., & Dick, D. M. (2011). Predicting alcohol consumption in adolescence from alcohol-specific and general externalizing genetic risk factors, key environmental exposures and their interaction. *Psychological Medicine*, *41*(7), 1507–1516. https://doi.org/10.1017/S003329171000190X

Kendler, K. S., Gardner, C. O., Neale, M. C., Aggen, S., Heath, A., Colodro-Conde, L., Couvyduchesne, B., Byrne, E. M., Martin, N. G., & Gillespie, N. A. (2019). Shared and specific genetic risk factors for lifetime major depression, depressive symptoms and neuroticism in three population-based twin samples. *Psychological Medicine*, *49*(16), 2745–2753. https://doi.org/10.1017/S003329171800377X

Kendler, K. S., Gardner, C. O., & Prescott, C. A. (2001). Panic syndromes in a population-based sample of male and female twins. *Psychological Medicine*, *31*(6), 989–1000. https://doi.org/10.1017/S0033291701004226

Kendler, K. S., Neale, M. C., & Walsh, D. (1995). Evaluating the spectrum concept of schizophrenia in the Roscommon Family Study. *American Journal of Psychiatry*, *152*(5), 749–754.

Kim, J. J., Vitale, D., Otani, D. V., Lian, M. M., Heilbron, K., Iwaki, H., Lake, J., Solsberg, C. W., Leonard, H., Makarious, M. B., Tan, E.-K., Singleton, A. B., Bandres-Ciga, S., Noyce, A. J., Blauwendraat, C., Nalls, M. A., Foo, J. N., & Mata, I. (2024). Multi-ancestry genome-wide association meta-analysis of Parkinson's disease. *Nature Genetics*, *56*(1), 27–36. https://doi.org/10.1038/s41588-023-01584-8

Kotov, R., Krueger, R. F., Watson, D., Achenbach, T. M., Althoff, R. R., Bagby, R. M., Brown, T. A., Carpenter, W. T., Caspi, A., Clark, L. A., Eaton, N. R., Forbes, M. K., Forbush, K. T., Goldberg, D., Hasin, D., Hyman, S. E., Ivanova, M. Y., Lynam, D. R., Markon, K., . . . Zimmerman, M. (2017). The Hierarchical Taxonomy of Psychopathology (HiTOP): A dimensional alternative to traditional nosologies. *Journal of Abnormal Psychology*, *126*(4), 454–477. https://doi.org/10.1037/abn0000258

Kushima, I., Aleksic, B., Nakatochi, M., Shimamura, T., Okada, T., Uno, Y., Morikawa, M., Ishizuka, K., Shiino, T., Kimura, H., Arioka, Y., Yoshimi, A., Takasaki, Y., Yu, Y., Nakamura, Y., Yamamoto, M., Iidaka, T., Iritani, S., Inada, T., . . . Ozaki, N. (2018). Comparative analyses of copy-number variation in autism spectrum disorder and schizophrenia reveal etiological overlap and biological insights. *Cell Reports*, *24*(11), 2838–2856. https://doi.org/10.1016/j.celrep.2018.08.022

Kwong, A. S. F., Morris, T. T., Pearson, R. M., Timpson, N. J., Rice, F., Stergiakouli, E., & Tilling, K. (2021). Polygenic risk for depression, anxiety and neuroticism are associated with the severity and rate of change in depressive symptoms across adolescence. *Journal of Child Psychology and Psychiatry*, *62*(12), 1462–1474. https://doi.org/10.1111/jcpp.13422

Lam, M., Chen, C.-Y., Li, Z., Martin, A. R., Bryois, J., Ma, X., Gaspar, H., Ikeda, M., Benyamin, B., Brown, B. C., Liu, R., Zhou, W., Guan, L., Kamatani, Y., Kim, S.-W., Kubo, M., Kusumawardhani, A. A. A. A., Liu, C.-M., Ma, H., . . . Huang, H. (2019). Comparative genetic architectures of schizophrenia in East Asian and European populations. *Nature Genetics*, *51*(12), 1670–1678. https://doi.org/10.1038/s41588-019-0512-x

Larsson, H., Anckarsater, H., Råstam, M., Chang, Z., & Lichtenstein, P. (2012). Childhood attention-deficit hyperactivity disorder as an extreme of a continuous trait: A quantitative genetic study of 8,500 twin pairs. *Journal of Child Psychology and Psychiatry*, *53*(1), 73–80. https://doi.org/10.1111/j.1469-7610.2011.02467.x

Lee, P. H., Feng, Y.-C. A., & Smoller, J. W. (2021). Pleiotropy and cross-disorder genetics among psychiatric disorders. *Biological Psychiatry*, *89*(1), 20–31. https://doi.org/10.1016/j.biopsych.2020.09.026

Lee, S. H., Ahn, W.-Y., Seweryn, M., & Sadee, W. (2018). Combined genetic influence of the nicotinic receptor gene cluster CHRNA5/A3/B4 on nicotine dependence. *BMC Genomics*, *19*(1), 826. https://doi.org/10.1186/s12864-018-5219-3

Lee, S. H., DeCandia, T. R., Ripke, S., Yang, J., Sullivan, P. F., Goddard, M. E., Keller, M. C., Visscher, P. M., & Wray, N. R. (2012). Estimating the proportion of variation in susceptibility to schizophrenia captured by common SNPs. *Nature Genetics*, *44*(3), 247–250. https://doi.org/10.1038/ng.1108

Legge, S. E., Jones, H. J., Kendall, K. M., Pardiñas, A. F., Menzies, G., Bracher-Smith, M., Escott-Price, V., Rees, E., Davis, K. A. S., Hotopf, M., Savage, J. E., Posthuma, D., Holmans, P., Kirov, G., Owen, M. J., O'Donovan, M. C., Zammit, S., & Walters, J. T. R. (2019). Association of genetic liability to psychotic experiences with neuropsychotic disorders and traits. *JAMA Psychiatry*, *76*(12), 1256–1265. https://doi.org/10.1001/jamapsychiatry.2019.2508

Legge, S. E., Santoro, M. L., Periyasamy, S., Okewole, A., Arsalan, A., & Kowalec, K. (2021). Genetic architecture of schizophrenia: A review of major advancements. *Psychological Medicine*, *51*(13), 2168–2177. https://doi.org/10.1017/S0033291720005334

Leppert, B., Millard, L. A. C., Riglin, L., Smith, G. D., Thapar, A., Tilling, K., Walton, E., & Stergiakouli, E. (2020). A cross-disorder PRS-pheWAS of 5 major psychiatric disorders in UK Biobank. *PLoS Genetics*, *16*(5), e1008185. https://doi.org/10.1371/journal.pgen.1008185

Levey, D. F., Stein, M. B., Wendt, F. R., Pathak, G. A., Zhou, H., Aslan, M., Quaden, R., Harrington, K. M., Nuñez, Y. Z., Overstreet, C., Radhakrishnan, K., Sanacora, G., McIntosh, A. M., Shi, J., Shringarpure, S. S., 23andMe Research Team, the Million Veteran Program, Concato, J., Polimanti, R., & Gelernter, J. (2021). Bi-ancestral depression GWAS in the Million Veteran Program and meta-analysis in >1.2 million individuals highlight new therapeutic directions. *Nature Neuroscience*, *24*(7), 954–963. https://doi.org/10.1038/s41593-021-00860-2

Li, J., & Zhang, Q. (2017). Insight into the molecular genetics of myopia. *Molecular Vision*, *23*, 1048–1080.

Loh, P.-R., Bhatia, G., Gusev, A., Finucane, H. K., Bulik-Sullivan, B. K., Pollack, S. J., de Candia, T. R., Lee, S. H., Wray, N. R., Kendler, K. S., O'Donovan, M. C., Neale, B. M., Patterson, N., & Price, A. L. (2015). Contrasting genetic architectures of schizophrenia and other complex diseases using fast variance-components analysis. *Nature Genetics*, *47*(12), 1385–1392. https://doi.org/10.1038/ng.3431

Martin, A. R., Kanai, M., Kamatani, Y., Okada, Y., Neale, B. M., & Daly, M. J. (2019). Clinical use of current polygenic risk scores may exacerbate health disparities. *Nature Genetics*, *51*(4), 584–591. https://doi.org/10.1038/s41588-019-0379-x

Martin, J., Taylor, M. J., & Lichtenstein, P. (2018). Assessing the evidence for shared genetic risks across psychiatric disorders and traits. *Psychological Medicine*, *48*(11), 1759–1774. https://doi.org/10.1017/S0033291717003440

Martin, N. G., & Eaves, L. J. (1977). The genetical analysis of covariance structure. *Heredity*, *38*(1), 79–95. https://doi.org/10.1038/hdy.1977.9

Maynard, T. M., Haskell, G. T., Peters, A. Z., Sikich, L., Lieberman, J. A., & LaMantia, A.-S. (2003). A comprehensive analysis of 22q11 gene expression in the developing and adult brain. *Proceedings of the National Academy of Sciences*, *100*(24), 14433–14438. https://doi.org/10.1073/pnas.2235651100

McDonald-McGinn, D. M., Sullivan, K. E., Marino, B., Philip, N., Swillen, A., Vorstman, J. A. S., Zackai, E. H., Emanuel, B. S., Vermeesch, J. R., Morrow, B. E., Scambler, P. J., & Bassett, A. S. (2015). 22q11.2 deletion syndrome. *Nature Reviews Disease Primers*, *1*(1), 1–19. https://doi.org/10.1038/nrdp.2015.71

McGuffin, P., Rijsdijk, F., Andrew, M., Sham, P., Katz, R., & Cardno, A. (2003). The heritability of bipolar affective disorder and the genetic relationship to unipolar depression. *Archives of General Psychiatry*, *60*(5), 497–502. https://doi.org/10.1001/archpsyc.60.5.497

McKee, K. L. (2020). *Phenotype extraction: Estimation and biometrical genetic analysis of individual dynamics* [Doctoral dissertation, Virginia Commonwealth University].

McKee, K. L. (2021). Hierarchical biometrical genetic analysis of longitudinal dynamics. *Behavior Genetics*, *51*(6), 654–664. https://doi.org/10.1007/s10519-021-10060-0

McKee, K., Russell, M., Mennis, J., Mason, M., & Neale, M. (2020). Emotion regulation dynamics predict substance use in high-risk adolescents. *Addictive Behaviors*, *106*, 106374. https://doi.org/10.1016/j.addbeh.2020.106374

Meehl, P. E. (1962). Schizotaxia, schizotypy, schizophrenia. *American Psychologist*, *17*(12), 827–838. https://doi.org/10.1037/h0041029

Meehl, P. E. (1977). Specific etiology and other forms of strong influence: Some quantitative meanings. *Journal of Medicine and Philosophy*, *2*(1), 33–53. https://doi.org/10.1093/jmp/2.1.33

Meehl, P. E. (1989). Schizotaxia revisited. *Archives of General Psychiatry*, *46*(10), 935. https://doi.org/10.1001/archpsyc.1989.01810100077015

Meehl, P. E. (1990). Toward an integrated theory of schizotaxia, schizotypy, and schizophrenia. *Journal of Personality Disorders*, *4*(1), 1–99. https://doi.org/10.1521/pedi.1990.4.1.1

Moore, T. M., Visoki, E., Argabright, S. T., DiDomenico, G. E., Sotelo, I., Wortzel, J. D., Naeem, A., Gur, R. C., Gur, R. E., Warrier, V., Guloksuz, S., & Barzilay, R. (2021). *The exposome and its associations with broad mental and physical health measures in early adolescence*. medRxiv, 2021-08. https://doi.org/10.1101/2021.08.11.21261918

Muramatsu, T., Zu-Cheng, W., Yi-Ru, F., Kou-Bao, H., Heqin, Y., Yamada, K., Higuchi, S., Harada, S., & Kono, H. (1995). Alcohol and aldehyde dehydrogenase genotypes and drinking behavior of Chinese living in Shanghai. *Human Genetics*, *96*(2), 151–154. https://doi.org/10.1007/BF00207371

Neale, M., & Cardon, L. R. (1992). *Methodology for genetic studies of twins and families*. Springer Science & Business Media.

Neale, M. C., & Kendler, K. S. (1995). Models of comorbidity for multifactorial disorders. *American Journal of Human Genetics*, *57*(4), 935–953.

Nguyen, T.-D., Harder, A., Xiong, Y., Kowalec, K., Hägg, S., Cai, N., Kuja-Halkola, R., Dalman, C., Sullivan, P. F., & Lu, Y. (2022). Genetic heterogeneity and subtypes of major depression. *Molecular Psychiatry*, *27*(3), 1667–1675. https://doi.org/10.1038/s41380-021-01413-6

Norton, B., & Pearson, E. S. (1976). A note on the background to, and refereeing of, R. A. Fisher's 1918 paper "On the Correlation between Relatives on the Supposition of Mendelian Inheritance." *Notes and Records of the Royal Society of London*, *31*(1), 151–162.

Park, J.-H., Wacholder, S., Gail, M. H., Peters, U., Jacobs, K. B., Chanock, S. J., & Chatterjee, N. (2010). Estimation of effect size distribution from genome-wide association studies and implications for future discoveries. *Nature Genetics*, *42*(7), 570–575. https://doi.org/10.1038/ng.610

Pergadia, M. L., Heath, A. C., Martin, N. G., & Madden, P. a. F. (2006). Genetic analyses of DSM-IV nicotine withdrawal in adult twins. *Psychological Medicine*, *36*(7), 963–972. https://doi.org/10.1017/S0033291706007495

Purcell, S., & Sham, P. (2002). Variance components models for gene–environment interaction in quantitative trait locus linkage analysis. *Twin Research and Human Genetics*, *5*(6), 572–576. https://doi.org/10.1375/twin.5.6.572

Rathouz, P. J., Van Hulle, C. A., Rodgers, J. L., Waldman, I. D., & Lahey, B. B. (2008). Specification, testing, and interpretation of gene-by-measured-environment interaction models in the presence of gene–environment correlation. *Behavior Genetics*, *38*(3), 301–315. https://doi.org/10.1007/s10519-008-9193-4

Rees, E., Walters, J. T. R., Georgieva, L., Isles, A. R., Chambert, K. D., Richards, A. L., Mahoney-Davies, G., Legge, S. E., Moran, J. L., McCarroll, S. A., O'Donovan, M. C., Owen, M. J., & Kirov, G. (2014). Analysis of copy number variations at 15 schizophrenia-associated loci. *The British Journal of Psychiatry*, *204*(2), 108–114. https://doi.org/10.1192/bjp.bp.113.131052

Reich, T., Cloninger, C. R., & Guze, S. B. (1975). The multifactorial model of disease transmission: I. Description of the model and its use in psychiatry. *The British Journal of Psychiatry*, *127*(1), 1–10. https://doi.org/10.1192/bjp.127.1.1

Reich, T., James, J. W., & Morris, C. A. (1972). The use of multiple thresholds in determining the mode of transmission of semi-continuous traits*. *Annals of Human Genetics*, *36*(2), 163–184. https://doi.org/10.1111/j.1469-1809.1972.tb00767.x

Reich, T., Rice, J., Cloninger, C. R., Wette, R., & James, J. (1979). The use of multiple thresholds and segregation analysis in analyzing the phenotypic heterogeneity of multifactorial traits. *Annals of Human Genetics*, *42*(3), 371–390. https://doi.org/10.1111/j.1469-1809.1979.tb00670.x

Reichborn-Kjennerud, T., Czajkowski, N., Røysamb, E., Ørstavik, R. E., Neale, M. C., Torgersen, S., & Kendler, K. S. (2010). Major depression and dimensional representations of DSM-IV personality disorders: A population-based twin study. *Psychological Medicine*, *40*(9), 1475–1484. https://doi.org/10.1017/S0033291709991954

Rende, R., Slomkowski, C., Lloyd-Richardson, E., Stroud, L., & Niaura, R. (2006). Estimating genetic and environmental influences on depressive symptoms in adolescence: Differing effects on higher and lower levels of symptoms. *Journal of Clinical Child & Adolescent Psychology*, *35*(2), 237–243. https://doi.org/10.1207/s15374424jccp3502_7

Rende, R., Slomkowski, C., McCaffery, J., Lloyd-Richardson, E., & Niaura, R. (2005). A twin-sibling study of tobacco use in adolescence: Etiology of individual differences and extreme scores. *Nicotine & Tobacco Research*, *7*(3), 413–419. https://doi.org/10.1080/14622200500125609

Ripke, S., Neale, B. M., Corvin, A., Walters, J. T., Farh, K.-H., Holmans, P. A., Lee, P., Bulik-Sullivan, B., Collier, D. A., Huang, H., Pers, T. H., Agartz, I., Agerbo, E., Albus, M., Alexander, M., Amin, F., Bacanu, S. A., Begemann, M., Belliveau, R. A., . . . O'Donovan, M. C. (2014). Biological insights from

108 schizophrenia-associated genetic loci. *Nature*, *511*(7510), 421–427. https://doi.org/10.1038/nature13595

Ripke, S., O'Dushlaine, C., Chambert, K., Moran, J. L., Kähler, A. K., Akterin, S., Bergen, S. E., Collins, A. L., Crowley, J. J., Fromer, M., Kim, Y., Lee, S. H., Magnusson, P. K. E., Sanchez, N., Stahl, E. A., Williams, S., Wray, N. R., Xia, K., Bettella, F., . . . Sullivan, P. F. (2013). Genome-wide association analysis identifies 13 new risk loci for schizophrenia. *Nature Genetics*, *45*(10), 1150–1159. https://doi.org/10.1038/ng.2742

Robinson, E. B., Koenen, K. C., McCormick, M. C., Munir, K., Hallett, V., Happé, F., Plomin, R., & Ronald, A. (2011). Evidence that autistic traits show the same etiology in the general population and at the quantitative extremes (5%, 2.5%, and 1%). *Archives of General Psychiatry*, *68*(11), 1113–1121. https://doi.org/10.1001/archgenpsychiatry.2011.119

Saccone, N. L., Culverhouse, R. C., Schwantes-An, T.-H., Cannon, D. S., Chen, X., Cichon, S., Giegling, I., Han, S., Han, Y., Keskitalo-Vuokko, K., Kong, X., Landi, M. T., Ma, J. Z., Short, S. E., Stephens, S. H., Stevens, V. L., Sun, L., Wang, Y., Wenzlaff, A. S., . . . Bierut, L. J. (2010). Multiple independent loci at chromosome 15q25.1 affect smoking quantity: A meta-analysis and comparison with lung cancer and COPD. *PLoS Genetics*, *6*(8), e1001053. https://doi.org/10.1371/journal.pgen.1001053

Saito, R., Koebis, M., Nagai, T., Shimizu, K., Liao, J., Wulaer, B., Sugaya, Y., Nagahama, K., Uesaka, N., Kushima, I., Mori, D., Maruyama, K., Nakao, K., Kurihara, H., Yamada, K., Kano, M., Fukada, Y., Ozaki, N., & Aiba, A. (2020). Comprehensive analysis of a novel mouse model of the 22q11.2 deletion syndrome: A model with the most common 3.0-Mb deletion at the human 22q11.2 locus. *Translational Psychiatry*, *10*(1), 1–13. https://doi.org/10.1038/s41398-020-0723-z

Sanchez-Roige, S., Palmer, A. A., Fontanillas, P., Elson, S. L., the 23andMe Research Team, the Substance Use Disorder Working Group of the Psychiatric Genomics Consortium, Adams, M. J., Howard, D. M., Edenberg, H. J., Davies, G., Crist, R. C., Deary, I. J., McIntosh, A. M., & Clarke, T.-K. (2019). Genome-wide association study meta-analysis of the Alcohol Use Disorders Identification Test (AUDIT) in two population-based cohorts. *American Journal of Psychiatry*, *176*(2), 107–118. https://doi.org/10.1176/appi.ajp.2018.18040369

Schizophrenia Working Group of the Psychiatric Genomics Consortium, Ripke, S., Walters, J. T., & O'Donovan, M. C. (2020). *Mapping genomic loci prioritises genes and implicates synaptic biology in schizophrenia*. medRxiv, 2020-09. https://doi.org/10.1101/2020.09.12.20192922

Seddon, J. M. (2005). The US twin study of age-related macular degeneration: Relative roles of genetic and environmental influences. *Archives of Ophthalmology*, *123*(3), 321. https://doi.org/10.1001/archopht.123.3.321

Shi, J., Levinson, D. F., Duan, J., Sanders, A. R., Zheng, Y., Pe'er, I., Dudbridge, F., Holmans, P. A., Whittemore, A. S., Mowry, B. J., Olincy, A., Amin, F., Cloninger, C. R., Silverman, J. M., Buccola, N. G., Byerley, W. F., Black, D. W., Crowe, R. R., Oksenberg, J. R., . . . Gejman, P. V. (2009). Common variants on chromosome 6p22.1 are associated with schizophrenia. *Nature*, *460*(7256), 753–757. https://doi.org/10.1038/nature08192

Sieradzka, D., Power, R. A., Freeman, D., Cardno, A. G., McGuire, P., Plomin, R., Meaburn, E. L., Dudbridge, F., & Ronald, A. (2014). Are genetic risk factors for psychosis also associated with dimension-specific psychotic experiences in adolescence? *PloS one*, *9*(4), e94398. https://doi.org/10.1371/journal.pone.0094398

Simms, L. J., Wright, A. G. C., Cicero, D., Kotov, R., Mullins-Sweatt, S. N., Sellbom, M., Watson, D., Widiger, T. A., & Zimmermann, J. (2022). Development of measures for the Hierarchical Taxonomy of Psychopathology (HiTOP): A collaborative scale development project. *Assessment*, *29*(1), 3–16. https://doi.org/10.1177/10731911211015309

Slutske, W. S., Eisen, S., True, W. R., Lyons, M. J., Goldberg, J., & Tsuang, M. (2000). Common genetic vulnerability for pathological gambling and alcohol dependence in men. *Archives of General Psychiatry*, *57*(7), 666–673.

Tackett, J. L., Lahey, B. B., Hulle, C. V., Waldman, I., Krueger, R. F., & Rathouz, P. J. (2013). Common genetic influences on negative emotionality and a general psychopathology factor in childhood and adolescence. *Journal of Abnormal Psychology*, *122*(4), 1142–1153. https://doi.org/10.1037/a0034151

Taylor, M. J., Martin, J., Lu, Y., Brikell, I., Lundström, S., Larsson, H., & Lichtenstein, P. (2019). Association of genetic risk factors for psychiatric disorders and traits of these disorders in a Swedish population twin sample. *JAMA Psychiatry, 76*(3), 280–289. https://doi.org/10.1001/jamapsychiatry.2018.3652

Thapar, A., Harrington, R., & McGuffin, P. (2001). Examining the comorbidity of ADHD-related behaviours and conduct problems using a twin study design | *The British Journal of Psychiatry, 179*(3), 224–229. https://doi.org/10.1192/bjp.179.3.224

The AMD Gene Consortium. (2013). Seven new loci associated with age-related macular degeneration. *Nature Genetics, 45*(4), 433. https://doi.org/10.1038/ng.2578

Torgersen, S., Czajkowski, N., Jacobson, K., Reichborn-Kjennerud, T., Røysamb, E., Neale, M. C., & Kendler, K. S. (2008). Dimensional representations of DSM-IV cluster B personality disorders in a population-based sample of Norwegian twins: A multivariate study. *Psychological Medicine, 38*(11), 1617–1625. https://doi.org/10.1017/S0033291708002924

Torgersen, S., Myers, J., Reichborn-Kjennerud, T., Røysamb, E., Kubarych, T. S., & Kendler, K. S. (2012). The heritability of Cluster B personality disorders assessed both by personal interview and questionnaire. *Journal of Personality Disorders, 26*(6), 848–866. https://doi.org/10.1521/pedi.2012.26.6.848

Trubetskoy, V., Pardiñas, A. F., Qi, T., Panagiotaropoulou, G., Awasthi, S., Bigdeli, T. B., Bryois, J., Chen, C.-Y., Dennison, C. A., Hall, L. S., Lam, M., Watanabe, K., Frei, O., Ge, T., Harwood, J. C., Koopmans, F., Magnusson, S., Richards, A. L., Sidorenko, J., . . . O'Donovan, M. C. (2022). Mapping genomic loci implicates genes and synaptic biology in schizophrenia. *Nature, 604*(7906), 502–508. https://doi.org/10.1038/s41586-022-04434-5

Visscher, P. M., & Goddard, M. E. (2019). From R.A. Fisher's 1918 paper to GWAS a century later. *Genetics, 211*(4), 1125–1130. https://doi.org/10.1534/genetics.118.301594

Visscher, P. M., Wray, N. R., Zhang, Q., Sklar, P., McCarthy, M. I., Brown, M. A., & Yang, J. (2017). 10 Years of GWAS discovery: Biology, function, and translation. *The American Journal of Human Genetics, 101*(1), 5–22. https://doi.org/10.1016/j.ajhg.2017.06.005

Waszczuk, M. A., Jonas, K. G., Bornovalova, M., Breen, G., Bulik, C. M., Docherty, A. R., Eley, T. C., Hettema, J. M., Kotov, R., Krueger, R. F., Lencz, T., Li, J. J., Vassos, E., & Waldman, I. D. (2023). Dimensional and transdiagnostic phenotypes in psychiatric genome-wide association studies. *Molecular Psychiatry, 28*(12), 4943–4953. https://doi.org/10.1038/s41380-023-02142-8

Welter, D., MacArthur, J., Morales, J., Burdett, T., Hall, P., Junkins, H., Klemm, A., Flicek, P., Manolio, T., Hindorff, L., & Parkinson, H. (2014). The NHGRI GWAS Catalog, a curated resource of SNP-trait associations. *Nucleic Acids Research, 42*(D1), D1001–D1006. https://doi.org/10.1093/nar/gkt1229

Wray, N. R., Ripke, S., Mattheisen, M., Trzaskowski, M., Byrne, E. M., Abdellaoui, A., Adams, M. J., Agerbo, E., Air, T. M., Andlauer, T. M. F., Bacanu, S.-A., Bækvad-Hansen, M., Beekman, A. F. T., Bigdeli, T. B., Binder, E. B., Blackwood, D. R. H., Bryois, J., Buttenschøn, H. N., Bybjerg-Grauholm, J., . . . Sullivan, P. F. (2018). Genome-wide association analyses identify 44 risk variants and refine the genetic architecture of major depression. *Nature Genetics, 50*(5), 668–681. https://doi.org/10.1038/s41588-018-0090-3

Yang, J., Bakshi, A., Zhu, Z., Hemani, G., Vinkhuyzen, A. A. E., Lee, S. H., Robinson, M. R., Perry, J. R. B., Nolte, I. M., van Vliet-Ostaptchouk, J. V., Snieder, H., Esko, T., Milani, L., Mägi, R., Metspalu, A., Hamsten, A., Magnusson, P. K. E., Pedersen, N. L., Ingelsson, E., . . . Visscher, P. M. (2015). Genetic variance estimation with imputed variants finds negligible missing heritability for human height and body mass index. *Nature Genetics, 47*(10), 1114–1120. https://doi.org/10.1038/ng.3390

Yang, J., Benyamin, B., McEvoy, B. P., Gordon, S., Henders, A. K., Nyholt, D. R., Madden, P. A., Heath, A. C., Martin, N. G., Montgomery, G. W., Goddard, M. E., & Visscher, P. M. (2010). Common SNPs explain a large proportion of the heritability for human height. *Nature Genetics, 42*(7), 565–569. https://doi.org/10.1038/ng.608

Yang, J., Lee, S. H., Goddard, M. E., & Visscher, P. M. (2011). GCTA: A tool for genome-wide complex trait analysis. *The American Journal of Human Genetics, 88*(1), 76–82.

Zaso, M. J., Goodhines, P. A., Wall, T. L., & Park, A. (2019). Meta-analysis on associations of alcohol metabolism genes with alcohol use disorder in East Asians. *Alcohol and Alcoholism, 54*(3), 216–224. https://doi.org/10.1093/alcalc/agz011

Zavos, H. M. S., Freeman, D., Haworth, C. M. A., McGuire, P., Plomin, R., Cardno, A. G., & Ronald, A. (2014). Consistent etiology of severe, frequent psychotic experiences and milder, less frequent manifestations: A twin study of specific psychotic experiences in adolescence. *JAMA Psychiatry*, *71*(9), 1049–1057. https://doi.org/10.1001/jamapsychiatry.2014.994

Zheutlin, A. B., Dennis, J., Karlsson Linnér, R., Moscati, A., Restrepo, N., Straub, P., Ruderfer, D., Castro, V. M., Chen, C.-Y., Ge, T., Huckins, L. M., Charney, A., Kirchner, H. L., Stahl, E. A., Chabris, C. F., Davis, L. K., & Smoller, J. W. (2019). Penetrance and pleiotropy of polygenic risk scores for schizophrenia in 106,160 patients across four health care systems. *American Journal of Psychiatry*, *176*(10), 846–855. https://doi.org/10.1176/appi.ajp.2019.18091085

Zhou, H., Sealock, J. M., Sanchez-Roige, S., Clarke, T.-K., Levey, D. F., Cheng, Z., Li, B., Polimanti, R., Kember, R. L., Smith, R. V., Thygesen, J. H., Morgan, M. Y., Atkinson, S. R., Thursz, M. R., Nyegaard, M., Mattheisen, M., Børglum, A. D., Johnson, E. C., Justice, A. C., . . . Gelernter, J. (2020). Genome-wide meta-analysis of problematic alcohol use in 435,563 individuals yields insights into biology and relationships with other traits. *Nature Neuroscience*, *23*(7), 809–818. https://doi.org/10.1038/s41593-020-0643-5

CHAPTER 18

Computational Psychiatry and Transdiagnostic Models of Mental Disorders

Confluences and Conflicts

MICHAEL N. HALLQUIST, TIMOTHY A. ALLEN, AYSENUR OKAN, SOPHIE PAOLIZZI, AND ALEXANDRE Y. DOMBROVSKI

Introduction

Although opinions vary on how best to describe the nature of mental illness, there is widespread agreement regarding the value of a scientifically grounded nosology that informs diagnosis and treatment (Zachar & Kendler, 2017). Indeed, for many medical conditions, an accurate diagnosis goes beyond summarizing signs and symptoms by conveying information about their causes and potential treatments. For example, knowing that a patient has sickle cell disease yields an understanding of why he is anemic—a genetic mutation leads to "sickled" hemoglobin cells, which die more quickly than typical hemoglobin cells. Moreover, this diagnosis informs treatments, including modern gene therapies that edit blood stem cell DNA to reduce the likelihood of sickling in hemoglobin cells.

Yet, what is a diagnosis? Modern medicine typically proceeds from the assumption that there are distinct diseases whose biological mechanisms can be identified. Thus, a primary goal of diagnosis is to judge whether a patient's symptoms are attributable to the presence of a disease. Although this discrete disease approach has proven effective in describing and treating many conditions, its track record in describing mental illness is mixed. Inspired by successes in neurology in localizing strokes and tumors and diagnosing cell-level pathology such as Parkinson's disease, early psychiatrists such as Charcot sought to identify physiological causes of putatively distinct syndromes such as hysteria (Goetz, 2016). In contrast, Kraepelin did not view symptoms as specific to a given psychiatric disease, positing that different forms of mental illness could be delineated by characterizing symptom evolution over time (Engstrom & Kendler, 2015)[1].

Modern psychiatric classification, most recently in the DSM-5 (American Psychiatric Association, 2013), has largely extended this view, emphasizing that cognitive, emotional, and behavioral problems can be organized in terms of categorical diagnoses such as social

[1] As Engstrom and Kendler (2015) note, despite the influence of the so-called neo-Kraepelinian movement on psychiatry, Kraepelin was skeptical about whether psychiatric illness could be best described in terms of discrete diseases.

anxiety disorder or schizophrenia. Building on this, biological psychiatry was founded on the idea that mental diseases are caused by dysfunction in body systems, particularly the brain. Indeed, it is hard to argue with the notion that if an illness manifests in psychological experience and behavioral problems, then the brain is the right organ to study! Proponents of a biological perspective often go further, however, emphasizing that mental illnesses should be conceptualized as brain diseases, whereas, "diagnosis in psychiatry is based on clustering enigmatic symptoms, rather than biological ground truths" (Totah et al., 2016, p. 47).

In search of such ground truths, researchers over the past 75 years have studied numerous molecules, genes, cells, circuits, functional brain networks, and physiological indices in people diagnosed with psychiatric illness. This work has been aided by remarkable advances in biology, neuroscience, technology, and data science. For example, neuroscientists now have the ability to drive neural population activity in vivo in non-human animals using techniques like optogenetics (Fenno et al., 2011). Such approaches can identify the circuitry responsible for the effects of drugs such as ketamine (Alexander et al., 2021; Fuchikami et al., 2015). Yet, the idea that mental disorders are fundamentally brain diseases, while increasingly common (e.g., Volkow et al., 2016), encounters objections (Fried, 2022; Troisi, 2022). Moreover, many reductionist accounts of mental illness that emerged in part from pharmacological trials have failed to withstand empirical scrutiny. For example, in a recent systematic review, the widespread idea that depression is caused by a deficit in serotonin signaling received little, if any, support (Moncrieff et al., 2023).

Even as biological psychiatry and translational neuroscience have advanced our understanding of brain circuits and systems, biological approaches effective in somatic medicine such as imaging-based diagnosis have struggled to provide direct benefits to individuals with mental illness (e.g., Voineskos et al., 2024). A full examination of the challenges could easily fill the pages of another volume; here we focus on two central concerns. First, the relationship between biological systems and psychological experience is complex, thwarting efforts to connect these levels theoretically and using current technology (Huys et al., 2016). Second, the model of mental illness as a set of disorders fails to explain robust evidence of overlap between putative syndromes, as well as the continuum of symptom severity that spans from health to illness (Krueger & Markon, 2006). Motivated by these concerns, computational psychiatry has emerged as a new discipline that uses computational models and machine learning methods to connect across levels of analysis and provide more mechanistic accounts of mental illness (Montague et al., 2012). Crucially, however, the failings of categorical models of diagnosis have long been on the minds of psychopathology researchers who study the hierarchical dimensional structure of psychiatric symptoms (e.g., Watson, 2005). The broader question of how best to develop and validate a modern psychiatric nosology is considered in detail elsewhere in this volume. This chapter offers an introduction to computational psychiatry and considers the largely unrealized potential of integrating computational approaches with transdiagnostic dimensional models of psychopathology.

What Is Computational Psychiatry?

Over the past decade, computational psychiatry has become an increasingly popular term linked to numerous review papers (here is just a subset: Hitchcock et al., 2021; Huys et al., 2015, 2016; Montague et al., 2012; Stephan & Mathys, 2014; Wiecki et al., 2015), funding opportunities (e.g., through the National Institute of Mental Health's Translational Digital and Computational Psychiatry Program), and training programs (e.g., the Translational Neuromodeling Unit's Computational Psychiatry Course, hosted annually in Zürich since 2015). Yet, it is difficult to answer succinctly the question, "What is computational psychiatry?"

Computational psychiatry uses analytic tools and conceptual frameworks from cognitive neuroscience, computer science, and decision science to understand mental computations in psychopathology (Huys et al., 2016). The goal of these endeavors is to uncover complex brain-behavior relationships using advanced mathematical and computational approaches, particularly those that traditional methods might miss.

Computationally intensive approaches have been proposed to address the four central goals of psychological science, namely: description (e.g., Patzelt et al., 2018), explanation (e.g., Brown et al., 2018), prediction (e.g., Weigard et al., 2023), and classification (e.g., Kaczkurkin et al., 2020). With respect to description and classification, some computational psychiatry advocates have argued that psychiatry erred in focusing primarily on observable signs and symptoms of illness (inspired in part by Kraepelin). Perhaps instead we could describe illness in terms of "computational phenotypes," the parameters of computational model fit to neural and/or behavioral data that putatively quantify cognitive mechanisms (Montague et al., 2012; Patzelt et al., 2018). This could be achieved by developing batteries of experimental tasks and neurobiological assays that are married with validated computational models to provide the mechanistic glue between brain and behavior. This view also aligns broadly with psychopathology research that uses intermediate phenotypes (e.g., neurobiological measures or cognitive indices) to bridge between observable disease characteristics and the hypothesized causes of disease (Cuthbert, 2014).

Although it is appealing to imagine a descriptive taxonomy of psychopathology based on cognitive mechanisms that are causally linked to signs and symptoms, the field is still far from reaching this goal. In practice, most studies of computational phenotypes have relied on parameter estimates from a preferred model fit to a single experiment. To advance a taxonomy that incorporates computational phenotypes, more focused studies of convergent and construct validity must be conducted that incorporate many models and experimental tasks (for a more detailed treatment of this topic, see Karvelis et al., 2023). Nevertheless, extant studies of computational phenotypes can support the goal of explanation by testing theory-related computational models that account for relationships among brain, cognition, and behavior. As we detail in the next section, explanatory computational approaches seek to provide formal mathematical accounts of the processes that generate behavior and cognition in psychopathology.

Prediction approaches in computational psychiatry support the complementary goal of statistically linking a large array of markers—from computational phenotypes to biological indices to self-reported traits—with clinical outcomes. The intention here is to understand *how* various measures are related to psychopathology without necessarily understanding *why* this is so. As discussed below, prediction-focused studies often build on machine learning methods that can combine large, multimodal data to form predictions regarding diagnosis, prognosis, or important clinical outcomes. Although psychological science has long prioritized explanatory approaches, there is increasing recognition that many putatively explanatory studies focus on the fit of a model to sample data without seeking to predict future outcomes or behavior in an independent sample (Yarkoni & Westfall, 2017). Additionally, predicting clinical outcomes—for example, how well a treatment will work for a particular patient (Webb et al., 2019)—is often valuable even if we lack a clear explanation for how a prediction was derived.

Although computational psychiatry broadly involves computationally intensive methods, its dual emphasis on explanation and prediction is confounding. Whereas explanatory approaches ultimately seek to test models of cognitive and neural processes that could specify the causes of mental illness in terms of neural computations, predictive approaches are better suited to forecasting clinical outcomes. Bennett and colleagues (2019) have referred to this divide as the "two cultures" of computational psychiatry, noting that explanatory and predictive approaches serve different, but important, goals (also see Huys et al., 2016). In the following section, we consider the contribution of each culture to understanding psychopathology, as well as their relations to transdiagnostic dimensional models.

Explanatory Approaches in Computational Psychiatry

Measures of systematic, stable individual differences that underlie human behavior go back to 19th-century studies of intelligence and memory (Ebbinghaus, 1913; Galton, 1883). Yet, after 150 years of research, cognitive performance measures still capture only a final behavioral outcome, not the process that led to it. Some performance measures are easier to interpret than others: For example, working memory capacity can be related to neural dynamics in frontoparietal networks (Jacob et al., 2018). A measure of working memory may help diagnose dementia, but otherwise offers no insight into why buffer size varies among individuals, to say nothing of individual differences in its neural implementation.

Turning to psychopathology, performance on cognitive tasks does little to explain phenomena seen in the clinic—anxious avoidance, lack of energy, delusions, binge-eating, or interpersonal aggression—or broader dimensions of psychopathology such as detachment or antagonism. On the other hand, data-driven models of individual differences are often hard to interpret and unlikely to advance our mechanistic understanding of functional neuroanatomy and neurophysiology. For example, models of functional connectivity between brain regions can predict psychological traits but do not capture the information represented in trait-predicting regions or connections (Kriegeskorte & Douglas, 2018), thus offering limited insight into *how* traits are determined. Such insights require process models founded on a theory that specifies the sources of these individual differences.

Psychiatrists and psychologists have long seen value in studying the processes involved in psychopathology. Kendler (2008, p. 696) summarized this motivation well: "Our task is to clarify the mechanisms that underlie and have an impact on central mind/brain processes such as mood, perception, belief formation, and hedonic processes so that we can understand the causal processes whereby they become disordered in psychiatric illness." For example, Freud (1923) proposed that illness emerges from unconscious conflicts originating in early development that could be revealed through psychoanalysis, while early behaviorists linked anxiety to Pavlovian fear conditioning (Jones, 1924). As noted in the previous section, biological psychiatry has approached the questions of mechanisms in terms of the development and function of brain systems associated with illness.

Computational psychiatry addresses these questions by building mathematical models that simulate mental processes thought to underlie behavioral and neural dysfunction. In this section, we consider generative modeling approaches to understanding internalizing psychopathology, psychosis, and antagonism. Although the form of generative models varies, they share an emphasis on specifying the latent processes and dynamics that map inputs—primarily sensory information—to relevant outputs—typically, behavior or neural activity. Crucially, such models are generative because they can simulate plausible outputs (e.g., behavior) based on essentially the same inputs provided to subjects in the laboratory. If a model generates data that closely mirror empirical observations, it provides a plausible explanation of the cognitive or biological mechanisms involved. Model-building requires researchers to attend to many technical considerations including identification, parameter estimation, model recovery, and model comparison. We have elected to keep our treatment of generative models largely at the conceptual level, but readers interested in implementing these models are encouraged to review literature on this topic (Forstmann & Wagenmakers, 2015; Hallquist & Dombrovski, 2020; He et al., 2020; Wilson & Collins, 2019).

To build generative models, computational cognitive neuroscience has historically focused on pragmatic problems that an organism must solve, such as visual perception, movement control, or—of relevance to psychopathology—behavioral adaptation to maximize rewards and minimize punishments (Forstmann & Wagenmakers, 2015). David Marr noted that these problems can be evaluated productively across three levels, namely the computational (the general problem, e.g., maximizing food rewards), algorithmic (a set of steps or procedures, e.g., incremental learning from reinforcement), and implementational (instantiation of this algorithm in a biological system, e.g., dopaminergic meso-striatal circuit). Computational theory is essential if we want to move beyond simple descriptions of neural and behavioral data. As Marr says in his 1982 book, *Vision*: "trying to understand perception by studying only neurons is like trying to understand bird flight by studying only feathers . . . we have to understand aerodynamics; only then do the structure of feathers and the different shapes of birds' wings make sense" (Marr, 1982, p. 27). By extension, Marr's levels provide a useful framework for considering how high-level goals (computational level), specific cognitive processes (algorithmic level), and biological systems (implementational level) each contribute to maladaptive patterns of thinking and behavior.

Reinforcement learning (RL) is a prototypical generative model, and here we discuss how RL models can capture individual differences and dimensions of psychopathology. RL algorithms have been widely successful in explaining behavior across many learning paradigms and have provided important insights into signals in the dopaminergic meso-striatal system (Gureckis & Love, 2015). Moreover, many psychiatric symptoms and pathological behaviors point to maladaptive learning from rewards and aversive stimuli (Halahakoon et al., 2020; Ng et al., 2019). We then review the contributions of explanatory computational psychiatry approaches to understanding internalizing psychopathology and psychosis, concluding with an illustrative example of explanatory models in relation to antagonism.

Reinforcement Learning. RL models learn to maximize gains and minimize losses in an environment without being explicitly instructed on what actions are right or wrong. They do so by integrating the unfolding experience of rewards and punishments into learned values of actions or stimuli, which approximate the true expected reward or punishment rate. The three basic components of RL models are a representation of the environment, a learning rule, and a policy or choice rule.

Most RL models simplify decision problems by considering current values of actions or stimuli, rather than representing more remote experiences (e.g., using an episodic buffer). The agent's interaction with the environment is viewed as a Markov decision process (MDP), in which in each state (e.g., a rat's position in a maze) the agent chooses an action (e.g., move left) taking it to the next state (position). Rewards (finding the cheese) and consequently the actions to obtain them depend only on the current state and are conditionally independent of the preceding sequence of states. We can also imagine a more intuitive example: Upon the patron sitting down at a restaurant, the waiter first offers a choice between two unfamiliar wines, let's say Riesling and Zinfandel. Based on the action (wine) selected, one transitions to a new state in which new actions become available (e.g., ordering the appetizer). Thus, it may be useful to distinguish the Riesling-ordered state from the Zinfandel-ordered state, because smoked mackerel may be great with Riesling but have a metallic taste with Zinfandel. Our restaurant MDP has a reward function, which we can simply define as the taste (from bad to good) of menu items or, if we want to be realistic, a weighted sum of taste, quantity, and healthfulness minus the price, a negative reward.

Having assigned distinct action values to menu items, we must update these values based on experience, using a learning rule. Many RL models use the delta rule, which in the restaurant example may be written as:

$$Q_{\text{Riesling}}(t+1) = \begin{cases} Q_{\text{Riesling}}(t) + \alpha\left[r(t) - Q_{\text{Riesling}}(t)\right] & \text{if action}(t) = \text{Riesling} \\ Q_{\text{Riesling}}(t) & \text{if action}(t) = \text{Zinfandel} \end{cases}$$

$$Q_{\text{Zinfandel}}(t+1) = \begin{cases} Q_{\text{Zinfandel}}(t) + \alpha\left[r(t) - Q_{\text{Zinfandel}}(t)\right] & \text{if action}(t) = \text{Zinfandel} \\ Q_{\text{Zinfandel}}(t) & \text{if action}(t) = \text{Riesling} \end{cases}$$

For simplicity, let t represent the current meal at the restaurant, $t + 1$ being the next meal, and $r(t)$, the taste reward. The update of an action value estimate, Q_{Riesling} or $Q_{\text{Zinfandel}}$, depends on the *learning rate* parameter, α, bounded between zero and one, which scales the effect of the discrepancy between the reinforcement received, $r(t)$, and the expected reinforcement, $Q(t)$. This discrepancy, $r(t) - Q(t)$, is the prediction error, and reflects the magnitude and direction of surprise, indicating how unexpected the outcome was. As one gains experience in a stable environment, prediction errors diminish as one's expectations approach the true expected values of the actions.

Finally, our RL model needs a policy to map states and their values onto choices. If one likes Zinfandel better than Riesling, should one always order Zinfandel? And what if one has never tried Riesling before? Generally, should one always take advantage of or exploit the currently preferred option or explore alternatives that may look less attractive now but may prove superior in the future? To balance exploration versus exploitation, policies must be stochastic (i.e., probabilistic rather than deterministic). A simple stochastic policy is ε-greedy, which allocates a fixed proportion of choices, ε, to exploring (here, trying less preferred or unfamiliar drinks), exploiting the preferred option (Zinfandel) the rest of the time. For example, if we set ε to 0.1, then one would order Zinfandel on 90% of meals and Riesling (or another, unfamiliar drink) on the remaining 10%. However, if one definitely dislikes Riesling, why order it at all? The softmax policy not only exploits preferred actions, but, unlike ε-greedy, also avoids non-preferred ones, weighting choice probabilities by action values:

$$p(\text{action}(t) = i) = \frac{\exp(Q_i / \beta)}{\sum_{j=1}^{J} \exp(Q_j / \beta)}$$

In our restaurant example, i would denote one of the possible actions (e.g., Zinfandel) and J, all available actions: $J = \{\text{Zinfandel, Riesling}\}$. The temperature parameter β controls the exploration rate: at higher temperatures, alternative options approach equiprobability (more exploratory). At lower temperatures, the probability of the best option approaches one (more exploitative).

How Can Generative Models Help Us Understand Dimensions of Psychopathology and Individual Differences in General? Computational psychiatry researchers have used generative models in three ways to understand individual differences in psychopathology. The first is to relate individual differences in model parameters, such as the learning rate in RL, to symptom dimensions or diagnoses. The second is to argue that different people rely on different computational models (algorithms), either by estimating the posterior probability that a given model best characterizes a person's behavior or by allowing for variation in mixing parameters that blend cognitive processes (e.g., relative reliance on a working memory-like buffer versus a slowly evolving representation of learned value). The third approach tests the degree to which model-predicted signals (e.g., reward prediction errors) correspond to dynamics of neural activity, including how such relationships relate to features of psychopathology.

The first two approaches are conceptually distinct, yet both rely directly on the estimation of model parameters, usually from behavioral data. While the direct approach is intuitive and transparent, it depends heavily on how accurately the model captures the neural or behavioral processes that vary between individuals. And since our closed-form models are heuristic approximations of the mechanisms underlying observed behavior, this correspondence is often uncertain, particularly with complex processes such as learning. The free parameters of generative models offer a formal perspective on individual differences in behavior. For example, higher learning rates in RL models push the representation of value toward the latest reinforcement relative to the preceding reinforcement history. Moreover, the parameters of the choice process are often easy to interpret—for example, lower temperature parameters are associated with a stronger preference for high-value options—whereas learning parameters such as learning rate shape how the model's hidden states (e.g., subjective value) evolve, so their interpretation is contingent on those dynamics. However, most generative models offer no formal account of the mechanisms that set their free parameters. Thus, by conceptualizing individual differences as free parameters of a computational model, we specify the cognitive or behavioral mechanism subject to individual differences but not the mechanism that gives rise to them.

The third approach employs the generative model as an analytic tool to uncover individual differences in physiological and neural processes. For example, in a neuroimaging study of reward learning in people with and without depressive symptoms, a researcher could compare the effects of model-derived prediction errors on striatal fMRI signals across individuals, relating them to depression symptom severity (Dombrovski et al., 2015). Estimating the extent to which neural dynamics in a person's brain conform to idealized learning dynamics predicted by the model, we obtain an individual neural index of reward learning. In addition to mapping individual differences to anatomical structures (or bands of cortical oscillations), this approach can compare the fit of various models to neural data at individual and group levels. One caveat with this approach is its interpretative flexibility, where weaker brain-model correspondences in people with clinical traits can be seen as evidence of disrupted computation and stronger brain-model correspondences, as evidence of inefficient computation (cf. Poldrack, 2015). Further, individual differences in the scaling or variance of model-predicted signals such as prediction errors—often due to differences in individual parameter estimates—may induce spurious differences in the strength of model-brain relationships across people (Lebreton et al., 2019). The gravity of this problem has been debated (Katahira & Toyama, 2021; Wilson & Niv, 2015), but it can be mitigated by conducting sensitivity analyses and using sample mean computational model parameter estimates for individual differences analyses.

Reinforcement Learning Models in the Study of Internalizing Psychopathology. Early studies using the first of the aforementioned approaches, parameter estimation, suggested that people with depression and specifically anhedonia (decreased positive affect) display lower learning rates or reward sensitivity (Chase et al., 2010; Dombrovski et al., 2010; Huys et al., 2013). Results of subsequent larger studies proved to be heterogeneous, although diminished appetitive learning is often selectively associated with anhedonia (Brown et al., 2021; Mukherjee et al., 2020). Parameters sensitive to depression vary by task and sample, and the most consistent parameter alteration observed in depressed people is higher choice temperature, a marker of generally poorer learning performance (meta-analysis reported in Pike & Robinson, 2022). Another set of parameter estimation studies sought to explain anxious avoidance in terms of uncertainty aversion or, in RL terms, lower exploration of uncertain options. Findings were again mixed (Aberg et al., 2022; Charpentier et al., 2022; Krypotos et al., 2022;

Morriss et al., 2021; Smith et al., 2022; Zbozinek et al., 2021). Some depression studies took the alternative approach, examining the extent to which RL model-derived reward prediction errors (RPEs) modulated striatal responses. While early studies found blunted striatal RPE responses (Gradin et al., 2011; Kumar et al., 2008), subsequent findings varied across tasks and samples (Dombrovski et al., 2015; Kumar et al., 2018; Rutledge et al., 2017; Ubl et al., 2015). Altogether, these conflicting studies portray a field in need of better descriptive models of psychopathology as we argued above, as well as improved methods for fitting models to individual behavior (Brown et al., 2020), larger samples (Marek et al., 2022; Szucs & Ioannidis, 2017), and, most important, new theoretical insights and formal models that afford a better conceptual match to the aspects of psychopathology they seek to explain (Brown et al., 2023). Finally, almost all extant studies failed to distinguish pathological traits from within-person state changes, tacitly implying that these would have the same neurobehavioral underpinnings. Formal models of within-person evolution of learning and affect and intensive longitudinal studies (Eldar et al., 2018) are needed to test this assumption.

Psychoticism and Models of Perceptual Inference. Descriptive psychopathology has long considered psychosis as a disruption of inference processes (Jaspers, 1913). More recently, computational psychiatry researchers have suggested that the positive symptoms of psychosis—delusions and hallucinations—involve an altered precision of prior beliefs relative to sensory input data (reviewed in Sterzer et al., 2018). In Bayesian models of perception, cortical networks integrate noisy perceptual inputs with prior expectations or inputs from other modalities to make inferences about the environment (Knill & Pouget, 2004; Ma, 2012; Pouget et al., 2013). These models draw on Helmholtz's (1860) idea of filling in visual information to make sense of a scene and Bruner's (1947) concept of top-down influences on perception. In a hierarchy of representations, lower levels receive ever-changing noisy perceptual inputs whereas at higher levels representations are increasingly abstract and stable. Predictive coding is an influential formal treatment of such perceptual systems that specifies how prior representations from upper levels provide top-down predictive inputs, and discrepancies between these predictions and bottom-up sensory signals trigger prediction error updates across the hierarchy (Huang & Rao, 2011).

Hallucinatory experiences—even without clinical psychosis—may involve abnormally strong perceptual priors (Powers et al., 2017). Delusions, on the other hand, may emerge from weak perceptual priors (Corlett et al., 2010) and persist through increased memory consolidation and abnormally strong priors at the highest levels. These hypotheses can be tested using generative models of perception, paired with neural data to understand the role of different circuits in perceptual aberrations. For example, Schmack and colleagues (2021) recently paired an auditory detection experiment with a Bayesian computational model of belief-updating to reveal that elevated dopamine levels in the striatum prior to an auditory stimulus were associated with hallucination-like false alarms. The computational model confirmed that these false detections occurred when prior expectations (of a sound) outweighed sensory input.

Illustrative Example of an Explanatory Approach in Computational Psychiatry: Antagonism and Models of Social Perception and Cooperation

Computational models have also been used to understand individual differences in human social behavior. As an example of an explanatory approach in computational psychiatry, we examine whether differences in the traits of callousness and exploitativeness can be explained by how individuals learn to cooperate during social exchanges. For further details on this study, please see the published manuscript and supplement (Allen et al., 2024). Below, we introduce the scientific background, describe our experimental procedure, and show how a neurocomputational approach can help to build mechanistic theories of the structure of personality and psychopathology.

Scientific Motivation. Humans began living in loose social groups over 50 million years ago to harness the benefits of collective foraging, rearing, and defense (Shultz et al., 2011). The computational demands imposed by this new social environment likely contributed to a rapid expansion of the cortex and the emergence of sophisticated social cognitive abilities (Dunbar, 2009). Nonetheless, there remain important individual differences in the extent to which humans cooperate with one another, in part because defection can be advantageous so long as it remains rare, and the few defectors deal mostly with cooperative counterparts (Avilés, 2002). In contemporary dimensional models of psychopathology, individual differences in cooperation are captured by a trait known as antagonism versus agreeableness, which encompasses two lower-order facets: callousness versus compassion and exploitativeness versus politeness (Allen & DeYoung, 2017). Compassion-callousness reflects empathy and generosity as opposed to cruelty and indifference, whereas politeness-exploitativeness reflects honesty and humility as opposed to selfishness and manipulativeness (Allen et al., 2020). Interestingly, callousness is associated with inferior social cognition, whereas the opposite is true of exploitativeness (Allen et al., 2017). We examined whether callousness and exploitativeness are differentially related to neural and learning processes that allow us to predict others' cooperative behavior during social interactions, a basic form of social cognition.

How do humans decide whether to cooperate in social interactions? If you are like us, the holiday season brings a familiar dilemma every year: should I buy that neighbor down the street a present, or are we not that close (Figure 18.1A)? To make this decision, you probably consider information from at least two different sources. First, you might weigh the person's reputation: does the neighborhood gossip portray them as generous or tightfisted? Second, you might consider your direct experience with the neighbor: Did they lend you a ladder last time you needed one, or buy you a gift last year? The stakes are high, because if one party purchases a gift and the other does not, the result can be embarrassment, shame, or even feelings of rejection. However, if you assume the neighbor will not buy you a gift and you are right, then you might walk away relieved at having correctly inferred the nature of the relationship, even though you received no present! This example shows how, in social interactions, it can be reinforcing to correctly predict others' cooperation (or lack thereof). In RL terms, the strategy one employs when trying to make such cooperation/defection decisions is called a "policy." In previous work, we found that learning signals in the striatum and default network track the expected return (value) of one's interpersonal policy: neural activation increased following both correctly anticipated cooperation and defection (Vanyukov et al., 2019; Fig. 7).

The default network—encompassing the medial prefrontal cortex, posterior cingulate, inferior parietal lobule, and medial and lateral temporal regions (Andrews-Hanna et al., 2014; Buckner et al., 2008)—is a strong candidate for encoding learning signals that track the value of one's policy toward others. This network expanded disproportionately with the evolution of social living (Buckner & Krienen, 2013; Hill et al., 2010), and both its structure and connectivity scale with the size of an individual's social network (Noonan et al., 2018). Activity of the default network has also been linked to agreeableness and to performance on standard social cognition tasks (Allen et al., 2017; Udochi et al., 2022).

In this study, we tested the hypothesis that callousness and exploitativeness would be differentially associated with learning signals tracking the value of one's interpersonal policy

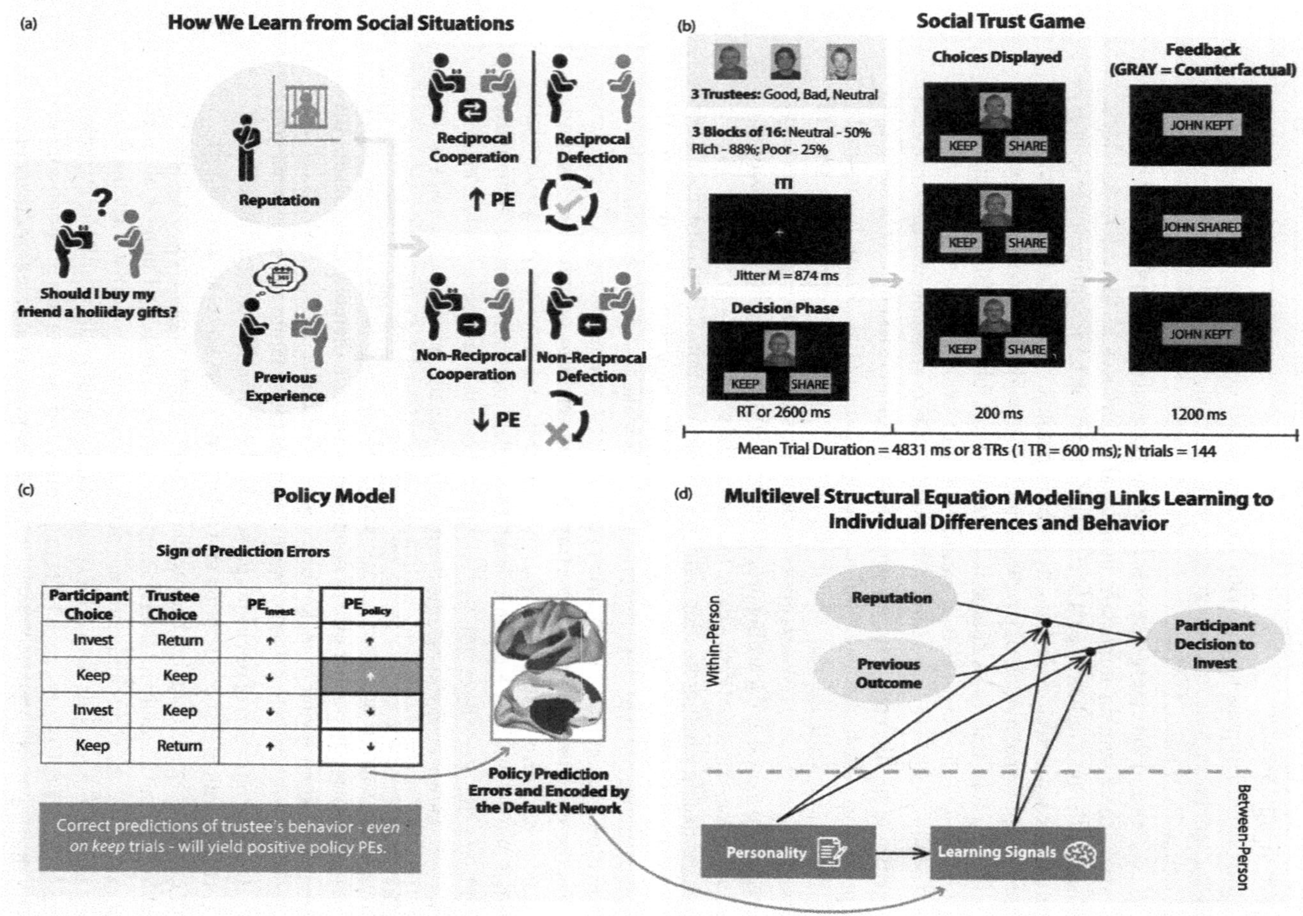

FIGURE 18.1 Rationale, design, and analytic approach. Individuals learn from experience by selecting an action, observing its outcome, and updating the expected reward value of future actions. Value updates are made using prediction errors (PEs), which reflect the discrepancy between expected and obtained outcomes such that better-than-expected outcomes lead to positive PEs and worse-than-expected outcomes lead to negative PEs. Other salient social information can also be integrated with experience to influence social decision-making, as when the reputation of one's partner predicts decisions to trust them even when reputation is unrelated to the partner's actual behavior.

during a modified social trust task in which participants used reputational information and previous experience to guide cooperative decision-making. We expected that these learning signals, encoded within the default network, would explain the relationship among callousness, exploitativeness, and trial-level reciprocity (i.e., reciprocal cooperation or reciprocal defection) on the task. We tested these hypotheses in a sample of 168 participants, 113 of whom were diagnosed with borderline personality disorder, ensuring that we included callousness and exploitativeness in the clinical range.

Modified Social Trust Task (Figure 18.1B). Participants interacted with three different trustees of varying reputation (good, bad, neutral). In each exchange, participants received $1.00, which they could elect to either keep or invest (i.e., share) with the trustee. If participants chose to keep, they retained their dollar. If participants chose to invest, the outcome was contingent on the trustee: if the trustee returned, the participant received $1.50, whereas if the trustee kept, they were left with nothing. Trustees returned 50% of the time at the start of each interaction, but then became very untrustworthy (returning 25% of the time) and then very trustworthy (88%), or vice versa. By manipulating the reinforcement rate in this way, we were able to observe individual differences in how participants responded to social feedback (i.e., learning). Critically, participants were shown the trustee's decision even if they chose to keep the $1.00, which allowed them to experience predicted defections (as when your decision not to buy the neighbor a gift is reinforced by them not buying you one, either). Behaviorally, we found that participants were more likely to share with the good and neutral trustees than with the bad trustee, though this effect was dampened in individuals high on callousness. This is consistent with literature showing that callousness is related to a broad insensitivity to social signals (Brislin et al., 2018). Importantly, there was also a robust reciprocity effect on the task, such that participants were more likely to share if the trustee had returned on the preceding trial.

Generative Computational Model: The Policy Model (Figure 18.1C). We considered several computational RL models, all of which extended Q-learning, updating the expected value of investing on a given trial:

$$Q(invest)_t = Q(invest)_{t-1} + \alpha\left[\text{reward}_t - Q(invest)_{t-1}\right]$$

where α is the learning rate parameter and $\text{reward}_t - Q(invest)_{t-1}$ is the prediction error. Choices were modeled using a softmax function that included four free parameters:

$$p(invest)_t = \frac{1}{1 + \exp\left[\kappa_s + \kappa_{t(good)} + \kappa_{t(bad)} + \beta Q(invest)_t\right]}$$

β is a temperature parameter capturing choice stochasticity, κ_s is a participant-level parameter that reflects a general bias to invest (vs. keep) regardless of reinforcement history, and $\kappa_{t(good)}$ and $\kappa_{t(bad)}$ represent the shift in the participant's sharing observed with the good and bad trustees relative to the neutral trustee. Critically, we tested competing models that differed in how they represented outcomes (i.e., rewards) in a payoff matrix (trustee decision x participant decision; Figure 18.1C). Bayesian comparison supported a "policy model," which tracked the participant's interpersonal policy toward the trustee, distinguishing itself by assigning a positive reward value to trials in which participants correctly predicted a trustee's defection compared to trials with incorrect defection predictions. This means that when participants correctly predicted the trustee's defection, we expected them to experience a positive prediction error, reflecting a better-than-expected outcome. This contrasts with a more traditional

RL model that tracks actual rewards, in which any defection is indicative of a lower reward rate and would be expected to generate a negative prediction error.

We then extracted participant-level parameter estimates from the policy model and related them to individual differences in personality. We found that antagonistic individuals were slower to update the value of investing based on trustee's choices, as reflected in a lower learning rate. Moreover, callousness was positively associated with the κ_t parameter for the bad trustee, which converged with our behavioral analyses showing that callous individuals were less sensitive to the effects of reputation.

Next, in model-based fMRI analyses, we tested the relationship of prediction error (PE) signals from the policy model with whole-brain BOLD activity. We found signed policy prediction errors in the canonical reward network (i.e., ventral and dorsal striatum, putamen), but also throughout the brain's default network.

From Trait to rain to Behavior. How do policy prediction errors relate to personality and behavior? To answer this question, we used multilevel structural equation modeling, a flexible latent variable modeling technique that allows for the simultaneous examination of multiple predictors and outcomes in hierarchically structured data (Sadikaj et al., 2019). Specifically, we tested whether policy PE signals in the default network mediated the effect of callousness and/or exploitativeness on decisions to reciprocate during the trust game. We found that PEs in the default network were differentially related to callousness and exploitativeness, and positively related to reciprocity on the task (Figure 18.1D). Further, blunted policy PEs accounted for the association between callousness and lower reciprocal cooperation, whereas amplified policy PEs accounted for the association between exploitativeness and higher reciprocal cooperation.

Our findings demonstrate how computational modeling of trait-relevant behavioral processes can enrich neurobiological dimensional models of psychopathology, explaining how lower-order traits emerge from higher-order factors. By focusing on latent cognitive processes, such as policy prediction errors in social learning, we identified mechanisms distinguishing callousness from exploitativeness, providing a theoretical and biological basis for their divergence from higher-order antagonism. We gained further confidence in our account by evaluating its predictions in behavioral data, neural activity, and comparative model performance. Altogether, this example highlights how dimensional models can provide a road map for computational inquiries by highlighting important patterns of covariance in traits and symptoms. In turn, computational approaches support formal theories of traits and symptoms, offering external validation for dimensional models across levels of analysis.

Prediction Approaches in Computational Psychiatry

Explanatory approaches are fundamentally tied to the premise that the complexity of mental illness can be reduced across levels of analysis (behavior, cognitive process, neural system, etc.) using formal models that specify how dynamics at one level are connected to adjacent levels (this relates to reductionism in neuroscience more generally; Craver, 2001). Such approaches have proven remarkably productive in molecular biology and other basic sciences. For example, understanding mutations of the CFTR gene at the molecular level has greatly advanced our understanding of *why* the symptoms of cystic fibrosis (e.g., the buildup of thick mucus) occur and has guided the development of targeted treatments that directly improve the function of the CFTR protein, dramatically improving respiratory function (Despotes & Donaldson, 2022). Yet, genomic studies of mental illness consistently reveal that both symptom dimensions and categorical diagnoses are influenced by many genetic variants of small effect and that genetic associations often overlap substantially across disorders (O'Donovan & Owen, 2016). Moreover, psychiatric symptoms are multidetermined, spanning social, environmental, lifestyle, genomic, and biological influences (Lynch et al., 2021). In view of this complexity, psychological researchers increasingly embrace the reality that mental illness is typically the product of interactions among many interdependent dynamic systems at different levels of analysis (Fried & Robinaugh, 2020; Kendler, 2019).

Whereas explanatory approaches in computational psychiatry seek to clarify the nature of such interactions, prediction approaches focus more on the outcomes of these interactions. Many efforts to date aim to predict clinically relevant outcomes, such as suicide risk (Su et al., 2020) or treatment response (Chekroud et al., 2016) using a large array of predictors. Machine learning techniques aid these efforts by generating robust, generalizable predictions from complex, high-dimensional data (for a didactic introduction to this topic, see Coutanche & Hallion, 2020). Recent reviews have highlighted the promise of machine learning in handling large, multimodal datasets with inter-correlated features (Bzdok & Meyer-Lindenberg, 2018; Chekroud et al., 2021; Yarkoni & Westfall, 2017).

Importantly, machine learning prediction approaches are not cleanly separated from more conventional methods such as linear regression (Iniesta et al., 2016). For example, we might use bivariate correlation to find the association between depression severity and the size of the hippocampus, or use multiple regression to consider whether hippocampal versus amygdala volume is a stronger predictor. However, as the number of predictors increases substantially (sometimes called the "$p \gg n$" problem, where p is the number of predictors and n is the number of observations), conventional methods quickly break down, often overfitting the sample data and producing predictions that do not generalize to new datasets (Hastie et al., 2009). In addition, when researchers lack a clear theory for which of many possible variables should be included, or even what prediction method is best, they may fall prey to overusing "researcher degrees of freedom" in exploring the data, undermining reproducibility (Whelan & Garavan, 2014). The difficulties are especially prevalent in the era of big data, where many datasets include whole-brain activity, behavior, daily experience, personality traits, electronic health records, and so on (Gillan & Whelan, 2017).

Although machine learning approaches vary widely in their objectives, we focus particularly on high-dimensional prediction algorithms that can largely be thought of as extensions of regression that accommodate many predictors and many outcomes. Exemplars include variants of regularized regression such as elastic net, least absolute shrinkage and selection operator (LASSO), and ridge regression (Hastie et al., 2009). These methods are particularly well suited to predicting clinical outcomes in rich datasets where (a) we have only weak causal evidence linking a given predictor and the outcome, and/or (b) where we believe the outcome is influenced by many predictors. Returning to the example above, we might reason that if the brain is the most important organ to study in mental illness, then we should use as many brain indices as possible in predicting a clinical outcome such as depression severity. Yet, if we enter, say, MRI-based volume measurements of hundreds of brain regions into a standard regression model, we are likely to overfit the noise and produce an inflated (i.e., overly optimistic) prediction.

Regularized regression models address the problem of overfitting by penalizing coefficient estimates for each predictor, shifting them toward zero. Although the technical details are beyond the scope of this chapter, coefficient penalization helps to automate feature selection (i.e., determine which subset of predictors is best) and reduces overfitting by discouraging large coefficients and model complexity (a detailed introduction is provided in Hastie et al., 2009). In addition, these models are typically paired with internal cross-validation to increase the generalizability of their predictions. This procedure involves splitting the dataset into "training" and "test" subsets. Then, model parameters are estimated on the training data alone. This best-fitting model is then tasked with predicting the outcome of interest in the "unseen" test dataset. This process is repeated until the set of parameters that minimizes cross-validation error, rather than fit to the training data, is found. More complex versions of this process, such as *k*-fold cross-validation, allow all data to be used for both training and test data by dividing the data into *k* number of folds, and training the model *k* times (Coutanche & Hallion, 2020). Each time, a different fold is used for the test set and the others as the training set. Altogether, regularization and cross-validation are two essential components of computational psychiatry prediction approaches that reduce the influence of researcher degrees of freedom and increase generalizability.

Compared to explanatory approaches, most prediction models de-emphasize the importance of any one variable, instead focusing on how well a set of features predicts relevant outcomes. For example, we could ask whether the prediction of incident suicide attempts in a longitudinal study is aided by including functional connectivity among 100 brain regions measured at baseline, relative to symptom measures alone. Or, consider the recent findings of Shafiei and colleagues (2024), who found that the pattern of functional connectivity among 400 brain regions predicted variation in borderline personality disorder features and that more predictive regions were also more likely to change as a function of age. The goal of such analyses is often not to derive an explanatory model of which brain regions, clinical measures, or computational indices are most closely related to a clinical outcome, but instead to show the overall value of some data modality (e.g., computational model parameters) for producing robust predictions. Finally, proponents of machine learning in psychiatry suggest that robust prediction algorithms could forecast outcomes for the *individual* (Bzdok & Meyer-Lindenberg, 2018; Monosov et al., 2024; Rutledge et al., 2019) using intensively sampled personal data or observations across people (though see Molenaar, 2004).

Predicting Treatment Outcomes. Machine learning approaches have already demonstrated promise for predicting treatment selection and response. Initial reviews and meta-analyses highlight several cases in which prediction algorithms can forecast treatment response and illness remission reliably above chance (Lee et al., 2018; Sajjadian et al., 2021). For example, using elastic net regression, Iniesta and colleagues (2018) combined genetic and clinical data to predict individual differences in the response to escitalopram (an antidepressant) for depression. Interestingly, the best models differed for escitalopram versus nortriptyline, suggesting that such algorithms may be able to inform antidepressant selection. As another treatment example, in a large dataset from college counseling centers, Kilcullen and colleagues (2021) used LASSO regression to identify which psychotherapy clients were likely to return for additional courses of therapy, finding that factors like initial duration of therapy, academic distress, and social anxiety predicted the likelihood of seeking additional treatment.

Predicting Psychiatric Symptoms from Other Measures and Domains. Another prototypical prediction approach in computational psychiatry is the use of non-clinical variables to predict clinical outcomes, such as the prediction of borderline personality symptoms from brain functional connectivity data mentioned above. The goal of such analyses is often to demonstrate that neurocognitive, neurobiological, or ambulatory data can predict symptom dimensions (or diagnosis) in isolation, or in addition to other clinical variables. For example, we may believe that neurocognition is fundamental to the development of attention deficit hyperactivity disorder (ADHD) symptoms (Pievsky & McGrath, 2018), yet we may not know whether variation in ADHD symptoms can be adequately decoded from a battery of neurocognitive tests. In a large sample of youth, Weigard and colleagues (2023) used regularized regression models to test whether ADHD symptoms could be prospectively predicted from a large set of measures encompassing neurocognition, demographics, and family and child characteristics. By looking at the feature weights from these models (analogous to partial regression coefficients), they found that neurocognitive measures contributed to ADHD prediction above and beyond more conventional measures such as self-reported impulsivity.

Integrating Computational Psychiatry and Hierarchical Dimensional Models of Psychopathology

Categorical approaches to psychiatric diagnosis have been useful in clinical and research settings, enhancing communication among healthcare providers, researchers, patients, and their families by using standardized terminology. Furthermore, categorical systems provide a common framework for diagnosis and assist in matching patients with evidence-based treatments (Lilienfeld & Treadway, 2016). Despite their utility, categorical approaches to diagnosing psychopathology have major shortcomings. They tend to oversimplify the complexity of mental health disorders and fail to account for the dimensional structure of psychopathology (Borsboom, 2008). Detailed critiques of categorical models can be found elsewhere in this volume (also see Lilienfeld & Treadway, 2016; Widiger & Sankis, 2000), but suffice it to say that these approaches suffer from at least five serious challenges: (1) symptom heterogeneity within people who share a diagnosis; (2) surprisingly high levels of diagnostic co-occurrence; (3) unclear boundaries between health and illness; (4) limited evidence of diagnosis-treatment specificity; and (5) remarkably overlapping genetic and neurobiological risk factors (Goodkind et al., 2015; O'Donovan & Owen, 2016).

Dimensional models of psychopathology emerged in part as a response to these anomalies and seek to organize mental illness in terms of broad liability factors such as fear sensitivity that are evident in several psychiatric diagnoses such as panic disorder and specific phobia (Krueger & Markon, 2006; Watson, 2005). Psychometric analyses of psychiatric symptoms increasingly converge on the conclusion that psychopathology can be understood in terms of a hierarchy of symptom dimensions that vary from broad, such as internalizing symptoms including depressed mood and anxiety, to specific, such as maladaptive social withdrawal (Forbes et al., 2025; Kotov et al., 2017). Such thinking is evident in the DSM-5's Alternative Model of Personality Disorders, which requires clinicians to consider a number of maladaptive dimensional traits in assessment and treatment planning (Clark & Watson, 2022).

More comprehensive dimensional models of psychopathology can be found in the Research Domain Criteria (RDoC) and the Hierarchical Taxonomy of Psychopathology (HiTOP; though there are important differences between them; see Michelini et al., 2021). Proponents of these models highlight robust evidence supporting the validity of major dimensions of psychopathology (e.g., Krueger et al., 2021). They also note that genetic, neurobiological, and clinical data better align with a hierarchical dimensional model than with a categorical taxonomy (Conway et al., 2019). Compared to diagnostic categories, dimensions are better at predicting impairment, risk of mortality (Kim et al., 2021), the development of psychopathology over time (Kessler et al., 2011), and longitudinal links among disorders (Eaton et al., 2013). Furthermore, they show better structural validity and statistical fit to real-world data (Kotov et al., 2017; Forbes et al., 2021; Greene et al., 2019).

Computational Psychiatry and Transdiagnostic Dimensional Models: Similar Concerns, Different Approaches. In the broadest sense, computational psychiatry and modern dimensional approaches to psychopathology grew out of the same dilemma: Categorical psychiatric taxonomy failed to provide a satisfactory system for understanding how symptoms relate to one another and what causes them. From this common point of departure, these approaches have evolved largely independently (though with notable exceptions such as Fox et al., 2024; Wise et al., 2023). Computational psychiatry has roundly criticized the lack of mechanistic specificity in psychiatric taxonomy, hoping to find computational phenotypes that could inform diagnosis (e.g., Stephan & Mathys, 2014). Several critiques have also pointed out that biological psychiatry has produced many candidate "biomarkers" that either failed to replicate or did not provide a compelling account of the mechanisms linking neurobiology, behavior, and cognition. In addition, some computational psychiatry theorists (and for that matter, biological psychiatrists; Kapur et al., 2012) have hoped for taxonomies that are based not on observable signs and symptoms, but on underlying cognitive mechanisms and neurocomputational systems that putatively play a more causal role (Patzelt et al., 2018; Wiecki et al., 2015).

Conversely, dimensional models of psychopathology have primarily focused on the relationships among observable signs and symptoms, often using self-report and clinical interview data (Krueger & Markon, 2006). The goal of many studies in this area, particularly seminal early contributions, was to provide a more satisfactory model of the latent structure of symptom covariance patterns using hierarchical factor models (Achenbach, 2020; Markon et al., 2005; Markon & Krueger, 2005). If descriptive psychopathology can find latent dimensions such as internalizing and externalizing that explain symptom patterns better than discrete diagnoses can, it could guide researchers toward constructs that are more fruitful in developing effective treatments for mental illness (Conway et al., 2019). Recent reviews also highlight evidence for many of the transdiagnostic dimensions in various data modalities including temperament, genetics, neuroimaging, neurophysiology, and treatment response (Krueger et al., 2021, 2021; Watson et al., 2022).

Any generalities about the similarities or differences between computational psychiatry and transdiagnostic dimensional models necessarily invite objections regarding overgeneralization—some may find that we consider too few points of overlap, whereas others may think our treatment does not emphasize the philosophical differences enough. We take the middle ground: although these approaches have significant potential to converge in scientifically productive ways, the potential remains largely latent. We note three critical challenges that have created obstacles to further integration and provide suggestions for overcoming them.

First, much of computational psychiatry research remains implicitly tied to the epistemology of biological psychiatry, namely that we should seek lower-level mechanisms of psychiatric disease that *explain* the manifestation of mental illness. Computational psychiatry advocates argue that generative models provide an "algorithmic bridge" between brain and behavior (Love, 2015), allowing us to identify not merely biological correlates of illness, but also formal accounts of cognitive mechanisms that cause these relationships (Montague et al., 2012). We are sympathetic to this view, yet many explanatory studies largely overlook the definition and measurement of psychopathology. Simply put, many computational studies are remarkably innovative in their approach to cognitive modeling but remain being surprisingly conventional in their reliance on traditional diagnostic categories. This can give rise to problems familiar in biological psychiatry research, such as the inclusion of heterogeneous patients who share a diagnosis or the use of extreme group designs that are inconsistent with dimensional realities (Preacher et al., 2005). Basic neuroscientists are likewise led to seek a neurocomputational model of, say, obsessive-compulsive disorder (OCD), even as genetic (Strom et al., 2021) and neuroimaging (Grazioplene et al., 2022) measures point toward the dimensional structure of risk for OCD symptoms. Thus, computational psychiatry could benefit substantially from focusing on transdiagnostic symptom dimensions whose construct validity is often far better than related diagnostic categories (for a more detailed treatment, see Allen et al., 2020).

Relatedly, although computational psychiatry advocates have proposed the development of a psychiatric nosology based on cognitive mechanisms, not signs and symptoms, we are pessimistic that such an approach will ultimately prove clinically and scientifically useful. The lack of a "gold standard" definition of psychiatric illness has long plagued psychopathology researchers (Kapur et al., 2012). We might wish for definitive tests that reveal whether a person is sick or well, yet our theories of mental illness are inherently tied to social constructions of psychological health (Maddux et al., 2019) and operational definitions of constructs that are subject to revision (i.e., open concepts; see Zachar et al., 2020). Even if we hope for "biotypes" of a given illness (e.g., of psychosis; Clementz et al., 2016), we must consider deeply how we define illness in terms of cognition, emotion, and behavior, as well as whether illness is categorical or dimensional in nature. These are longstanding conceptual, not mathematical, problems that cannot be surmounted using modern computational machinery.

Second, even as computational psychiatry has struggled to distance itself from the disease model of its biological psychiatry predecessors, transdiagnostic dimensional studies of psychopathology have made more progress on the question of *how* people vary than *why* they do so. Efforts such as RDoC grew out of discussions among clinical neuroscience experts about the brain-based systems most relevant to psychopathology, such as negative and positive valence systems, which can be studied across many levels of analysis (e.g., behavior and genes). Although such biology-first approaches often build on both robust theory (e.g., dopamine's role in positive emotion and motivation; Depue & Collins, 1999) and empirical evidence (Smillie, 2013), they nevertheless lack clarity on clinically relevant targets at the psychological level of measurement (e.g., symptoms). Conversely, transdiagnostic models based on symptom covariance patterns, such as HiTOP, provide a useful framework for clinical description but have not been closely informed by insights gained from biology and neuroscience (for a useful cross-walk between RDoC and HiTOP, see Michelini et al., 2021).

Symptom-based transdiagnostic models increasingly aim to validate their dimensions by considering evidence from genetic, neurophysiological, neuroimaging, and cognitive studies, with promising initial reviews (Kotov et al., 2020; Krueger et al., 2021; Watson et al., 2022). As we have argued previously (Allen et al., 2020, 2022), identifying cross-level correlations is an important exploratory step toward building more robust theories of *why* psychopathology varies across people. However, if this work stops at correlating symptom dimensions and biological measures, it risks falling into the same trap that inspired the ascendence of computational psychiatry: the need for formal cognitive models linking brain and behavior.

We see significant potential for transdiagnostic dimensional models to benefit from explanatory approaches in computational psychiatry. With convergent evidence supporting many transdiagnostic dimensions (Conway et al., 2019) and their neurobiological correlates, computational models can now be developed to dissect these dimensions into underlying cognitive processes (e.g., Robbins et al., 2012). This would encourage researchers to think about their dimensional questions more formally in terms of Marr's levels: (Computational) What is the normative function of the dimension and what evolutionarily relevant problems does it solve? (Algorithmic) What cognitive processes underlie variation in the dimension and how can we formally specify and test them? (Implementational) How are these processes instantiated in the brain and how can we validate our biological inferences using experimental manipulation? (See DeYoung & Krueger, 2018 for a cybernetic perspective.) For example, impulsivity is a well-known transdiagnostic construct relevant to various forms of externalizing psychopathology such as harmful substance use and antisocial personality (Beauchaine et al., 2017). Yet, computational modeling approaches have helped uncover a number of cognitive mechanisms (Dalley et al., 2011), such as decreased motor inhibition (Chamberlain et al., 2006), discounting of future rewards, reduced sensitivity to negative outcomes compared to positive ones (Cockburn & Holroyd, 2010; Frank et al., 2007), and problems in adjusting decision thresholds appropriately (Cavanagh et al., 2011; Mulder et al., 2010).

Third, although computational psychiatry hopes to uncover cognitive mechanisms, the success of this aspiration depends on the validity of the computational models that instantiate our formal mathematical predictions. Moreover, computational models are ultimately quantitative tools that produce numbers including estimates of parameters and latent processes such as subjective value or receptor conductance (Murray et al., 2014). This gives rise to three related concerns: construct validity, reliability, and model specificity (for a more detailed treatment, see Karvelis et al., 2023; Paulus et al., 2016).

To date, generative computational models have largely been developed to explain data collected in experimental contexts (especially behavior). Thus, with respect to construct validity, an assertion that "blunted learning rate on a reward task is a computational marker of anhedonia" is not fundamentally different from other non-computational claims like, "commission errors on a go-no go task are a sensitive measure of inattention." That is, we must validate our computational constructs in the same way as any other hypothetical construct, through convergent validation with related computational and non-computational measures, testing their ability to predict relevant outcomes, investigating their external validity in other populations and settings, and so on, thereby pulling the construct up by its "bootstraps" (Cronbach & Meehl, 1955). Relatedly, we must demonstrate that important indices derived from generative models are reliable—producing consistent results under consistent conditions (Nunnally & Bernstein, 1994). This is no small matter, as experiments often tap into multiple cognitive processes (the task impurity problem; Miyake et al., 2000). Moreover, summary measures from experiments are often unreliable or only weakly related to individual differences measured using self-report (Hedge et al., 2018; Sharma et al., 2014), and computational models do not necessarily have an inherent advantage (Hedge et al., 2020). Recent work has found that using hierarchical methods when testing generative models can lead to more reliable estimates than conventional summary statistics and support robust tests of individual differences (Brown et al., 2020; Haines et al., 2023).

Finally, as noted above, our computational models instantiate our *beliefs* about the cognitive processes that give rise to other measures, including brain activity and behavior. Even for a well-fitting model, the reality of the underlying computation could be surprisingly different. When we fit computational models to data, we often rely on relative evidence in forming our conclusions—does this model fit better than that one? Model comparison is an important step in bolstering our confidence (Hallquist & Dombrovski, 2020; Stephan et al., 2009), but it can often be valuable to examine how closely the model's predictions match the data (sometimes called a "posterior predictive check"). Nevertheless, even if our candidate model fits better than competitors and its predictions closely match the data, computational models can differ in their flexibility to fit different datasets, and more complex generative models can sometimes capture data that were generated by another model altogether (He et al., 2020). Our point is not to claim that "all models are wrong" but to highlight that even successful computational models that generate plausible data and fit empirical observations should be viewed as heuristic approximations of the true cognitive processes.

What about Data-driven Approaches? As we have devoted considerable space to the links between generative models and transdiagnostic dimensions, the reader may be wondering about the data-driven culture of computational psychiatry. In short, most of the machine learning techniques used in clinical prediction and classification studies have close counterparts in conventional psychometrics and statistics (Urban & Gates, 2021).

As noted above, many prediction algorithms can be viewed as extensions of regression that better handle big data. In the realm of classification, traditional mixture modeling approaches long used to search for latent classes in clinical populations (e.g., Lenzenweger et al., 2008) are one of several "unsupervised learning" approaches regularly used in machine learning settings (Alloghani et al., 2020). Likewise, we have seen factor analysis, the engine of most structural dimensional analyses of psychopathology, described as a "computational model" in grant applications. Factor analysis is closely related to a larger family of dimension reduction techniques that have been studied and expanded in the machine learning literature (Sorzano et al., 2014). Altogether, data-driven approaches in computational psychiatry answer familiar questions of prediction and classification using modern machine learning methods that better accommodate datasets with many observations and many variables.

Given this, what can machine learning bring to our structural understanding of psychopathology? Although dimension reduction techniques like factor analysis scale well to reasonably large datasets, machine learning approaches may aid in situations in which there are many variables, which can lead both to estimation problems and slow computation (Urban & Bauer, 2021). As the field aims to scale up transdiagnostic models to virtually all psychiatric symptoms (e.g., Simms et al., 2022), we may benefit from techniques that can handle the large number of symptom dimensions that will necessarily emerge at finer levels of the hierarchy. In addition, the machine learning convention of seeking parameter estimates based on internal cross-validation procedures may increase the generalizability of our latent structure models across samples (this topic has been approached in the psychological literature, but it is not standard; MacCallum et al., 1994). Such considerations are already beginning to emerge in analyses that use a hold-out sample to test the robustness of structural models of psychopathology (e.g., Forbes et al., 2025).

Conclusion

Computational psychiatry and transdiagnostic dimensional models have emerged from the desire to describe the underlying structure of psychopathology and to understand why psychopathology symptoms vary across people. Despite common motivations, communication between these scientific communities has been limited. Our hope is that the strengths of each can be combined to support more mechanistic studies of psychopathology that focus on construct-valid clinical targets. Efforts to develop computational phenotypes are in their infancy and further progress requires a strong focus on the construct validity of these measures (Karvelis et al., 2023). Likewise, dimensional models of psychopathology have successfully demonstrated cross-level associations with genetics and brain measures, yet the cognitive mechanisms that link symptom dimensions and neurobiology are not yet clear. In a nutshell, computational psychiatry needs better clinical targets, and dimensional models need better explanations.

References

Aberg, K. C., Toren, I., & Paz, R. (2022). A neural and behavioral trade-off between value and uncertainty underlies exploratory decisions in normative anxiety. *Molecular Psychiatry*, *27*, 1573–1587. https://doi.org/10.1038/s41380-021-01363-z

Achenbach, T. M. (2020). Bottom-up and top-down paradigms for psychopathology: A half-century odyssey. *Annual Review of Clinical Psychology*, *16*(1), 1–24. https://doi.org/10.1146/annurev-clinpsy-071119-115831

Alexander, L., Jelen, L. A., Mehta, M. A., & Young, A. H. (2021). The anterior cingulate cortex as a key locus of ketamine's antidepressant action. *Neuroscience & Biobehavioral Reviews*, *127*, 531–554. https://doi.org/10.1016/j.neubiorev.2021.05.003

Allen, T. A., Hall, N. T., Schreiber, A. M., & Hallquist, M. N. (2022). Explanatory personality science in the neuroimaging era: The map is not the territory. *Current Opinion in Behavioral Sciences*, *43*, 236–241.

Allen, T. A., Hallquist, M. N., & Dombrovski, A. Y. (2024). Callousness, exploitativeness, and tracking of cooperation incentives in the human default network. *Proceedings of the National Academy of Sciences*, *121*(29), e2307221121. https://doi.org/10.1073/pnas.2307221121

Allen, T. A., Rueter, A. R., Abram, S. V., Brown, J. S., & DeYoung, C. G. (2017). Personality and neural correlates of mentalizing ability. *European Journal of Personality*, *31*(6), 599–613. https://doi.org/10.1002/per.2133

Allen, T. A., Schreiber, A. M., Hall, N. T., & Hallquist, M. N. (2020). From description to explanation: Integrating across multiple levels of analysis to inform neuroscientific accounts of dimensional personality pathology. *Journal of Personality Disorders*, *34*(5), 650–676. https://doi.org/10.1521/pedi.2020.34.5.650

Alloghani, M., Al-Jumeily, D., Mustafina, J., Hussain, A., & Aljaaf, A. J. (2020). A systematic review on supervised and unsupervised machine learning algorithms for data science. In M. W. Berry, A. Mohamed, & B. W. Yap (Eds.), *Supervised and unsupervised learning for data science* (pp. 3–21). Springer International Publishing. https://doi.org/10.1007/978-3-030-22475-2_1

American Psychiatric Association. (2013). *Diagnostic and statistical manual of mental disorders: DSM-5* (5th ed.). American Psychiatric Publishing.

Andrews-Hanna, J. R., Smallwood, J., & Spreng, R. N. (2014). The default network and self-generated thought: Component processes, dynamic control, and clinical relevance. *Annals of the New York Academy of Sciences*, *1316*(1), 29–52. https://doi.org/10.1111/nyas.12360.The

Avilés, L. (2002). Solving the freeloaders paradox: Genetic associations and frequency-dependent selection in the evolution of cooperation among nonrelatives. *Proceedings of the National Academy of Sciences*, *99*(22), 14268–14273. https://doi.org/10.1073/pnas.212408299

Beauchaine, T. P., Zisner, A. R., & Sauder, C. L. (2017). Trait impulsivity and the externalizing spectrum. *Annual Review of Clinical Psychology*, *13*(1), 343–368. https://doi.org/10.1146/annurev-clinpsy-021815-093253

Bennett, D., Silverstein, S. M., & Niv, Y. (2019). The two cultures of computational psychiatry. *JAMA Psychiatry*, *76*(6), 563–564. https://doi.org/10.1001/jamapsychiatry.2019.0231

Borsboom, D. (2008). Psychometric perspectives on diagnostic systems. *Journal of Clinical Psychology*, *64*(9), 1089–1108. https://doi.org/10.1002/jclp.20503

Brislin, S. J., Yancey, J. R., Perkins, E. R., Palumbo, I. M., Drislane, L. E., Salekin, R. T., Fanti, K. A., Kimonis, E. R., Frick, P. J., Blair, R. J. R., & Patrick, C. J. (2018). Callousness and affective face processing in adults: Behavioral and brain-potential indicators. *Personality Disorders: Theory, Research, and Treatment*, *9*(2), 122–132. https://doi.org/10.1037/per0000235

Brown, V. M., Chen, J., Gillan, C. M., & Price, R. B. (2020). Improving the reliability of computational analyses: Model-based planning and its relationship with compulsivity. *Biological Psychiatry: Cognitive Neuroscience and Neuroimaging*, *5*(6), 601–609. https://doi.org/10.1016/j.bpsc.2019.12.019

Brown, V. M., Price, R., & Dombrovski, A. Y. (2023). Anxiety as a disorder of uncertainty: Implications for understanding maladaptive anxiety, anxious avoidance, and exposure therapy. *Cognitive, Affective, & Behavioral Neuroscience*, *23*(3), 844–868. https://doi.org/10.3758/s13415-023-01080-w

Brown, V. M., Zhu, L., Solway, A., Wang, J. M., McCurry, K. L., King-Casas, B., & Chiu, P. H. (2021). Reinforcement learning disruptions in individuals with depression and sensitivity to symptom change following cognitive behavioral therapy. *JAMA Psychiatry*, *78*(10), 1113–1122. https://doi.org/10.1001/jamapsychiatry.2021.1844

Brown, V. M., Zhu, L., Wang, J. M., Frueh, B. C., King-Casas, B., & Chiu, P. H. (2018). Associability-modulated loss learning is increased in posttraumatic stress disorder. *eLife*, *7*, e30150. https://doi.org/10.7554/eLife.30150

Buckner, R. L., Andrews-Hanna, J. R., & Schacter, D. L. (2008). The brain's default network: Anatomy, function, and relevance to disease. *Annals of the New York Academy of Sciences, 1124*, 1–38. https://doi.org/10.1196/ANNALS.1440.0113

Buckner, R. L., & Krienen, F. M. (2013). The evolution of distributed association networks in the human brain. *Trends in Cognitive Sciences, 17*(12), 648–665. https://doi.org/10.1016/j.tics.2013.09.017

Bzdok, D., & Meyer-Lindenberg, A. (2018). Machine learning for precision psychiatry: Opportunities and challenges. *Biological Psychiatry: Cognitive Neuroscience and Neuroimaging, 3*(3), 223–230. https://doi.org/10.1016/j.bpsc.2017.11.007

Cavanagh, J. F., Wiecki, T. V., Cohen, M. X., Figueroa, C. M., Samanta, J., Sherman, S. J., & Frank, M. J. (2011). Subthalamic nucleus stimulation reverses mediofrontal influence over decision threshold. *Nature Neuroscience, 14*(11), 1462–1467. https://doi.org/10.1038/nn.2925

Chamberlain, S. R., Fineberg, N. A., Blackwell, A. D., Robbins, T. W., & Sahakian, B. J. (2006). Motor inhibition and cognitive flexibility in obsessive-compulsive disorder and trichotillomania. *The American Journal of Psychiatry, 163*(7), 1282–1284. https://doi.org/10.1176/ajp.2006.163.7.1282

Charpentier, C. J., Cogliati Dezza, I., Vellani, V., Globig, L. K., Gädeke, M., & Sharot, T. (2022). Anxiety increases information-seeking in response to large changes. *Scientific Reports, 12*(1), 7385. https://doi.org/10.1038/s41598-022-10813-9

Chase, H. W., Frank, M. J., Michael, A., Bullmore, E. T., Sahakian, B. J., & Robbins, T. W. (2010). Approach and avoidance learning in patients with major depression and healthy controls: Relation to anhedonia. *Psychological Medicine, 40*(3), 433–440. https://doi.org/10.1017/S0033291709990468

Chekroud, A. M., Bondar, J., Delgadillo, J., Doherty, G., Wasil, A., Fokkema, M., Cohen, Z., Belgrave, D., DeRubeis, R., & Iniesta, R. (2021). The promise of machine learning in predicting treatment outcomes in psychiatry. *World Psychiatry, 20*(2), 154–170.

Chekroud, A. M., Zotti, R. J., Shehzad, Z., Gueorguieva, R., Johnson, M. K., Trivedi, M. H., Cannon, T. D., Krystal, J. H., & Corlett, P. R. (2016). Cross-trial prediction of treatment outcome in depression: A machine learning approach. *The Lancet Psychiatry, 3*(3), 243–250.

Clark, L. A., & Watson, D. (2022). The trait model of the DSM-5 alternative model of personality disorder (AMPD): A structural review. *Personality Disorders: Theory, Research, and Treatment, 13*(4), 328–336. https://doi.org/10.1037/per0000568

Clementz, B. A., Sweeney, J. A., Hamm, J. P., Ivleva, E. I., Ethridge, L. E., Pearlson, G. D., Keshavan, M. S., & Tamminga, C. A. (2016). Identification of distinct psychosis biotypes using brain-based biomarkers. *American Journal of Psychiatry, 173*(4), 373–384. https://doi.org/10.1176/appi.ajp.2015.14091200

Cockburn, J., & Holroyd, C. B. (2010). Focus on the positive: Computational simulations implicate asymmetrical reward prediction error signals in childhood attention-deficit/hyperactivity disorder. *Brain Research, 1365*, 18–34. https://doi.org/10.1016/j.brainres.2010.09.065

Conway, C. C., Forbes, M. K., Forbush, K. T., Fried, E. I., Hallquist, M. N., Kotov, R., Mullins-Sweatt, S. N., Shackman, A. J., Skodol, A. E., South, S. C., Sunderland, M., Waszczuk, M. A., Zald, D. H., Afzali, M. H., Bornovalova, M. A., Carragher, N., Docherty, A. R., Jonas, K. G., Krueger, R. F., . . . Eaton, N. R. (2019). A Hierarchical Taxonomy of Psychopathology can transform mental health research. *Perspectives on Psychological Science, 14*(3), 419–436. https://doi.org/10.1177/1745691618810696

Corlett, P. R., Taylor, J. R., Wang, X.-J., Fletcher, P. C., & Krystal, J. H. (2010). Toward a neurobiology of delusions. *Progress in Neurobiology, 92*(3), 345–369. https://doi.org/10.1016/j.pneurobio.2010.06.007

Coutanche, M. N., & Hallion, L. S. (2020). Machine learning for clinical psychology and clinical neuroscience. In A. G. C. Wright & M. N. Hallquist (Eds.), *Handbook of research methods in clinical psychology* (pp. 467–481). Cambridge University Press.

Craver, C. F. (2001). Role functions, mechanisms, and hierarchy. *Philosophy of Science, 68*(1), 53–74. https://doi.org/10.1086/392866

Cronbach, L. J., & Meehl, P. E. (1955). Construct validity in psychological tests. *Psychological Bulletin, 52*(4), 281–302.

Cuthbert, B. N. (2014). Translating intermediate phenotypes to psychopathology: The NIMH Research Domain Criteria. *Psychophysiology, 51*(12), 1205–1206. https://doi.org/10.1111/psyp.12342

Dalley, J. W., Everitt, B. J., & Robbins, T. W. (2011). Impulsivity, compulsivity, and top-down cognitive control. *Neuron, 69*(4), 680–694. https://doi.org/10.1016/j.neuron.2011.01.020

Depue, R. A., & Collins, P. F. (1999). Neurobiology of the structure of personality: Dopamine, facilitation of incentive motivation, and extraversion. *The Behavioral and Brain Sciences, 22*(3), 491–517; discussion 518–569.

Despotes, K. A., & Donaldson, S. H. (2022). Current state of CFTR modulators for treatment of cystic fibrosis. *Current Opinion in Pharmacology, 65*, 102239. https://doi.org/10.1016/j.coph.2022.102239

DeYoung, C. G., & Krueger, R. F. (2018). A cybernetic theory of psychopathology. *Psychological Inquiry, 29*(3), 117–138. https://www-tandfonline-com.ezaccess.libraries.psu.edu/doi/abs/10.1080/1047840X.2018.1513680

Dombrovski, A. Y., Clark, L., Siegle, G. J., Butters, M. A., Ichikawa, N., Sahakian, B. J., & Szanto, K. (2010). Reward/punishment reversal learning in older suicide attempters. *American Journal of Psychiatry, 167*(6), 699–707. https://doi.org/10.1176/appi.ajp.2009.09030407

Dombrovski, A. Y., Szanto, K., Clark, L., Aizenstein, H. J., Chase, H. W., Reynolds, C. F., & Siegle, G. J. (2015). Corticostriatothalamic reward prediction error signals and executive control in late-life depression. *Psychological Medicine, 45*(7), 1413–1424. https://doi.org/10.1017/S0033291714002517

Dunbar, R. I. M. (2009). The social brain hypothesis and its implications for social evolution. *Annals of Human Biology, 36*(5), 562–572. https://doi.org/10.1080/03014460902960289

Eaton, N. R., Krueger, R. F., Docherty, A. R., & Sponheim, S. R. (2013). Toward a model-based approach to the clinical assessment of personality psychopathology. *Journal of Personality Assessment, 96*(3), 283–292. https://doi.org/10.1080/00223891.2013.830263

Ebbinghaus, H. (1913). *Memory; A contribution to experimental psychology*. Teachers College, Columbia University. http://archive.org/details/memorycontributiooebbiuoft

Eldar, E., Roth, C., Dayan, P., & Dolan, R. J. (2018). Decodability of reward learning signals predicts mood fluctuations. *Current Biology, 28*(9), 1433–1439.e7. https://doi.org/10.1016/j.cub.2018.03.038

Engstrom, E. J., & Kendler, K. S. (2015). Emil Kraepelin: Icon and reality. *American Journal of Psychiatry, 172*(12), 1190–1196. https://doi.org/10.1176/appi.ajp.2015.15050665

Fenno, L., Yizhar, O., & Deisseroth, K. (2011). The development and application of optogenetics. *Annual Review of Neuroscience, 34*(1), 389–412. https://doi.org/10.1146/annurev-neuro-061010-113817

Forbes, M. K., Sunderland, M., Rapee, R. M., Batterham, P. J., Calear, A. L., Carragher, N., Ruggero, C., Zimmerman, M., Baillie, A. J., Lynch, S. J., Mewton, L., Slade, T., & Krueger, R. F. (2021). A detailed hierarchical model of psychopathology: From individual symptoms up to the general factor of psychopathology. *Clinical Psychological Science, 9*(2), 139–168. https://doi.org/10.1177/2167702620954799

Forbes, M. K., Baillie, A., Batterham, P. J., Calear, A., Kotov, R., Krueger, R. F., Markon, K. E., Mewton, L., Pellicano, E., Roberts, M., Rodriguez-Seijas, C., Sunderland, M., Watson, D., Watts, A. L., Wright, A. G. C., & Anna Clark, L. (2025). Reconstructing psychopathology: A data-driven reorganization of the symptoms in the Diagnostic and Statistical Manual of Mental Disorders. *Clinical Psychological Science, 13*(3), 462–488. https://doi.org/10.1177/21677026241268345

Forstmann, B. U., & Wagenmakers, E.-J. (Eds.). (2015). *An introduction to model-based cognitive neuroscience*. Springer New York. https://doi.org/10.1007/978-1-4939-2236-9

Fox, C. A., Teckentrup, V., Donegan, K. R., Seow, T., Benwell, C., Tervo-Clemmens, B., & Gillan, C. (2024). *Cognitive arbitration between candidate dimensions of psychopathology*. Open Science Framework. https://doi.org/10.31234/osf.io/7waey

Frank, M. J., Samanta, J., Moustafa, A. A., & Sherman, S. J. (2007). Hold your horses: Impulsivity, deep brain stimulation, and medication in Parkinsonism. *Science, 318*(5854), 1309–1312. https://doi.org/10.1126/science.1146157

Freud, S. (1923). *The ego and the id* (J. Strachey, Ed.; J. Riviere, Trans.). Norton; WorldCat.

Fried, E. I. (2022). Studying mental health problems as systems, not syndromes. *Current Directions in Psychological Science, 31*(6), 500–508. https://doi.org/10.1177/09637214221114089

Fried, E. I., & Robinaugh, D. J. (2020). Systems all the way down: Embracing complexity in mental health research. *BMC Medicine, 18*(1), 205, s12916-020-01668-w. https://doi.org/10.1186/s12916-020-01668-w

Fuchikami, M., Thomas, A., Liu, R., Wohleb, E. S., Land, B. B., DiLeone, R. J., Aghajanian, G. K., & Duman, R. S. (2015). Optogenetic stimulation of infralimbic PFC reproduces ketamine's rapid and sustained antidepressant actions. *Proceedings of the National Academy of Sciences, 112*(26), 8106–8111. https://doi.org/10.1073/pnas.1414728112

Galton, S. F. (1883). *Inquiries into human faculty and its development*. Macmillan.

Gillan, C. M., & Whelan, R. (2017). What big data can do for treatment in psychiatry. *Current Opinion in Behavioral Sciences, 18*, 34–42. https://doi.org/10.1016/j.cobeha.2017.07.003

Goetz, C. G. (2016). Chapter 2—Charcot, hysteria, and simulated disorders. In M. Hallett, J. Stone, & A. Carson (Eds.), *Handbook of clinical neurology* (Vol. 139, pp. 11–23). Elsevier. https://doi.org/10.1016/B978-0-12-801772-2.00002-3

Goodkind, M., Eickhoff, S. B., Oathes, D. J., Jiang, Y., Chang, A., Jones-Hagata, L. B., Ortega, B. N., Zaiko, Y. V., Roach, E. L., Korgaonkar, M. S., Grieve, S. M., Galatzer-Levy, I., Fox, P. T., & Etkin, A. (2015). Identification of a common neurobiological substrate for mental illness. *JAMA Psychiatry, 72*(4), 305–315. https://doi.org/10.1001/jamapsychiatry.2014.2206

Gradin, V. B., Kumar, P., Waiter, G., Ahearn, T., Stickle, C., Milders, M., Reid, I., Hall, J., & Steele, J. D. (2011). Expected value and prediction error abnormalities in depression and schizophrenia. *Brain, 134*(Pt 6), 1751–1764. https://doi.org/10.1093/brain/awr059

Grazioplene, R. G., DeYoung, C. G., Hampson, M., Anticevic, A., & Pittenger, C. (2022). Obsessive compulsive symptom dimensions are linked to altered white-matter microstructure in a community sample of youth. *Translational Psychiatry, 12*(1), 1–10. https://doi.org/10.1038/s41398-022-02013-w

Greene, A. L., Eaton, N. R., Li, K., Forbes, M. K., Krueger, R. F., Markon, K. E., Waldman, I. D., Cicero, D. C., Conway, C. C., Docherty, A. R., Fried, E. I., Ivanova, M. Y., Jonas, K. G., Latzman, R. D., Patrick, C. J., Reininghaus, U., Tackett, J. L., Wright, A. G. C., & Kotov, R. (2019). Are fit indices used to test psychopathology structure biased? A simulation study. *Journal of Abnormal Psychology*, 128(7), 740–764. https://doi.org/10.1037/abn0000434

Gureckis, T. M., & Love, B. C. (2015). Computational reinforcement learning. In J. R. Busemeyer, Z. Wang, J. T. Townsend, & A. Eidels (Eds.), *The Oxford handbook of computational and mathematical psychology* (pp. 99–120). Oxford University Press. http://www.oxfordhandbooks.com/view/10.1093/oxfordhb/9780199957996.001.0001/oxfordhb-9780199957996-e-5

Haines, N., Sullivan-Toole, H., & Olino, T. (2023). From classical methods to generative models: Tackling the unreliability of neuroscientific measures in mental health research. *Biological Psychiatry: Cognitive Neuroscience and Neuroimaging, 8*(8), 822–831. https://doi.org/10.1016/j.bpsc.2023.01.001

Halahakoon, D. C., Kieslich, K., O'Driscoll, C., Nair, A., Lewis, G., & Roiser, J. P. (2020). Reward-processing behavior in depressed participants relative to healthy volunteers: A systematic review and meta-analysis. *JAMA Psychiatry, 77*(12), 1286–1295. https://doi.org/10.1001/jamapsychiatry.2020.2139

Hallquist, M. N., & Dombrovski, A. (2020). Reinforcement learning approaches to computational clinical neuroscience. In A. G. C. Wright & M. N. Hallquist (Eds.), *Handbook of research methods in clinical psychology* (pp. 168–189). Cambridge University Press.

Hastie, T., Tibshirani, R., & Friedman, J. (2009). *The elements of statistical learning: Data mining, inference, and prediction* (2nd ed.). Springer.

He, L., Zhao, W. J., & Bhatia, S. (2020). An ontology of decision models. *Psychological Review, 129*(1), 49–72. https://doi.org/10.1037/rev0000231

Hedge, C., Bompas, A., & Sumner, P. (2020). Task reliability considerations in computational psychiatry. *Biological Psychiatry: Cognitive Neuroscience and Neuroimaging, 5*(9), 837–839. https://doi.org/10.1016/j.bpsc.2020.05.004

Hedge, C., Powell, G., & Sumner, P. (2018). The reliability paradox: Why robust cognitive tasks do not produce reliable individual differences. *Behavior Research Methods, 50*(3), 1166–1186. https://doi.org/10.3758/s13428-017-0935-1

Hill, J., Inder, T., Neil, J., Dierker, D., Harwell, J., & Van Essen, D. (2010). Similar patterns of cortical expansion during human development and evolution. *Proceedings of the National Academy of Sciences of the United States of America, 107*(29), 13135–13140. https://doi.org/10.1073/pnas.1001229107

Hitchcock, P., Fried, E. I., & Frank, M. (2021). *Computational psychiatry needs time and context*. PsyArXiv. https://doi.org/10.31234/osf.io/xf2u3

Huang, Y., & Rao, R. P. N. (2011). Predictive coding. *WIREs Cognitive Science*, *2*(5), 580–593. https://doi.org/10.1002/wcs.142

Huys, Q. J. M., Guitart-Masip, M., Dolan, R. J., & Dayan, P. (2015). Decision-theoretic psychiatry. *Clinical Psychological Science*, *3*(3), 400–421. https://doi.org/10.1177/2167702614562040

Huys, Q. J. M., Maia, T. V., & Frank, M. J. (2016). Computational psychiatry as a bridge from neuroscience to clinical applications. *Nature Neuroscience*, *19*(3), 404–413. https://doi.org/10.1038/nn.4238

Huys, Q. J. M., Pizzagalli, D. A., Bogdan, R., & Dayan, P. (2013). Mapping anhedonia onto reinforcement learning: A behavioural meta-analysis. *Biology of Mood & Anxiety Disorders*, *3*(1), 12. https://doi.org/10.1186/2045-5380-3-12

Iniesta, R., Hodgson, K., Stahl, D., Malki, K., Maier, W., Rietschel, M., Mors, O., Hauser, J., Henigsberg, N., Dernovsek, M. Z., Souery, D., Dobson, R., Aitchison, K. J., Farmer, A., McGuffin, P., Lewis, C. M., & Uher, R. (2018). Antidepressant drug-specific prediction of depression treatment outcomes from genetic and clinical variables. *Scientific Reports*, *8*(1), 5530. https://doi.org/10.1038/s41598-018-23584-z

Iniesta, R., Stahl, D., & McGuffin, P. (2016). Machine learning, statistical learning and the future of biological research in psychiatry. *Psychological Medicine*, *46*(12), 2455–2465. https://doi.org/10.1017/S0033291716001367

Jacob, S. N., Hähnke, D., & Nieder, A. (2018). Structuring of abstract working memory content by fronto-parietal synchrony in primate cortex. *Neuron*, *99*(3), 588–597.e5. https://doi.org/10.1016/j.neuron.2018.07.025

Jaspers, K. (1913). *General psychopathology*. Johns Hopkins University Press.

Jones, M. C. (1924). The elimination of children's fears. *Journal of Experimental Psychology*, *7*(5), 382–390. https://doi.org/10.1037/h0072283

Kaczkurkin, A. N., Sotiras, A., Baller, E. B., Barzilay, R., Calkins, M. E., Chand, G. B., Cui, Z., Erus, G., Fan, Y., Gur, R. E., Gur, R. C., Moore, T. M., Roalf, D. R., Rosen, A. F. G., Ruparel, K., Shinohara, R. T., Varol, E., Wolf, D. H., Davatzikos, C., & Satterthwaite, T. D. (2020). Neurostructural heterogeneity in youths with internalizing symptoms. *Biological Psychiatry*, *87*(5), 473–482. https://doi.org/10.1016/j.biopsych.2019.09.005

Kapur, S., Phillips, A. G., & Insel, T. R. (2012). Why has it taken so long for biological psychiatry to develop clinical tests and what to do about it? *Molecular Psychiatry*, *17*(12), 1174–1179. https://doi.org/10.1038/mp.2012.105

Karvelis, P., Paulus, M. P., & Diaconescu, A. O. (2023). Individual differences in computational psychiatry: A review of current challenges. *Neuroscience & Biobehavioral Reviews*, *148*, 105137. https://doi.org/10.1016/j.neubiorev.2023.105137

Katahira, K., & Toyama, A. (2021). Revisiting the importance of model fitting for model-based fMRI: It does matter in computational psychiatry. *PLOS Computational Biology*, *17*(2), e1008738. https://doi.org/10.1371/journal.pcbi.1008738

Kendler, K. S. (2008). Explanatory models for psychiatric illness. *American Journal of Psychiatry*, *165*(6), 695–702. https://doi.org/10.1176/appi.ajp.2008.07071061

Kendler, K. S. (2019). From many to one to many—The search for causes of psychiatric illness. *JAMA Psychiatry*, *76*(10), 1085. https://doi.org/10.1001/jamapsychiatry.2019.1200

Kessler, R. C., Ormel, J., Petukhova, M., McLaughlin, K. A., Green, J. G., Russo, L. J., Stein, D. J., Zaslavsky, A. M., Aguilar-Gaxiola, S., Alonso, J., Andrade, L., Benjet, C., de Girolamo, G., de Graaf, R., Demyttenaere, K., Fayyad, J., Haro, J. M., Hu, Cy., Karam, . . . Ustün T. B. (2011). Development of lifetime comorbidity in the World Health Organization world mental health surveys. *Archives of General Psychiatry*, *68*(1), 90–100. https://doi.org/10.1001/archgenpsychiatry.2010.180

Kilcullen, R. J., Castonguay, L. G., Janis, R. A., Hallquist, M. N., Hayes, J. A., & Locke, B. D. (2021). Predicting future courses of psychotherapy within a grouped LASSO framework. *Psychotherapy Research*, *31*(1), 63–77. https://doi.org/10.1080/10503307.2020.1762948

Kim, H., Turiano, N. A., Forbes, M. K., Kotov, R., Krueger, R. F., Eaton, N. R., Conway, C. C., Docherty, A. R., Dretsch, M., Forbush, K. T., Goghari, V. M., Markon, K. E., Mullins-Sweatt, S. N., Nelson,

B., Olino, T. M., & Slade, T. (2021). Internalizing psychopathology and all-cause mortality: A comparison of transdiagnostic vs. diagnosis-based risk prediction. *World Psychiatry*, *20*(2), 276–282. https://doi.org/10.1002/WPS.20859

Knill, D. C., & Pouget, A. (2004). The Bayesian brain: The role of uncertainty in neural coding and computation. *Trends in Neurosciences*, *27*(12), 712–719. https://doi.org/10.1016/j.tins.2004.10.007

Kotov, R., Jonas, K. G., Carpenter, W. T., Dretsch, M. N., Eaton, N. R., Forbes, M. K., Forbush, K. T., Hobbs, K., Reininghaus, U., Slade, T., South, S. C., Sunderland, M., Waszczuk, M. A., Widiger, T. A., Wright, A. G. C., Zald, D. H., Krueger, R. F., Watson, D., & HiTOP Utility Workgroup. (2020). Validity and utility of Hierarchical Taxonomy of Psychopathology (HiTOP): I. Psychosis superspectrum. *World Psychiatry*, *19*(2), 151–172. https://doi.org/10.1002/wps.20730

Kotov, R., Krueger, R. F., Watson, D., Achenbach, T. M., Althoff, R. R., Bagby, R. M., Brown, T. A., Carpenter, W. T., Caspi, A., Clark, L. A., Eaton, N. R., Forbes, M. K., Forbush, K. T., Goldberg, D., Hasin, D., Hyman, S. E., Ivanova, M. Y., Lynam, D. R., Markon, K., . . . Zimmerman, M. (2017). The Hierarchical Taxonomy of Psychopathology (HiTOP): A dimensional alternative to traditional nosologies. *Journal of Abnormal Psychology*, *126*(4), 454–477. http://dx.doi.org/10.1037/abn0000258

Kriegeskorte, N., & Douglas, P. K. (2018). Cognitive computational neuroscience. *Nature Neuroscience*, *21*(9), 1148. https://doi.org/10.1038/s41593-018-0210-5

Krueger, R. F., Hobbs, K. A., Conway, C. C., Dick, D. M., Dretsch, M. N., Eaton, N. R., Forbes, M. K., Forbush, K. T., Keyes, K. M., Latzman, R. D., Michelini, G., Patrick, C. J., Sellbom, M., Slade, T., South, S. C., Sunderland, M., Tackett, J., Waldman, I., Waszczuk, M. A., . . . HiTOP Utility Workgroup. (2021). Validity and utility of Hierarchical Taxonomy of Psychopathology (HiTOP): II. Externalizing superspectrum. *World Psychiatry*, *20*(2), 171–193. https://doi.org/10.1002/wps.20844

Krueger, R. F., & Markon, K. E. (2006). Reinterpreting comorbidity: A model-based approach to understanding and classifying psychopathology. *Annual Review of Clinical Psychology*, *2*(1), 111–133. https://doi.org/10.1146/annurev.clinpsy.2.022305.095213

Krypotos, A.-M., Alves, M., Crombez, G., & Vlaeyen, J. W. S. (2022). The role of intolerance of uncertainty when solving the exploration-exploitation dilemma. *International Journal of Psychophysiology*, *181*, 33–39. https://doi.org/10.1016/j.ijpsycho.2022.08.001

Kumar, P., Goer, F., Murray, L., Dillon, D. G., Beltzer, M. L., Cohen, A. L., Brooks, N. H., & Pizzagalli, D. A. (2018). Impaired reward prediction error encoding and striatal-midbrain connectivity in depression. *Neuropsychopharmacology*, *43*(7), 1581–1588. https://doi.org/10.1038/s41386-018-0032-x

Kumar, P., Waiter, G., Ahearn, T., Milders, M., Reid, I., & Steele, J. D. (2008). Abnormal temporal difference reward-learning signals in major depression. *Brain*, *131*(Pt 8), 2084–2093. https://doi.org/10.1093/brain/awn136

Lebreton, M., Bavard, S., Daunizeau, J., & Palminteri, S. (2019). Assessing inter-individual differences with task-related functional neuroimaging. *Nature Human Behaviour*, *3*(9), 897–905. https://doi.org/10.1038/s41562-019-0681-8

Lee, Y., Ragguett, R.-M., Mansur, R. B., Boutilier, J. J., Rosenblat, J. D., Trevizol, A., Brietzke, E., Lin, K., Pan, Z., Subramaniapillai, M., Chan, T. C. Y., Fus, D., Park, C., Musial, N., Zuckerman, H., Chen, V. C.-H., Ho, R., Rong, C., & McIntyre, R. S. (2018). Applications of machine learning algorithms to predict therapeutic outcomes in depression: A meta-analysis and systematic review. *Journal of Affective Disorders*, *241*, 519–532. https://doi.org/10.1016/j.jad.2018.08.073

Lenzenweger, M. F., Clarkin, J. F., Yeomans, F. E., Kernberg, O. F., & Levy, K. N. (2008). Refining the phenotype of borderline personality disorder using finite mixture modeling: Implications for classification. *Journal of Personality Disorders*, *22*(4), 313–331.

Lilienfeld, S. O., & Treadway, M. T. (2016). Clashing diagnostic approaches: DSM-ICD versus RDoC. *Annual Review of Clinical Psychology*, *12*(1), 435–463. https://doi.org/10.1146/annurev-clinpsy-021815-093122

Love, B. C. (2015). The algorithmic level is the bridge between computation and brain. *Topics in Cognitive Science*, *7*(2), 230–242. https://doi.org/10.1111/tops.12131

Lynch, S. J., Sunderland, M., Newton, N. C., & Chapman, C. (2021). A systematic review of transdiagnostic risk and protective factors for general and specific psychopathology in young people. *Clinical Psychology Review*, *87*, 102036. https://doi.org/10.1016/j.cpr.2021.102036

Ma, W. J. (2012). Organizing probabilistic models of perception. *Trends in Cognitive Sciences, 16*(10), 511–518. https://doi.org/10.1016/j.tics.2012.08.010

MacCallum, R. C., Roznowski, M., Mar, C. M., & Reith, J. V. (1994). Alternative strategies for cross-validation of covariance structure models. *Multivariate Behavioral Research, 29*(1), 1–32. https://doi.org/10.1207/s15327906mbr2901_1

Maddux, J. E., Gosselin, J. T., & Winstead, B. A. (2019). Conceptions of psychopathology. In J. E. Maddux & B. A. Winstead (Eds.), *Psychopathology* (5th ed., pp. 3–18). Routledge. https://doi.org/10.4324/9780429028267-1

Marek, S., Tervo-Clemmens, B., Calabro, F. J., Montez, D. F., Kay, B. P., Hatoum, A. S., Donohue, M. R., Foran, W., Miller, R. L., Feczko, E., Miranda-Dominguez, O., Graham, A. M., Earl, E. A., Perrone, A. J., Cordova, M., Doyle, O., Moore, L. A., Conan, G., Uriarte, J., . . . Dosenbach, N. U. F. (2022). Reproducible brain-wide association studies require thousands of individuals. *Nature, 603*, 654–660. https://doi.org/10.1038/s41586-022-04492-9

Markon, K. E., & Krueger, R. F. (2005). Categorical and continuous models of liability to externalizing disorders: A direct comparison in NESARC. *Archives of General Psychiatry, 62*(12), 1352–1359.

Markon, K. E., Krueger, R. F., & Watson, D. (2005). Delineating the structure of normal and abnormal personality: An integrative hierarchical approach. *Journal of Personality and Social Psychology, 88*(1), 139–157.

Marr, D. (1982). *Vision: A computational investigation into the human representation and processing of visual information.* MIT Press.

Michelini, G., Palumbo, I. M., DeYoung, C. G., Latzman, R. D., & Kotov, R. (2021). Linking RDoC and HiTOP: A new interface for advancing psychiatric nosology and neuroscience. *Clinical Psychology Review, 86*, 102025. https://doi.org/10.1016/j.cpr.2021.102025

Miyake, A., Emerson, M. J., & Friedman, N. P. (2000). Assessment of executive functions in clinical settings: Problems and recommendations. *Seminars in Speech and Language, 21*(2), 169–183. https://doi.org/10.1055/s-2000-7563

Molenaar, P. C. M. (2004). A manifesto on psychology as idiographic science: Bringing the person back into scientific psychology, this time forever. *Measurement: Interdisciplinary Research & Perspective, 2*(4), 201–218. https://doi.org/10.1207/s15366359mea0204_1

Moncrieff, J., Cooper, R. E., Stockmann, T., Amendola, S., Hengartner, M. P., & Horowitz, M. A. (2023). The serotonin theory of depression: A systematic umbrella review of the evidence. *Molecular Psychiatry, 28*, 3243–3256. https://doi.org/10.1038/s41380-022-01661-0

Monosov, I. E., Zimmermann, J., Frank, M. J., Mathis, M. W., & Baker, J. T. (2024). Ethological computational psychiatry: Challenges and opportunities. *Current Opinion in Neurobiology, 86*, 102881. https://doi.org/10.1016/j.conb.2024.102881

Montague, P. R., Dolan, R. J., Friston, K. J., & Dayan, P. (2012). Computational psychiatry. *Trends in Cognitive Sciences, 16*(1), 72–80. https://doi.org/10.1016/j.tics.2011.11.018

Morriss, J., Zuj, D. V., & Mertens, G. (2021). The role of intolerance of uncertainty in classical threat conditioning: Recent developments and directions for future research. *International Journal of Psychophysiology, 166*, 116–126. https://doi.org/10.1016/j.ijpsycho.2021.05.011

Mukherjee, D., Filipowicz, A. L. S., Vo, K., Satterthwaite, T. D., & Kable, J. W. (2020). Reward and punishment reversal-learning in major depressive disorder. *Journal of Abnormal Psychology, 129*(8), 810–823. https://doi.org/10.1037/abn0000641

Mulder, M. J., Bos, D., Weusten, J. M. H., van Belle, J., van Dijk, S. C., Simen, P., van Engeland, H., & Durston, S. (2010). Basic impairments in regulating the speed-accuracy tradeoff predict symptoms of attention-deficit/hyperactivity disorder. *Biological Psychiatry, 68*(12), 1114–1119. https://doi.org/10.1016/j.biopsych.2010.07.031

Murray, J. D., Anticevic, A., Gancsos, M., Ichinose, M., Corlett, P. R., Krystal, J. H., & Wang, X.-J. (2014). Linking microcircuit dysfunction to cognitive impairment: Effects of disinhibition associated with schizophrenia in a cortical working memory model. *Cerebral Cortex, 24*(4), 859–872. https://doi.org/10.1093/cercor/bhs370

Ng, T. H., Alloy, L. B., & Smith, D. V. (2019). Meta-analysis of reward processing in major depressive disorder reveals distinct abnormalities within the reward circuit. *Translational Psychiatry, 9*(1), 1–10. https://doi.org/10.1038/s41398-019-0644-x

Noonan, M. P., Mars, R. B., Sallet, J., Dunbar, R. I. M., & Fellows, L. K. (2018). The structural and functional brain networks that support human social networks. *Behavioural Brain Research*, *355*, 12–23. https://doi.org/10.1016/J.BBR.2018.02.019

Nunnally, J. C., & Bernstein, I. H. (1994). *Psychometric theory* (3rd ed.). McGraw-Hill.

O'Donovan, M. C., & Owen, M. J. (2016). The implications of the shared genetics of psychiatric disorders. *Nature Medicine*, *22*(11), 1214–1219. https://doi.org/10.1038/nm.4196

Patzelt, E. H., Hartley, C. A., & Gershman, S. J. (2018). Computational phenotyping: Using models to understand individual differences in personality, development, and mental illness. *Personality Neuroscience*, *1*, e18. https://doi.org/10.1017/pen.2018.14

Paulus, M. P., Huys, Q. J. M., & Maia, T. V. (2016). A roadmap for the development of applied computational psychiatry. *Biological Psychiatry: Cognitive Neuroscience and Neuroimaging*, *1*(5), 386–392. https://doi.org/10.1016/j.bpsc.2016.05.001

Pievsky, M. A., & McGrath, R. E. (2018). The neurocognitive profile of attention-deficit/hyperactivity disorder: A review of meta-analyses. *Archives of Clinical Neuropsychology*, *33*(2), 143–157. https://doi.org/10.1093/arclin/acx055

Pike, A. C., & Robinson, O. J. (2022). Reinforcement learning in patients with mMood and anxiety disorders vs control individuals: A systematic review and meta-analysis. *JAMA Psychiatry*, *79*(4), 313–322. https://doi.org/10.1001/jamapsychiatry.2022.0051

Poldrack, R. A. (2015). Is "efficiency" a useful concept in cognitive neuroscience? *Developmental Cognitive Neuroscience*, *11*, 12–17. https://doi.org/10.1016/j.dcn.2014.06.001

Pouget, A., Beck, J. M., Ma, W. J., & Latham, P. E. (2013). Probabilistic brains: Knowns and unknowns. *Nature Neuroscience*, *16*(9), 1170–1178. https://doi.org/10.1038/nn.3495

Powers, A. R., Mathys, C., & Corlett, P. R. (2017). Pavlovian conditioning–induced hallucinations result from overweighting of perceptual priors. *Science*, *357*(6351), 596–600. https://doi.org/10.1126/science.aan3458

Preacher, K. J., Rucker, D. D., MacCallum, R. C., & Nicewander, W. A. (2005). Use of the extreme groups approach: A critical reexamination and new recommendations. *Psychological Methods*, *10*(2), 178–192. https://doi.org/10.1037/1082-989X.10.2.178

Robbins, T. W., Gillan, C. M., Smith, D. G., de Wit, S., & Ersche, K. D. (2012). Neurocognitive endophenotypes of impulsivity and compulsivity: Towards dimensional psychiatry. *Trends in Cognitive Sciences*, *16*(1), 81–91.

Rutledge, R. B., Chekroud, A. M., & Huys, Q. J. (2019). Machine learning and big data in psychiatry: Toward clinical applications. *Current Opinion in Neurobiology*, *55*, 152–159.

Rutledge, R. B., Moutoussis, M., Smittenaar, P., Zeidman, P., Taylor, T., Hrynkiewicz, L., Lam, J., Skandali, N., Siegel, J. Z., Ousdal, O. T., Prabhu, G., Dayan, P., Fonagy, P., & Dolan, R. J. (2017). Association of neural and emotional impacts of reward prediction errors with major depression. *JAMA Psychiatry*, *74*(8), 790–797. https://doi.org/10.1001/jamapsychiatry.2017.1713

Sadikaj, G., Wright, A. G. C., Dunkley, D. M., Zuroff, D. C., & Moskowitz, D. S. (2021). Multilevel structural equation modeling for intensive longitudinal data: A practical guide for personality researchers. In J. F. Rauthmann (Ed.), *The handbook of personality dynamics and processes* (pp. 855–885). Elsevier Academic Press. https://doi.org/10.1016/B978-0-12-813995-0.00033-9

Sajjadian, M., Lam, R. W., Milev, R., Rotzinger, S., Frey, B. N., Soares, C. N., Parikh, S. V., Foster, J. A., Turecki, G., Müller, D. J., Strother, S. C., Farzan, F., Kennedy, S. H., & Uher, R. (2021). Machine learning in the prediction of depression treatment outcomes: A systematic review and meta-analysis. *Psychological Medicine*, *51*(16), 2742–2751. https://doi.org/10.1017/S0033291721003871

Schmack, K., Bosc, M., Ott, T., Sturgill, J. F., & Kepecs, A. (2021). Striatal dopamine mediates hallucination-like perception in mice. *Science*, *372*(6537), eabf4740. https://doi.org/10.1126/science.abf4740

Shafiei, G., Keller, A. S., Bertolero, M., Shanmugan, S., Bassett, D. S., Chen, A. A., Covitz, S., Houghton, A., Luo, A., Mehta, K., Salo, T., Shinohara, R. T., Fair, D., Hallquist, M. N., & Satterthwaite, T. D. (2024). Generalizable links between borderline personality traits and functional connectivity. *Biological Psychiatry*, *96*(6), 486–494. https://doi.org/10.1016/j.biopsych.2024.02.1016

Sharma, L., Markon, K. E., & Clark, L. A. (2014). Toward a theory of distinct types of "impulsive" behaviors: A meta-analysis of self-report and behavioral measures. *Psychological Bulletin*, *140*(2), 374–408. http://dx.doi.org/10.1037/a0034418

Shultz, S., Opie, C., & Atkinson, Q. D. (2011). Stepwise evolution of stable sociality in primates. *Nature, 479*(7372), 219–222. https://doi.org/10.1038/nature10601

Simms, L. J., Wright, A. G. C., Cicero, D., Kotov, R., Mullins-Sweatt, S. N., Sellbom, M., Watson, D., Widiger, T. A., & Zimmermann, J. (2022). Development of measures for the Hierarchical Taxonomy of Psychopathology (HiTOP): A collaborative scale development project. *Assessment, 29*(1), 3–16. https://doi.org/10.1177/10731911211015309

Smillie, L. D. (2013). Extraversion and reward processing. *Current Directions in Psychological Science, 22*(3), 167–172. https://doi.org/10.1177/0963721412470133

Smith, R., Taylor, S., Wilson, R. C., Chuning, A. E., Persich, M. R., Wang, S., & Killgore, W. D. S. (2022). Lower levels of directed exploration and reflective thinking are associated with greater anxiety and depression. *Frontiers in Psychiatry, 12*, 782136. https://doi.org/10.3389/fpsyt.2021.782136

Sorzano, C. O. S., Vargas, J., & Montano, A. P. (2014). *A survey of dimensionality reduction techniques* (No. arXiv:1403.2877). arXiv. https://doi.org/10.48550/arXiv.1403.2877

Stephan, K. E., & Mathys, C. (2014). Computational approaches to psychiatry. *Current Opinion in Neurobiology, 25*, 85–92. https://doi.org/10.1016/j.conb.2013.12.007

Stephan, K. E., Penny, W. D., Daunizeau, J., Moran, R. J., & Friston, K. J. (2009). Bayesian model selection for group studies. *NeuroImage, 46*(4), 1004–1017. https://doi.org/10.1016/j.neuroimage.2009.03.025

Sterzer, P., Adams, R. A., Fletcher, P., Frith, C., Lawrie, S. M., Muckli, L., Petrovic, P., Uhlhaas, P., Voss, M., & Corlett, P. R. (2018). The predictive coding account of psychosis. *Biological Psychiatry, 84*(9), 634–643. https://doi.org/10.1016/j.biopsych.2018.05.015

Strom, N. I., Soda, T., Mathews, C. A., & Davis, L. K. (2021). A dimensional perspective on the genetics of obsessive-compulsive disorder. *Translational Psychiatry, 11*(1), 1–11. https://doi.org/10.1038/s41398-021-01519-z

Su, C., Aseltine, R., Doshi, R., Chen, K., Rogers, S. C., & Wang, F. (2020). Machine learning for suicide risk prediction in children and adolescents with electronic health records. *Translational Psychiatry, 10*(1), 1–10. https://doi.org/10.1038/s41398-020-01100-0

Szucs, D., & Ioannidis, J. P. A. (2017). Empirical assessment of published effect sizes and power in the recent cognitive neuroscience and psychology literature. *PLOS Biology, 15*(3), e2000797. https://doi.org/10.1371/journal.pbio.2000797

Totah, N., Akil, H., Huys, Q. J. M., Krystal, J. H., MacDonald, A. W., Maia, T. V., Malenka, R. C., & Pauli, W. M. (2016). Complexity and heterogeneity in psychiatric disorders: Opportunities for computational psychiatry. In A. D. Redish & J. A. Gordon (Eds.), *Computational psychiatry: New perspectives on mental illness* (pp. 33–60). MIT Press. https://doi.org/10.7551/mitpress/9780262035422.003.0003

Troisi, A. (2022). Biological psychiatry is dead, long live biological psychiatry! *Clinical Neuropsychiatry, 19*(6), 351–354. https://doi.org/10.36131/cnfioritieditore20220601

Ubl, B., Kuehner, C., Kirsch, P., Ruttorf, M., Diener, C., & Flor, H. (2015). Altered neural reward and loss processing and prediction error signalling in depression. *Social Cognitive and Affective Neuroscience, 10*(8), 1102–1112. https://doi.org/10.1093/scan/nsu158

Udochi, A. L., Blain, S. D., Sassenberg, T. A., Burton, P. C., Medrano, L., & DeYoung, C. G. (2022). Activation of the default network during a theory of mind task predicts individual differences in agreeableness and social cognitive ability. *Cognitive, Affective and Behavioral Neuroscience, 22*(2), 383–402. https://doi.org/10.3758/S13415-021-00955-0/TABLES/4

Urban, C. J., & Bauer, D. J. (2021). A deep learning algorithm for high-dimensional exploratory item factor analysis. *Psychometrika, 86*(1), 1–29. https://doi.org/10.1007/s11336-021-09748-3

Urban, C. J., & Gates, K. M. (2021). Deep learning: A primer for psychologists. *Psychological Methods, 26*(6), 743.

Vanyukov, P. M., Hallquist, M. N., Delgado, M., Szanto, K., & Dombrovski, A. Y. (2019). Neurocomputational mechanisms of adaptive learning in social exchanges. *Cognitive, Affective, & Behavioral Neuroscience, 19*, 985–997. https://doi.org/10.3758/s13415-019-00697-0

Voineskos, A. N., Hawco, C., Neufeld, N. H., Turner, J. A., Ameis, S. H., Anticevic, A., Buchanan, R. W., Cadenhead, K., Dazzan, P., Dickie, E. W., Gallucci, J., Lahti, A. C., Malhotra, A. K., Öngür, D., Lencz, T., Sarpal, D. K., & Oliver, L. D. (2024). Functional magnetic resonance imaging in schizophrenia:

Current evidence, methodological advances, limitations and future directions. *World Psychiatry*, *23*(1), 26–51. https://doi.org/10.1002/wps.21159

Volkow, N. D., Koob, G. F., & McLellan, A. T. (2016). Neurobiologic advances from the brain disease model of addiction. *New England Journal of Medicine*, *374*(4), 363–371. https://doi.org/10.1056/NEJMra1511480

Watson, D. (2005). Rethinking the mood and anxiety disorders: A quantitative hierarchical model for DSM-V. *Journal of Abnormal Psychology*, *114*(4), 522–536. https://doi.org/10.1037/0021-843X.114.4.522

Watson, D., Levin-Aspenson, H. F., Waszczuk, M. A., Conway, C. C., Dalgleish, T., Dretsch, M. N., Eaton, N. R., Forbes, M. K., Forbush, K. T., Hobbs, K. A., Michelini, G., Nelson, B. D., Sellbom, M., Slade, T., South, S. C., Sunderland, M., Waldman, I., Witthöft, M., Wright, A. G. C., . . . Zinbarg, R. E. (2022). Validity and utility of Hierarchical Taxonomy of Psychopathology (HiTOP): III. Emotional dysfunction superspectrum. *World Psychiatry*, *21*(1), 26–54. https://doi.org/10.1002/wps.20943

Webb, C. A., Trivedi, M. H., Cohen, Z. D., Dillon, D. G., Fournier, J. C., Goer, F., Fava, M., McGrath, P. J., Weissman, M., Parsey, R., Adams, P., Trombello, J. M., Cooper, C., Deldin, P., Oquendo, M. A., McInnis, M. G., Huys, Q., Bruder, G., Kurian, B. T., . . . Pizzagalli, D. A. (2019). Personalized prediction of antidepressant v. placebo response: Evidence from the EMBARC study. *Psychological Medicine*, *49*(7), 1118–1127. https://doi.org/10.1017/S0033291718001708

Weigard, A., McCurry, K. L., Shapiro, Z., Martz, M. E., Angstadt, M., Heitzeg, M. M., Dinov, I. D., & Sripada, C. (2023). Generalizable prediction of childhood ADHD symptoms from neurocognitive testing and youth characteristics. *Translational Psychiatry*, *13*(1), 1–11. https://doi.org/10.1038/s41398-023-02502-6

Whelan, R., & Garavan, H. (2014). When optimism hurts: Inflated predictions in psychiatric neuroimaging. *Biological Psychiatry*, *75*(9), 746–748. https://doi.org/10.1016/j.biopsych.2013.05.014

Widiger, T. A., & Sankis, L. M. (2000). Adult psychopathology: Issues and controversies. *Annual Review of Psychology*, *51*(1), 377. https://doi.org/10.1146/annurev.psych.51.1.377

Wiecki, T. V., Poland, J., & Frank, M. J. (2015). Model-based cognitive neuroscience approaches to computational psychiatry: Clustering and classification. *Clinical Psychological Science*, *3*(3), 378–399. https://doi.org/10.1177/2167702614565359

Wilson, R. C., & Collins, A. G. (2019). Ten simple rules for the computational modeling of behavioral data. *eLife*, *8*, e49547. https://doi.org/10.7554/eLife.49547

Wilson, R. C., & Niv, Y. (2015). Is model fitting necessary for model-based fMRI? *PLOS Computational Biology*, *11*(6), e1004237. https://doi.org/10.1371/journal.pcbi.1004237

Wise, T., Robinson, O. J., & Gillan, C. M. (2023). Identifying transdiagnostic mechanisms in mental health using computational factor modeling. *Biological Psychiatry*, *93*(8), 690–703. https://doi.org/10.1016/j.biopsych.2022.09.034

Yarkoni, T., & Westfall, J. (2017). Choosing prediction over explanation in psychology: Lessons from machine learning. *Perspectives on Psychological Science*, *12*(6), 1100–1122.

Zachar, P., & Kendler, K. S. (2017). The philosophy of nosology. *Annual Review of Clinical Psychology*, *13*(1), 49–71. https://doi.org/10.1146/annurev-clinpsy-032816-045020

Zachar, P., Turkheimer, E., & Schaffner, K. F. (2020). Defining and redefining phenotypes: Operational definitions as open concepts. In A. G. C. Wright & M. N. Hallquist (Eds.), *The Cambridge handbook of research methods in clinical psychology* (1st ed., pp. 5–17). Cambridge University Press. https://doi.org/10.1017/9781316995808.003

Zbozinek, T. D., Charpentier, C. J., Qi, S., & Mobbs, D. (2021). Economic decisions with ambiguous outcome magnitudes vary with low and high stakes but not trait anxiety or depression. *Computational Psychiatry*, *5*(1), 119. https://doi.org/10.5334/cpsy.79

CHAPTER 19

Dynamical Systems Approaches to Modeling Psychopathological Processes

LINDLEY R. SLIPETZ AND TEAGUE R. HENRY

Introduction

Psychological disorders are not static. They evolve over time, transitioning between different states and severities of the disease. For example, major depressive disorder is characterized by episodes of depressive symptoms, rather than one uniform level of depression. As such, dynamical systems analysis is particularly situated as a gold standard method for capturing these dynamic changes in psychopathology. Dimensional views of psychopathology, such as those articulated in Hopwood, Morey, and Markon (2023), are particularly amenable, both methodologically and theoretically, to this dynamical systems representation of disorders. Describing psychological disorders not as binary diagnoses, but rather as constellations of related symptoms and constructs, allows for questions such as, How do the dimensions of psychopathology related to one another over time, and What specific dimensions of psychopathology are most amenable to intervention? Increasingly, researchers see a greater need for dynamical models that can capture the intricacies of psychological trajectories. The options for adequate models of this kind are myriad, and this chapter sets out to explain and clarify the variety of models that are available for the use in modeling dimensional perspectives of psychopathology dynamically.

We begin with an explanation of dynamical systems, setting the stage for the over-arching modeling schema. We then differentiate between traditional data-driven models and more recent work on formal modeling in which psychological theory drives model creation. Overall, our goal is to articulate how these types of dynamical models are consistent and can be utilized with dimensional views of psychopathology.

What Are Dynamical Systems?

The term "dynamical system" covers a multitude of possible definitions, and is so expansive as to be near useless as a scientific specification. Put simply, a dynamical system is a mathematical description of how a variable or set of variables changes over time with respect to previous values of the variables. The dependency on previous values distinguishes the general class of dynamical systems from other models of longitudinal data such as growth models and developmental trajectory models. Here, growth models refer to modeling strategies similar to latent growth curves (Bollen & Curran, 2006), where the change in a variable over time is simply a function of time, rather than a function of previous values of a variable. In psychological research, growth models are often used to model change in constructs over a longer period of time (i.e., over several years, over a developmental period), where the time frame is large enough that any potential temporal relation among values of the studied constructs is small relative to the overall trajectory of that construct. However, in intensive longitudinal data, data collected many times over the course of a few days or weeks, due to the smaller time frame of measurement, temporal relations between variables are a stronger driver for the evolution of the system, and modeling those takes priority. It does need to be said that dynamical systems models can contain growth type processes, in which some aspect of the change is due to an exogenous variable such as time or seasonality, but at their core, dynamical systems are focused on how variables evolve with respect to their histories, and we adopt that property as the central theme of these models.

While dynamical systems distinguish themselves from other models of longitudinal data by focusing on temporal dependence of the component variables, this definition covers a variety of vastly different modeling scenarios. Figure 19.1 contains visualizations of four dynamical systems that differ both in their mathematical properties and in how they are used. Panel A contains a visualization of the Lorenz system (Lorenz, 1963), a widely studied example of a chaotic dynamical system (we will elaborate on these terms later), and, due to its simplicity,

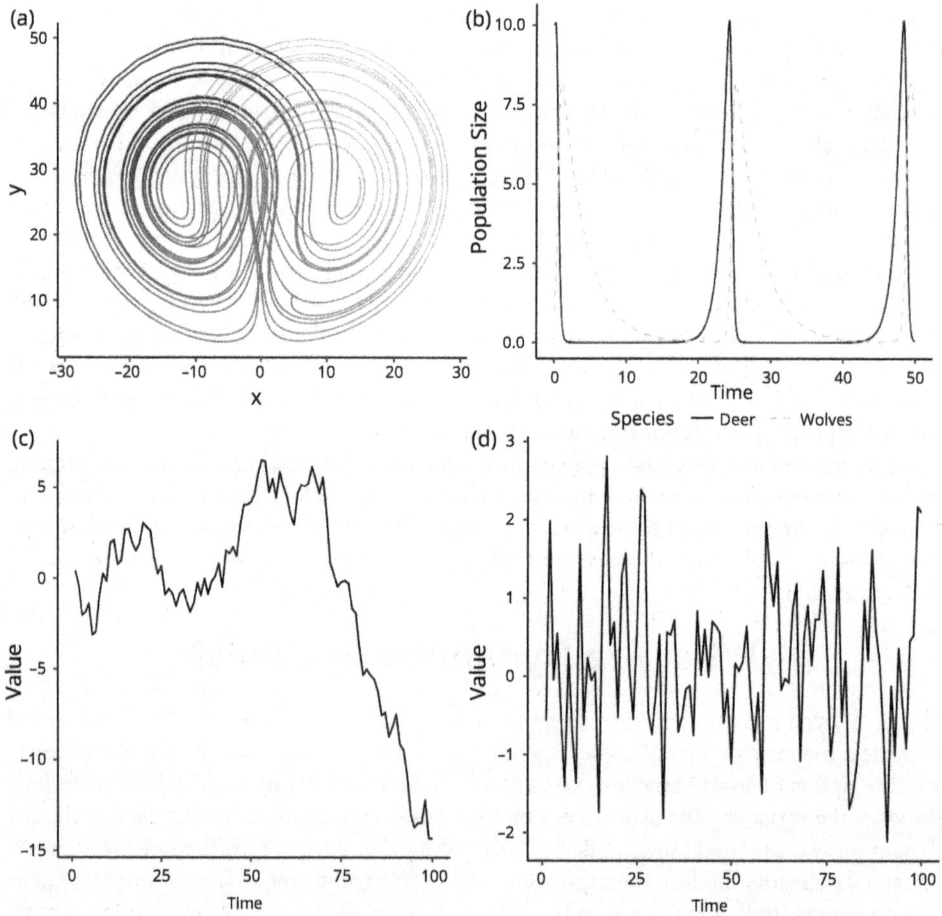

FIGURE 19.1 Examples of Dynamical Systems. A) Lorenz. B) Lokta-Volterra. C) Random Walk Autoregressive. D) Stationary Autoregressive.

usually the first example of a dynamical system readers might encounter when they start investigating the topic. Panel B contains a visualization of the Lokta-Volterra system, a non-chaotic system, that originally described the population dynamics between predator and prey species, and has been used to model infectious diseases (Hethcote, 2000) and language dynamics (Abrams & Strogatz, 2003). Panels C and D are two examples of an autoregressive system, $x_t = ax_{t-1} + \epsilon_t$, that have radically different properties depending on the value of the autoregressive parameter a. In panel C, $a = 1$, corresponding to a random walk process where the variable does not return to any equilibrium over time. Panel D, with $a = .25$, corresponds to a stationary system, in which any changes in the value of the variables will dissipate over time and the variables will fluctuate around an equilibrium point. Autoregressive systems are extensively used in the study of psychopathology, and we will describe them in further detail later in this section.

The point of the above comparison is to emphasize that these four systems, each with different properties and use cases, all fall under the blanket term of "dynamical systems." We break this class of models down further into the following, more useful, categories.

The first distinction in the class of dynamical systems is if the system is continuous- time or discrete-time. From a technical perspective, a continuous-time system is modeled using differential equations, while a discrete-time system is modeled using difference or autoregressive equations. Conceptually, continuous-time systems can be evaluated at any point in time, and the time interval between observations can differ. For example, a continuous-time model of the dynamics of depression symptoms measured multiple times a day would be able to appropriately model differences in data collection times, and, in theory, would be able to provide a prediction for any specific time (including a time without collected data). The Lorenz and Lokta-Volterra systems in Figure 19.1 are two examples of continuous-time dynamical systems. Discrete-time systems do not account for the specific time interval between observations, instead modeling the relation between time points directly (which implicitly makes the assumption that the interval between time points is equal). Discrete-time systems are expressed using difference equations and/or autoregressive equations, and the two autoregressive systems presented in Figure 19.1 are examples of discrete-time systems.

The utility of a continuous-time system versus a discrete-time system generally depends on the timescale of studied process and the ability to gather data on that timescale. Continuous-time systems tend to be best suited for the modeling of continuously measured processes, such as physical measurements (e.g., readings from passive sensors such as heart rate, light exposure, etc.), and are less suitable for the more common self-reported data collected in intensive longitudinal psychological research. The important exception here is when the specific time-interval is vital to the understanding of a process. Take, for example, a study of how the urge to engage in a disordered eating behavior relates to the actual disordered eating behavior. Here, the relationship between urge and behavior with respect to the specific amount of time between an urge and a behavior is the primary relation of interest. Because the specific time interval is important to the question, a continuous-time model would be warranted. Contrast this with a study of how daily stress and mood are related between days, with data being collected at the same time each day. Here, not only are the time intervals between data collections the same by design, the scientific question of interest does not relate to the specific time intervals between collections. As such, a discrete-time model would be more appropriate here. A full review of the differences between continuous-time and discrete-time approaches to modeling psychological data is beyond the scope of this chapter, and we refer interested readers to Voelkle, Gische, Driver, and Lindenberger (2018) as an overview, Voelkle, Oud, Davidov, and Schmidt (2012) as an interesting application of continuous time models, and to Boker, Tiberio, and Moulder (2018) for work on the impact of time-interval misspecification.

The next distinction to discuss is that of chaotic versus non-chaotic systems. Unlike with the distinction between continuous-time and discrete-time systems, chaotic versus non-chaotic are, at least in application to psychological research, a matter of degree. A chaotic system, by traditional definitions, is one in which the behavior of the system is extremely sensitive to initial conditions[1]. This in turn implies that chaotic systems are extremely sensitive to perturbations, as minute changes in the system will lead to radically different future trajectories. However, it must be noted that chaotic systems are not random in any sense. Indeed, chaotic systems are wholly deterministic, but, due to the sensitivity of the system, impossible to predict. Chaotic systems exhibit large-scale patterns of behavior, like the two lobes of the Lorenz system in Figure 19.1, but it is difficult to predict when chaotic systems might exhibit one of those patterns of behavior or switch among multiple distinct patterns. Contrast this with a non-chaotic dynamical system like that of the Lokta-Volterra system in Figure 19.1 where there are consistent, predictable patterns of behavior, here representing the population dynamics of a prey and predator species.

While the technical properties of chaotic systems are less relevant for the study of psychological systems, simply due to the fact that specific examples of chaotic systems tend to involve some level of abstraction, conceptually there are two properties that do apply to the theoretical understanding of psychological systems. First, the sensitivity to initial conditions captures the notion that the trajectory of a given person's psychological system (of any kind) will be highly dependent on the life history of the individual. Second, the sensitivity to disturbances captures the notion that an individual's psychological system does not evolve in a vacuum, and will be heavily impacted (perhaps even wholly driven by) life events. Bringing these considerations back to practical advice, they suggest that in any study of psychological systems, researchers should take care to collect relevant trait and life history information, so as to control for potential variations due to differences, as well as collect markers of relevant life events during the data collection time frame (for example, daily stressors).

The next important property of dynamical systems is the notion of stationarity. On a technical level, a stationary system is one in which its statistical properties (e.g., the mean, covariance, etc.) do not change over time. However, this rather dry definition does not adequately capture the consequences of a stationary system. In a strictly stationary system, no permanent meaningful change is possible. Any fluctuation, any external perturbation to the system, might cause a change in the system, but that change will quickly dissipate as the system returns to equilibrium. From the perspective of psychopathology research, a stationary representation of a psychopathological process would both be impossible to permanently intervene on as well as never able to exhibit the sort of transitions between pathological states that characterize most disorders. This in turn makes stationary models an inappropriate choice for representing the data-generating process of these sorts of systems. The autoregressive process in Panel D of Figure 19.1 is one example of a stationary process, where the values of the process fluctuate around the mean value. Non-stationary processes are a wide class of models, as all it means for a process to be non-stationary is for the statistical properties to change in some way. Common non-stationary models used in psychopathology research include regime-switching autoregressive processes (Hamaker, Grasman, & Kamphuis, 2010), where, for example, discrete shifts in the severity of symptoms are explicitly modeled; time-varying parameter

[1] There are two other properties that define a chaotic system, topological mixing (where the system is guaranteed to visit any given point in the space eventually), and dense periodic orbits (Strogatz, 2024). While these properties are important to understand chaotic systems mathematically, they are less useful in understanding the conceptual implications of chaotic systems for psychological research.

processes, where the relationships between variables are allowed to change over time (Fisher et al., 2022); and random walk processes, where perturbations in the system are permanent (Henry, Robinaugh, & Fried 2022). Panel C in Figure 19.1 shows an example of a random walk process. Note that in contrast to the stationary process shown in Panel D, the random walk process does not fluctuate around any specific point.

There are several other terms used in the dynamical systems modeling of psychopathology that are useful to review. The notion of "attractor states" refers to points in the system's space in which the process might become trapped in, orbit around permanently, or, in chaotic systems, orbit temporally before transitioning to a new attractor. Psychopathology research tends to use the term more colloquially, describing psychopathological (i.e., high symptom severity) and healthy (i.e., low symptom severity) states as attractors. The term "phase transition" is closely related to attractor states, and originally referred to the behavior of matter as it transitions among solid, liquid, and gas phases. In psychopathology research, phase transition refers to a sudden qualitative change in the overall behavior of the system, for example, the transition to a manic state in a patient with bipolar disorder. The key feature of a phase transition is that the behavior of the system changes *suddenly*. Phase transitions are closely related to the concept of "criticality," which refers how phase transitions occur when control parameters (i.e., aspects of the dynamical system that are not the variables under study) reach certain points. The classic example of criticality is found in the phase transition behavior of the Ising model, which originally was used to model magnetization in ferrous materials. Ferrous materials transition suddenly from a magnetic state, where the atoms' spins are aligned, to a para-magnetic state, where the atoms' spins are not aligned, once the temperature of the material reaches its critical point. In psychopathology research, an example of a critical point and corresponding phase transition can be found in the seminal work of Robinaugh et al. (2019). There, the authors present a formal model of panic disorder and show that changing an individual's arousal schema (i.e., how one interprets and reacts to their own physiological arousal) leads to a phase transition in the occurrence of panic attacks, where a small change in arousal schema at the critical value leads to the presence or absence of panic attacks. Criticality is an important property in the study of dynamical systems conceptualizations of psychopathology as parameters that lead to phase transitions provide potential intervention targets with large impacts on behavior.

With the terminology of dynamical system modeling established, we can now turn to the central theme of this chapter, that of how dynamical systems models have been used to study dimensional views of psychopathology.

Dynamical Systems and Dimensional Views of Psychopathology

While modern dynamical systems approaches to psychopathology research are firmly rooted in the empirical tradition, the notion that psychopathology arises from the interaction between the system that is the patient, and the system that is the environment originates with Freud (Breuer & Freud, 1895). Psychotherapists have characterized psychopathology using language very close to that of more modern dynamical systems. In Delmonte (1989), "People with relatively stable but 'maladaptive' behavioral repertories have arrived at a certain equilibrium. Their symptoms make sense in as far as they are attempted solutions to problems and they thus help create systemic balance" (p. 120). However, there is an important conceptual distinction to be made between the systems view espoused in the psychotherapeutic tradition and the modern dynamical systems view. The psychotherapeutic view tends to conceptualize psychopathology as arising from the interaction of the person with their environment, and that in order to treat a disorder, one must understand what role psychopathology plays in that interaction. Less discussed is how specific symptoms of a given disorder interact with one another over time to, at least in part, give rise to psychopathological states. While environment and external events play an important role in current work, it is this notion of causally interacting symptoms that underlies much of the current use of dynamical systems methods in psychopathology research.

Modern dynamical systems approaches to psychopathology primarily originated with the rise of network psychometrics, which is both (1) a theoretical orientation regarding the underlying nature of psychopathology and psychological constructs, and (2) a set of analysis techniques. Network psychometrics conceptualizes psychopathology as a set of causally interacting symptoms, behaviors, or issues, the collective dynamics of which lead to an individual's psychological system entering a psychopathological attractor state (Borsboom & Cramer, 2013; Epskamp, 2020; Marsman et al., 2018). This is in sharp contrast to the historical conceptualization of psychopathology, which has been termed the "medical model" or "common cause" model of psychopathology. Traditionally, the symptoms of psychopathology were thought to arise from a common cause, for example, the symptoms of depression are all indicators of the underlying condition. This way of describing the underlying structure of psychopathology fits neatly into the way that symptoms are described for physical medical disorders. For example, the symptoms of measles arise from the underlying cause, the measles virus. Network psychometrics rejects this conceptualization that complex mental disorders such as depression can be reduced to a latent common cause comparable to a measles virus. Instead, network psychometrics proposes that the symptoms of a psychological disorder are in part the interacting "causes" from which the disorder emerges. From Borsboom and Cramer (2013), "psychopathology symptoms are not symptoms in the strict sense of the word. Instead of passive receptors of the causal influence of a medical condition, symptoms are causally active ingredients of the mental disorders themselves" (p. 96).

Readers will already notice that the network psychometric conceptualization of psychopathology has a great deal of synergy with the dynamical systems perspective described previously, and indeed, the two strongly support one another. Network psychometrics, with the focus on the causal relations between symptoms, allows for the application of dynamical systems approaches at the level of the symptoms, while the dynamical systems perspective lends itself well to describing and quantifying how causally interacting sets of symptoms can transition between healthy functioning and psychopathological dysfunction. Dimensional views of psychopathology can also synergize well with dynamical systems approaches, but dimensional views of psychopathology need to be better conceptually reconciled with the network psychometric perspective to fully link the three approaches, and that task is what we turn to now.

At the simplest level, the dimensional view of psychopathology, as summarized by Hopwood et al. (2023), can be defined in contrast to the categorical view of psychopathology. While the categorical view of psychopathology provides binary determinations of disorder status (i.e., one either has or does not have a given disorder based on a count of symptoms), a dimensional view allows for a continuous spectrum of psychopathology severity. For example, a categorical view of depression would specify that an individual is depressed if they exhibit a certain number of symptoms, while the dimensional view cares less about a threshold for diagnosis and more about the *number* of symptoms present. This is the simplest possible definition of the dimensional view and is wholly compatible with the dynamical systems approach to modeling, and partially compatible with the network psychometric perspective. Dynamical systems can be used to model the changes in disorder severity over time and with respect to external predictors like stress and mood, while the focus on severity of a disorder rather than categorical diagnoses aligns this perspective with network psychometrics, though without focus on the causal dynamics of individual symptoms/behaviors/issues this alignment is incomplete.

Dimensional views of psychopathology do not stop at the focus on continuous severity of disorders, however, and instead propose transdiagnostic organizing principles for sets of symptoms. For example, the Hierarchical Taxonomy of Psychopathology (HiTOP) uses data-driven methods to organize symptoms into conceptually cohesive continuous spectra, such as internalizing and externalizing symptoms (Kotov et al., 2017), while the Research Domain Criteria (RDoC) initiative organizes behaviors into different biologically based systems, such as negative/positive valence systems and social processes (Insel et al., 2010). That both HiTOP and RDoC exist simultaneously illustrates an important property of dimensional views of psychopathology: they are systems of measurement, fundamentally related to the organization of behavioral data for specific purposes, rather than purporting to establish the "true" structure of psychopathology. In the case of HiTOP, the guiding principle is to organize psychopathological behaviors into common spectra. This in turn serves to enrich our delineations of mental disorders beyond simple categories, in particular enabling research on common patterns of behavior across diagnostic categories and their transdiagnostic treatment. RDoC, on the other hand, seeks to organize psychopathological behaviors (as well as normative behaviors) into categories that correspond to basic biological/neural processes. This in turn serves to guide research as to how these basic processes might be understood to relate to the behaviors, and how treatments might be based on these processes.

In contrast to dimensional views, the dynamical system perspective of psychopathology is not a system of measurement, as it is agnostic to the specific way of organizing data. Rather, dynamical systems applied to psychopathology provide a means to quantify how psychopathology, its behavioral expressions, and its etiological factors, change together over time. Fundamentally, dynamical systems are a framework with which researchers can posit causal systems that can explain how pathological behavior emerges, evolves, and interacts with other factors such as treatment or external events. While it is certainly analytically possible to construct dynamical systems in which categorical diagnoses are changing together over time, the very nature of categorical diagnoses make this sort of dynamical system less useful for understanding the dynamics of psychopathology than a dimensional view. The reason for this is that categorical diagnoses are summarizations of collections of symptoms and lack the granularity necessary to provide scientifically or clinically useful information about the dynamics of a disorder. For example, a dynamical model of the presence/absence of depressive episodes might, at most, provide information as to external drivers of those episodes, but would provide no information as to which specific symptoms are being impacted by those external drivers. Applied across multiple individuals, potential heterogeneity in the definition of a diagnosis is also a problem. If depressive episodes are modeled for two individuals who share no overlapping symptoms, what can be said about the predictors of those episodes? In both cases, the question is why model a categorical summarization of potentially non-overlapping symptoms, when one can apply the same approach to the symptoms themselves? If necessary, the dynamics of the categorical diagnoses can be directly calculated from the dynamics of the symptoms. Put simply, dimensional views of psychopathology are necessary for dynamical systems models of psychopathology because dimensional views provide a sufficiently rich measurement structure for subsequent dynamical systems models to explore.

Data-driven Models versus Formal Models

With terminology now established, and an overview of the intersections between dynamical systems and dimensional views of psychopathology provided, we can now discuss specific dynamical systems methodologies and how they can be, and have been, applied to psychopathology research. Broadly speaking, we can divide dynamical systems models into two types based on their use of data or not. Dynamical systems models that are fit to datasets we refer to as data-driven models. Dynamical systems models that are constructed to reflect a substantive theory of a disorder, rather than being estimated from data, are formal models. In either case, as we describe the model types below, we will focus on high-level understanding of these models rather than specific technical details, and in each case provide references to more technical work.

Data-driven Models

Data-driven models are the most commonly used within the context of psychology, as empirical data serves as the basis for model construction and testing. The most basic data-driven dynamical systems model is that of the vector autoregressive model (VAR; Sims, 1980), and a detailed understanding of this model type is important to understand subsequent elaborations.

The VAR Family of Models

Consider an intensive longitudinal dataset that has a set of symptom/behavior (or composite measures of behavior) variables, **x**, evaluated at each time point, *t*, for a single participant, *i*. A VAR model represents the temporal dynamics, that is, how each variable is related to one another over time, as a linear system:

$$\mathbf{x}i,t+1 = \mu i + \mathbf{A}\mathbf{x}i,t + \varepsilon i,t+1 \tag{1}$$

where μi is a vector of means, **A** is a matrix of regression coefficients representing how each variable in $\mathbf{x}_{i,t}$ is related to each variable in $\mathbf{x}_{i,t+1}$, and $\boldsymbol{\varepsilon}$ is a vector of normally distributed error. The above VAR model is a VAR model at lag-1, commonly denoted as VAR(1), which means it posits that the temporal relation between variables is relevant only for consecutive timepoints. VAR models with greater lags can also be modeled, such as a VAR(2), which would posit that x_t depends on both x_{t-1} and x_{t-2}, but the most common VAR model applied to psychopathology data is the VAR(1) model. The use of VAR models or their extensions are often justified via an appeal to Granger causality (Shojaie & Fox, 2022), and it is important to understand what this concept means in the context of analyzing intensive longitudinal (ILD) data. A variable *X* is said to Granger-cause a different variable *Y* if *X* precedes *Y*, and *X* provides unique information as to values of *Y*. In the context of VAR models, based on these two criteria, a significant lagged relation between two variables can be interpreted as Granger causality. However, Granger causality is not the same as causality, and its developer later specified Granger causality as simply showing that variables are temporally related and therefore useful in forecasting applications (Granger & Newbold, 1986).

A VAR model is a simplistic model of the dynamics of psychopathology, positing that symptoms at time *t* are linearly related to symptoms at time *t* + 1 and that this is the whole of their temporal relation. Due to this linear setup, VAR models carry with them an assumption of stationarity (i.e., the means and parameters are indexed to individuals and not to time)[2],

[2] As a technical aside, a linear VAR model could be non-stationary. However, there are only two forms of non-stationarity it could achieve: explosive, where the variables increase/decrease exponentially; or random walk, which is only achieved at very specific parameter values. More to the point, the estimation of VAR models assume stationarity, so any VAR model fit to empirical data will result in a stationary model.

which in turn implies that interesting non-linear relations among symptoms, such as chaotic behavior, attractor states, and phase transitions, do not occur. Conceptually, VAR models can be thought of as exploratory dynamical systems models, suitable for uncovering broad patterns of temporal relations between symptoms. However, the basic VAR model described above has a number of methodological weaknesses that have been addressed in subsequent extensions. Primary to these, the basic VAR model is suitable for analysis at either a purely idiographic level (i.e., fitting a separate model to each participant), or a purely nomothetic level (i.e., fitting a single model to all participants data). The multi-level VAR (mlVAR; Bringmann et al., 2013) addresses this issue.

The mlVAR model is a multi-level extension of the VAR model, where both fixed effects, quantifying the aggregate temporal relations between variables, and random effects, quantifying the inter-individual differences in those temporal relations, are modeled. The mlVAR model is the first model described here that we consider to be universally usable for the analysis of typical intensive longitudinal psychopathology data. This is to say that mlVAR has a simple to use implementation, its behaviors are well understood (as the model is fundamentally a series of mixed effects models), and can appropriately account for multiple participants' time series data. It is important to note however, that mlVAR retains the same weaknesses as the basic VAR model, in that it is still a linear, stationary model incapable of demonstrating emergent dynamical systems properties that arise from non-linearity (i.e., transitions, permanent change, etc.). mlVAR has been implemented in the mlvar R package as outlined by Epskamp, Deserno, and Bringmann (2019).

The mlVAR model has been further extended by the generalized VAR modeling framework (GVAR; Epskamp, 2020). In a GVAR model, the contemporaneous relations, controlling for the temporal relations, between variables are modeled as a Gaussian graphical model, resulting in partial correlation estimates of the relations within a given time point. The GVAR model also estimates the relations between the mean values of variables, representing how different variables are related to one another at a between-subjects level. Between these three sets of effects, the temporal relations of variables, the relations between variables within a time point controlling for the temporal relations, and the between-subject relations among the means of the variables, the GVAR model provides a comprehensive view of the linear dynamics between the analyzed variables. However, the extension to contemporaneous effects and addition of the between-subjects effects does not change the linear, stationary nature of the VAR model, and therefore the GVAR approach carries with it the same concerns as previously noted. GVAR has also been implemented in the mlVAR R package (Epskamp et al., 2019).

The VAR type models discussed so far involve the estimation of every pairwise temporal relation between variables. If there are p symptoms being analyzed in a traditional GVAR model, then there will be p^2 lag-1 relations estimated. Not only does accurately estimating this number of parameters require large amounts of ILD data, estimating every single temporal relation is not parsimonious and can result in overfitting the model to the data. There are two approaches to VAR modeling that result in more parsimonious models, regularized VAR and Group Iterative Multiple Model Estimation (GIMME; Gates & Molenaar, 2012). Regularized VAR uses a method called graphical LASSO (Friedman, Hastie, & Tibshirani, 2008) to "shrink" small temporal relations to 0, resulting in a sparse set of temporal relations between variables. The advantage of this approach is that, once properly tuned, regularized models are often more generalizable than unregularized models as they avoid the issue of overfitting. The disadvantage of regularized methods is that they must be *tuned*, in that there are user-specified parameters in the model that must be chosen to maximize the performance of the regularization. Lack of appropriate tuning will result in models that are either overfit, or too harshly regularized and therefore underfit. There are a number of methods for tuning regularized models, and a review of them is beyond the scope of this chapter. Additionally, while regularized mlVAR models are possible to estimate using more general R packages such as glmnet, turnkey implementations are not available in popular network psychometrics packages like mlvar or psychonetrics. As such, using regularized VAR models requires substantial technical expertise to both implement and tune appropriately.

The GIMME algorithm (Gates & Molenaar, 2012) provides a simple to use alternative to regularized VAR. Briefly, GIMME fits separate GVAR models to each participant's ILD data, modifying them in a stepwise fashion. Effects that are common for some large percentage of the participants are classified as group level effects, and are estimated for all participants, while individual participants also have individual level paths. This results in a group level model that reflects common patterns of temporal relations between variables, as well as individual level models that can capture inter-individual differences in the temporal relations. While there are a number of technical differences between GIMME and regularized VAR or GVAR, the end point is ultimately very similar: VAR models that describe common temporal relations between the analyzed variables while accounting for inter-individual differences in those temporal relations. GIMME has the added advantage of having an easy-to-use implementation (Lane et al., 2024), with added capabilities of subgroup detection (Gates, Lane, Varangis, Giovanello, & Guiskewicz, 2017), confirmatory subgroup testing (Henry et al., 2019), and integration of latent variables (Gates, Fisher, & Bollen, 2020).

At this point, we have reviewed a number of types of VAR models, and it is worth emphasizing that all of the model types reviewed thus far have similar advantages and disadvantages from the perspective of dynamical systems models of psychopathology. The advantage of these VAR-based methods is that they are ready to use exploratory models capable of testing if different variables are related to one another over time. Very little model building, apart from choosing which variables to include in the model, is needed, which in turn allows these approaches to be applied in an atheoretical way. There are two major disadvantages to these models that are, for the most part, common for each approach described. First, as previously mentioned, each of these previously described models are linear and stationary, and therefore cannot exhibit any interesting dynamical systems behaviors such as phase transitions or attractor states. This in turn implies that these models, while useful in exploring psychopathology from an atheoretical perspective, should not be used as confirmatory analysis models for theoretical models that hypothesize this sort of behavior. Second, each of the models described previously (with the exception of GIMME) are observed variable models. While using observed variables such as individual symptom severity is consistent with the dimensional view of psychopathology, this means these models are not able to directly model higher order dimensions of psychopathology as latent variables. Before moving on to describing different modeling techniques that do allow for dynamical systems behaviors and/or latent variable representations, it is useful to summarize recent work in psychopathology that have used the previously described modeling approaches.

Applications of VAR Models in Psychopathology Research

VAR models have been applied broadly within psychopathology research, as they excel as a first, exploratory step in determining how particular symptoms relate and change over time. It is a burgeoning area of research that currently has approximately 120 citations across psychology covering topics from differences in fear and avoidance in those with and without social anxiety (Heeren & McNally, 2018) to the relationship between anxiety and functional somatic symptoms (Groen, van Gils, Emerencia, Bos, & Rosmalen, 2021) to identifying the process characteristics for successful therapeutic interventions into PTSD (Leonhard Kratzer

& Karatzias, 2022). In a study of the treatment of depression, Snippe et al. (2015) explored the efficacy of mindfulness-based treatments in six women with depressive symptoms with idiographic VAR models with mindfulness, repetitive thinking, and depressive symptoms as variables. Snippe et al. (2015) found that changes in mindfulness and repetitive thinking did precede changes in depressive symptoms in some participants, though the reverse chain did not hold. In addition, there were strong contemporaneous links between the variables for all participants. Overall, VAR models are capable of capturing the trajectories of psychopathological symptoms; but many researchers rely solely on idiographic modeling (as opposed to the above partially idiographic choices), and they are limited to stationary processes.

Time-varying, Regime-switching, and Latent Variable Dynamical Systems Models

Methodologists working in the dynamical systems modeling field or the network psychometrics field have recognized the inherent limitations of the simple linear VAR models, and have proposed a number of extensions that each attempt to capture other aspects of dynamical behavior. Here, we divide these efforts into a number of broad categories: time-varying parameter models, in which the model might specify linear relations over time, but these linear relations also change over time and can therefore capture how the psychopathological process itself is changing as a result of treatment or exogenous stressors; regime-switching models, in which change points that correspond to sudden changes in the modeled variables, or sudden changes in the temporal relations, are automatically detected; and latent variable models, in which dimensional representations of higher order spectra can be integrated into the dynamical systems model. Each of these categories of model extensions represent the cutting edge of dynamical systems models applied to psychological science, with most of the literature developing these models appearing in the last 5 to 10 years. Here, we will describe specific examples within each category while focusing on how each category of model can be used to study different properties of dynamical systems.

Time-Varying Parameter Models

Time-varying parameter models allow for the temporal relations between variables to change smoothly as a function of time and/or other exogenous predictors. Because the temporal relations are allowed to change over the timecourse, these models can capture how psychopathological processes change over the course of treatment or simply with respect to time. This is an important capability of these models, as without allowing the parameters to change, the only change possible in the system is with respect to the levels of the analyzed variables. Applied to the study of psychopathology, time-invariant models would be able to potentially capture the effects of modelled treatments on the severity of the symptoms, but a time-varying parameter model would be able to capture how a treatment changes the causal relations between symptoms.

Time-varying parameter models have been developed in a number of different fields, from econometrics to neuroscience. Here, we will focus on time-varying parameter VAR models, as they have the most accessible implementations, but note that time-varying parameter models have also been developed in the context of dynamic factor models (see Fisher et al., 2022; Molenaar, Beltz, Gates, & Wilson, 2016). The two most accessible time-varying parameter VAR models are the Generalized Additive Model VAR of Bringmann, Ferrer, Hamaker, Borsboom, & Tuerlinckx (2018); Bringmann et al. (2017) (GAM-VAR) and the kernel smoothed VAR model of Haslbeck and Waldorp (2020) (KS-VAR). These methods have R implementations in the tvarGAM (Bringmann, 2023) and mgm (Haslbeck & Waldorp,

2020) packages, respectively. While it is beyond the scope of this chapter to go into detail as to the specific technical differences between these two model types, a brief description of the differences is useful to illustrate what researchers need to be concerned with while fitting these types of models. Both the GAM-VAR and KS-VAR are turn-key implementations that do not require the analyst to specify the model structure; rather, each model has a tuning parameter that impacts how the parameters can vary over time. In the GAM-VAR model, parameters vary non-linearly as a function of time, which is achieved under the GAM framework by use of spline functions. The specific technical details are beyond the current scope, but it is important to note that the correct application of GAM models requires careful tuning. For more details on the use and tuning of the GAM-VAR model, see Bringmann et al. (2018) and Haslbeck, Bringmann, & Waldorp (2021). KS-VAR uses a kernel smoothing approach to estimate how parameters vary over time. Like with GAM models, this approach requires careful tuning. Haslbeck and Waldorp (2020) describe a cross-validation procedure for tuning, and this procedure is included in the mgm package. Finally, we note that both GAM-VAR and KS-VAR have regularized implementations, but neither are implemented in a multi-level context. This means that these models must be applied idiographically (i.e., separately for each participant).

As the family of time-varying parameter VAR models are relatively new, they have not yet gained widespread application; however, using Bringmann et al. (2018), we see the utility of time-varying approaches for the study of different aspects of dynamical systems. Bringmann et al. (2018) estimate the trajectory of emotions, using a 91-day dataset of a dyad responding to 10 positive items ranked on a five-point Likert scale from the Positive and Negative Affective Schedule. They compared model fit, measured by AIC and BIC, of a variety of VAR models, ranging from fixed parameters to all parameters varying for each member of the dyad. Whether the model should use time-varying parameters depended on the fit index used and which member of the dyad was being considered, though, ultimately, they chose a model in which the intercept and cross-lagged effect were time-varying and the autoregressive effect was not. The way this model was interpreted was that the male's positive emotions from the previous day stably effected the following day, while the effect of the female's emotions on the male's emotions varied over time.

Regime Switching Models

Unlike time-varying parameter models, regime switching is characterized by abrupt changes in the means or dynamic parameters followed by a period of stability. These changes can be one-time changes (e.g., a shift in socialization variables in a sample taken pre- and during the pandemic) or recurrent, in which individuals fluctuate between regimes and back continually (e.g., individuals with bipolar disorder transitioning between depression and mania throughout the course of their life). The assumption of a regime switching framework is that an observation comes from one of these particular distributions or regimes (Hamaker & Grasman, 2012; C.-j. Kim & Nelson, 1999).

Regime switching models are widely applicable across psychological phenomena that show steady phases to the trajectories, for instance, in capturing sudden changes in drinking tendencies (Chow, Witkiewitz, Grasman, Hutton, & Maisto, 2014) or investigating dysregulated affect in bipolar disorder (Hamaker, Grasman, & Kamphuis, 2016). Hamaker et al. (2010) use Positive and Negative Affect Schedule (PANAS) data self-reported over 91 days for an individual with rapid cycling bipolar disorder. Comparing four models, they conclude that the patient's bipolar disorder can be modeled with two regimes in which the switch between regimes is influenced by an exogenous mechanism, that is, not by affect. Even so, they could not immediately conclude that the regimes coincided with mania and depression without further investigation into the specific values of positive and negative affect within each regime. With this additional information, an accurate interpretation of the character of the regimes could be given.

Latent Variable Models

The previously described modeling frameworks, with the exception of one extension of the GIMME model, are observed variable models: they assume that all variables entered into the model are measured without error. This, of course, is a problematic assumption to make in the context of any form of psychological research. Psychological measurements are prone to measurement error, and this is why the field has moved to develop measurement error modeling approaches such as confirmatory factor analysis and item response theory. Dynamical systems modeling has several approaches that allow for latent variables to be used.

Epskamp (2020) presents the ts-lvgvar (time-series latent-variable graphical VAR) model, a dynamic latent variable idiographic model appropriate for both continuous and discrete intensive time series, based on the work of Epskamp, Rhemtulla, & Borsboom (2017). Like traditional graphical VAR, temporal and contemporaneous networks are estimated; however, for ts-lvgvar, the networks are defined between latent variables rather than observed variables. In Epskamp (2020), he analyzes a one-subject data set of a man with depression measured over 239 days. Using an EFA, the author found five factors to utilize within the network that, within the temporal network, showed strong positive autoregressive effects and changes in the second factor predicted lower levels of the first factor. For the contemporaneous network (i.e., the partial correlations between variables that capture relationships within a given timepoint), the first factor played a central role as at high levels it corresponded to lower levels of all other factors.

State-space modeling is another form of dynamic latent variable modeling in which measured variables serve as indicators of unobserved states (Kalman, 1960). State-space models are comprised of a measurement model (akin to a factor model, though it can be even more flexible) and a model of how the latent variables (states) change together over time. One simple example of a state-space model would be a VAR of latent variables. A more elaborate state-space model might consist of a differential equation model that describes the change in states in continuous time, with a non-linear measurement model for those states. While this framework is extremely flexible, there are a number of technical caveats that make applying the more elaborate varieties to data generated by psychological studies difficult. For example, while traditional VAR models might erroneously treat Likert scale items as continuous, under a state space modeling framework, one can specify an ordinal variable measurement model. Henry, Slipetz, Falk, Qiu, and Chen (2024) do precisely that, developing ordinal state-space models that accommodate ordinal variables by using a graded response model (Samejima, 1969) as the underlying measurement model. However, estimating this class of models is difficult, requiring a number of identifying assumptions. For applied research, state-space modeling can be viewed as a generalized set of tools for estimating arbitrary types of dynamical systems.

One particular use case for state-space models is in estimating the trajectories of latent constructs as measured by symptom variables. These models have found use as such in evaluating the dynamics of attention bias (Takano, Taylor, Wittekind, Sakamoto, & Ehring, 2021) and assessing the relationship between depressive symptoms and temperament characteristics (Elovainio et al., 2015). As an example of state-space modeling applied to psychological data, McKee, Russell, Mennis, Mason, and Neale (2020) presented a continuous time model with the state being affect, which was measured by the observed affect measures. In addition, there were an autoregressive regulation parameter as the index of emotion regulation (which was defined as the percent recovery to equilibrium over each time period), a standard deviation of exogenous disturbances (which was defined as the unmeasured influences on the individuals), and total counts of nicotine, alcohol, and cannabis use. They found significant between-person relationships between affective state and substance use, perhaps indicating bidirectional temporal feedback cycles in which, for example, higher negative affect was associated with a higher tendency to use substances. This study demonstrates the ability of state-space models to track affective regulation over time, specifically, or regulation of psychological phenomena, generally, over time.

Non-Linear Models

Most of the modeling approaches described previously are extensions or generalizations of a linear model, in that variables relate to one another over time in a linear fashion. However, as mentioned previously, linear models do not allow one to capture emergent behaviors that a true dynamical system might exhibit. For example, data generated from a VAR model cannot exhibit sudden transitions in dynamics the way data generated from a dynamical systems model such as the Lorentz attractor can. Non-linear models are vital for the study of psychological dynamics (e.g., complex systems analyses of psychopathology in which the disorder is an emergent property of the model; see Cramer et al. (2016) or Wichers, Wigman, & Myin-Germeys (2015)), but they are considerably more difficult to specify (as non-linear refers to a infinite number of possible relations) and more difficult to estimate with empirical data.

Generalized Additive Models (GAM) are a type of semiparametric generalization of linear regression models in which the models are linear in the parameters, though the distribution of the parameters and the link between the parameters need not be (T.J. Hastie, 1990). They are semiparametric in that they combine both parametric and non-parametric terms within one model (Mckeown & Sneddon, 2013; T. J. Hastie, 1990). Key to these non-parametric elements is a smoothing function that often takes the form of splines, piecewise polynomial functions that are joined smoothly by what are termed "knots." (Bringmann et al., 2017; Sullivan, Shadish, & Steiner, 2015). This allows the predictors to change in non-linear ways (Brown, 1993). In practice, these models have found a variety of uses, including in work on markers of reassurance (J. J. Kim, Henderson, Best, Cunnington, & Kirby, 2020), patterns in hallucinogen use (Chilcoat & Schu¨tz, 1996), the dynamics of emotion (Mckeown & Sneddon, 2013), and the relationship between fear of childbirth and sleep quality (Mei et al., 2023). Bringmann et al. (2017) used a GAM model to assess emotional inertia, or the temporal dependence of emotions, in an isolation study meant to mimic the experience and duration of a Mars mission. Using this approach, the authors were able to depart from analyzing inertia at the trait level and, instead, had access to values of inertia at every timepoint. They fit idiographic models, which showed differing results for each participant, that is, a non-stationary model without autoregressive effects for Participant 1 and a model with significant autoregressive effects for Participant 2. Overall, the authors stress that these results would not have been uncovered if alternative models like a time-invariant model had been used.

Formal Models

Formal models are mathematical instantiations of a specific theory of psychopathology. For example, consider the relationship between negative affect and the symptoms of psychosis. This relationship has been found to be moderated by symptoms including stress sensitivity and depression levels (Kramer et al., 2013), and negative affect has also been found to moderate the relationship between insomnia and psychosis (Reeve, Nickless, Sheaves, & Freeman, 2018) and negative-self-schemas and psychosis symptoms (Jaya, Ascone, & Lincoln, 2018). Consider the translation of these theoretical claims into a formal model, for instance, the relation between high arousal negative affect and auditory hallucinations, a symptom of psychosis.

In our toy model, we follow the results of So et al. (2021) and say that negative affect (NA) predicts an increase in auditory hallucinations (AH), and auditory hallucinations predict an increase in negative affect. Beliefs about the alignment of the voices (i.e., if malevolent and omnipotent) moderated the cross-sectional relationship and increased hallucinatory experiences in the proceeding moments. This is a verbal theory of this relation that can be simplified and translated into the following quantitative model:

$$dNA = (\alpha NA + \gamma AH(\frac{AH}{AH_{thres}})^2)(1 - \frac{NA}{K_{NA}}) - \zeta NA \quad (2)$$

$$dAH = (-\delta AH + \varepsilon NA)(1 - \frac{AH}{K_{AH}}) \quad (3)$$

The model described by these equations has both NA and AH as self-limiting processes that are coupled together in a feedback loop. α represents the strength of self excitation for NA with ζ as the inhibitory effect. The rate of increase in NA is determined by both the current value of NA, as well as the current value of AH. The effect of AH on dNA(γ) is moderated by a soft threshold $(AH\frac{AH}{thres})^2$ that acts as a limiting factor on the effectiveness of AH in the model, entailing that at low levels of AH below the threshold (i.e., AH_{thres}), the coupling between NA and AH is weak, though strengthens when AH is greater than the threshold. The definition of dAH is an equation for a self-limiting system in which the only increase in AH is due to its coupling with NA (parameterized by ϵ). The system is stabilized against non-realistic behaviors by the terms $(1-\frac{NA}{K_{NA}})$ and $(1-\frac{AH}{K_{AH}})$.

This system is simulated in Figure 19.2 holding all parameters the same while varying the value of AH_{thres}. At a high threshold, when NA and AH only become coupled at high levels of psychosis, there is an overall decrease in in both NA and AH, with AH briefly increasing then dropping off. At a low threshold, when there is a strong feedback loop between NA and AH, there is an explosive relationship between NA and AH, which, in a real patient, would be indicative of the emergence of severe psychosis.

Further examples of formal models of psychopathology appear in Robinaugh et al. (2019) and Wang, Robinaugh, Millner, Fortgang, and Nock (2023). Using the network theoretical framework that claims that psychopathology is a complex system and clinical theory as a jumping-off point, Robinaugh et al. (2019) offers a computational model of panic disorder. They identify five core building blocks of panic disorder as their variables (physiological arousal, perceived threat, escape behavior, anxiety sensitivity, and avoidance behavior).

The components of the model are that there must be a positive feedback loop between physiological arousal and perceived threat (which represents the theoretically proposed "vicious cycle" of panic disorder), a negative feedback loop between perceived threat and escape behavior, and a learning feedback loop in which the panic attacks can either increase the belief in the danger of the arousal or disconfirm this belief (a positive feedback loop in the former case and a negative feedback loop in the latter case). While the model generally performed as expected via simulation, the authors identify two potential limitations to the model. First, it cannot account for non-clinical panic attacks. Second, if the participant is sufficiently elevated on the variables in the model, this will always result in a panic attack in the model; however, in reality, subjects can do things to lessen the possibility of panic attack onset.

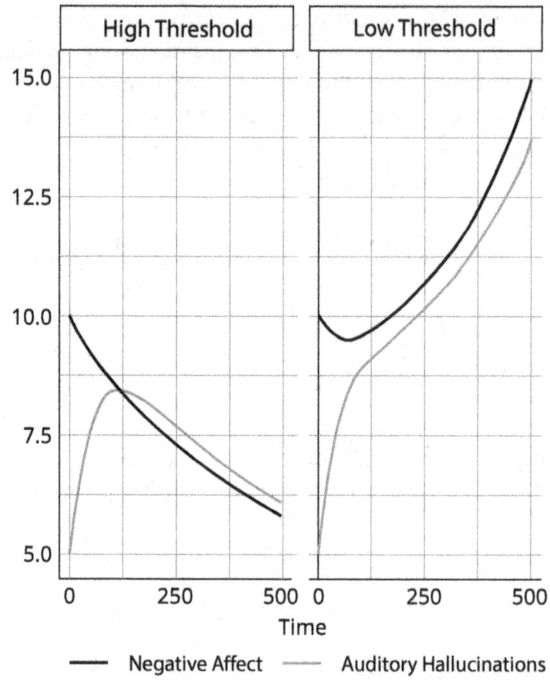

FIGURE 19.2 Simulated Trajectories. Left panel has a high AH_{thres}, right panel has a low AH_{thres}. All other parameters have the same values. Note: Units of X and Y axis are arbitrary.

Wang et al. (2023) propose a formal model of the General Escape Theory of Suicide, which asserts that suicidality arises from the urge to escape and eliminate what the authors call aversive internal states. It is a more complex model than the one cited in the previous section, with seven variables (suicidal thoughts, escape behaviors, urge to escape, aversive interval state, external-focused strategies, external stressors, and internal-focused strategies), with each variable with an autoregressive component. The proposed path is that external stressors lead to aversive internal states, resulting in escape behaviors. However, there is also a dampening feedback loop between the aversive internal states and the escape behaviors, which is a short-term strategy. Longer term strategies of external-focused strategies and internal-focused strategies may, in the long term, diminish the escape behaviors, and suicidality occurs when these strategies fail.

Formal modeling of psychopathology is a nascent but rapidly developing field, brought on by both an increase in the methodological sophistication of researchers and the availability of intensive longitudinal *and* dimensional data. The approach of formal modeling, summarized by Haslbeck, Ryan, Robinaugh, Waldorp, and Borsboom (2022), allows researchers to precisely quantify hypotheses by formalizing theoretical models into mathematical equations. This approach has great promise to the study of psychopathology, meshing the theoretical and methodological sides of research, but there are a number of issues that must be addressed in the near future. Core to these issues is that, as of now, formal models are divorced from empirical data. This is to say that formal models are developed from empirically supported theory, and the behaviors of the dynamical systems described are compared against previous empirical findings, but empirical data is not directly integrated into the estimation of these formal models. This is an important step in validating these models, as without a direct connection to empirical data, we can only qualitatively compare findings. Related to this issue are concerns about measurement and timescale. Formal models simulate at the level of the constructs rather than at the level of individual items that might be collected in a study. Integrating measurement into formal models is a necessary step for both generating reasonable data, as well as integrating empirical data into the specification and estimation of these models. Timescale is another methodological concern with formal models. Empirical data has a collection limit, for example, it is not possible to collect psychological data at every moment of every day. As such, empirical studies of psychopathology dynamics need to think carefully about when and how often to collect the necessary information. Contrast this to formal models, which can simulate an unlimited amount of data that does not necessarily take into account a reasonable timescale for the modeled process. This can be easily resolved by reparameterizing the formal models to operate on an empirical timescale, but this in turn will change how these models function. Resolving both the measurement and timescale issues with formal modeling will open the door to estimating the parameters of these models using empirically collected data, and this can be relatively easily achieved using the previously described state-space framework. Once empirical data can be directly linked to formal models, this will provide a way for researchers to close the scientific loop: Specify a formal model based on theory, directly evaluate the performance of the model on empirical data, accept or falsify the proposed model based on that performance.

Summary, Conclusions, and Future Directions

Dynamical systems applied to the study of psychopathology portray mental disorders not as a static entity, but rather as a collection of symptoms, problems, and behaviors that cause and change together over time. Under this conceptualization, psychopathology is a form of pathological state of the underlying psychological system, which is driven to pathology by a combination of external factors and the dynamics of the system itself. It is clear where the dimensional view of psychopathology fits into dynamical systems: it provides a rich characterization of psychopathology that allows for these dynamical systems models to be defined in a way that would be near impossible using a more traditional diagnosis-based view of psychopathology.

In this chapter we have provided a technical grounding for the various features of dynamical systems (i.e., phase transitions, chaotic behavior, non-linear dynamics) that are most applicable to the study of psychopathology. Following that, we presented an overview of the most common data-driven modeling approaches, from the humble VAR model to the more flexible state-space modeling approach. These model types capture the most common data-driven dynamical systems modeling techniques in psychological science, and are, for the most part, available in easy to use software packages. The specific use of each modeling type is highly dependent on the scientific question being posed, and researchers need to consider the use of each of these models carefully. We also presented a brief overview of formal modeling, an approach to constructing complex mathematical models of psychological phenomena based on existing theory. These formal models allow researchers to study psychopathology *in silico*, performing simulation studies to evaluate how changes in different constructs might lead to changes in behavior.

We end this chapter with a call for researchers interested in applying dynamical systems methods to psychopathology, and to methodologists interested in developing new tools for studying psychopathology: the dynamical systems modeling approach has a great deal of promise for the study of psychopathology, but is still in its infancy. Core methodological questions of integrating measurement, of appropriately modeling non-linear dynamics, and of formally testing dynamical hypotheses using data still need to be answered. On the theoretical side of psychopathology, researchers must work to understand the specifics of disorders in a way that is amenable to the use of dynamical systems. In part, researchers are already achieving this through the collection of intensive longitudinal data, but questions remain, such as: Over what timescale do pathological behaviors evolve? What is the role of lived experience (i.e., stressors, events) in the momentary experience of psychopathology? What is the role of physiological factors in the momentary experience of psychopathology? Beginning to answer these questions will inform future dynamical systems work in this area, creating a virtuous cycle of theory to model to theory development. But this work must be done with both methodological sophistication and deep understanding of the theory of psychopathology, necessitating that applied scientists work hand in hand with methodologists. There is great promise in the application of dynamical systems to psychopathology, from deepening our understanding of mental health to allowing us to develop personalized interventions, but there is a great deal of work to be done before these gains will be fully realized.

References

Abrams, D. M., & Strogatz, S. H. (2003). Modelling the dynamics of language death. *Nature, 424* (6951), 900–900. (Nature Publishing Group)

Boker, S. M., Tiberio, S. S., & Moulder, R. G. (2018). Robustness of time delay embedding to sampling interval misspecification. In K. van Montfort, J. H. L. Oud, & M. C. Voelkle (Eds.), *Continuous time modeling in the behavioral and related sciences* (pp. 239–258).Springer International Publishing.

Bollen, K. A., & Curran, P. J. (2006). *Latent curve models: A structural equation perspective.* Wiley-Interscience.

Borsboom, D., & Cramer, A. O. (2013). Network analysis: An integrative approach to the structure of psychopathology. *Annual Review of Clinical Psychology, 9*(1), 91–121.

Breuer, J., & Freud, S. (1895). *Studies on hysteria* (Standard Edition 2nd ed.). Hogarth.

Bringmann, L. F., Ferrer, E., Hamaker, E. L., Borsboom, D., & Tuerlinckx, F. (2018). Modeling nonstationary emotion dynamics in dyads using a time-varying vector-autoregressive model. *Multivariate Behavioral Research, 53*(3), 293–314. (Routledge eprint: https://doi.org/10.1080/00273171.2018.1439722)

Bringmann, L. F., Hamaker, E. L., Vigo, D. E., Aubert, A., Borsboom, D., & Tuerlinckx, F. (2017). Changing dynamics: Time-varying autoregressive models using generalized additive modeling. *Psychological Methods, 22*(3), 409–425.

Bringmann, L. F., Vissers, N., Wichers, M., Geschwind, N., Kuppens, P., Peeters, F., . . . Tuerlinckx, F. (2013). A network approach to psychopathology: New insights into clinical longitudinal data. *PLOS ONE, 8*(4), e60188. (Public Library of Science)

Brown, C. H. (1993). Analyzing preventive trials with generalized additive models. *American Journal of Community Psychology, 21*(5), 635–664.

Chilcoat, H. D., & Schütz, C. G. (1996). Age-specific patterns of hallucinogen use in the us population: An analysis using generalized additive models. *Drug and Alcohol Dependence, 43*(3), 143–153.

Chow, S.-M., Witkiewitz, K., Grasman, R., Hutton, R., & Maisto, S. (2014). A regime-switching longitudinal model of alcohol lapse-relapse. In *Handbook of developmental systems theory & methodology* (pp. 397–424). Guilford Press.

Cramer, A. O. J., van Borkulo, C. D., Giltay, E. J., van der Maas, H. L. J., Kendler, K. S., Scheffer, M., & Borsboom, D. (2016). Major depression as a complex dynamic system. *PloS one, 11*(12), e0167490.

Delmonte, M. M. (1989). Systems theory and psychotherapy. *Journal of Contemporary Psychotherapy, 19*(2), 117–135.

Elovainio, M., Jokela, M., Rosenstr¨om, T., Pulkki-R˚ab¨ack, L., Hakulinen, C., Josefsson, K., . . . Keltikangas-J¨arvinen, L. (2015, January). Temperament and depressive symptoms: What is the direction of the association? *Journal of Affective Disorders, 170*, 203–212. https://www.sciencedirect.com/science/article/pii/S0165032714005291

Epskamp, S. (2020). Psychometric network models from time-series and panel data. *Psychometrika*, *85*(1), 206–231.

Epskamp, S., Deserno, M. K., & Bringmann, L. F. (2019). *mlVAR: Multi-level vector autoregression.*

Epskamp, S., Rhemtulla, M., & Borsboom, D. (2017). Generalized network psychometrics: Combining network and latent variable models. *Psychometrika*, *82*(4), 904–927.

Fisher, Z. F., Chow, S.-M., Molenaar, P. C. M., Fredrickson, B. L., Pipiras, V., & Gates, K. M. (2022). A square-root second-order extended kalman filtering approach for estimating smoothly time-varying parameters. *Multivariate Behavioral Research*, *57*(1), 134–152.

Friedman, J., Hastie, T., & Tibshirani, R. (2008). Sparse inverse covariance estimation with the graphical lasso. *Biostatistics*, *9*(3), 432–441. (tex.ids=friedmanSparseInverseCovariance2008, friedmanSpar- seInverseCovariance2008a)

Gates, K. M., Fisher, Z. F., & Bollen, K. A. (2020). Latent variable GIMME using model implied instrumental variables (MIIVs). *Psychological Methods*, *25*(2), 227–242. (American Psychological Association)

Gates, K. M., Lane, S. T., Varangis, E., Giovanello, K., & Guiskewicz, K. (2017). Unsupervised classification during time-series model building. *Multivariate Behavioral Research*, *52*(2), 129–148. (Routledge eprint: https://doi.org/10.1080/00273171.2016.1256187)

Gates, K. M., & Molenaar, P. C. (2012). Group search algorithm recovers effective connectivity maps for individuals in homogeneous and heterogeneous samples. *NeuroImage*, *63*(1), 310–319.

Granger, C. W. J., & Newbold, P. (1986). *Forecasting economic time series* (2nd ed.). Academic Press.

Groen, R., van Gils, A., Emerencia, A., Bos, E., & Rosmalen, J. (2021, July). Exploring temporal relationships among worrying, anxiety, and somatic symptoms. *Journal of Psychosomatic Research*, *146*, 110293. https://www.sciencedirect.com/science/article/pii/ S0022399920308552

Hamaker, E. L., & Grasman, R. P. P. P. (2012). Regime switching state-space models applied to psychological processes: Handling missing data and making inferences. *Psychometrika*, *77*(2), 400– 422.

Hamaker, E. L., Grasman, R. P. P. P., & Kamphuis, J. H. (2010). Regime-switching models to study psychological processes. In Peter C. M. Molenaar & Karl M. Newell (Eds.), *Individual pathways of change: Statistical models for analyzing learning and development* (pp. 155–168). American Psychological Association.

Hamaker, E. L., Grasman, R. P. P. P., & Kamphuis, J. H. (2016). Modeling bas dysregulation in bipolar disorder: Illustrating the potential of time series analysis. *Assessment*, *23*(4), 436–446. https://doi.org/10.1177/1073191116632339 (PMID: 26906639)

Haslbeck, J. M. B., Bringmann, L. F., & Waldorp, L. J. (2021). A tutorial on estimating time-varying vector autoregressive models. *Multivariate Behavioral Research*, *56*(1), 120–149. (Routledge eprint: https://doi.org/10.1080/00273171.2020.1743630)

Haslbeck, J. M. B., Ryan, O., Robinaugh, D. J., Waldorp, L. J., & Borsboom, D. (2022). Modeling psychopathology: From data models to formal theories. *Psychological Methods*, *27*(6), 930–957. (US Publisher: American Psychological Association)

Haslbeck, J. M. B., & Waldorp, L. J. (2020). mgm: Estimating time-varying mixed graphical models in high-dimensional data. *Journal of Statistical Software*, *93*, 1–46.

Heeren, A., & McNally, R. J. (2018, February). Social anxiety disorder as a densely interconnected network of fear and avoidance for social situations. *Cognitive Therapy and Research*, *42*(1), 103–113. https://doi.org/10.1007/s10608-017-9876-3

Henry, T. R., Feczko, E., Cordova, M., Earl, E., Williams, S., Nigg, J. T., . .. Gates, K. M. (2019). Comparing directed functional connectivity between groups with confirmatory subgrouping GIMME. *NeuroImage*, *188*, 642–653.

Henry, T. R., Robinaugh, D. J., & Fried, E. I. (2022). On the control of psychological networks. *Psychometrika*, *87*(1), 188–213.

Henry, T. R., Slipetz, L. R., Falk, A., Qiu, J., & Chen, M. (2024). Ordinal outcome state-space models for intensive longitudinal data. *Psychometrika*, *89*(4), 1203–1229.

Hethcote, H. W. (2000). The mathematics of infectious diseases. *SIAM Review*, *42*(4), 599–653. (Society for Industrial and Applied Mathematics)

Hopwood, C. J., Morey, L. C., & Markon, K. E. (2023). What is a psychopathology dimension? *Clinical Psychology Review*, *106*, 102356.

Insel, T., Cuthbert, B., Garvey, M., Heinssen, R., Pine, D. S., Quinn, K., . . . Wang, P. (2010). Research domain criteria (RDoC): Toward a new classification framework for research on mental disorders. *The American Journal of Psychiatry*, *167*(7), 748–751. (American Psychiatric Assn)

Jaya, E. S., Ascone, L., & Lincoln, T. M. (2018). A longitudinal mediation analysis of the effect of negative-self-schemas on positive symptoms via negative affect. *Psychological Medicine*, *48*(8), 1299–1307.

Kalman, R. E. (1960). A new approach to linear filtering and prediction problems. *Journal of Basic Engineering*, *82*(1), 35–45.

Kim, C.-j., & Nelson, C. R. (1999). *State-space models with regime switching: Classical and Gibbs- sampling approaches with applications*. MIT Press.

Kim, J. J., Henderson, T., Best, T., Cunnington, R., & Kirby, J. N. (2020). Neural and self-report markers of reassurance: A generalized additive modelling approach. *Frontiers in Psychiatry*, *11*, 566141.

Kotov, R., Krueger, R. F., Watson, D., Achenbach, T. M., Althoff, R. R., Bagby, R. M., . . . Zimmerman, M. (2017). The Hierarchical Taxonomy of Psychopathology (HiTOP): A dimensional alternative to traditional nosologies. *Journal of Abnormal Psychology*, *126*(4), 454–477.

Kramer, I., Simons, C. J. P., Wigman, J. T. W., Collip, D., Jacobs, N., Derom, C., . . . Wichers, M. (2013, 02). Time-lagged moment-to-moment interplay between negative affect and paranoia: New insights in the affective pathway to psychosis. *Schizophrenia Bulletin*, *40*(2), 278–286. fromhttps://doi.org/10.1093/schbul/sbs194

Lane, S., Gates, K., Fisher, Z., Arizmendi, C., Molenaar, P., Merkle, E., . . . Alvarez, S. C. (2024). *gimme: Group iterative multiple model estimation.* Laura Bringmann. (2023). *LauraBringmann/tvvarGAM.* (original-date: 2017-08-07T10:04:56Z)

Kratzer, L., Schiepek, G., Heinz, P., Schöller, H., Knefel, M., Haselgruber, A., & Karatzias, T. (2022). What makes inpatient treatment for PTSD effective? Investigating daily therapy process factors. *Psychotherapy Research*, *32*(7), 847–859. https://doi.org/10.1080/10503307.2022.2050830 (PMID: 35285787)

Lorenz, E. N. (1963). Deterministic onperiodic flow. *Journal of the Atmospheric Sciences*, *20*(2), 130–141.

Marsman, M., Borsboom, D., Kruis, J., Epskamp, S., Van Bork, R., Waldorp, L. J., . . . Maris, G. (2018). An introduction to network psychometrics: Relating ising network models to item response theory models. *Multivariate Behavioral Research*, *53*(1), 15–35.

McKee, K., Russell, M., Mennis, J., Mason, M., & Neale, M. (2020). Emotion regulation dynamics predict substance use in high-risk adolescents. *Addictive Behaviors*, *106*, 106374.

Mckeown, G., & Sneddon, I. (2013). Modeling continuous self-report measures of perceived emotion using generalized additive mixed models. *Psychological Methods*, *19*(1), 155–174.

Mei, X., Du, P., Li, Y., Mei, R., Wang, X., Chen, Q., & Ye, Z. (2023). Fear of childbirth and sleep quality among pregnant women: a generalized additive model and moderated mediation analysis. *BMC Psychiatry*, *23*(1), 931.

Molenaar, P. C., Beltz, A. M., Gates, K. M., & Wilson, S. J. (2016). State space modeling of time-varying contemporaneous and lagged relations in connectivity maps. *NeuroImage*, *125*, 791–802.

Reeve, S., Nickless, A., Sheaves, B., & Freeman, D. (2018). Insomnia, negative affect, and psychotic experiences: Modelling pathways over time in a clinical observational study. *Psychiatry Research*, *269*, 673–680.

Robinaugh, D., Haslbeck, J., Waldorp, L., Kossakowski, J., Fried, E. I., Millner, A., . . . Borsboom, D. (2019). *Advancing the network theory of mental disorders: A computational model of panic disorder.* Open Science Framework.

Samejima, F. (1969). Estimation of latent ability using a response pattern of graded scores. *Psychometrika Monograph Supplement*, *34*, 100–100.

Shojaie, A., & Fox, E. B. (2022). Granger causality: A review and recent advances. *Annual Review of Statistics and Its Application*, *9*, 289–319. (Annual Reviews)

Sims, C. A. (1980). Macroeconomics and reality. *Econometrica*, *48*(1), 1.

Snippe, E., Bos, E. H., van der Ploeg, K. M., Sanderman, R., Fleer, J., & Schroevers, M. J. (2015). Time-series analysis of daily changes in mindfulness, repetitive thinking, and depressive symptoms during mindfulness-based treatment. *Mindfulness*, *6*(5), 1053–1062.

So, S. H.-w., Chung, L. K.-h., Tse, C.-Y., Chan, S. S.-m., Chong, G. H.-c., Hung, K. S.-y., & Sommer, I. E. C. (2021). Moment-to-moment dynamics between auditory verbal hallucinations and negative affect and the role of beliefs about voices. *Psychological Medicine*, *51*(4), 661–667.

Strogatz, S. (2024). *Nonlinear dynamics and chaos: With applications to physics, biology, chemistry, and engineering* (3rd ed.). CRC Press, Taylor & Francis Group.

Sullivan, K. J., Shadish, W. R., & Steiner, P. M. (2015). An introduction to modeling longitudinal data with generalized additive models: Applications to single-case designs. *Psychological methods*, *20*(1), 26—42.

Takano, K., Taylor, C. T., Wittekind, C. E., Sakamoto, J., & Ehring, T. (2021, February). Disentangling temporal dynamics in attention bias from measurement error: A state-space modeling approach. *Journal of Abnormal Psychology*, *130*(2), 198—210. https://doi.org/ 10.1037/abn0000657

Hastie, T. J. (1990). *Generalized additive models* (1st ed.). Chapman and Hall/CRC.

Voelkle, M. C., Gische, C., Driver, C. C., & Lindenberger, U. (2018). The role of time in the quest for understanding psychological mechanisms. *Multivariate Behavioral Research*, *53*(6), 782–805. (Taylor & Francis)

Voelkle, M. C., Oud, J. H. L., Davidov, E., & Schmidt, P. (2012). An SEM approach to continuous time modeling of panel data: Relating authoritarianism and anomia. *Psychological Methods*, *17*(2), 176–192.

Wang, S., Robinaugh, D., Millner, A., Fortgang, R., & Nock, M. K. (2023). *Mathematical and computational modeling of suicide as a complex dynamical system*. Open Science Framework.

Wichers, M., Wigman, J. T. W., & Myin-Germeys, I. (2015, October). Micro-level affect dynamics in psychopathology viewed from complex dynamical system theory. *Emotion Review* , *7*(4), 362–367. Retrieved 2022-04-08, from https://doi.org/10.1177/1754073915590623 (SAGE Publications)

CHAPTER 20

Longitudinal Modeling of Developmental Dimensional Models of Psychopathology

THOMAS M. OLINO AND SYLIA WILSON

Introduction

Dimensional models of psychopathology are increasingly the dominant organizational framework of psychopathology in the adult literature. However, dimensional models have long been considered in studies of youth psychopathology, given historical skepticism that children are capable of meeting diagnostic criteria for specific disorders. Since the 1950s, studies of children show broad organization of psychopathology into internalizing and externalizing dimensions. In the decades that followed, studies of later adolescents and adults have shown similar dimensions of internalizing and externalizing problems. More recently, there has been greater elaboration in the number and nuance of these dimensions described in the literature, with multiple narrower dimensions being identified within the broad internalizing and externalizing dimensions, as well as identifying multiple other dimensions, including thought disorder.

It is now clear that there is continuity of psychopathology across the lifespan and that manifestations of psychopathology in childhood presage disorders observed in adolescence and adulthood. Longitudinal approaches are necessary to understand developmental models of psychopathology. However, research on lifespan dimensional models of psychopathology, grounded in developmental theory, must grapple with several important methodological challenges in order to understand how development and longitudinal changes are implicated in the organization and manifestation of psychopathology. These considerations involve addressing the stability and change in the overall structure of psychopathology, mean levels of dimensions of psychopathology, and how individual dimensions of psychopathology manifest and influence other dimensions across time and development. Addressing each of these important conceptual research questions requires specific study designs and quantitative methods.

In this chapter, we provide a brief overview of key concepts that underpin examining psychopathology in a developmental and longitudinal context. These connections between development and psychopathology lead to key principles about how questions about longitudinal changes in psychopathology are organized. We then provide a survey of the literature examining questions about the structure of psychopathology, how these structures are consistent or inconsistent across time or development, relationships between dimensions of psychopathology, and changes in levels of dimensions of psychopathology in developmental contexts, and include an overview of quantitative methods to address these questions.

We close with suggestions on how the field will move forward in addressing novel, timely questions.

A Developmental Perspective to Longitudinal Dimensional Models of Psychopathology

Taking a developmental perspective when considering dimensional models of psychopathology incorporates fundamental developmental processes that underlie psychopathology—consistency and change—and developmental psychopathology theory to inform our understanding of the organization, dynamic development, and changes in psychopathology across the lifespan. These issues are inherent to extending dimensional models of psychopathology that were built on cross-sectional methods and findings.

Consistency and Change. There are multiple ways of considering development and change in psychopathology across the lifespan. One approach focuses on the consistency in overall similarity of organization of psychopathology over time and development. Another approach focuses on longitudinal changes in the severity of psychopathology across time. Consistency encompasses both continuity and stability, whereas change encompasses both discontinuity and instability (Bornstein et al., 2017). Continuity (versus discontinuity) refers to whether there is change in mean levels of a characteristic over time. Stability (versus instability) refers to whether there is change in the relative order or rank of individuals in a group on a characteristic over time. Continuity and stability can be homotypic (of the same type) or heterotypic (of different types). Homotypic continuity refers to a characteristic predicting itself later on, whereas heterotypic continuity refers to a characteristic predicting a different characteristic later on. Conversely, homotypic stability refers to maintaining individual order in the same characteristic measured in the same metric over time, whereas heterotypic stability refers to maintaining individual order on different manifest characteristics over time when the different characteristics are theoretically related and presumed to reflect the same trait. These fundamental developmental principles help frame the understanding of, guide research on, and inform the quantitative methods used to examine developmental dimensional models of psychopathology.

The developmental psychopathology perspective incorporates theory and research from both normal and abnormal developmental processes (Cicchetti, 1993). Two key principles in developmental psychopathology relevant for developmental dimensional models of psychopathology are those of equifinality and multifinality (Cicchetti & Rogosch, 1996). Equifinality refers to the phenomenon of multiple initial states leading to a single outcome. Multifinality refers to a single initial state leading to multiple different outcomes. These principles map onto the principles of etiological and phenotypic heterogeneity, respectively, with etiological heterogeneity meaning heterogeneity in etiology or origin, and phenotypic heterogeneity meaning heterogeneity in phenotypic manifestation. Temporal heterogeneity is less often considered than etiological and phenotypic heterogeneity, but also is critical for understanding the manifestation of psychopathology (Elison, 2020). Temporal heterogeneity reflects observed variability in developmental timing and may represent a specific feature of phenotypic heterogeneity and/or the evolving patterns of environmental contexts and demands and pressures that temporally coincide and interact with changes. The developmental psychopathology principles of equifinality and multifinality have been applied to psychopathology and, in particular, to how forms of psychopathology might stay the same or change over development and time.

Methods of Testing Longitudinal Developmental Dimensional Models

Empirical tests of our theories require appropriate study designs and analytical approaches. Likewise, specific questions about developmental dimensional models of psychopathology require complementary, specific methods.

Structural Models of Psychopathology Dimensions in Youth and Adults. There is extensive interest in how psychopathology is organized in a coherent structure (Kotov et al., 2017) in expectation that the dimensional structure will lead to more precise understanding of etiology and appropriate treatments. This work is largely informed by a latent disease conceptualization, wherein an underlying latent factor is the causal influence on the manifestation of symptoms (e.g., a depression diagnosis is thought to reflect an underlying latent construct that is causally related to manifest depressive symptoms). In practice, psychopathology dimensions are modeled using exploratory factor analysis and confirmatory factor analysis, with factor loadings reflecting the strength of the associations between the factors and symptom indicators.

Using factor analytic methods, early studies of youth psychopathology showed that psychopathology could be organized by correlated broad internalizing and externalizing dimensions (Achenbach, 1966, 2011; see Copeland et al., this volume, for a review of this literature). In these studies, internalizing problems reflect depression, anxiety, withdrawal, and somatic complaints, whereas externalizing problems reflect aggression and rule-breaking. More recent studies examining the structure of psychopathology in youth largely find support for organizing symptoms into internalizing and externalizing dimensions (Lahey et al., 2004, 2011).

Investigations of the structure of psychopathology in older adolescents and adults followed. Factor analytic studies of adults using diagnoses and symptoms of psychiatric disorders largely replicated the dimensional structure first identified in youth. Some studies examined internalizing problems (e.g., Krueger & Finger, 2001) and externalizing problems (e.g., Krueger et al., 2002, 2005, 2007) in isolation of the other dimension. These studies supported single latent dimensions of internalizing and externalizing dimensions. Studies also tested the structure of psychopathology inclusive of both internalizing and externalizing problems in the same model (e.g., Krueger et al., 2001), with results showing that these are correlated, but separable, dimensions. Across cross-sectional studies, an early meta-analytic review of structural models of psychopathology in adults included a wider array of disorder indicators than did individual studies (Krueger & Markon, 2006). This review found that the optimal structure included broad dimensions of externalizing and internalizing, with the latter dimension being comprised of sub-dimensions of distress and fear disorders. More recent work in adults has expanded to include additional dimensions (e.g., psychosis/thought disorder, detachment).

Psychopathology Dimensions across Ages and Developmental Periods. Initial cross-sectional studies provide a foundation for similarity in structural dimensional models of psychopathology among youth and adults. However, questions quickly arise about whether the dimensional structure of psychopathology changes or differs across development or age. Early work in this area relied on very weak tests that showed consistency in gross factor analytic model structure across samples from different developmental periods. Harris, Swanson, and Petersen (2024) conducted a meta-analysis of variance explained by a general factor of psychopathology, estimated as a general or higher-order factor, in samples of youth ages 2 to 17. They found that age was not significantly associated with explained common variance, suggesting that the strength of the common factor is consistent across time. However, the focus on the explained variance is heavily influenced by the magnitude of factor loadings, but is agnostic to whether loadings are weaker, stronger, or the same across time. Thus, although this meta-analysis provides supportive evidence about developmental continuity in the variance explained in the indicators, this does not demonstrate that the latent psychopathology factor is associated with each of the specific indicators similarly across time. Murray et al. (2016) examined the broad structural organization of psychopathology dimensions in youth initially assessed at age 7 and then repeatedly assessed annually until age 15. Their final model included a general factor, as well as specific dimensions of aggression, ADHD, pro-sociality, and internalizing. Factor reliability was assessed using omega hierarchical (McDonald, 1999). This method focuses on the overall strength of loadings, without consideration as to whether the specific loadings show the same values across time as with tests of measurement invariance. They found longitudinal stability of the reliability of each factor, with the highest degree of stability demonstrated for the general factor. These results lend support that the general organization of psychopathology is the same across middle childhood to mid-adolescence. However, as this study did not formally test longitudinal stability, it is not clear whether model parameters are invariant across time. Well-fitting models across different samples may be found, despite the pattern of associations substantially differing among the diagnostic or symptom indicators (i.e., the co-variance structures; Bonifay et al., 2025; Levin-Aspenson et al., 2021).

Stronger tests of consistency and change in dimensional models of psychopathology rely on methods that directly compare the statistical fit of models across development and require longitudinal study designs. Formal tests of equivalence of modeling measurement structure are broadly referred to as measurement invariance (Millsap, 2011). Briefly, this family of methods, within the broad application of confirmatory factor analysis, imposes increasingly restrictive constraints on the model across some identifiable unit (e.g., time, reporter) to examine whether the factor has the same configuration of indicators on a common factor (i.e., configural invariance), that the factor loadings to indicators are equivalent (i.e., metric invariance), and that the expected mean level of an indicator is equivalent given the same level of the latent dimension across that unit (i.e., scalar invariance). In developmental studies, measurement invariance in the structure of psychopathology can be tested by examining models fit to data from subsamples of participants at different ages or developmental ranges, that is, between-group comparisons. Alternatively, more rigorous approaches rely on longitudinal assessments of the same participants, that is, within-person comparisons (Millsap, 2011; Widaman et al., 2010). Whether invariance is supported is largely based on reduction in model fit when constraints are applied (Chen, 2007), and invariance can be considered fully or partially met (Byrne et al., 1989). Equivalence of factor loadings (i.e., metric invariance) provides support for the construct having relative order comparisons (i.e., evaluating rank-ordering) and can be full (i.e., all factor loadings can be constrained to be equivalent) or partial (i.e., some factor loadings need to be freed to vary across different ages or developmental stages) metric invariance. Equivalence of intercepts for continuous indicators or thresholds for categorical indicators (i.e., scalar invariance) provides support for the construct having absolute level comparisons (i.e., evaluating mean-levels).

Cross-sectional Developmental Measurement Invariance. Studies that rely on cross-sectional designs to test invariance of the developmental structure of psychopathology typically include participants spanning age ranges that are coded into specific bands of age or developmental periods for analysis. These studies directly test whether the factor loadings of indicators on their specified factors do or do not significantly differ across age. Using data from National Epidemiologic Survey on Alcohol and Related Conditions (NESARC; Grant et al., 2003, 2009), Hoertel et al. (2015) tested invariance of a model including internalizing, with subfactors of distress and fear, and externalizing problems across participants aged 18–24, 25–34, 35–44, 45–55, 55–64, 65–74, and older than 75 years. Their results showed that the structure of psychopathology was invariant from late adolescence to late life.

Longitudinal Developmental Measurement Invariance Models. Although cross-sectional approaches provide good information about consistency in measurement across ages or developmental periods, because development is fundamentally a within-person process, focal tests using longitudinal approaches are necessary to address questions about development and change. There have been only a small number of longitudinal studies that test for invariance in psychopathology structure across youth development. These studies have varied in the age at baseline and time interval between assessments. Gluschkooff, Jokela, and Rosenstrom (2019) examined the long-term stability of the structure of psychopathology in the National Comorbidity Study (NCS; Kessler et al., 1994) and the follow-up survey that took place approximately 10 years after the initial assessment. The authors tested a correlated three-factor model, including fear, distress, and externalizing dimensions, and a bifactor model, including a general factor and specific internalizing and externalizing factors. They found that both longitudinal models showed excellent fit to the data and supported full measurement invariance. These results offer some assurances that there is consistency in the dimensional structure of psychopathology across relatively long follow-up intervals. However, given the wide age range of participants in this study, it is not possible to evaluate whether invariance is supported in specific developmental windows but not in others, which may be masked when evaluated in the context of a wider age range.

Some longitudinal studies have focused on examining invariance of the structure of dimensions of psychopathology. Olino et al. (2018) examined the structure of psychopathology in youth at age three and again when reassessed at age six. At each time point, the same model with a general factor with loadings to all indicators (except to specific phobia) and group internalizing and externalizing factors with loadings to specific internalizing and externalizing indicators was fit to the data. This model demonstrated the best fit to the data, relative to a correlated two-factor (internalizing and externalizing) and a single-factor model, meeting configural invariance. However, metric invariance of factor loadings across time was not met. Thus, while the factors encompassed the same indicators across separate assessments, the specific inter-correlations between the disorder indicators differed at age three and age six, raising questions about whether the factors reflect the same meaning across time. Snyder et al. (2017) examined the stability of a similar general, internalizing, and externalizing dimension factor model across 18 months in a sample ranging in age from 9 to 17 at the initial assessment. In contrast to Olino et al. (2018), Snyder et al. (2017) found that, across this time interval, the model supported invariance of the loadings defining each of the factors. These disparate findings raise questions about when in development and across what time interval the structure and measurement of psychopathology may be consistent.

To summarize, initial studies of the structure of psychopathology across development have taken multiple forms. Studies have been motivated by somewhat different questions leading to different implications of their findings. Overall, studies have converged on the organization of broad dimensions of psychopathology in youth and adults. However, studies have differed in their ability to draw conclusions about the continuity of the structure of psychopathology over development and time. Studies that have focused on developmental change in the structure of psychopathology have provided preliminary tests of measurement invariance with a need for more work in this area, as results have been inconsistent. Studies have differed widely on the ages and developmental periods; duration of follow-up assessments; and specific indicators, measurement, and informants of psychopathology, all of which may be potent influences on the replicability of findings. Establishing metric and scalar invariance has fundamental implications for evaluating tests of rank-order and mean-level stability, respectively, of dimensions of psychopathology. Further testing of longitudinal invariance across focal periods of development, in youth and adults (including older adults), is sorely needed.

Longitudinal Models of Psychopathology Dimensions over Time and Development. Beyond consistency in the structure of dimensional models of psychopathology, longitudinal studies also examine stability and continuity of individual dimensions of psychopathology. That is, are there patterns of stability such that individuals show the same standing on dimensions of psychopathology, or change in dimension levels across time? Additionally, is there continuity in dimensions of psychopathology, such that individuals higher on dimensions on one occasion tend to also be higher on the same, or different dimensions on another occasion? These questions of continuity encompass those of rank-order stability.

Drawing from principles of developmental psychopathology, there is interest in how specific dimensions of psychopathology are consistent across time (i.e., homotypic continuity) and how specific dimensions of psychopathology predict different dimensions of psychopathology (i.e., heterotypic continuity) across time. Multiple longitudinal studies testing the consistency of broad measurement structure have tested homotypic continuity. With few exceptions, these studies have reported significant homotypic paths showing stability of broad dimensions of psychopathology across time, in models of correlated internalizing-externalizing dimensions and models involving general and specific factors (Greene & Eaton, 2017; Krueger et al., 1998; Olino, Bufferd et al., 2018; Snyder et al., 2017; Vollebergh et al., 2001). Somewhat surprisingly, fewer studies have reported on heterotypic continuity in structural models of psychopathology. However, notable exceptions have different findings. Olino et al. (2018) found homotypic continuity of dimensions in the preschool years and heterotypic continuity in that the general factor of psychopathology predicted externalizing problems. However, Snyder et al. (2017) did not find evidence of heterotypic continuity across an approximate 18-month follow-up in adolescence. Notably, it is unclear whether other studies tested for heterotypic continuity, but did not report findings of these tests.

Much of the work on homotypic and heterotypic continuity relies on studies within a relatively narrow developmental window, or the same instrument without substantial changes in the measures used and particular kinds of behaviors assessed. Examinations of homotypic and heterotypic continuity can be challenged by developmental changes in symptomatic expression. Homotypic continuity is suggestive that the same construct is reflected across development and shows some degree of rank-order consistency. When a construct changes across time, this inference may not be valid. For example, the construct of externalizing problems includes different content at age 3 (e.g., oppositionality, irritability, rule-breaking) than it does at age 21 (e.g., oppositionality, irritability, rule breaking, substance use). We return to challenges of longitudinal and developmental work such as this below.

Developmental Trajectories of Psychopathology. In addition to tests of rank-order consistency in dimensions of psychopathology, studies have examined mean-level changes in levels (i.e., severity) of dimensions of psychopathology (latent dimensions or measured scale scores). Much of this work relies on growth curve modeling methods, which characterize trajectories of dimensions of psychopathology (Biesanz et al., 2004; Bollen & Curran, 2006; Singer et al., 2003). These models operationalize trajectories based on initial levels (although this can be shifted to any time point in the study time frame) and rates of change across time. In addition to point estimates of levels and rates of change, growth models include random effects that reflect individual differences in these parameters. Studies differ in their focus on variability across the full range of the dimension, or dividing variability into group-based trajectories (with or without within-group variability; B. L. Jones & Nagin, 2007; Muthén & Muthén, 2000). Beyond the description of developmental trajectories, growth models can also be extended to examine how other characteristics, frequently at or preceding the first assessment occasion, are associated with the initial levels or rates of change in the dimension. Thus, there are complementary interests in describing the patterns of change in dimensions of psychopathology and examining predictors of differences in those trajectories. Growth curve modeling methods focus on explaining mean-level changes in dimension severity. Notably, there is flexible utility of these models to permit examining predictors (i.e., causes), correlates, or outcomes of the developmental trajectories that may inform prevention or intervention.

Growth models require at least three assessment occasions to estimate linear developmental trajectories and individual differences in trajectories. When additional assessments are available, developmental trajectories of continuous non-linear (e.g., quadratic, cubic) or discontinuous (e.g., piecewise growth) forms are possible. These functional forms of change permit testing of different possibilities of developmental trajectories. Moreover, when considering two dimensions of psychopathology, parallel process (or bivariate) growth modeling can be applied. In these models, growth parameters of two outcomes are permitted to correlate, reflecting the expectation that the intercepts (initial levels) and slopes (rates of change) of each dimension are associated over time.

Methods of modeling more than two outcomes with correlated change include related models that have very different theoretical underpinnings (Estabrook, 2018; McArdle, 1988). One form of model is a curve of factors, also referred to as a multiple indicator or second-order growth curve model. In this approach, multiple dimensions of psychopathology are reflective of a first-order factor at each time point and the first-order factors function as the indicators of the growth (i.e., intercept and slope) factors. This approach assumes that the modeling of the first-order factor is invariant across time. The modeling structure is guided by the overall trajectory influencing the higher-order factor that, in turn, influences the change in the lower-order factors. An alternative approach is the factor of curves model. In this model, growth models are estimated for individual dimensions of psychopathology. Second-order factors are then specified to account for co-variation among intercepts, slopes, or both parameters. Thus, there could be multiple factors that account for the associations among the intercepts and separate factors that account for the associations among the slopes. Both of these approaches have been sparingly used in the literature (Duncan et al., 2000; Duncan & Duncan, 1996; Laceulle et al., 2023; Mann et al., 2020). This may be due to a need for fairly large, longitudinal studies with relatively consistent measures of constructs across time. These models may also have challenges in convergence if multiple dimensions show very similar patterns of change, leading to inadmissible model solutions.

Studies of the developmental trajectories of broad internalizing or externalizing dimensions have reported mixed results. Wang et al. (2018) found that there was an increasing developmental trajectory of internalizing dimensions from age four to seven. Using data from the U.K. Millenium Cohort Study, Papachristou and Flouri (2020) found that there were significant increases in internalizing problems and decreases in externalizing problems from age 3 to 14. Moreover, there were significant associations between initial levels and rates of change of internalizing and externalizing problems. Studies of narrow-band dimensions within broader dimensions, such as depression, anxiety, or irritable behaviors within the internalizing dimension, have been mixed. Olino et al. (2014) examined parallel development of depression and anxiety symptoms in girls from ages 10 to 17, finding that depressive symptoms decreased, on average, whereas anxiety symptoms did not show a significant change over this interval. Moreover, they found that initial levels and rates of change were significantly correlated between depression and anxiety, but initial levels of depression and anxiety were inversely associated with rates of change of the other construct. In a study spanning participant ages 15 to 30 with up to 11 assessments, Pettit et al. (2010) found decelerating reductions (lower rate of change) in depressive symptoms. In youth from age 2 to 10 years, Sorcher et al. (2023) found that irritability decreased over this time span.

In addition to quantitative approaches (i.e., individual differences in starting points and rates of change), studies have taken qualitative approaches (i.e., identifying groups that differ in their trajectories) to understand developmental trajectories of psychopathology. Testing Moffitt (1993)'s developmental typologies of adolescent limited and life course persistent antisocial behavior, studies using group-based developmental trajectory models have identified some classes that are consistent with this model, as well as other trajectories that were not previously predicted, such as childhood desisting. Across multiple prospective studies, results have varied tremendously with respect to the number of profiles, as well as the prevalence of each profile (Jolliffe et al., 2017). Thus, there are challenges in identifying which trajectory profiles reflect more normative experiences. Davis, Votruba-Drzal, and Silk (2015) used longitudinal mixture models to examine subtypes of longitudinal trajectories of internalizing symptoms in youth from age 4 to 15 in the National Institute of Child Health and Human Development Study of Early Child Care and Youth Development. Their results suggested four trajectory classes noted as low stable, mean stable, moderate stable, and moderate increasing. That is, the identified classes were largely characterized by individual differences in symptom severity across development, rather than differences in rates of change across development.

Currently, the majority of work examining developmental trajectories of psychopathology has been conducted with studies of youth. However, there is an important need to examine the continued trajectories into adulthood, mid-life, and late-life in order to have a more complete understanding of the life course trajectories of psychopathology. In addition, theories about sensitive periods of development of psychopathology require researchers to be mindful in selecting time intervals in their longitudinal studies that correspond with the appropriate time scale to provide the greatest leverage to support or refute the theory.

Direct longitudinal associations between dimensions of psychopathology. The previously discussed models focus on the organization of broad dimensions of psychopathology and how normative developmental processes undergird the development of those dimensions. However, there is considerable interest in alternative and complementary models of interrelations between dimensions of psychopathology. That is, how specific dimensions are directly associated with other dimensions, which may or may not involve latent dimensions.

Studies also have considered longitudinal interrelations among multiple dimensions of psychopathology using traditional cross-lagged panel models. These models include autoregressive stability paths within each outcome and cross-domain paths modeling temporally lagged associations. This method was used for studies of internalizing and externalizing problems, as broad domains, as well as other studies examining associations between two constructs, such as depression and anxiety, depression and conduct problems (Brensilver et al., 2011; Van der Giessen et al., 2013), and depression and paranoia (Moritz et al., 2017), and other studies examining the longitudinal associations among three constructs (e.g., depression, anxiety, and delinquency; Fanti et al., 2019). Across the range of studies, results have typically found autoregressive effects, but inconsistently found lagged, cross-time associations between dimensions of psychopathology. Authors desire to infer that these models show within-person directional associations, with temporal precedence, from the cross-lagged paths. However, recent work has shown that these inferences are not possible using this method, but have also presented analytic methods that support more valid inferences (Berry & Willoughby, 2017; Hamaker et al., 2015; Lucas, 2023; Mulder & Hamaker, 2021).

A significant challenge of the traditional cross-lagged panel model is that the regression associations conflate both between- and within-person variance, preventing inferences about within-person effects (Berry & Willoughby, 2017). Within the traditional cross-lagged panel model, individuals high on one domain may also be high on the other domain consistently across time. Thus, time-invariant associations may capture person- or trait-level associations. The inclusion of a trait factor for each psychopathology domain, specified as a random intercept, partitions variance into between-person (i.e., trait) and within-person (i.e., occasion) variance. The application of these models permits testing and drawing inferences about the directional, longitudinal associations between the constructs. These have been termed random intercept, cross-lagged panel models (Hamaker et al., 2015). Recently, Richards et al. (2024) examined the longitudinal associations among internalizing, externalizing, and attention problems across six waves of data collection in the TRacking Adolescents' Individual Lives Survey (TRAILS). They found substantial associations among intercepts of all processes ($rs > .57$), but found little consistent evidence for within-person lagged associations among dimensions of psychopathology.

Within a longitudinal and developmental context, the RI-CLPM may not be fully satisfactory (for a critique of RI-CLPMs, see Orth et al., 2021). Across time in youth, there may be normative developmental trends in one or each of the outcomes that are not included in the standard RI-CLPM (or CLPM). However, when there are expected, or observed, changes in outcomes' sample mean levels, generalizations of this model can estimate these changes in outcomes by including a random slope effect (Curran, Howard et al., 2014). For example, Murray, Eisner, and Ribeaud (2020) estimated an autoregressive latent trait model with structured residuals (ALT-SR), amounting to an RI-CLPM with the inclusion of a random slope, examining the associations between internalizing and externalizing problems. They found that, beyond the between-person level associations between intercepts and slopes of internalizing and externalizing, there were some cross-domain associations across several intervals. These models permit drawing distinct inferences for between- and within-person associations, while also considering trajectories in change of the outcomes.

Challenges in Longitudinal and Developmental Work

Evaluating overall consistency in model structure, mean-level changes in dimensions, and associations among dimensions of psychopathology is fairly straightforward within narrow developmental timeframes or phases of development. However, research conducted during sensitive periods or over long periods of development when change is expected to occur introduces several challenges to examining and testing questions about stability and change. These challenges include reliance on multiple informants, differences in behaviors relevant to dimensions of psychopathology that change over time, and the fact that dimensions of psychopathology change on different timescales.

Reporters. Studies of infants and toddlers require informant reporters, such as parents, day care providers, or teachers, as target participants cannot provide information on their levels of functioning. In childhood and adolescence, youth are better able to report on their experiences and behaviors and multiple investigations rely on their self-reports. Younger children, however, may require additional scaffolding for providing responses and/or require fairly crude options for their responses. At the same time, the child and adolescent self-reports are frequently complemented by reports by parents, teachers, or peers. In adulthood, there is a near uniform reliance on self-reports, with only a small number of studies including informant reports. However, the reliance on informant reports becomes more common with participants as they approach and enter into late life. The availability of multi-informant designs offers opportunities and challenges for studies in these phases of development.

Reliance on different informants leads to important questions about the psychometric comparability of reports. There is a rich history of examining correspondence among informants. Across multiple decades of work, meta-analyses show that there are more robust associations among adult informants, but modest associations between adult and youth informants (Achenbach et al., 1987; De Los Reyes et al., 2015). In the more recent meta-analysis, inter-informant associations between co-parents were stronger than associations between other informant pairs (i.e., parent-child; parent-teacher; child-teacher) for both broad internalizing and externalizing problems. This meta-analysis also found that the magnitude of the inter-informant associations was consistent across youth ages. This work does not diminish the importance of information from each informant being useful for predicting important outcomes. Beyond dimensional assessments of symptoms, diagnostic assessments frequently rely on combining information assessed from both the youth and their caregiver (e.g., Birmaher et al., 2009). Given the different responses provided by each informant, interviewers use their judgment to evaluate if individual symptoms, and, ultimately, disorder diagnoses, are present or absent.

Studies of inter-informant agreement in adulthood and mid-life are rarer. In a sample of patients with a history of chronic depression, Klein et al. (1994) found substantial reliability of multiple forms of psychopathology, inclusive of mood, anxiety, substance use, and personality disorders, as assessed via interviews with patients, as well as with informants. Oltmanns et al. (2014) examined correspondence in the evaluation of personality disorder dimensional ratings using self-report, interviews, and informant interviews. Across all dimensions, the overall associations among informants and methods were within the small–moderate range.

Gold et al. (2020) examined the role of cognitive impairment on correspondence of ratings of depression in a sample that included individuals from 18 to 104 years of age. They found that higher levels of cognitive impairment were associated with poorer correspondence between self- and informant reports of depressive symptoms. Although cognitive impairment is not directly tied to chronological age, this illustrates how other developmental processes impact decisions about the methods to use in assessing psychopathology across the lifespan.

There are multiple explanations for modest inter-informant agreement. Some of these models focus on perspectives suggesting that each perspective is useful and may demonstrate value in understanding functioning (De Los Reyes et al., 2013; De Los Reyes & Kazdin, 2005; Makol et al., 2020). However, this perspective is based on the premise that the psychometric construct being reported on by individual informants is the same. Thus, there is important work testing whether the psychometric constructs are equivalent across informants, which tests for measurement invariance. The sequence and testing of invariance across informants is comparable to that when testing longitudinal invariance, as the target of the assessment is the same (Olino, 2020).

These tests of invariance have yielded mixed results across informants. Studies have also found mixed results for testing invariance across development (Olino et al., 2018). Olino et al. (2018) tested invariance between self- and maternal reports of anxiety dimensions in youth ages 9 and 12. For analyses focusing on youth at age 9, the authors found support for partial scalar invariance for symptoms of generalized anxiety and full scalar invariance for symptoms of social anxiety. However, models for panic/somatic symptoms and separation anxiety did not show adequate enough fit between informants to pursue further tests of invariance. For analyses at age 12, the authors found support for a partial scalar invariant model for generalized anxiety, panic/somatic, and social anxiety symptoms. Like tests at age nine, separation anxiety did not show adequate enough fit among informants to pursue further tests of invariance at age 12. These mixed findings require further scrutiny to better understand this phenomenon, or to refine measures that are not compromised by differences in psychometric functioning across informants. Much of this work has focused on only single syndrome dimensions. Future work will benefit from examining how higher-order dimensional models of psychopathology are consistent across informants.

Changes in Symptom Expression over Time. Much of the previous work on tests of cross-sectional structure, longitudinal structure, longitudinal mean-level changes, and comparability across informants focuses on assessing the same constructs using the same measures. This provides clear opportunities to examine continuities in structure and levels across development. However, across development, the behaviors or symptoms of specific dimensions of psychopathology may change. These changes reflect critical issues in modeling the development of dimensions of psychopathology. These may be reflected by heterotypic continuity, differentiation of constructs, or temporal heterogeneity.

Early in development, youth manifest psychological distress as a general presentation. In this developmental phase, parent informants are not fully able to distinguish among types of distress. However, as youth develop greater cognitive, motor, and affective abilities, their behaviors are easier to describe with more fine-grain components of internalizing or externalizing broad spectra.

Similarly, the externalizing spectrum is reflected by both disinhibited and antagonistic externalizing behaviors. However, distinguishing aspects of those dimensions involves content about substance use. Typically, childhood behavior problems are reflected more strongly by antagonistic behaviors. As youth develop into and through adolescence, social norms and opportunity to engage in substance use begins, leading to more engagement in disinhibited externalizing problems. Thus, these symptoms appear to emerge with development. Likewise, sexual problems are located within the broad internalizing spectrum. This specific symptom dimension may only become apparent as youth develop into adolescence when sexual debut occurs, or in adulthood when sexual relationships for childbearing or maintaining relationships leads to distress over performance or functionality. Inasmuch as neurodegenerative disorders are relevant to dimensions of psychopathology, the role of those dimensions would have relevance in late life, but not earlier in development. The changes in the developmentally normative indicators of psychopathology leads to challenges in evaluating structural models longitudinally. For example, longitudinal studies of externalizing problems across youth through mid-life would have substantial differences in the behaviors assessing the dimension across the life of the study, leading to questions about whether the observed changes are attributable to development or to measurement differences.

Multiple processes could explain the changes in behavioral expression of a single dimension across development. The emergence of specific phenotypes could reflect heterotypic continuity, such that earlier, broader dimensions predict different, narrower dimensions later in development. This could suggest that the individual dimensions are distinct, but prospectively associated across development, such that the earlier dimension is a predisposition for the development of the other dimension. Further, this may also suggest that the earlier and later manifesting dimensions of psychopathology are etiologically distinct. Alternatively, a differentiation hypothesis has also been proposed (Weiss & Nurcombe, 1992; Werner, 2004). Within this perspective, broader dimensions of psychopathology earlier in development may give rise to narrower dimensions later in development. Thus, these models may suggest that the broad dimensions are causally related to the novel dimensions later in development. Thus, behaviors reflective of internalizing and externalizing problems are hypothesized to be more highly correlated early in development and then become distinguished over time.

In contrast to other models, the temporal heterogeneity model suggests that different dimensions of psychopathology may develop at different rates over time or emerge in distinct developmental windows. That is, rather than being influenced by other dimensions of psychopathology, each dimension of psychopathology will develop according to its own developmental time scale. However, the course of its manifestation could still result in associations with other dimensions of psychopathology.

Changes in symptomatic expression of behavior problems raise conceptual questions about their underlying latent processes involved in leading to those behaviors. For example, does the apparent single latent externalizing dimension in childhood reflect latent liability for only the observed externalizing behaviors that are directly assessed? In childhood, these are focally centered on antagonistic behavior problems. Or, despite not being assessed, does the latent vulnerability reflect the spectrum of all relevant behaviors, inclusive of antagonistic and disinhibited behaviors, the latter of which includes liability for problematic substance use? If the latter, the liability for disinhibited behaviors would suggest that if given the opportunity, youth would demonstrate them. That is, even if not directly assessed, the underlying latent dimension could still predict some liability of engaging in the behavior.

A Way Forward

Despite these important challenges, there have been innovations in study design and data analysis that permit examining critical issues in longitudinal structure, stability, differentiation, and course of psychopathology. These methods permit inclusion of diverse psychopathology dimensions across development and reporters. Moreover, newer methods also permit flexible options of studying the structure of psychopathology, including challenging the reliance on latent dimensional models, as well as testing symptom trajectories across multiple distinct time scales.

Integrative Data Analysis

As noted above, there are multiple challenges in the study of dimensions of psychopathology across development. Studies rely on different reporters, behaviors, and times of assessment across development. In previous decades, models would be substantially simplified, or very strong assumptions about the functioning of different behaviors across development would need to be made to permit model testing. However, in the past decade, there have been tremendous advances made in integrating information across time, reporters, and specific measures used.

Integrative data analysis (Bauer, 2017; Curran, McGinley et al., 2014; Curran & Hussong, 2009) is a set of statistical methods developed to estimate latent dimensional scores from data from different studies, measures, and across time. There are rigorous data harmonization efforts to map similar content and response options together to reduce heterogeneity across measures and to estimate dimensional scores. However, the method is flexible, permitting inclusion of distinct measures and measures that are used only in some—but not all—studies, and at some—but not all—waves of assessments. The analytic backbone of these methods is moderated non-linear factor analysis (MNLFA; Bauer, 2017; Curran, McGinley et al., 2014). This method permits specifying an a priori measurement structure for latent factors. The initial implementations have focused on unidimensional constructs, but could be extended to multidimensional, hierarchical, or higher-order factor structures. These models are well suited to testing for effects of co-variates on item intercepts (or thresholds, depending on item scaling) and factor loadings. These are identical principles of testing MI, but are generalized for the use of a continuous variable's influences on measurement functioning. Moreover, whereas application of MI nearly always relies on measurement differences across a single unit (e.g., time; other grouping variable), MNLFA can be flexibly implemented to include multiple predictors, as well as interactions among predictors, to identify unique and interactive influences on measurement properties. As these can lead to a very large number of analyses, there have been adaptations to these methods to include regularization to focus on likely true and more reliable effects (Bauer et al., 2020). Although initially developed for use with integrating data from different studies, the principles can be directly applied within a single longitudinal study in which measures change over time.

The most frequent application of integrative data analysis is to estimate latent scores for a single latent dimension to estimate scores for use in subsequent analyses. Magee et al. (2023) used MNLFA to estimate trajectories of depression, externalizing problems, and inhibitory control spanning ages 2 to 30, including individual participant data from four primary studies. The authors provide information about their data harmonization processes across the instruments used in their study. That is, despite there being no fully common instruments across the individual studies, the authors fit factor models, with multiple predictors to allow for study and individual participant level co-variates to influence the functioning of the latent construct. After estimating the latent factor score estimates, the authors found linear growth in each of the processes. Moreover, they found that the externalizing problems intercept predicted the slopes of depression and inhibitory control; the depression intercept predicted the slopes of externalizing and inhibitory control; and the inhibitory control intercept predicted the slope of depression.

These models offer tremendous promise, but they have important limitations. First, they can model quantitative differences in loadings and thresholds for a consistent factor structure, but these models cannot be as flexibly implemented in contexts where the factor structure changes. That is, if the optimal model consists of a single factor at one assessment, but two-factors at a subsequent assessment or time in development, models are not able to consider time continuously and include gradual changes in overall structure. Second, the frequent implementation of the MNLFA models is to estimate factor scores for use in describing trajectories of symptoms, which is intended to model within-person change. However, the recommended practice is to randomly select single assessments per participant and estimate the effects of time and other effects (e.g., main effects of co-variates; non-linear effects of time; time by co-variate interactions). Then, those model parameters are used to estimate the factor scores across all participants, across all assessments. This approach focuses on using between-person model parameters to estimate within-person effects, which would be warranted if the parameters generalize from the group to individuals (Molenaar, 2004). However, this is an untested assumption in this context.

Network Analysis. Whereas there has been a long-standing tradition of focusing on latent disease models of psychopathology, in the past decade, the use of network models has grown considerably. Network models fundamentally challenge the assumptions of the latent disease model (see Slipetz and Henry, this volume). Thus, whereas factor analysis is built on the premise that a latent disease construct formally causes the manifest indicators, network analysis suggests that the presence of symptoms reflects a dynamic system. Within this approach, symptoms are thought to directly influence other symptoms within the system (although see Forbes et al., 2017 for important concerns). These are routinely estimated as partial correlation networks, with associations among observed variables (i.e., nodes) being quantified by edge weights. Broader network properties are summarized by an array of indices that quantify how individual items influence multiple other symptoms (i.e., centrality).

Networks are frequently estimated with variables in a single system either cross-sectionally, which reflects psychonetrics, or longitudinally, which better reflects the influence of single symptoms on the dynamics of a network (Epskamp, 2020; Epskamp et al., 2017). Using data from the Adolescent Brain Cognitive Development (ABCD) Study, Funkhouser et al. (2021) examined cross-lagged panel networks involving youth self-reports of internalizing, externalizing, and attention problems. In longitudinal associations, they found that depressed mood, inattention, and worry were associated with a range of follow-up symptoms.

However, studies of single psychopathological dimensions have modest impact on understanding the larger structure of psychopathology. Other studies have estimated networks of related, but conceptually distinct, networks. Work with bridge symptoms (P. J. Jones et al., 2021) has shown the value in modeling relationships among disorders based on shared, linking symptoms. For example, Groen et al. (2020) examined symptoms of anxiety and depressive symptoms during an ecological momentary assessment study of individuals with depression, anxiety, and comorbid depression and anxiety. In their work, they found that experience of worry linked symptoms across depression and anxiety, which was stronger among individuals with both depression and anxiety. Thus, identification of specific symptoms that functionally bridge associations among sets of symptoms, rather than are merely common to multiple disorders, may be important for developing and refining interventions.

Ambulatory Assessments. Using either latent variable modeling or network models, studies frequently rely on fairly few assessment occasions that are frequently used to describe psychopathology over fairly broad periods of time. As contacting research participants has become easier via email and smartphones, ambulatory assessments have become much more readily implemented. With the use of these methods, participants provide responses about their experiences and symptoms on a daily basis, or on multiple occasions throughout the day. Thus, these more intensive longitudinal designs can characterize patterns of symptoms over shorter-term time intervals. Other flexible implementations of these studies may administer intensive longitudinal assessments at multiple follow-up occasions, providing a combination of precise experiences in short bursts and longer-term development. Studies with more specific, fine-grained hypotheses about development or change may benefit from more intensive, time-limited assessments (Kaurin et al., 2025), whereas slower, more protracted development may benefit from assessments that are more widely spaced out (Abitante et al., 2022).

A key related issue is that studies conducting ambulatory assessments are frequently concerned with participant burden. As part of these studies, a relatively small number of items are administered per contact, which frequently leads to focusing on only one or two substantive domains of inquiry. However, in the context of psychopathology, there are many dimensions of signs and symptoms of interest. To permit assessing a wider span of items, inspired by planned missingness designs (Little & Rhemtulla, 2013; Rioux et al., 2020), individual assessment occasions could have random subsets of items administered to participants. This strategy could permit examining momentary structure of psychopathology, which may not necessarily be the same structure at an aggregate, person level.

Future Directions

The cross-sectional studies of age differences in measurement structure have relied on a priori age groups. However, these investigations can be extended to test age as a continuous moderator of the loadings. More exploratory and flexible modeling approaches may be particularly useful for delineating when in development gross or nuanced changes in model structure may be found. For example, rather than focusing solely on a singular a priori age cutoff, models could be iteratively estimated using single or multiple cut points for age and testing for invariance across the multiple different groups. Alternatively, with cross-sectional studies, investigations could consider age continuously and use higher-order polynomial terms to consider non-linear influences on the magnitude of loadings. As noted earlier, a related challenge is that there are not yet methods developed to evaluate gradual changes in gross measurement structure.

Conclusions

Studies of the longitudinal development of psychopathology require careful attention to the specific questions being addressed. There are considerations about the overall structure, longitudinal changes in symptoms, and how these are reflected in longitudinal consistency. These different kinds of questions rely on different methods. Moreover, in the context of development, there are important challenges in integrating information from different sources, which have been adapted using novel measurement models. Although factor analytic methods are frequently used to describe the dimensions of psychopathology, alternative kinds of models, such as network models, can provide valuable information about dynamics among dimensions of psychopathology within individuals and advance our understanding of these dimensions across time.

References

Abitante, G., Haraden, D. A., Pine, A., Cole, D., & Garber, J. (2022). Trajectories of positive and negative affect across adolescence: Maternal history of depression and adolescent sex as predictors. *Journal of Affective Disorders, 315*, 96–104. https://doi.org/10.1016/j.jad.2022.07.038

Achenbach, T. M. (1966). The classification of children's psychiatric symptoms: A factor-analytic study. *Psychological Monographs: General and Applied, 80*(7), 1–37. https://doi.org/10.1037/h0093906

Achenbach, T. M. (2011). Commentary: Definitely more than measurement error: But how should we understand and deal with informant discrepancies? *Journal of Clinical Child & Adolescent Psychology, 40*(1), 80–86. https://doi.org/10.1080/15374416.2011.533416

Achenbach, T. M., McConaughy, S. H., & Howell, C. T. (1987). Child/adolescent behavioral and emotional problems: Implications of cross-informant correlations for situational specificity. *Psychological Bulletin, 101*(2), 213.

Bauer, D. J. (2017). A more general model for testing measurement invariance and differential item functioning. *Psychological Methods, 22*(3), 507. https://doi.org/10.1037/met0000077

Bauer, D. J., Belzak, W. C. M., & Cole, V. T. (2020). Simplifying the assessment of measurement invariance over multiple background variables: Using regularized moderated nonlinear factor analysis to detect differential item functioning. *Structural Equation Modeling: A Multidisciplinary Journal, 27*(1), 43–55. https://doi.org/10.1080/10705511.2019.1642754

Berry, D., & Willoughby, M. T. (2017). On the practical interpretability of cross-lagged panel models: Rethinking a developmental workhorse. *Child Development, 88*(4), 1186–1206. https://doi.org/10.1111/cdev.12660

Biesanz, J. C., Deeb-Sossa, N., Papadakis, A. A., Bollen, K. A., & Curran, P. J. (2004). The role of coding time in estimating and interpreting growth curve models. *Psychological Methods, 9*(1), 30–52.

Birmaher, B., Ehmann, M., Axelson, D. A., Goldstein, B. I., Monk, K., Kalas, C., Kupfer, D., Gill, M. K., Leibenluft, E., & Bridge, J. (2009). Schedule for affective disorders and schizophrenia for school-age children (K-SADS-PL) for the assessment of preschool children: A preliminary psychometric study. *Journal of Psychiatric Research, 43*(7), 680–686.

Bollen, K. A., & Curran, P. J. (2006). *Latent curve models: A structural equation perspective*. John Wiley & Sons.

Bonifay, W., Winter, S. D., Skoblow, H. F., & Watts, A. L. (2025). Good fit is weak evidence of replication: Increasing rigor through prior predictive similarity checking. *Assessment, 32*(2), 170–189. https://doi.org/10.1177/10731911241234118

Bornstein, M. H., Putnick, D. L., & Esposito, G. (2017). Continuity and stability in development. *Child Development Perspectives, 11*(2), 113–119.

Brensilver, M., Negriff, S., Mennen, F. E., & Trickett, P. K. (2011). Longitudinal relations between depressive symptoms and externalizing behavior in adolescence: Moderating effects of maltreatment experience and gender. *Journal of Clinical Child & Adolescent Psychology, 40*(4), 607–617. https://doi.org/10.1080/15374416.2011.581618

Byrne, B. M., Shavelson, R. J., & Muthén, B. (1989). Testing for the equivalence of factor covariance and mean structures: The issue of partial measurement invariance. *Psychological Bulletin, 105*(3), 456.

Chen, F. F. (2007). Sensitivity of goodness of fit indexes to lack of measurement invariance. *Structural Equation Modeling, 14*(3), 464–504.

Cicchetti, D. (1993). Developmental psychopathology: Reactions, reflections, projections. *Developmental Review, 13*(4), 471–502. https://doi.org/10.1006/drev.1993.1021

Cicchetti, D., & Rogosch, F. A. (1996). Equifinality and multifinality in developmental psychopathology. *Development and Psychopathology, 8*, 597–600.

Curran, P. J., Howard, A. L., Bainter, S. A., Lane, S. T., & McGinley, J. S. (2014). The separation of between-person and within-person components of individual change over time: A latent curve model with structured residuals. *Journal of Consulting and Clinical Psychology, 82*(5), 879–894. https://doi.org/10.1037/a0035297

Curran, P. J., & Hussong, A. M. (2009). Integrative data analysis: The simultaneous analysis of multiple data sets. *Psychological Methods, 14*(2), 81–100.

Curran, P. J., McGinley, J. S., Bauer, D. J., Hussong, A. M., Burns, A., Chassin, L., Sher, K., & Zucker, R. (2014). A moderated nonlinear factor model for the development of commensurate measures in integrative data analysis. *Multivariate Behavioral Research, 49*(3), 214–231. https://doi.org/10.1080/00273171.2014.889594

Davis, S., Votruba-Drzal, E., & Silk, J. S. (2015). Trajectories of internalizing symptoms from early childhood to adolescence: Associations with temperament and parenting. *Social Development, 24*(3), 501–520. https://doi.org/10.1111/sode.12105

De Los Reyes, A., Augenstein, T. M., Wang, M., Thomas, S. A., Drabick, D. A., Burgers, D. E., & Rabinowitz, J. (2015). The validity of the multi-informant approach to assessing child and adolescent mental health. *Psychological Bulletin, 141*(4), 858–900. https://doi.org/10.1037/a0038498

De Los Reyes, A., & Kazdin, A. E. (2005). Informant discrepancies in the assessment of childhood psychopathology: A critical review, theoretical framework, and recommendations for further study. *Psychological Bulletin, 131*(4), 483–509.

De Los Reyes, A., Thomas, S. A., Goodman, K. L., & Kundey, S. M. (2013). Principles underlying the use of multiple informants' reports. *Annual Review of Clinical Psychology, 9*, 123–149.

Duncan, S. C., & Duncan, T. E. (1996). A multivariate latent growth curve analysis of adolescent substance use. *Structural Equation Modeling: A Multidisciplinary Journal, 3*(4), 323–347. https://doi.org/10.1080/10705519609540050

Duncan, S. C., Duncan, T. E., & Strycker, L. A. (2000). Risk and protective factors influencing adolescent problem behavior: A multivariate latent growth curve analysis. *Annals of Behavioral Medicine, 22*(2), 103–109. https://doi.org/10.1007/BF02895772

Elison, J. T. (2020). Considering transient instantiators. *Development and Psychopathology, 32*(4), 1173–1174.

Epskamp, S. (2020). Psychometric network models from time-series and panel data. *Psychometrika, 85*(1), 206–231. https://doi.org/10.1007/s11336-020-09697-3

Epskamp, S., Rhemtulla, M., & Borsboom, D. (2017). Generalized network psychometrics: Combining network and latent variable models. *Psychometrika, 82*(4), 904–927. https://doi.org/10.1007/s11336-017-9557-x

Estabrook, R. (2018). From factors of curves to factors of change. In E. Ferrer, S. M. Boker, & K. J. Grimm (Eds.), *Longitudinal multivariate psychology* (1st ed., pp. 240–260). Routledge. https://doi.org/10.4324/9781315160542-12

Fanti, K. A., Colins, O. F., & Andershed, H. (2019). Unraveling the longitudinal reciprocal associations between anxiety, delinquency, and depression from early to middle adolescence. *Journal of Criminal Justice, 62*, 29–34. https://doi.org/10.1016/j.jcrimjus.2018.09.004

Forbes, M. K., Wright, A. G. C., Markon, K. E., & Krueger, R. F. (2017). Evidence that psychopathology symptom networks have limited replicability. *Journal of Abnormal Psychology, 126*(7), 969–988. https://doi.org/10.1037/abn0000276

Funkhouser, C. J., Chacko, A. A., Correa, K. A., Kaiser, A. J. E., & Shankman, S. A. (2021). Unique longitudinal relationships between symptoms of psychopathology in youth: A cross-lagged panel network analysis in the ABCD study. *Journal of Child Psychology and Psychiatry*, *62*(2), 184–194. https://doi.org/10.1111/jcpp.13256

Gluschkoff, K., Jokela, M., & Rosenström, T. (2019). The general psychopathology factor: Structural stability and generalizability to within-individual changes. *Frontiers in Psychiatry*, *10*. https://doi.org/10.3389/fpsyt.2019.00594

Gold, D., Rosowsky, E., Piryatinsky, I., & Sinclair, S. J. (2020). Comparing patient and informant ratings of depressive symptoms in various stages of Alzheimer's disease. *Neuropsychology*, *34*(5), 535–550. https://doi.org/10.1037/neu0000630

Grant, B. F., Dawson, D. A., Stinson, F. S., Chou, P. S., Kay, W., & Pickering, R. (2003). The Alcohol Use Disorder and Associated Disabilities Interview Schedule-IV (AUDADIS-IV): Reliability of alcohol consumption, tobacco use, family history of depression and psychiatric diagnostic modules in a general population sample. *Drug and Alcohol Dependence*, *71*(1), 7–16. https://doi.org/10.1016/S0376-8716(03)00070-X

Grant, B. F., Goldstein, R. B., Chou, S. P., Huang, B., Stinson, F. S., Dawson, D. A., Saha, T. D., Smith, S. M., Pulay, A. J., & Pickering, R. P. (2009). Sociodemographic and psychopathologic predictors of first incidence of DSM-IV substance use, mood and anxiety disorders: Results from the Wave 2 National Epidemiologic Survey on Alcohol and Related Conditions. *Molecular Psychiatry*, *14*(11), 1051–1066.

Greene, A. L., & Eaton, N. R. (2017). The temporal stability of the bifactor model of comorbidity: An examination of moderated continuity pathways. *Comprehensive Psychiatry*, *72*, 74–82. https://doi.org/10.1016/j.comppsych.2016.09.010

Groen, R. N., Ryan, O., Wigman, J. T. W., Riese, H., Penninx, B. W. J. H., Giltay, E. J., Wichers, M., & Hartman, C. A. (2020). Comorbidity between depression and anxiety: Assessing the role of bridge mental states in dynamic psychological networks. *BMC Medicine*, *18*(1), 308. https://doi.org/10.1186/s12916-020-01738-z

Hamaker, E. L., Kuiper, R. M., & Grasman, R. P. P. P. (2015). A critique of the cross-lagged panel model. *Psychological Methods*, *20*(1), 102–116. https://doi.org/10.1037/a0038889

Harris, J. L., Swanson, B., & Petersen, I. T. (2024). A developmentally informed systematic review and meta-analysis of the strength of general psychopathology in childhood and adolescence. *Clinical Child and Family Psychology Review*, *27*(1), 130–164. https://doi.org/10.1007/s10567-023-00464-1

Hoertel, N., McMahon, K., Olfson, M., Wall, M. M., Rodríguez-Fernández, J. M., Lemogne, C., Limosin, F., & Blanco, C. (2015). A dimensional liability model of age differences in mental disorder prevalence: Evidence from a national sample. *Journal of Psychiatric Research*, *64*, 107–113. https://doi.org/10.1016/j.jpsychires.2015.03.017

Jolliffe, D., Farrington, D. P., Piquero, A. R., MacLeod, J. F., & van de Weijer, S. (2017). Prevalence of life-course-persistent, adolescence-limited, and late-onset offenders: A systematic review of prospective longitudinal studies. *Aggression and Violent Behavior*, *33*, 4–14. https://doi.org/10.1016/j.avb.2017.01.002

Jones, B. L., & Nagin, D. S. (2007). Advances in group-based trajectory modeling and an SAS procedure for estimating them. *Sociological Methods & Research*, *35*(4), 542–571.

Jones, P. J., Ma, R., & McNally, R. J. (2021). Bridge centrality: A network approach to understanding comorbidity. *Multivariate Behavioral Research*, *56*(2), 353–367. https://doi.org/10.1080/00273171.2019.1614898

Kaurin, A., Vize, C. E., & Wright, A. G. C. (2025). The resolution of affective reactivity to stressful events. *Emotion*. https://doi.org/10.1037/emo0001598

Kessler, R. C., McGonagle, K. A., Zhao, S., Nelson, C. B., Hughes, M., Eshleman, S., Wittchen, H. U., & Kendler, K. S. (1994). Lifetime and 12-month prevalence of DSM-III-R psychiatric disorders in the United States. *Archives of General Psychiatry*, *51*(1), 8–19.

Klein, D. N., Ouimette, P. C., Kelly, H. S., Ferro, T., & et al. (1994). Test-retest reliability of team consensus best-estimate diagonses of Axis I and II disorders in a family study. *American Journal of Psychiatry*, *151*(7), 1043–1047.

Kotov, R., Krueger, R. F., Watson, D., Achenbach, T. M., Althoff, R. R., Bagby, R. M., Brown, T. A., Carpenter, W. T., Caspi, A., Clark, L. A., Eaton, N. R., Forbes, M. K., Forbush, K. T., Goldberg, D., Hasin, D., Hyman, S. E., Ivanova, M. Y., Lynam, D. R., Markon, K., . . . Zimmerman, M. (2017). The Hierarchical Taxonomy of Psychopathology (HiTOP): A dimensional alternative to traditional nosologies. *Journal of Abnormal Psychology, 126*(4), 454–477. https://doi.org/10.1037/abn0000258

Krueger, R. F., Caspi, A., Moffitt, T. E., & Silva, P. A. (1998). The structure and stability of common mental disorders (DSM-III-R): A longitudinal-epidemiological study. *Journal of Abnormal Psychology, 107*(2), 216–227.

Krueger, R. F., & Finger, M. S. (2001). Using item response theory to understand comorbidity among anxiety and unipolar mood disorders. *Psychological Assessment, 13*(1), 140–151.

Krueger, R. F., Hicks, B. M., Patrick, C. J., Carlson, S. R., Iacono, W. G., & McGue, M. (2002). Etiologic connections among substance dependence, antisocial behavior, and personality: Modeling the externalizing spectrum. *Journal of Abnormal Psychology, 111*(3), 411–424.

Krueger, R. F., & Markon, K. E. (2006). Reinterpreting comorbidity: A model-based approach to understanding and classifying psychopathology. *Annual Review of Clinical Psychology, 2*, 111–133. https://doi.org/10.1146/annurev.clinpsy.2.022305.095213

Krueger, R. F., Markon, K. E., Patrick, C. J., Benning, S. D., & Kramer, M. D. (2007). Linking antisocial behavior, substance use, and personality: An integrative quantitative model of the adult externalizing spectrum. *Journal of Abnormal Psychology, 116*(4), 645.

Krueger, R. F., Markon, K. E., Patrick, C. J., & Iacono, W. G. (2005). Externalizing psychopathology in adulthood: A dimensional-spectrum conceptualization and its implications for DSM-V. *Journal of Abnormal Psychology, 114*(4), 537–550.

Krueger, R. F., McGue, M., & Iacono, W. G. (2001). The higher-order structure of common DSM mental disorders: Internalization, externalization, and their connections to personality. *Personality and Individual Differences, 30*(7), 1245–1259.

Laceulle, O. M., Rienks, K., Meijer, L., de Moor, E. L., & Karreman, A. (2023). A developmental approach to youth maladaptive personality traits: Variable- versus person-centered change in the transition from childhood to adolescence. *European Journal of Personality, 37*(6), 649–668. https://doi.org/10.1177/08902070221130116

Lahey, B. B., Applegate, B., Waldman, I. D., Loft, J. D., Hankin, B. L., & Rick, J. (2004). The structure of child and adolescent psychopathology: Generating new hypotheses. *Journal of Abnormal Psychology, 113*(3), 358–385.

Lahey, B. B., Van Hulle, C. A., Singh, A. L., Waldman, I. D., & Rathouz, P. J. (2011). Higher-order genetic and environmental structure of prevalent forms of child and adolescent psychopathology. *Archives of General Psychiatry, 68*(2), 181–189. https://doi.org/10.1001/archgenpsychiatry.2010.192

Levin-Aspenson, H. F., Watson, D., Clark, L. A., & Zimmerman, M. (2021). What is the general factor of psychopathology? Consistency of the p factor across samples. *Assessment, 28*(4), 1035–1049. https://doi.org/10.1177/1073191120954921

Little, T. D., & Rhemtulla, M. (2013). Planned missing data designs for developmental researchers. *Child Development Perspectives, 7*(4), 199–204. https://doi.org/10.1111/cdep.12043

Lucas, R. E. (2023). Why the cross-lagged panel model is almost never the right choice. *Advances in Methods and Practices in Psychological Science, 6*(1), 25152459231158378. https://doi.org/10.1177/25152459231158378

Magee, K. E., Connell, A., Hipwell, A. E., Shaw, D., Westling, E., Keenan, K., Stormshak, E., Ha, T., & Stepp, S. (2023). Developmental models of depression, externalizing problems, and self-regulatory processes: Integrated data analysis across four longitudinal studies of youth. *Prevention Science, 24*(8), 1499–1509. https://doi.org/10.1007/s11121-022-01441-w

Makol, B. A., Youngstrom, E. A., Racz, S. J., Qasmieh, N., Glenn, L. E., & De Los Reyes, A. (2020). Integrating multiple informants' reports: How conceptual and measurement models may address long-standing problems in clinical decision-making. *Clinical Psychological Science, 8*(6), 953–970. https://doi.org/10.1177/2167702620924439

Mann, F. D., Atherton, O. E., DeYoung, C. G., Krueger, R. F., & Robins, R. W. (2020). Big five personality traits and common mental disorders within a hierarchical taxonomy of psychopathology:

A longitudinal study of Mexican-origin youth. *Journal of Abnormal Psychology, 129*(8), 769–787. https://doi.org/10.1037/abn0000633

McArdle, J. J. (1988). Dynamic but structural equation modeling of repeated measures data. In J. R. Nesselroade & R. B. Cattell (Eds.), *Handbook of multivariate experimental psychology* (pp. 561–614). Springer US. https://doi.org/10.1007/978-1-4613-0893-5_17

McDonald, R. P. (1999). *Test theory: A unified treatment*. Psychology Press. https://doi.org/10.4324/9781410601087

Millsap, R. E. (2011). *Statistical approaches to measurement invariance*. Taylor and Francis Group.

Moffitt, T. E. (1993). Adolescence-limited and life-course-persistent antisocial behavior: A developmental taxonomy. *Psychological Review, 100*(4), 674–701.

Molenaar, P. C. M. (2004). A manifesto on psychology as idiographic science: Bringing the person back into scientific psychology, this time forever. *Measurement: Interdisciplinary Research & Perspective, 2*(4), 201–218. https://doi.org/10.1207/s15366359mea0204_1

Moritz, S., Göritz, A. S., McLean, B., Westermann, S., & Brodbeck, J. (2017). Do depressive symptoms predict paranoia or vice versa? *Journal of Behavior Therapy and Experimental Psychiatry, 56*, 113–121. https://doi.org/10.1016/j.jbtep.2016.10.002

Mulder, J. D., & Hamaker, E. L. (2021). Three extensions of the random intercept cross-lagged panel model. *Structural Equation Modeling: A Multidisciplinary Journal, 28*(4), 638–648. https://doi.org/10.1080/10705511.2020.1784738

Murray, A. L., Eisner, M., & Ribeaud, D. (2016). The development of the general factor of psychopathology 'p Factor' through childhood and adolescence. *Journal of Abnormal Child Psychology, 44*(8), 1–14. https://doi.org/10.1007/s10802-016-0132-1

Murray, A. L., Eisner, M., & Ribeaud, D. (2020). Within-person analysis of developmental cascades between externalising and internalising problems. *Journal of Child Psychology and Psychiatry, 61*(6), 681–688. https://doi.org/10.1111/jcpp.13150

Muthén, B. O., & Muthén, L. K. (2000). Integrating person-centered and variable-centered analyses: Growth mixture modeling with latent trajectory classes. *Alcoholism: Clinical and Experimental Research, 24*(6), 882–891.

Olino, T. M. (2020). Clinical applications of measurement invariance. *Journal of Personality Assessment, 102*(5), 727–729. https://doi.org/10.1080/00223891.2020.1793766

Olino, T. M., Bufferd, S. J., Dougherty, L. R., Dyson, M. W., Carlson, G. A., & Klein, D. N. (2018). The development of latent dimensions of psychopathology across early childhood: Stability of dimensions and moderators of change. *Journal of Abnormal Child Psychology, 46*, 1373–1383.

Olino, T. M., Finsaas, M., Dougherty, L. R., & Klein, D. N. (2018). Is parent–child disagreement on child anxiety explained by differences in measurement properties? An examination of measurement invariance across informants and rime. *Frontiers in Psychology, 9*. https://doi.org/10.3389/fpsyg.2018.01295

Olino, T. M., Stepp, S. D., Keenan, K., Loeber, R., & Hipwell, A. (2014). Trajectories of depression and anxiety symptoms in adolescent girls: A comparison of parallel trajectory approaches. *Journal of Personality Assessment, 96*(3), 316–326.

Oltmanns, T. F., Rodrigues, M. M., Weinstein, Y., & Gleason, M. E. J. (2014). Prevalence of personality disorders at midlife in a community sample: Disorders and symptoms reflected in interview, self, and informant reports. *Journal of Psychopathology and Behavioral Assessment, 36*(2), 177–188. https://doi.org/10.1007/s10862-013-9389-7

Orth, U., Clark, D. A., Donnellan, M. B., & Robins, R. W. (2021). Testing prospective effects in longitudinal research: Comparing seven competing cross-lagged models. *Journal of Personality and Social Psychology, 120*(4), 1013–1034. https://doi.org/10.1037/pspp0000358

Papachristou, E., & Flouri, E. (2020). The codevelopment of internalizing symptoms, externalizing symptoms, and cognitive ability across childhood and adolescence. *Development and Psychopathology, 32*(4), 1375–1389. https://doi.org/10.1017/S0954579419001330

Pettit, J. W., Lewinsohn, P. M., Seeley, J. R., Roberts, R. E., & Yaroslavsky, I. (2010). Developmental relations between depressive symptoms, minor hassles, and major events from adolescence through age 30 years. *Journal of Abnormal Psychology, 119*(4), 811.

Richards, J. S., Hartman, C. A., Ormel, J., & Oldehinkel, A. J. (2024). Continuity of psychopathology throughout adolescence and young adulthood. *Journal of Clinical Child & Adolescent Psychology*, *53*(4), 623–636. https://doi.org/10.1080/15374416.2022.2042695

Rioux, C., Lewin, A., Odejimi, O. A., & Little, T. D. (2020). Reflection on modern methods: Planned missing data designs for epidemiological research. *International Journal of Epidemiology*, *49*(5), 1702–1711. https://doi.org/10.1093/ije/dyaa042

Singer, J. D., Willett, J. B., & Willett, J. B. (2003). *Applied longitudinal data analysis: Modeling change and event occurrence*. Oxford University Press.

Snyder, H. R., Young, J. F., & Hankin, B. L. (2017). Strong homotypic continuity in common psychopathology-, internalizing-, and externalizing-specific factors over time in adolescents. *Clinical Psychological Science*, *5*(1), 98–110. https://doi.org/10.1177/2167702616651076

Sorcher, L. K., Mennies, R. J., Robeson, M., Seeley, J. R., Klein, D. N., Dougherty, L. R., & Olino, T. M. (2023). Offspring irritability: Associations with parental psychopathology and personality. *European Child & Adolescent Psychiatry*, *32*(9), 1691–1699. https://doi.org/10.1007/s00787-022-01985-w

Van der Giessen, D., Branje, S., Overbeek, G., Frijns, T., van Lier, P. A. C., Koot, H. M., & Meeus, W. (2013). Co-occurrence of aggressive behavior and depressive symptoms in early adolescence: A longitudinal multi-informant study. *European Review of Applied Psychology*, *63*(4), 193–201. https://doi.org/10.1016/j.erap.2013.03.001

Vollebergh, W. A. M., Iedema, J., Bijl, R. V., de Graaf, R., Smit, F., & Ormel, J. (2001). The structure and stability of common mental disorders: The NEMESIS study. *Archives of General Psychiatry*, *58*(6), 597–603.

Wang, C., Williams, K. E., Shahaeian, A., & Harrison, L. J. (2018). Early predictors of escalating internalizing problems across middle childhood. *School Psychology Quarterly*, *33*(2), 200–212. https://doi.org/10.1037/spq0000218

Weiss, B., & Nurcombe, B. (1992). Age, clinical severity, and the differentiation of depressive psychopathology: A test of the orthogenetic hypothesis. *Development and Psychopathology*, *4*(1), 113–124. https://doi.org/10.1017/S0954579400005599

Werner, H. (2004). *Comparative psychology of mental development*. ISD. https://www.torrossa.com/it/resources/an/5391498

Widaman, K. F., Ferrer, E., & Conger, R. D. (2010). Factorial invariance within longitudinal structural equation models: Measuring the same construct across time. *Child Development Perspectives*, *4*(1), 10–18. https://doi.org/10.1111/j.1750-8606.2009.00110.x

PART IV

Mechanics and Sociology of Paradigm Change in Diagnosis

CHAPTER 21

A Comparison of the Clinical Utility of Dimensional and Categorical Diagnostic Systems for Use in Clinical Practice

CHARLIE CHUNG-YIH SU, THOMAS BART, AND DAVID CICERO

Introduction

NOSOLOGISTS have long debated whether psychopathology is better conceptualized as categorical or dimensional constructs (Clark et al., 1995). In recent years, there is growing consensus that psychopathology is better understood in dimensional terms (i.e., it varies along a continuum throughout the population), even among psychologists, psychiatrists, and researchers who believe categorical systems are more effective for use in clinical practice (Zimmerman, 2021). In most clinical settings, clinicians are mandated by their employers or third-party payers to use traditional categorical systems for various clinical activities, such as billing for services, and training of future psychologists and psychiatrists is dominated by categorical systems (First, 2005). For example, the *Diagnostic and Statistical Manual of Mental Disorders* (DSM-5-TR; American Psychiatric Association, 2022) and International Classification of Diseases (ICD-11; World Health Organization, 2019) are far and away the most commonly used systems for diagnosis in the United States and internationally, respectively. The content of both systems is similar, and the manuals are harmonized such that ICD codes may be used for billing, regardless of whether the clinician is using the DSM or ICD to make the diagnoses (First, 2009).

Despite the ubiquity of the DSM and ICD, researchers and clinicians have proposed several alternative diagnostic systems, many of which conceptualize psychopathology dimensionally. These diagnostic systems include (1) the Alternative Model of Personality Disorders (AMPD) in the DSM-5, (2) the Personality Disorders and Related Traits section of the ICD-11, (3) the Hierarchical Taxonomy of Psychopathology (Kotov et al., 2017), (4) the *Psychodynamic Diagnostic Manual Second Edition* (Lingiardi & McWilliams, 2017), (5) *Operationalized Psychodynamic Diagnosis* (OPD Task Force, 2008), and (6) *Power Threat Meaning Framework* (PTMF; Johnstone & Boyle, 2018). In addition to these systems that aim to revolutionize nosology, others can be described as approaches to improve the accuracy of assessment while not explicitly being described as a diagnostic system, including the Achenbach System of Evidence-Based Assessment (Achenbach, 2009; Achenbach & Rescorla, 2001, 2003), the National Institute of Mental Health's (NIMH) Research Domain Criteria (Insel et al., 2010), Clinical Staging (McGorry et al., 2006), and network theory (Borsboom, 2017).

Arguably, the strongest case to be made in favor of categorical over dimensional systems is related to clinical utility (i.e., the systems' usefulness in clinical practice). The current chapter aims to compare the evidence for the clinical utility of dimensional and categorical diagnostic systems. Specifically, we will (1) describe commonly used diagnostic systems, (2) discuss how dimensional systems may be used by busy clinicians in clinical practice using HiTOP as an example, (3) define clinical utility, (4) review the empirical evidence for the clinical utility of categorical and dimensional systems, and (5) explore potential barriers to implementing dimensional systems in practice. Readers who are familiar with contemporary diagnostic frameworks and/or have read part III of the present volume on "Dimensional Approaches to Psychopathology" may prefer to skip to the next section to go straight to our consideration of clinical applications.

Major Diagnostic Systems: *The Diagnostic and Statistical Manual of Mental Disorders* and International Classification of Diseases

Before reviewing the clinical utility of categorical and dimensional diagnostic systems, it is important to first briefly describe the systems that will be discussed and explain how they are meant to be used in clinical practice. As mentioned, the two most used diagnostic systems in the United States and internationally are the DSM and the ICD, respectively. The first edition of the DSM was published in 1952 by the American Psychiatric Association and is currently in its fifth edition, for which a text revision was published in 2022. The ICD is published by the World Health Organization (WHO) and includes a chapter related to psychopathology, titled "Mental, Behavioural, and Neurodevelopmental Disorders." The 11th edition of the ICD was released in 2022, but many clinicians are still required to use the 10th edition for important clinical tasks, such as reimbursement for services.

Most clinicians and researchers acknowledge that these traditional categorical systems have considerable flaws related to construct validity. First, diagnoses based on these models have excessive comorbidity, much more than would be expected if the latent constructs these labels represent were actually discrete disorders (e.g., Caspi et al., 2020; Kessler et al., 2005). Second, the DSM criteria are polythetic, creating extensive heterogeneity among individuals diagnosed with the same disorder (Clark et al., 1995; Hasler et al., 2004; Olbert et al., 2014). Third, there are unclear and fuzzy boundaries between disorder and non-disorder, as well as between specific disorders (Cooper, 2013; Spitzer & Wakefield, 1999). Fourth, the DSM and ICD fail to account for subthreshold traits and symptoms that may still be clinically significant and impactful in treatment outcomes (Johnson et al., 2022). Finally, despite being criticized for an excessive number of categorical diagnoses, the DSM and ICD have also been criticized for lacking complete coverage of psychopathology, resulting in many individuals being diagnosed with "unspecified" diagnoses (Wakefield, 2016).

As mentioned, the DSM and ICD were "harmonized" by their developers (Widiger et al., this volume). A small number of individuals served on work groups for both manuals, with the goal of making the manuals similar to facilitate clinical work, billing, and research (First, 2009). As a result, the DSM and ICD are similar in many ways but deviate in others as a function of differing approaches (Clark et al., 2017). First, both systems have lists of features or symptoms that make up a disorder but differ in the way these features are used to make a diagnosis. In the DSM, diagnosticians count symptoms, and an individual is diagnosed with a disorder if they exceed a specified number of symptoms. The Clinical Descriptions and Diagnostic Requirements for the ICD-11 mental, behavioral, and neurodevelopmental disorders (CDDR) take a similar, albeit more flexible, approach. It includes "essential (required) features" that resemble symptom counts in the DSM, but exact symptom counts required for diagnosis are generally avoided.

Second, both the DSM and ICD are primarily categorical systems, with some notable exceptions. The development of the DSM-5 and the ICD-11 both saw workgroups strongly consider incorporating more dimensional constructs into their manuals (McCabe & Widiger, 2020). The workgroups dealing with personality disorders came the closest to converting to fully dimensional systems. For example, the DSM-5 Personality and Personality Disorders Workgroup originally proposed a fully dimensional model of personality disorders (Skodol, 2012) but ultimately retained the categorical model in the main body (called Section II) of the manual and included the dimensional/hybrid model in Section III, "Emerging Measures and Models," as the Alternative Model of Personality Disorders (AMPD). In contrast, the ICD-11 now includes a dimensional system as its main approach to the diagnosis of personality disorders. Thus, the newest edition of the ICD went much further than the DSM in incorporating dimensional approaches to diagnosis. In addition to personality disorders, both manuals saw the addition of spectra to describe disorders thought to exist on a continuum, such as schizophrenia spectrum disorders and autistic spectrum disorder.

The Hierarchical Taxonomy of Psychopathology

Another prominent dimensional model of psychopathology, in the same mold as DSM-5's AMPD and ICD-11 personality disorders, is the Hierarchical Taxonomy of Psychopathology (see Figure 21.1). HiTOP conceptualizes psychopathology dimensionally and hierarchically, with broad psychopathology at the top of the hierarchy and more specific factors and individual symptoms as one moves down the hierarchy (Kotov et al., 2017). The p factor, a general psychopathology factor that represents the shared aspects of psychopathology, rests at the top of the hierarchy. Below the p factor are the psychosis, externalizing, and emotional dysfunction superspectra. The externalizing superspectrum can be further broken down into disinhibited and antagonistic externalizing spectra, the psychosis superspectrum into thought disorder and detachment spectra, and emotional dysfunction into the internalization and somatoform spectra. Thus, there are six spectra in the HiTOP model, which roughly correspond to the five domains in the AMPD. The internalizing spectrum is similar to negative affectivity, antagonistic externalizing to antagonism, disinhibited externalizing to disinhibition, thought disorder to psychoticism, and detachment has the same name in both systems. Below the spectra are subfactors. For example, the internalizing spectrum includes subfactors of sexual problems, eating pathology, fear, distress, and mania. Next, subfactors are composed of homogenous symptom components/maladaptive traits, which are in turn composed of individual signs and symptoms. In the current chapter, HiTOP is more thoroughly described in the section below on applying HiTOP to clinical practice (see also Pham and Forbes, this volume).

Psychodynamic Dimensional Systems: The *Psychodynamic Diagnostic Manual* and *Operationalized Psychodynamic Diagnosis*

The original DSM classified psychopathology based on psychodynamic theory, which was the leading explanatory framework at the time (Shorter, 2008). However, the DSM-III, IV, and 5 have taken an atheoretical approach that aims to describe rather than explain the etiology of psychopathology. In the last 20 years, psychodynamic theorists, in partnership with international organizations, such as the International Psychoanalytic Association and American

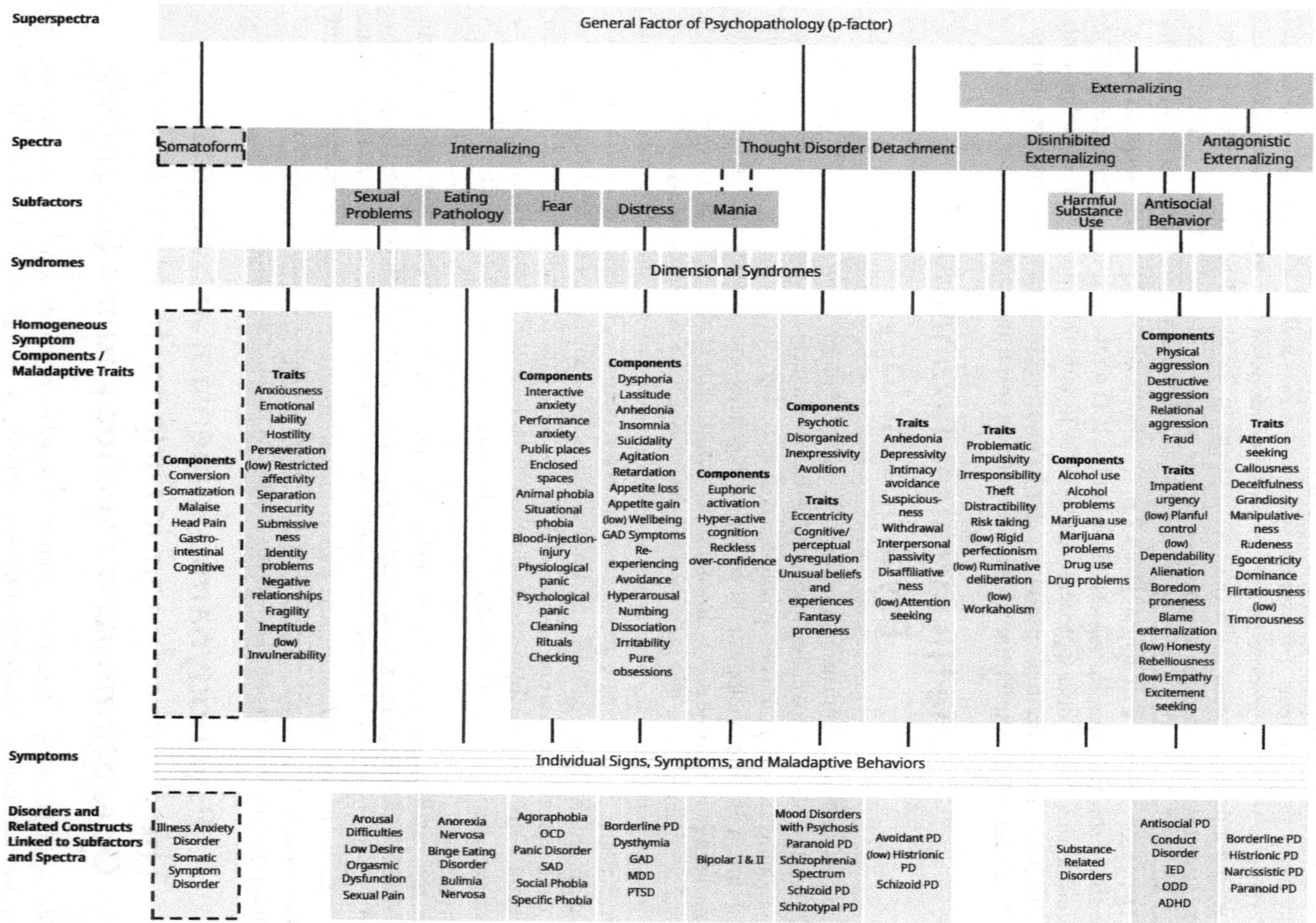

FIGURE 21.1 Official HiTOP Framework

Psychoanalytic Association, have developed a new manual based on psychodynamic principles called the *Psychodynamic Diagnostic Manual*, currently in its second edition (PDM-2; Lingiardi & McWilliams, 2017).

The PDM-2 is meant to be a complement to existing diagnostic systems rather than serve as a replacement. Like editions of the DSM prior to the fifth, the PDM is multiaxial, including a P-Axis (Personality Syndromes), M-Axis (Profile of Mental Functioning), and S Axis (Symptom Patterns: The Subjective Experience). The PDM includes separate sections for Adulthood, Adolescence, Childhood, Infancy and Early Childhood, and Later Life. The PDM begins with personality syndromes, because the authors view personality as more central than are symptoms to case conceptualization and treatment planning (McWilliams et al., 2018). Psychodynamic theorists make a distinction between personality organization (i.e., an individual's functioning and adaptation) and personality style (i.e., an individual's relatively stable response patterns to self and others). This is similar to the AMPD's Criterion A and B in that the former is meant to indicate level of personality functioning, and the latter describes personality traits experienced by the individual.

When conceptualizing a patient with the PDM-2, the psychoanalyst categorizes the client's personality organization into high, neurotic, borderline, and psychotic categories along a continuum of functioning from high to low. The P-Axis then includes 12 personality syndromes, similar to traditional categorical personality disorders in the DSM/ICD. The M-Axis includes an evaluation of 12 "capacities" for mental functioning organized into four domains, including cognitive and affective processes, identity and relationships, defense and coping, and self-awareness and self-direction. Individuals are rated on a 1–5 scale for each capacity, resulting in a 12–60 score with healthy (54–60), neurotic (40–53), borderline (19–39), and psychotic (12–18) levels of mental functioning. Finally, the S-Axis includes symptom patterns and the subjective experience of individuals using similar terms as the DSM/ICD. For example, the disorders in this section are grouped into classifications, including (1) predominantly psychotic-disorders, (2) mood disorders, (3) disorders related primarily to anxiety, (4) event- and stressor-related disorders, (5) somatic symptoms and related disorders, (6) specific symptom disorders, and (7) disorders related to addiction and to other medical conditions.

In addition to the PDM-2, a second manual available to psychodynamic clinicians is the *Operationalized Psychodynamic Diagnosis* (OPD Task Force, 2008). Originally developed in 1992 and first translated into English in 2008, the OPD aims to operationalize psychodynamic constructs and provide a framework by which clinicians can use these concepts in clinical practice. The OPD is similar to the PDM in some ways. For example, both (1) are meant to complement the DSM/ICD rather than replace them altogether, (2) conceptualize psychopathology dimensionally, and (3) are multiaxial. Axis I refers to the individual's relationship patterns, which may be adaptive or maladaptive. Axis II deals with inner conflicts, which can be further broken down into (1) closeness versus distance, (2) submission versus control, (3) taking care of oneself versus being cared for, (4) self-worth conflict, (5) guilt conflict, (6) Oedipal conflict, and (7) identity conflict. Axis III assesses mental structures as good, limited, poor, or disintegrated levels across four dimensions, including control, identity, interpersonality, and attachment. Finally, Axis IV, The Prerequisites for Treatment Axis, is mostly outside of the formulation of the client and focuses on treatment planning.

Power Threat Meaning Framework

Another diagnostic system is the *Power Threat Meaning Framework* (PTMF; Johnstone & Boyle, 2018), which conceptualizes psychopathology as a response to adverse environmental stressors. The PTMF was developed by the Division of Clinical Psychology (DCP) of the British Psychological Society and aims to understand the etiology of emotional distress and maladaptive behavior through a holistic framework (Gallagher et al., 2024). The PTMF pushes back on what the developers consider to be biological reductionism in traditional diagnostic systems and psychopathology research more broadly, which arguably overemphasize biological mechanisms/explanations of psychopathology. In contrast, the PTMF conceptualizes psychopathology in terms of (1) the operation of power, which may be within the body, legal, economic, ideological, social/cultural, or interpersonal systems, (2) the threat, often experienced as emotional distress, that an individual faces in response to this operation of power, (3) the meaning drawn from this power, threat, and response within the social/cultural contexts that is mediated by biological responses, and (4) the response of the individual, family, or cultural group to the operation of power to ensure adaptive functioning in a variety of contexts.

Research Domain Criteria

Although not meant for use in clinical practice, the National Institute of Mental Health developed the Research Domain Criteria (RDoC; Insel et al., 2010) in an effort to accelerate research into the etiology of psychopathology, noting significant problems with the DSM in research contexts, such as excessive comorbidity, problems with heterogeneity, and arbitrary boundaries between disorder and non-disorder. RDoC divides psychopathology processes into six domains, including arousal/regulatory, positive valence, negative valence, social processes, sensorimotor, and cognitive domains, and encourages researchers to measure these domains across different units of analyses, including genes, molecules, cells, circuits, physiology, behavior, self-report, and paradigms. RDoC is fully dimensional, but unlike these other dimensional systems, RDoC was not developed for use in clinical practice, and questions about clinical utility are therefore not relevant currently. Thus, RDoC is not covered in detail in the current chapter (see Sanislow et al., this volume).

Clinical Staging

Clinical staging takes a developmental and transdiagnostic approach to assessment and treatment, acknowledging that disorders develop over time, especially in youth, and fluctuate in terms of illness severity (McGorry et al., 2006; Mei et al., this volume). Arguably, clinical staging has the most promise in youth mental health, where individuals are still developing mental illness, as opposed to in adult mental health, where symptoms may change and fluctuate over time but generally present as fully formed disorders as outlined in the DSM/ICD (Nelson et al., 2021). Clinical staging models conceptualize illness progression as unidirectional as patients progress from less to more severe stages. Critically, this does not assume that progression is predetermined, and the clinical staging approach provides a framework for prevention services (Scott et al., 2024). Early stages typically have lower severity levels and low rates of progression to more severe diagnoses, while later stages are associated with higher severity levels and higher probability of progression to even more severe presentations (Scott & Henry, 2017). This approach enables clinicians to tailor treatment to the individual by providing the least invasive treatment appropriate for that stage of the illness. For example, a psychiatrist using a clinical staging model may decide to avoid antipsychotic medication for a prodromal patient, because there is a high probability they will not progress to an acute psychotic episode.

Network Theory

The network approach conceptualizes psychopathology as a dynamic system of interrelated symptoms that influence one another, emphasizing within-person processes and transitions between healthy and disordered states (Borsboom, 2017). Network models focus on how symptoms coalesce to form mental disorders, or systems (Robinaugh et al., 2020). The network perspective of transitions between healthy and disordered states can be illustrated by shifts in ecological systems. For example, lakes may exist in either clean or marshy states. The condition of the lakes depends on the presence of contaminants and may shift abruptly for some but more gradually for others, and the proposed dynamic relations between symptoms and systems is inconsistent with a purely dimensional approach (Borsboom, 2017).

This network approach has gained traction due to advances in statistical modeling, enabling the visualization of relations among symptoms at both the individual and group levels. It offers a novel perspective for understanding comorbidity, proposing that causal interactions among symptoms, rather than diagnostic categories, drive observed overlaps across disorders. While network theorists have not proposed a DSM replacement, they advocate for idiographic analyses and data-driven clustering of psychopathological processes (Beltz et al., 2016).

Notably, the network approach has utilized advanced statistical models to forecast transitions between states (Eaton et al., 2023). Preliminary evidence for these forecasting models shows promise in predicting a transition to disorder (Olthof et al., 2020; Wichers et al., 2020), though their utility in predicting prognosis for individual patients remains unclear (Helmich et al., 2024). Formal network theories aim to organize observed indicators into theory-based systems (e.g., components of major depression and the network relations across these components). These systems are entirely contingent on mathematical models that specify the network of relations across symptoms (Borsboom et al., 2017). Network metrics, such as node centrality (i.e., prominence of a given node within a network) and density (i.e., the connectedness among all nodes within a network), are then used to identify systems of psychopathology (Bringmann et al., 2019).

Despite its potential, the network approach faces challenges (Rodebaugh et al., this volume). The cross-sectional studies that support its utility are limited in causal inference, and longitudinal designs are necessary to better understand symptom dynamics (Fried, 2020). It is also currently unclear whether assumptions inherent in network statistical models may impact the interpretability of the output (Forbes et al., 2021), because non-linear phenomena central to network theory (e.g., feedback loops, phase transitions) may not align with linear assumptions in common models (Haslbeck et al., 2021). Over-interpretation of network graphs and reliance on small sample sizes further complicate conclusions (Epskamp et al., 2018). While the network approach offers invaluable insights into the interconnected dynamics of psychopathology, it falls short in providing a comprehensive framework for quantifying variations across individuals and populations. Comparatively, dimensional approaches offer robust, transdiagnostic models that systematically capture the continuum of psychopathology.

How Dimensional Systems Can Be Used in Practice

One of the most formidable barriers to clinicians switching from categorical to dimensional nosologies is a perceived lack of knowledge in how to use dimensional systems in practice (Gunderson, 2010). Most practicing clinicians were trained almost exclusively to use categorical systems, and although they report problems with these systems, they also report that the systems have clinical utility for most of the clinical tasks they engage in daily (First, 2010). At the present time, it is unclear how common the alternatives to the ICD and DSM are in actual clinical practice. A recent study asked 703 psychologists (mostly clinical and counseling) in the United States about their familiarity with, and support for, various alternatives to the DSM. Raskin and colleagues (2022) found that psychologists were familiar with the ICD (90%), but not with the other diagnostic systems, including the PDM (26%), RDoC (17%), HiTOP (6%), OPD (4%), and PTMF (1%). Although these dimensional nosologies are rarely explicitly used in practice, there are a number of assessment instruments that conceptualize psychopathology dimensionally that are used in practice. The next sections review some of the more commonly used instruments.

Pre-existing Dimensional Assessments

In the current chapter, we make a distinction between the "nosologies" reviewed in the previous section and "assessment instruments" reviewed in this section. If the assessment instruments (e.g., the ASEBA, PAI, MMPI) were viewed as diagnostic systems, then they would be defined by their operationalization with a single measure, whereas the nosologies are not dependent on a single measure. As a result, most of the "clinical utility" research on assessment instruments may be better categorized as "construct validity" research, in that it focuses on the psychometric properties of the scales rather than the effectiveness of the scale in improving treatment outcomes. Although clearly important, construct validity research is not the focus of the current chapter. At the same time, we acknowledge this may be an artificial distinction. These assessment systems may have more similarities to diagnostic systems than differences, and clinical utility research on diagnostic systems is also sparse (as described in the next section).

At first glance, changing from a categorical system to a dimensional system may feel like a dramatic shift in clinical practice. However, many clinicians, even those who are happy with the DSM, already use dimensional approaches to psychopathology as a matter of routine practice. For example, a relatively recent study showed that nearly 80% of psychologists recruited through the American Psychological Association Practice Organization reported using the Minnesota Multiphasic Personality Inventory (MMPI; Butcher et al., 2001), a dimensional measure, regularly in their work, and many more use other dimensional measures, such as the Personality Assessment Inventory (PAI; Morey, 1991; Wright et al., 2017). Clinicians who use these assessments are already familiar with how to collect and use dimensional information for a variety of clinical tasks, ranging from assigning a (categorical) diagnosis to treatment planning to billing for services. Thus, switching from a categorical nosology to a dimensional one may be more akin to formalizing their existing practices than a dramatic reconceptualization of their approach to treatment. At the same time, 20% of the potential participants in Wright et al. (2017) were screened out because they reported they were not conducting any formal assessments with their patients. Psychologists who do not do formal assessments or exclusively use categorical assessments with their patients may find it especially difficult to switch to dimensional systems that are based on thorough, dimensional assessments.

In the current section, we discuss three prominent assessment instruments, including the Achenbach System of Empirically Based Assessment (ASEBA; Achenbach & Rescorla, 2001, 2003), the PAI, and MMPI. Many other dimensional assessment instruments are not included due to space limitations (see Table 21.1 for a non-exhaustive list of dimensional assessment measures). First, the ASEBA represents a culmination of over 50 years of a research program led by Thomas Achenbach (Achenbach & Rescorla, 2001, 2003). This system includes the Child Behavior Checklist for children ages 1½ to 5 (CBCL 1 ½–5), Youth Self-report (YSR), the

CBCL for children ages 6–18 (CBCL/6-18), the Adult Self-Report (ASR) and Adult Behavior Checklist (ABCL) for adults 18–59, and the Older Adult Self-Report (OASR) and Older Adult Behavioral Checklist (OABCL). These instruments are for self- and informant-report, respectively. From its original development, the scales that would eventually comprise the ASEBA provided insights into the nature and structure of psychopathology, finding two or three dimensions, including internalizing, externalizing, and a factor later termed, thought disorder (Achenbach, 2013). The ASEBA has extensive support for the reliability and validity of its scale scores (for reviews, see Achenbach [2020] and Copeland, this volume). The original scoring of the ASEBA is based on these dimension/syndromes, and additional scales have been developed to mirror the DSM symptoms and categories (Achenbach, 2013). Clinicians using the ASEBA with their patients are already using a dimensional classification system, even if they ultimately translate these dimensional scores into ICD diagnoses to meet administrative requirements.

The PAI (Morey, 1991) is the second-most-used multiscale measure in the United States (behind the MMPI, discussed in this section) and assesses personality, broadly defined, through a dimensional approach (Piotrowski, 2017). It has extensive support for the reliability and validity of its scores in a variety of contexts (Slavin-Mulford et al., 2012). The measure includes 22 clinical scales (e.g., Depression, Borderline Features, Antisocial) and 31 subscales, with test items intending to capture a full range of personality functioning. Morey (1991) developed the PAI to be used in identifying clinically relevant constellations of symptoms (e.g., Social Detachment from the Schizophrenia scale, Cognitive Anxiety from the Anxiety scale) by comparing individual scores against normative data. Busch and colleagues (2017) reported evidence of convergent and discriminant validity of the clinical PAI scales with respect to scores on the PID-5 (Krueger et al., 2012) and the General Personality Pathology Scale (GPP; Morey et al., 2011) scale, providing evidence for the convergent validity of both dimensional measures. Notably, although some PAI items cross-loaded onto multiple factors, Busch and colleagues (2017) indicated that a five-factor model of the PAI converged well with the *AMPD*, particularly at a global level. Psychometric studies supporting the PAI present promising evidence that dimensional approaches to clinical assessment can be embraced by clinicians, particularly when considering the PAI's surge in popularity in a range of clinical settings (e.g., clinical, neuropsychology, forensic psychology; Piotrowski, 2017).

A third commonly used dimensional assessment is the MMPI-3 (Ben-Porath & Tellegen, 2020). The MMPI was originally developed in the 1930s and 1940s, the MMPI-2 was developed in the 1980s, and the MMPI-3 was published in 2020. The current version of the MMPI includes 335 items comprising three higher-order scales (Emotional/Internalizing Dysfunction, Thought Dysfunction, and Behavioral/Externalizing Dysfunction), nine Restructured Clinical Scales (e.g., Low Positive Emotions, Dysfunctional Negative Emotions, Antisocial Behavior), and 25 Specific Problems Scales across four domains, including Somatic/Cognitive Scales (e.g., Somatic Complaints, Cognitive Complaints), Internalizing Scales (e.g., Helplessness/Hopelessness, Self-Doubt), Externalizing Scales (e.g., Substance Abuse, Aggression), and Interpersonal Scales (e.g., Social Avoidance, Self-Importance). It also includes Personality Psychopathology Five (PSY-5) Scales (i.e., Aggressiveness, Psychoticism, Disconstraint, Negative Emotionality/Neuroticism, and Introversion/Low Positive Emotionality) and 10 validity scales (e.g., Adjustment Validity, Infrequent Responses). Like the ASEBA and PAI, the MMPI has considerable support for the reliability and validity of its scores across a variety of populations and settings (see Sellbom, 2019, for a review). For example, prior work has shown that MMPI scores accurately predict behavioral outcomes, including therapist ratings of therapeutic progress, treatment outcomes (Tylicki et al., 2019), and treatment engagement (Arbisi et al., 2023).

In addition to the ASEBA, PAI, and MMPI, several dimensional assessments are available for personality disorder sections of the DSM and ICD (Weekers, Hutsebaut, De Saeger et al., 2024). The most common measure of Criterion A in the AMPD is the Level of Personality Functioning Scale (LPFS-SR; Morey, 2017), which examines personality disorder presence/severity and provides impairment scores for the four Criterion A subdomains. Regarding Criterion B, the most widely used instrument is the Personality Inventory for the DSM-5 (PID-5; Krueger et al., 2012), which assesses the five domains and 25 personality facets of the maladaptive personality traits within the AMPD and has been shown to have stable psychometrics across a variety of cultures and contexts (Barchi-Ferreira et al., 2019). Like the AMPD, there are several measures available to assess dimensional ICD personality disorder constructs. These measures include the ICD-11 Personality Disorder Severity Scale (PDS-ICD-11; Bach et al., 2020), the Personality Inventory for the ICD-11 (Oltmanns & Widiger, 2018), and the Five-Factor Personality Inventory for the ICD-11 (Oltmanns & Widiger, 2020).

Using Dimensional Models in Clinical Practice: The Hierarchical Taxonomy of Psychopathology

In the previous sections, we defined traditional and alternative diagnostic systems and the dimensional assessment instruments that may be used to operationalize them as appropriate. The next step is to illustrate how these systems can be used in clinical practice. Rather than explicating this for every system reviewed, the next section uses one of these approaches, HiTOP, as an example of how to use a dimensional system in practice. We chose HiTOP because, of all the systems reviewed, it is the one with which the authors are most familiar.

Clinical activities from a HiTOP perspective begin with a thorough assessment of psychopathology. HiTOP's Clinical Translation Workgroup and Measure Development Workgroup have developed several tools to assist clinicians who are interested in using HiTOP in clinical practice. It is important to note that the HiTOP model is independent of any specific scale used to assess it. As can be seen in Table 21.1, there are already many measures in the public domain that assess small or large parts of the model. Clinicians wishing to use HiTOP in their practice can use any of these measures as part of an assessment battery.

In addition to the list of HiTOP-consistent measures, the Clinical Translation Workgroup has compiled the HiTOP-Digital Assessment Tracker (HiTOP-DAT; Jonas et al., 2022) as a self-report measure of the HiTOP model. The HiTOP-DAT includes open-access dimensional measures that assess parts of the model. It is composed of several measures, including (1) the Comprehensive Assessment of Traits relevant to Personality Disorder (CAT-PD; Simms et al., 2011), which measures maladaptive personality traits across all six HiTOP spectra; (2) the Inventory for Depression and Anxiety Symptoms-II (Watson et al., 2012); (3) the Community Assessment of Psychic Experiences (CAPE; Stefanis et al., 2002); (4) the Alcohol Use Disorder Identification Test (AUDIT; Babor et al., 1992); (5) Drug Use Disorder Identification Test (DUDIT; Berman et al., 2005); (6) the Personal Health Questionnaire Physical Symptoms (PHQ-15; Kroenke et al., 2002); and (7) the World Health Organization Disability Assessment Schedule (WHODAS 2.0; Ustun et al., 2010), which measures disability across six domains: cognition, mobility, self-care, getting along (i.e., interacting with other people), life activities, and participation in community activities.

The manual for the HiTOP-DAT is available at https://www.hitop-system.org/hitop-digital-assessment-and-tracker-hitop-dat, and Qualtrics and RedCap (two online survey administration platforms) versions of the inventory are available and free to use. The battery includes 405 items and takes 40–60 minutes to complete. Patients may complete the HiTOP-DAT at home or in the waiting room prior to their first session, and their clinician can be emailed the patient's (tabular and/or graphical) profile. Critically, all the measures chosen for the HiTOP-DAT have strong normative data, allowing for the calculation of *T*-scores for use in clinical decision making. If a patient is elevated on self-harm or suicidal ideation (i.e., a *T* score of 65 or higher), it is possible for the patient to be sent an email with information about local emergency services, and for the clinician to be sent an email alerting them to the patient's scores.

In addition to the HiTOP-DAT, the Measure Development Workgroup recently made an experimental version of the HiTOP Self-Report (HiTOP-SR) available for use in research and clinical work. Development of the scale began in 2017 under rigorous principles of construct-valid scale development (Clark & Watson, 1995, 2019; Loevinger, 1957) and involved classic and more modern quantitative methods (e.g., internal consistency, factor analysis, item response theory). First, the work groups operationally defined key constructs and developed over-inclusive item pools to represent them (Simms et al., 2022). Teams within the Measure Development Workgroup then used factor analytic methods to refine the items until each scale had 8–10 items. Next, a smaller analytic group finalized scale construction by addressing redundancies across domains in the joint structure of all preliminary scales and specifying broad scales to assess for each HiTOP spectrum. The HiTOP-SR represents an improvement over the HiTOP-DAT, because the HiTOP-SR is more comprehensive and is specifically keyed to the HiTOP model, as opposed to being a collection of pre-existing scales.

The HiTOP-SR is now freely accessible for researchers at https://www.hitop-system.org/measurement-of-the-hierarchical-taxonomy-of-psychopathology-hitop. The HiTOP-SR is still a work in progress, with additional analyses and potential modifications planned. The current version comprises 405 items that assess 87 unique dimensions of psychopathology across 76 primary scales and 17 nested subscales. The default reporting timeframe is the previous 12 months, but instructions are flexible so that clinicians/researchers can modify the timeframe (e.g., lifetime, last two years) for specific usages. Several additional analyses are planned, including (1) developing clinical interview and informant forms, (2) adapting and translating the measure for use internationally, (3) establishing norms to be used for scoring in a variety of populations, (4) creating shorter versions of the battery and modularized approaches for use in various clinical and research contexts, (5) embedding validity scales, (6) instituting an impairment scale, and (7) developing a version for children and adolescents.

One of the primary concerns about using HiTOP in clinical practice is that ICD codes, which are harmonized with DSM diagnoses, are required for administrative requirements, such as billing in the United States. The Clinical Translation Workgroup developed a crosswalk between elevations on HiTOP domains and ICD-10 codes. The crosswalk, and other clinical tools, is available at https://www.hitop-system.org/clinical-tools. In short, clinicians are encouraged to use "unspecified" codes for elevations on broad spectra (e.g., F39 unspecified mood [affective] disorder for patients with elevations on the internalizing spectrum broadly), subfactors (e.g., F41.9 anxiety disorder, unspecified for elevations on the fear subfactor within internalizing), and component/traits (e.g., F32.9 major depressive disorder, single episode, unspecified, for elevations on the narrow dysphoria symptom).

There are several features of HiTOP that are important to consider when using it in clinical practice. First, because HiTOP is dimensional, patients are not diagnosed with categorical disorders. Instead, patients are diagnosed with a profile of scores, as shown in Figure 21.2. HiTOP recommends using *T*-scores to identify mild (60–64), moderate (65–69), and severe (70+) elevations, although these suggested cutoff scores are not yet empirically validated (Jonas et al., 2022; Ruggero et al., 2019). Second, the hierarchical nature of the HiTOP model allows for treatment to target higher or lower levels of the hierarchy. A HiTOP assessment often begins with a broad screening of the six spectra: internalizing, antagonistic externalizing, disinhibited externalizing, thought disorder, detachment, and somatoform. However, there are times when a referral question may be narrower, and a clinician may choose to only screen for certain spectra. The clinician may then probe the next level of the hierarchy (i.e., subfactors) for spectra on which the patient has significant elevations. For example, a clinician working with a patient with elevations on the internalizing spectrum may use the Unified Protocol for Emotional Disorders (Barlow et al., 2017) to target the broad spectrum but use specific targeted adjunctive treatments for lower levels of the hierarchy (e.g., CBT for Insomnia for elevated insomnia on the symptom level of the hierarchy). Third, impairment is rated separately from symptoms, allowing clinicians to distinguish global impairment from symptom severity. This can be especially useful when a patient is dealing with multiple different elevations across spectra.

Figure 21.2 shows a sample HiTOP profile based on the HiTOP-DAT for a hypothetical patient who would meet DSM/ICD criteria for a schizophrenia spectrum disorder. We chose the constellation of symptoms comprising schizophrenia to illustrate how HiTOP-informed assessment works, because schizophrenia is a heterogeneous disorder that tends to involve elevations across multiple HiTOP spectra. As shown in Figure 21.2, this patient has elevations on four of the six spectra, including the spectra associated with positive symptoms (thought disorder) and negative symptoms (detachment), but also internalizing and disinhibited externalizing. This constellation of symptoms is common in people who could be described by the DSM/ICD's schizoaffective disorder, representing a combination of positive, negative, and affective symptoms. Noting the elevations in these four spectra, the clinician may choose to look at the next lowest level in the hierarchy. In the thought disorder spectrum, the patient has a severe elevation on positive symptoms (i.e., a *T*-score greater than 70) and moderate elevations on peculiarity, unusual experiences, and unusual beliefs. In terms of treatment planning, the clinician may consider medication management to target the thought disorder spectrum broadly and cognitive behavioral therapy for psychosis to target positive symptoms specifically (pCBT; Kingdon & Turkington, 2022; Morrison, 2017). Moving on to the detachment spectrum, the patient has severe elevations on anhedonia and social withdrawal, moderate elevations on romantic disinterest and depressiveness, and a mild elevation on mistrust. Similar to addressing the thought disorder spectrum, the clinician may use behavioral activation to target the lack of motivation and energy characteristic of the detachment spectrum broadly and social skills training (SST; Bellack et al., 2013) to more specifically target symptoms lower in the hierarchy, such as social withdrawal.

In addition to elevations on thought disorder and detachment, the patient has several significant elevations on the internalizing spectrum, such as severe elevations on lassitude (low energy), insomnia (trouble falling asleep, staying asleep, or getting high-quality sleep), cognitive problems (memory problems, disorientation, or confusion), and emotional detachment (being emotionally reserved or blunted experience and expression of emotions). Within HiTOP, disorganized symptoms of the psychosis spectrum are captured in the thought disorder spectrum. However, the HiTOP-SR development project has shown that there is significant overlap between disorganized thought/speech and cognitive problems (Cicero et al., 2022). Thus, this patient's elevation in the cognitive problems domain may be related to disorganization. The patient has a number of mild elevations as well on general depression (i.e., broad depressive symptoms, including low mood, hopelessness, pessimism about the future, pervasive guilt/shame, low self-worth, suicidal ideation), dysphoria (i.e., a narrower construct compared to general depression, with indicators including low mood, pessimism about the future, and tearfulness), and social anxiety (i.e., fear and avoidance related to social interactions).

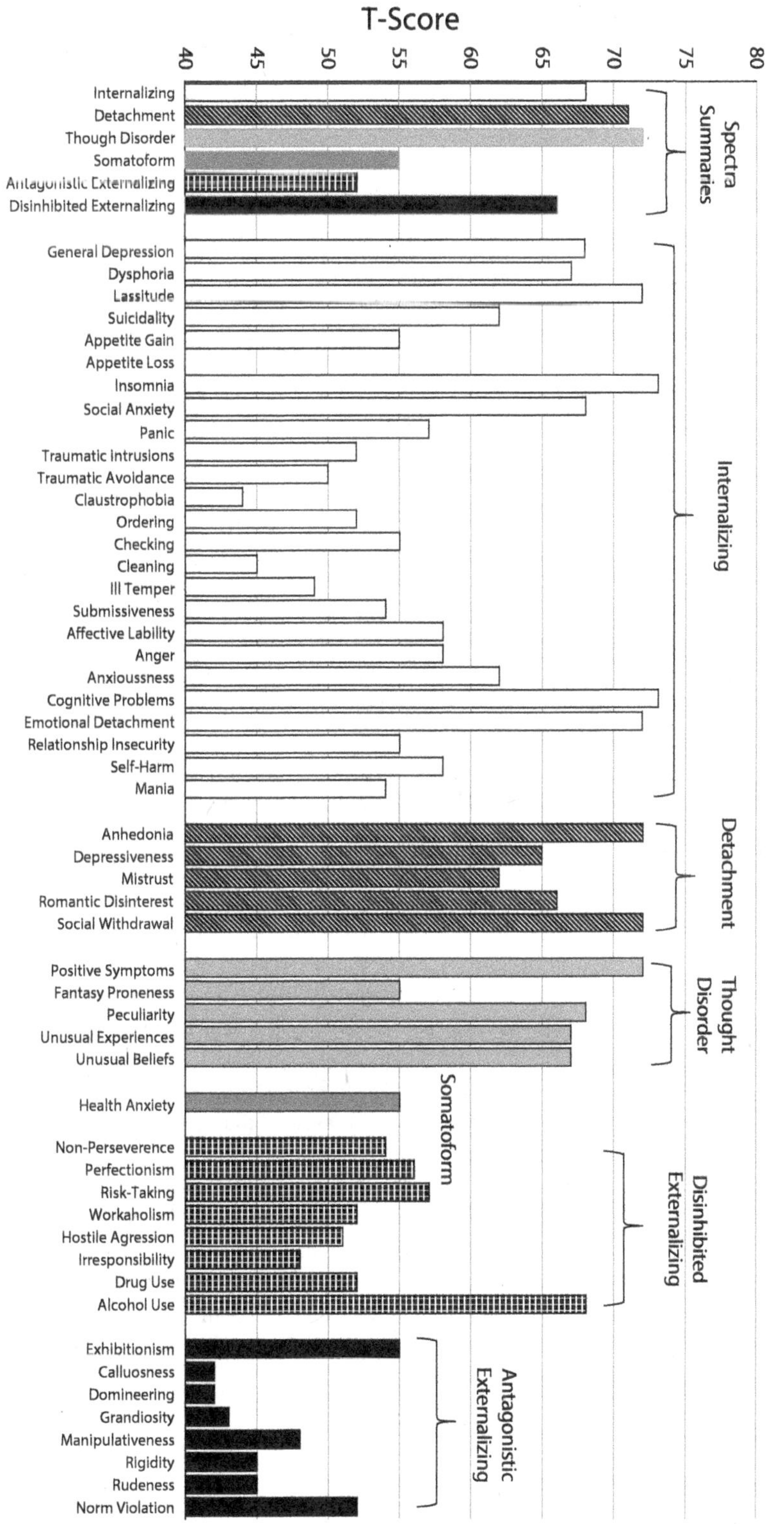

FIGURE 21.2 HiTOP T-Score Profiles

The clinician consults the HiTOP to ICD crosswalk and sees that there are several codes consistent with the patient's profile. The highest spectrum elevation is on thought disorder, so the clinician uses "F29 unspecified psychosis not due to a substance or known physiological condition" as the ICD code for administrative requirements. To target the internalizing spectrum, the clinician may again consider medication management in addition to broad treatments on the spectrum level, such as the Unified Protocol (Barlow et al., 2017). The patient's elevations on social anxiety and emotional detachment may benefit from the social skills training already in the treatment plan to address social withdrawal. Finally, the patient had elevations on the disinhibited externalizing spectrum. A closer look at the subscales suggests that this is primarily driven by a moderate elevation on alcohol use. Thus, the clinician may consider a dual diagnosis program to treat harmful substance use (Dixon, 1999).

Clinical Utility of Dimensional Nosologies

Defining Clinical Utility

We now review research examining the clinical utility of dimensional systems. As defined by the American Psychiatric Association, the clinical utility of a diagnostic system broadly refers to the usefulness of the system to complete a variety of clinical tasks, such as assigning diagnoses, planning treatment, communicating with patients and other mental health professionals, and predicting and monitoring treatment outcomes (First et al., 2004). The WHO has a similar definition of clinical utility, suggesting that its three primary aspects are its (1) utility in communication, (2) the ease of its use in practice, and (3) its value in planning treatment (Reed, 2010). Both the WHO and American Psychiatric Association have repeatedly stated that the primary goal in any new revision is to maintain or improve clinical utility, as the primary purpose of both manuals is to aid in clinical practice (American Psychiatric Association, 2000; Clark et al., 1995; First, 2005; Widiger et al., 1991).

When defining clinical utility, it is also important to define its boundaries. Mullins-Sweatt and colleagues (2016) have argued that some concepts commonly considered to be a part of clinical utility actually represent construct validity, a related but not completely overlapping concept. Within the context of diagnostic systems, construct validity refers to how well the operationalization of psychiatric disorders corresponds to latent psychopathology constructs (McGorry, 2019). Construct validity may be established by examining the observed relations among diagnoses and other variables in their nomological network (Cronbach & Meehl, 1955). The conclusion that a diagnostic system has adequate construct validity does not imply that the system also has clinical utility. For example, a system may perfectly predict prognosis in all cases but lack clinical utility if it is too complicated to be used in clinical practice or not useful when communicating with patients or other mental health professionals. Thus, Mullins-Sweatt and Widiger (2009) have noted that construct validity is a necessary but not sufficient prerequisite for establishing clinical utility and suggested a narrower definition of clinical utility more consistent with the WHO's definition that includes (1) communication, (2) ease of usage, and (3) treatment planning. This proposed definition suggests that the first step in establishing clinical utility is to examine the attitudes of clinicians, administrators, and patients themselves (Samuel & Widiger, 2006).

Communicative Value

For a system to be widely used in practice, clinicians must be able to readily apply it to communicate with other providers as well as with patients and their families (Ruggero et al., 2019).

As can be seen in Table 21.2, several studies have compared dimensional and categorical systems' clinical utility with respect to communicative value. Overall, results are mixed, with some study samples favoring dimensional systems (Bornstein & Natoli, 2019; Brown et al., 2023; Lowe & Widiger, 2009; Tracy et al., 2021a), others favoring categorical systems (Morey et al., 2014; Spitzer et al., 2008), and still others finding little evidence for a difference between systems (Cano & Sharp, 2023; Hansen et al., 2019; Milinkovic & Tiliopoulos, 2020; Samuel & Widiger, 2006; Weekers, Hutsebaut, Rovers et al., 2024).

Although it is difficult to draw firm conclusions based on studies with mixed conclusions, overall, there is some evidence that clinicians view dimensional models as at least as useful as categorical systems for communication, particularly with respect to communication with patients (Balling et al., 2023; Lowe & Widiger, 2009; Tracy et al., 2021a). Specifically, a meta-analysis comparing the utility of categorical and dimensional frameworks across 11 studies found support for using dimensional systems to describe personality pathology in a coherent and comprehensive way without losing important information or applying unclear diagnostic labels (Bornstein & Natoli, 2019). In a systematic review of 20 clinical utility studies, all eight studies that compared the communicative value of DSM-5's Section II with the AMPD found support for the AMPD in delivering helpful patient feedback (Milinkovic & Tiliopoulos, 2020). Furthermore, practicing psychologists and psychiatrists in Aotearoa/New Zealand rated the ICD-11 personality disorders section higher than the DSM Section II PDs due to its ability to better represent the complexity of personality pathology, which facilitates communication among providers through more informative descriptors (Brown et al., 2023). In a study investigating undergraduates' perceptions in the United States, Cano and Sharp (2023) found that participants rated DSM-5's Section II and AMPD as similarly useful in communicating with other non-professionals, but both were rated higher than the dimensional ICD-11 PDs.

Studies investigating the utility of dimensional systems in facilitating provider communication with patients' families are notably lacking (Milinkovic & Tiliopoulos, 2020), which may be important due to cultural differences in the level of family involvement in the recovery process. Many cultures hold stigmas toward psychopathology, which is particularly prominent among cultures with limited familiarity with mental health topics (Kirmayer & Ryder, 2016). Even for individuals with less understanding of psychopathology who are receptive to mental health diagnoses, traditional labels convey minimal information. For example, they do not convey which specific symptoms an individual is experiencing or information about the severity of symptoms or impairment. Moreover, individuals sharing a categorical diagnostic label may be assumed to be homogeneous as a group and distinct from others. This may carry substantial risks of prejudice and discrimination and promote stereotypes leading to public or self-stigmatization (Ben-Zeev et al., 2010; Lahey, 2021). Additionally, classification systems relying on unclear diagnostic labels may lead to patient/family retreat from appropriate interventions or the healthcare system altogether. The level of family involvement in medical and psychiatric decision-making highly varies by cultural background. Strong (and clear) communication between providers and family is imperative for individuals from cultural backgrounds in which families are more involved in patient care and experiences (Santisteban et al., 2002).

Diagnostic systems also play a key role in facilitating communication among providers, particularly in integrated healthcare systems and community health centers treating patients with acute presentations. Mental health professionals within these settings generally work within fast-paced environments alongside a multidisciplinary team (Bruffaerts et al., 2008). The level of urgency providers work with in these environments often demands efficient case formulation and cross-disciplinary consultation with minimal margin of error for miscommunication (Reinfeld et al., 2023). Even minor miscommunications may lead to prescription errors, misinformed risk assessment, decisional errors for psychiatric hospitalization, in addition to an increased burden of illness on the patient and the healthcare system. Extant studies have found that categorical systems are viewed more favorably when considering communication among mental health professionals, likely because all mental health professionals are already familiar with categorical labels. Although the ICD and DSM currently dominate these environments, the traditional diagnostic labels provide limited information about individual functioning. This may be particularly concerning due to the variable, often limited, familiarity with traditional diagnostic labels across provider disciplines and roles (e.g., social workers, psychiatry, nurses). A shift in focus toward a dimensional/symptoms-focused approach could potentially address needs for these settings.

Ease of Use

In clinical utility research, ease of use generally refers to a diagnostic system's perceived feasibility for integration into everyday practice when making clinical management decisions, such as whether to provide therapy and which treatment elements to use (Mullins-Sweatt et al., 2016). Practitioners often resist models that are cumbersome or difficult to implement in practice and choose systems that are easy to use and facilitate efficient diagnostic decision-making under the time constraints inherent in clinical settings. As shown in Table 21.2, most studies examining the ease of use of dimensional and categorical systems have found evidence that clinicians prefer dimensional systems (Balling et al., 2023; Brown et al., 2023; Hansen et al., 2019; Milinkovic & Tiliopoulos, 2020; Samuel & Widiger, 2006; Tracy et al., 2021a). As concerns with categorical systems and interest in dimensional systems grew over the past several decades, licensed practitioners are reporting increasingly positive ratings of dimensional models (e.g., AMPD, ICD-11, HiTOP) in ease of use compared to traditional models (Balling et al., 2023). For example, a diverse sample of mental health practitioners (i.e., psychologists, nurses, and medical doctors) rated the ICD-11 PD model easier to use, regardless of the clinician's years in practice (Hansen et al., 2019). In a review of eight clinical utility studies, the ICD-11 PD was rated highly because it required less time for application compared to the ICD-10 (Tracy et al., 2021).

In contrast to results favoring dimensional systems, three studies have either favored categorical systems or found non-significant differences. One study with a sample of 337 psychologists and psychiatrists reported a preference for the DSM-IV-TR personality disorder diagnoses over the AMPD (Morey et al., 2014), and another with a similar sample (N = 397) found that a prototype approach based on the DSM was easier to use than dimensional models or the traditional use of the DSM (Spitzer et al., 2008). A third study with a sample of 1,572 practicing psychologists found that, although clinicians rated dimensional models of personality functioning higher in ease of use than the DSM-IV, the differences did not reach conventional levels of statistical significance (Lowe & Widiger, 2009). It is important to note that the three studies favoring categorical approaches or finding no differences were published 10 or more years ago. Attitudes may have changed within the last 10 years, as more favorable attitudes toward dimensional systems are evident in recent research (e.g., Milinkovic & Tiliopoulos, 2020).

In addition to research concerning the ease of use of AMPD in clinicians, several studies have shown that the LPFS scales can be understood and potentially administered by laypersons. Zimmerman and colleagues (2014) asked undergraduates to view and rate videos of patient interviews conducted by psychodynamic clinicians. Undergraduates were able to use the system, showing adequate internal consistency, strong correlations with expert ratings, and elevated scores in patients with versus those without PDs. Similar results have been found with master's-level students using previously recorded diagnostic interviews (Preti et al., 2018). In other studies, undergraduates produced reliable scores on the LPFS across domains when reporting on acquaintances (Morey, 2018), using life story narratives (Roche et al., 2018) and vignettes (Garcia et al., 2018). Taken together, these results suggest that the AMPD can be easily understood by laypeople, which suggests that clinicians will also be able to easily use it in practicc.

There is very little research on clinician, patient, or family attitudes toward any of the other systems reviewed in the current chapter. Two studies have examined clinician attitudes about the "helpfulness" of the PDM in understanding clients. In the first study, 61 assessment "experts" were asked how helpful the PDM and DSM were in understanding patients. The plurality (44%) of clinicians identified as psychodynamic therapists, but more than half reported other orientations. Clinicians in this sample were more likely to report that the PDM Axes (50–79%) were helpful or very helpful than was the DSM diagnostic information (31%) in understanding clients (Gordon & Stoffey, 2014). In a second sample ($N = 510$) of clinicians attending PDM continuing education workshops, Gordon and Bornstein (2018) replicated these findings, showing that PDM Axes (41–75%) were viewed as more helpful than DSM/ICD symptom diagnoses (31%). Although all participants were attendees at PDM workshops, the plurality of clinicians (33%) reported CBT as their primary theoretical orientation, suggesting the PDM may be viewed as useful to psychotherapists from a variety of orientations.

Like psychodynamic manuals, there has been very little research on the clinical utility of the *PTMF* model, and most of this work has not been peer reviewed. Two dissertations have recently examined this topic, finding mixed results. Using Q-Sort methodology, the first identified four attitudes toward the *PTMF*, including that it: (1) "is an important development," (2) "is a possible adjunct to diagnoses," (3) "adds little to practice," and (4) "is a flawed attack on psychiatry" (Whetter, 2023). A second qualitative study found that some psychologists viewed the *PTMF* to be potentially useful in clinical practice while others thought it was inaccessible to both therapists and their patients and was too complicated to be used effectively in practice (Omur, 2023). These studies, coupled with recent findings indicating very few psychologists are aware of the *PTMF* (Raskin et al., 2022), suggest that more research is needed to properly evaluate its applications in practice.

Treatment Planning

The third important aspect of clinical utility is the usefulness of the system in planning treatment. Treatment planning is central to clinical utility, as classification systems exist to identify patient needs and match them to appropriate evidence-based interventions. As shown in Table 21.2, research comparing the utility of dimensional and categorical systems for treatment planning tend to favor dimensional systems (Balling et al., 2023; Bornstein & Natoli, 2019; Brown et al., 2023; Hansen et al., 2019; Lowe & Widiger, 2009; Milinkovic & Tiliopoulos, 2020; Morey et al., 2014;; Tracy et al., 2021a). However, one study found no significant differences (Weekers, Hutsebaut, Rovers et al., 2024), and one study found that undergraduates in the United States viewed both Section II and AMPD in the DSM to be equal, but both better than the fully dimensional ICD-11 personality disorders section (Cano & Sharp, 2023).

In a review of eight prior studies (Tracy et al., 2021), clinicians rated the ICD-11 PD and DSM AMPD, particularly Criterion A, as highly useful in treatment planning due to improved diagnostic accuracy. Ratings of the levels of personality functioning provide clinicians with an index of the severity of impairment, which they perceive as informative in defining clinical prognosis and identifying the intensity of treatment indicated for patients. Clinicians also rated the usefulness of Criterion B highly for directing the focus and style of treatment during case formulation.

In a comparison between classification systems, the hybrid AMPD model was favored over the purely dimensional ICD-11 PD model, which was, in turn, favored over the purely categorical ICD-10 PD model (Morey & Hopwood, 2020) by psychologists and psychiatrists of all ages and genders. Overall, the dimensional ICD-11 PD was rated more useful for clinical practice and for comprehensively describing global personality functioning compared to the categorical ICD-10 PD (Morey et al., 2014; Hansen et al., 2019; Tracy et al., 2021).

Case Illustration

We now return to the practical HiTOP tutorial from earlier in the chapter to explore how the HiTOP approach to clinical practice differs from the DSM method in terms of clinical utility (i.e., communication, ease of use, and treatment planning) for the patient described in Figure 21.2.

Communication

A fundamental goal of any classification system is to convey clear, succinct clinical information that allows multidisciplinary professionals to coordinate care. Within a categorical framework (e.g., DSM), communication among professionals generally relies on diagnostic labels (e.g., schizophrenia, schizoaffective disorder, unspecified psychotic disorder) that are virtually universally recognized. However, these labels can be imprecise, because many patients show a broad mixture of symptoms, and the label alone does not communicate which specific features are predominant (e.g., positive vs negative symptoms, affective disturbances, subtype of delusion, comorbid substance use, distrust). In contrast, HiTOP's dimensional profiles offer a more granular summary of symptom domains and severity. In the earlier vignette, describing a patient as elevated in thought disorder, detachment, internalizing, and disinhibited externalizing allows providers to clearly and efficiently communicate the broad range of the patient's functioning, including possible cognitive disorganization, social withdrawal, and problems with mood and impulse control. In addition to communicating prominent clinical needs, the HiTOP approach helps providers convey information about the clinical presentation that may impact the working alliance.

Dimensional profiles of psychopathology can be more intuitive for many patients. Instead of receiving a diagnostic label that may sound daunting or confusing, dimensional descriptions of psychological functioning provide information within individual contexts (e.g., "You seem to be experiencing difficulties in social settings, you have trouble with negative affect, and you notice unusual beliefs or sensations. All of these can be targets for treatment."). For our sample patient experiencing both psychotic and affective symptoms, describing the range of their elevations across the HiTOP domains can mitigate feelings of being misunderstood or mislabeled and provide reassurance that their experience is fully captured. In this way, HiTOP captures the unique symptom profiles of patients, addresses the relations among clinical domains, and provides a more intuitive segue into psychoeducation.

Communicating with patients' families may also benefit from using the HiTOP system. Families often play a significant role in the recovery process, particularly for child/adolescent, geriatric, or disabled patients. Explaining to the family of our sample patient that their loved one has "schizoaffective disorder" may convey the seriousness of the condition, but it may also foster stigma or misconceptions about prognosis. In contrast, emphasizing the presenting symptom constellation across HiTOP domains (e.g., difficulties with emotional expression, withdrawal from social activities, substance misuse) may enable family members to better understand how certain behaviors or symptoms fit together. They may also find it easier to accept and support targeted interventions for elevated domains (e.g., social skills training for withdrawal or family-based relapse prevention strategies for externalizing behaviors).

Ease of Use

Clinicians working with the DSM/ICD often follow extensive checklists to determine which diagnostic criteria a patient meets, a process that may feel cumbersome, particularly when symptoms overlap multiple categories and the underlying etiology is unclear. Our patient presented with positive and negative psychotic symptoms, affective symptoms, and comorbid substance misuse, which could complicate diagnostic decision-making during a comprehensive assessment. Using the DSM, a clinician may feel compelled to consider and explore multiple concurrent or differential diagnoses, spending time to chase a categorial label that best explains our patient's current functioning. This approach can lead to labels that (1) fail to capture the patient's full range of symptoms, (2) misrepresent their lived experience, and (3) lack severity estimates. Rather than assigning and reconciling a handful of diagnostic labels, HiTOP clinicians identify the relevant spectra and more specific components (e.g., anhedonia, unusual experiences, emotional detachment). This approach may help clinicians save time in case formulation, as it eliminates the demand for ruling out syndromes whose boundaries may be arbitrary.

Although adopting a dimensional system into clinical practice undoubtedly requires initial training, shifting to HiTOP may not be as challenging as anticipated. As previously discussed, several prominent assessment tools used nearly ubiquitously across clinical settings are dimensional in nature. This emphasizes that clinicians and trainees are already familiar with conceptualizing aspects of psychological functioning through a dimensional lens and that learning to use HiTOP in practice and in communication may be as straightforward as learning how to interpret a HiTOP scoring profile. HiTOP's use of normative data and *T*-scores to determine clinically significant elevations is also likely to not require novel training, given that basic statistics are a part of graduate training in most, if not all, mental health–related graduate training programs.

Treatment Planning

A key distinction between categorical and dimensional models is how they guide intervention choices. In the DSM approach, once the schizophrenia or schizoaffective label is assigned, treatment often proceeds via broad disorder-specific guidelines (e.g., anti-psychotic medication, cognitive-behavioral therapy for psychosis). Although empirically supported, such guidelines sometimes obscure the importance of co-occurring domains (e.g., internalizing, externalizing) that may benefit from adjunctive interventions. For our patient, HiTOP explicitly highlights multiple higher-order spectra and lower-level components to target. This allows the clinician to consider multiple evidence-based strategies. For example, they might integrate motivational enhancement interventions (i.e., simultaneously encourage medication adherence, quitting substance use, and engagement in treatment) with CBT for psychosis (i.e., address positive symptoms) to address more urgent needs, followed by behavioral activation and social skills training to address chronic, but less acute, needs (e.g., detachment and negative symptoms).

Tracking patient progression is also simpler with HiTOP. For example, if our patient's substance use improves over time while negative symptoms persist, the clinician may re-evaluate the patient's detachment elevations and decide on next steps (e.g., enhance behavioral activation or social skills training). Such dynamic, dimension-based monitoring can be invaluable, particularly for complex cases that do not fit neatly into diagnostic categories.

Practical Barriers in the Mental Health Community to Using Dimensional Systems

Although a compelling case can be made that dimensional systems have superior construct validity to categorical systems and equal or better clinical utility, many practical barriers to using dimensional systems in clinical practice remain. The Theory of Planned Behavior (TPB) provides a useful framework for understanding the decision-making processes of clinicians considering making a change in their assessments and provision of treatment (Ajzen, 1991). The TPB suggests that a clinician's intention to change behavior, in this case from a categorical to a dimensional system, is based on three factors: (1) attitudes toward dimensional systems, (2) subjective norms, and (3) perceived behavioral control. Clinicians are more likely to actually make a major change to their practice if they believe that (1) a dimensional system will assist in clinical tasks and ultimately lead to better patient outcomes, (2) other clinicians whom they respect already use dimensional systems, and (3) they are capable to actually make the change (e.g., they have the ability/knowledge and autonomy/institutional support to use a dimensional system in practice). The following sections describe the common barriers to clinicians using dimensional systems in clinical practice, including challenges to attitudes, subjective norms, and perceived behavioral control.

Attitudes to Dimensional Systems: Insufficient Evidence for Clinical Utility

Arguably, the most imposing barrier for practicing clinicians transitioning to dimensional diagnostic systems is the lack of clear evidence for the clinical utility of dimensional systems, particularly outside of personality disorders. As discussed above, the evidence for the clinical utility of dimensional systems is mixed but suggests that dimensional systems are at least equivalent to categorical systems, especially with respect to personality disorder assessment and treatment (e.g., Weekers, Hutsebaut, De Saeger et al., 2024; Weekers, Hutsebaut, Rovers et al., 2024). These studies have focused primarily on clinician attitudes, showing that many clinicians believe that dimensional models have superior clinical utility compared to categorical models. However, the ultimate evidence for the superiority of a dimensional system would be a randomized controlled trial showing that clinicians' use of a dimensional nosology leads to better therapeutic outcomes (Kamphuis et al., 2021). Very few studies have compared dimensional and categorical assessment systems using randomized controlled trials (RCTs), and these few studies have found no difference in patient outcomes between assessments (Haeffel et al., 2021). This lack of evidence is consistent with a long line of research that has failed to demonstrate the superiority of virtually any assessment compared to any other assessment in producing better patient outcomes (Kamphuis et al., 2021).

Given the lack of robust evidence for the superiority of dimensional diagnostic systems over categorical systems in leading to better patient outcomes, it is worth asking what strength of evidence would be needed for the modal clinician to undertake the formidable tasks of learning and implementing a new dimensional diagnostic system. Is the opinion that dimensional systems are more accurate enough to convince a clinician to make a major change in practice? Will clinicians require evidence of superior clinical utility, or will equivalent outcomes be sufficient if clinicians see other benefits for dimensional systems (e.g., more comprehensive description of psychopathology)? If they require evidence of superiority, how strong of an effect would be compelling? Would the new system need to result in substantially better outcomes, or would a modest improvement justify the cost associated with learning and implementing a new system? The answers to these questions are currently unclear, and future research will need to address them to provide answers based on empirical findings.

As mentioned, the gold standard method to determine the efficacy of any intervention, whether pharmacological or psychological, is an RCT. When exploring the clinical utility of dimensional models compared to categorical approaches, an RCT would include one group whose psychopathology is assessed via a dimensional system (e.g., HiTOP) and another whose psychopathology is assessed via a traditional categorical approach (e.g., DSM). In an ideal experiment, participants would then be assigned to a specific treatment modality based on the results of the assessment, as opposed to the assessment results being used to identify treatment targets within the same modality or less structured treatment as usual. To our knowledge, no RCTs to date have included all of these components. For example, Weekers, Hutsebaut, De Saeger et al. (2024) conducted an RCT in which 119 patients were randomly assigned to be assessed for Section II PDs with the SCID-5-PD or the AMPD with the SCID AMPD Module II. No differences in terms of clinical utility were found for the clinician or patient subjective judgments of the assessment, treatment motivation, or satisfaction. However, participants were not followed over time to determine whether the method of assessment led to improved treatment outcomes. The current literature surrounding the clinical utility of dimensional systems compared to categorical models, particularly outside of personality pathology, is nascent, and further evidence is necessary to convince mental health workers that using a dimensional approach can *improve* patient outcomes, which is likely necessary to implementing dimensional models in practice.

Subjective Norms

In addition to holding positive attitudes toward dimensional systems, the TPB suggests that clinicians are more likely to switch to dimensional diagnostic systems if they believe that other clinicians whom they respect also hold positive views of dimensional systems and are already using these systems in clinical practice. As described above, clinicians have used dimensional assessment instruments for decades but have to translate the data into categorical ICD/DSM diagnoses to meet administrative requirements, such as billing and insurance reimbursement in the United States (Reed, 2010; Ruggero et al., 2019). The use of dimensional nosologies is still relatively rare, and as a result, clinicians are unlikely to have trusted colleagues who already use them (Raskin et al., 2022). At the same time, there is evidence that clinicians believe dimensional systems are an improvement over categorical systems. Proponents of dimensional systems may focus their efforts on better dissemination of the results of clinical utility studies to influence subjective norms and encourage clinicians to use dimensional systems in practice (Cicero et al., 2024).

Perceived Behavioral Control

A third barrier to clinicians switching to dimensional models is a perceived lack of behavioral control. Perceived behavioral control refers to an individual's confidence in performing the desired behavior (i.e., using a dimensional nosology in practice). Two things that contribute to a lack of perceived behavioral control are (1) perceived lack of knowledge of how to use dimensional systems, and (2) perceived incompatibility between dimensional systems and administrative requirements.

Knowledge of Dimensional Models

Due to the ubiquity of the DSM and ICD in clinical practice, most curricula for mental health–related programs focus on these categorical systems, whereas dimensional systems are relegated to psychopathology courses that are divorced from clinical practicum experiences. As a result, the overwhelming majority of clinicians are not even aware that dimensional nosologies, such as HiTOP, exist (Raskin et al., 2022). Thus, one major barrier to clinicians using dimensional models in clinical practice is a lack of knowledge of these systems.

Despite the evidence that clinicians find dimensional systems easier to use than categorical systems, researchers have suggested that clinicians will find them too complicated to be used in practice (Shedler et al., 2010). For example, the AMPD requires clinicians to assess 25 different traits before determining the appropriate diagnosis. Proponents of dimensional systems have countered that dimensional symptoms often have fewer constructs that need to be assessed than do traditional systems (Widiger & Trull, 2007). Nevertheless, clinicians are unlikely to switch to dimensional models if they believe the models are too complicated to be useful in practice. Additionally, categorical models allow clinicians to assess diagnostic criteria and make a present/absent diagnosis, while dimensional models require clinicians to consider a more complex profile (see Figure 21.2) for which there are fewer clear guidelines for treatment planning.

Similarly, most treatment manuals and psychotherapy outcome research are based on categorical diagnoses. Clinicians working from an empirically supported treatment perspective can make a categorical diagnosis based on the DSM and then consult a list of empirically supported treatments, such as the American Psychological Association's Society of Clinical Psychology list, which is organized by DSM diagnoses. Thus, clinicians have access to a wide range of diagnostic manuals, assessments, and tools for categorical models but relatively few for dimensional diagnostic systems (Hopwood et al., 2020). As mentioned, some evidence suggests that psychologists believe dimensional systems have clinical utility for treatment planning (Bornstein & Natoli, 2019). However, providers can struggle with adapting treatment approaches to align with these models, likely a result of being trained in traditional, diagnosis-based interventions. To help clinicians overcome these barriers, proponents of dimensional models need to develop materials to assist clinicians in making the switch. As mentioned, the HiTOP Clinical Translation Workgroup has developed several tools that aim to help clinicians better understand how to use the model in clinical practice (Cicero et al., 2024; Kotov et al., 2021; Ruggero et al., 2019). Similar tools have been developed for the AMPD as well (e.g., Hopwood, 2018; Krueger et al., 2011; Morey et al., 2011).

Interpreting and integrating data from dimensional assessment tools requires additional training and resources that are difficult to access for the average full-time clinician who is likely already under-resourced and under strict time constraints. However, at the graduate level, research suggests that student clinicians can successfully interpret and apply diagnostic criteria of dimensional models. Garcia and colleagues (2018) found student clinicians have high inter-rater reliability regarding Criterion A of the DSM-5 AMPD and hold positive attitudes toward the AMPD's clinical utility. These findings suggest that incorporating training in dimensional models into graduate curricula will be necessary to disseminate the models for use in clinical practice.

When clinicians have adequate training in the use of dimensional models, they may then be presented with the conundrum of how to communicate their dimensional findings to their patients. Researchers have noted that the overwhelming majority of studies examining the clinical utility of dimensional versus categorical systems have focused on the attitudes of psychologists and psychiatrists rather than on patients and their families (Cano & Sharp, 2023; Milinkovic & Tiliopoulos, 2020). Thus, it is difficult to conclude with confidence whether patients and their families find categorical diagnoses to be easier to understand than dimensional ones. In a study of 154 people with borderline PD and their family members, participants rated categorical descriptions of hypothetical patients as easier to understand than those based on either the AMPD or ICD PD (Cano & Sharp, 2023). However, this was the only index of clinical utility that favored categorical diagnoses, and participants otherwise rated the AMPD and Section II to be equal, and both favorable to the ICD. Other research has found that treatment-seeking undergraduates and MTurk workers find personality feedback based on the PID-5 and a measure of Five-Factor personality traits to be accurate, relevant, and useful (Lengel & Mullins-Sweatt, 2017). Given the dearth of studies on patient preferences, more research is clearly needed to understand whether patients and their families appreciate dimensional approaches to diagnoses.

Institutional and Financial Barriers

Clinicians who (1) hold favorable attitudes toward the clinical utility of dimensional systems in practice, (2) believe other respected colleagues hold similar attitudes and are already using these systems in practice, and (3) are confident in their ability to use dimensional systems in practice still have formidable institutional and financial barriers to switching from categorical to dimensional systems. The DSM/ICD are embedded into nearly all aspects of our mental health–care system. For example, clinicians in the United States who bill for services are required to specify ICD codes, the Federal Drug Administration (FDA) requires pharmaceutical companies to use categorical diagnoses for the RCTs necessary to bring drugs to market, and many clinicians work in broader systems (e.g., hospitals or health maintenance organizations) in which the DSM/ICD are required by administrators. As described in the section "Using Dimensional Models in Clinical Practice," the HiTOP Clinical Translation Workgroup has worked to address the issue of billing by providing a crosswalk between HiTOP elevations and ICD codes (Ruggero et al., 2019).

In addition to complications with billing, clinicians who are not working in private practice are part of broader systems, where they often do not have the autonomy to use a diagnostic system other than the DSM or ICD. Clinicians may strongly believe that dimensional systems are superior for a variety of clinical tasks, but they will not make a change to these systems if prevented from doing so by their supervisors or other administrators. These changes would require the buy-in of many individuals working across different bureaucracies, and it is presently unclear if these changes are likely or even possible.

In summary, clinicians face significant challenges when considering dimensional diagnostic systems. Although these systems offer advantages, such as capturing a broader range of symptoms, their practical implementation encounters profound hurdles. At the graduate level, aspiring clinicians are typically trained with an approach based on the DSM and ICD. A lack of clear evidence for clinical utility and superiority over traditional, categorical models, stemming from an absence of RCTs that explore outcomes based on different assessment systems, can lead clinicians to question the practical benefits of dimensional models. Finally, dimensional nosologies may further complicate the insurance reimbursement process in the United States, which is an administrative burden that many psychologists already choose to avoid due to its time-consuming nature.

Conclusion

There is growing consensus that psychopathology is better understood as a set of dimensional rather than categorical constructs. Several dimensional nosologies are currently available for use, including the ones we focused on in this chapter (e.g., HiTOP, DSM's AMPD) and others that are discussed elsewhere in this volume. Assessment instruments have long been available to measure psychopathology from a dimensional perspective and are already commonly used in clinical practice. Recently, manuals, such as the HiTOP-DAT, have been developed to assist clinicians with using dimensional systems in practice. However, many questions remain about whether dimensional systems can be used as effectively as categorical systems in clinical practice. Research in this area is nascent, and there are no definitive studies that illustrate that dimensional systems lead to superior patient outcomes. Categorical systems remain entrenched in training and health care systems. It is incumbent on the proponents of dimensional systems to develop more tools to aid interested clinicians in switching to dimensional systems. Moreover, more research is needed to better explore the clinical utility of these systems.

References

Achenbach, T. M. (2009). *The Achenbach system of empirically based Assessment (ASEBA): Development, findings, theory, and applications.* University of Vermont Research Center for Children, Youth, and Families.

Achenbach, T. M. (2013). *DSM guide for the ASEBA.* University of Vermont, Research Center for Children, Youth, and Families.

Achenbach, T. M. (2020). Bottom-up and top-down paradigms for psychopathology: A half-century odyssey. *Annual Review of Clinical Psychology, 16*, 1–24. https://doi.org/10.1146/annurev-clinpsy-071119-115831

Achenbach, T. M., & Rescorla, L. A. (2001). *Manual for the ASEBA School-Age Forms and Profiles.* Burlington, VA: University of Vermont Research Center for Children, Youth, and Families.

Achenbach, T. M., & Rescorla, L. A. (2003). *Manual for the ASEBA Adult Forms and Profiles.* Burlington, VT: University of Vermont.

Ajzen, I. (1991). The theory of planned behavior. *Organizational Behavior and Human Decision Processes, 50*(2), 179–211. https://doi.org/10.1016/0749-5978(91)90020-T

American Psychiatric Association (Ed.). (2000). *Diagnostic and statistical manual of mental disorders: DSM-IV-TR* (4th ed., text revision). American Psychiatric Association.

American Psychiatric Association (Ed.). (2022). *Diagnostic and statistical manual of mental disorders: DSM-5-TR* (5th ed., text revision). American Psychiatric Association Publishing.

Arbisi, P. A., Finn, J. A., Polusny, M. A., & Erbes, C. R. (2023). The role of the MMPI-2-Restructured Form (MMPI-2-RF) in predicting and better understanding engagement in posttraumatic stress disorder treatment. *Psychological Services, 20*(3), 453–464. https://doi.org/10.1037/ser0000597

Babor, T. F., de la Fuente, J. R., Saunders, J. B., & Grant, M. (1992). *AUDIT: The Alcohol Use Disorders Identification Test: Guidelines for use in primary health care.* World Health Organization.

Bach, B., Kerber, A., Aluja, A., Bastiaens, T., Keeley, J. W., Claes, L., Fossati, A., Gutierrez, F., Oliveira, S. E. S., Pires, R., Riegel, K. D., Rolland, J.-P., Roskam, I., Sellbom, M., Somma, A., Spanemberg, L., Strus, W., Thimm, J. C., Wright, A. G. C., & Zimmermann, J. (2020). International assessment of DSM-5 and ICD-11 personality disorder traits: Toward a common nosology in DSM-5.1. *Psychopathology, 53*(3–4), 179–188. https://doi.org/10.1159/000507589

Balling, C. E., South, S. C., Lynam, D. R., & Samuel, D. B. (2023). Clinician perception of the clinical utility of the Hierarchical Taxonomy of Psychopathology (HiTOP) system. *Clinical Psychological Science, 11*(6) 21677026221138818. https://doi.org/10.1177/21677026221138818

Barchi-Ferreira, A. M., Loureiro, S. R., Torres, A. R., Da Silva, T. D. A., Moreno, A. L., DeSousa, D. A., Chagas, M. H. N., Dos Santos, R. G., Machado-de-Souza, J. P., & Chagas, N. M. de S. (2019). Personality inventory for DSM-5 (PID-5): Cross-cultural adaptation and content validity in the Brazilian context. *Trends in Psychiatry and Psychotherapy, 41*, 297–300.

Barlow, D. H., Farchione, T. J., Bullis, J. R., Gallagher, M. W., Murray-Latin, H., Sauer-Zavala, S., Bentley, K. H., Thompson-Hollands, J., Conklin, L. R., Boswell, J. F., Ametaj, A., Carl, J. R., Boettcher, H. T., & Cassiello-Robbins, C. (2017). The unified protocol for transdiagnostic treatment of emotional disorders compared with diagnosis-specific protocols for anxiety disorders. *JAMA Psychiatry*, *74*(9), 875–884. https://doi.org/10.1001/jamapsychiatry.2017.2164

Bellack, A. S., Mueser, K. T., Gingerich, S., & Agresta, J. (2013). *Social skills training for schizophrenia: A step-by-step guide*. Guilford Publications.

Beltz, A. M., Wright, A. G. C., Sprague, B. N., & Molenaar, P. C. M. (2016). Bridging the nomothetic and idiographic approaches to the analysis of clinical data. *Assessment*, 23(4), 447–458. https://doi.org/10.1177/1073191116648209

Ben-Porath, Y. S., & Tellegen, A. (2020). *Minnesota Multiphasic Personality Inventory-3 (MMPI-3) Manual for administration, scoring, and interpretation*. University of Minnesota Press.

Ben-Zeev, D., Young, M. A., & Corrigan, P. W. (2010). DSM-V and the stigma of mental illness. *Journal of Mental Health*, *19*(4), 318–327. https://doi.org/10.3109/09638237.2010.492484

Berman, A. H., Bergman, H., Palmstierna, T., & Schlyter, F. (2005). Evaluation of the Drug Use Disorders Identification Test (DUDIT) in criminal justice and detoxification settings and in a Swedish population sample. *European Addiction Research*, *11*(1), 22–31. https://doi.org/10.1159/000081413

Bornstein, R. F., & Natoli, A. P. (2019). Clinical utility of categorical and dimensional perspectives on personality pathology: A meta-analytic review. *Personality Disorders*, *10*(6), 479–490. https://doi.org/10.1037/per0000365

Borsboom, D. (2017). A network theory of mental disorders. *World Psychiatry*, *16*(1), 5. https://doi.org/10.1002/wps.20375

Bringmann, L. F., Elmer, T., Epskamp, S., Krause, R. W., Schoch, D., Wichers, M., Wigman, J. T. W., & Snippe, E. (2019). What do centrality measures measure in psychological networks? *Journal of Abnormal Psychology*, *128*(8), 892–903. https://doi.org/10.1037/abn0000446

Brown, T. A., Sellbom, M., Bach, B., & Newton-Howes, G. (2023). New Zealand (Aotearoa) clinicians' perspectives on the utility of the ICD-11 personality disorder diagnosis. *Personality and Mental Health*, *17*(3), 282–291. https://doi.org/10.1002/pmh.1582

Bruffaerts, R., Sabbe, M., & Demyttenaere, K. (2008). Emergency psychiatry in the 21st century: Critical issues for the future. *European Journal of Emergency Medicine*, *15*(5), 276. https://doi.org/10.1097/MEJ.0b013e3282fc7616

Busch, A. J., Morey, L. C., & Hopwood, C. J. (2017). Exploring the assessment of the *DSM*–*5* alternative model for personality disorders with the personality assessment inventory. *Journal of Personality Assessment*, *99*(2), 211–218. https://doi.org/10.1080/00223891.2016.1217872

Butcher, J. N., Graham, J. R., Ben-Porath, Y. S., Tellegen, A., Dahlstrom, W. G., & Kaemmer, B. (2001). *MMPI-2:Manual for administration and scoring. (Rev. Ed.)*. University of Minnesota Press.

Cano, K., & Sharp, C. (2023). A consumer perspective on personality diagnostic systems: One size does not fit all. *Journal of Personality Disorders*, 37(3), 263–284. https://doi.org/10.1521/pedi.2023.37.3.263

Caspi, A., Houts, R. M., Ambler, A., Danese, A., Elliott, M. L., Hariri, A., Harrington, H., Hogan, S., Poulton, R., Ramrakha, S., Rasmussen, L. J. H., Reuben, A., Richmond-Rakerd, L., Sugden, K., Wertz, J., Williams, B. S., & Moffitt, T. E. (2020). Longitudinal assessment of mental health disorders and cComorbidities across 4 decades among participants in the Dunedin Birth Cohort Study. *JAMA Network Open*, *3*(4), e203221. https://doi.org/10.1001/jamanetworkopen.2020.3221

Cicero, D. C., Jonas, K. G., Chmielewski, M., Martin, E. A., Docherty, A. R., Berzon, J., Haltigan, J. D., Reininghaus, U., Caspi, A., Graziolplene, R. G., & Kotov, R. (2022). Development of the thought disorder measure for the Hierarchical Taxonomy of Psychopathology. *Assessment*, 29(1), 46–61. https://doi.org/10.1177/10731911211015355

Cicero, D. C., Ruggero, C. J., Balling, C. E., Bottera, A. R., Cheli, S., Elkrief, L., Forbush, K. T., Hopwood, C. J., Jonas, K. G., Jutras-Aswad, D., Kotov, R., Levin-Aspenson, H. F., Mullins-Sweatt, S. N., Johnson-Munguia, S., Narrow, W. E., Negi, S., Patrick, C. J., Rodriguez-Seijas, C., Sheth, S., . . . Thomeczek, M. L. (2024). State of the science: The Hierarchical Taxonomy of Psychopathology (HiTOP). *Behavior Therapy*, 55(6), 1114–1129. https://doi.org/10.1016/j.beth.2024.05.001

Clark, L. A., Simms, L. J., Wu, K., & Casillas, A. (2014). *SNAP-2 Schedule for nonadaptive and adaptive personality—Second Edition: Manual for administration, scoring, and interpretation*. University of Notre Dame, Notre Dame, IN.

Clark, L. A., Cuthbert, B., Lewis-Fernández, R., Narrow, W. E., & Reed, G. M. (2017). Three approaches to understanding and classifying mental disorder: ICD-11, DSM-5, and the National Institute of Mental Health's Research Domain Criteria (RDoC). *Psychological Science in the Public Interest, 18*(2), 72–145.

Clark, L. A., & Watson, D. (2019). Constructing validity: New developments in creating objective measuring instruments. *Psychological Assessment, 31*(12), 1412–1427. https://doi.org/10.1037/pas0000626

Clark, L. A., Watson, D., & Reynolds, S. (1995). Diagnosis and classification of psychopathology: Challenges to the current system and future directions. *Annual Review of Psychology, 46*(1), 121–153.

Cooper, R. V. (2013). Avoiding false positives: Zones of rarity, the threshold problem, and the DSM clinical significance criterion. *The Canadian Journal of Psychiatry, 58*(11), 606–611. https://doi.org/10.1177/070674371305801105

Cronbach, L. J., & Meehl, P. E. (1955). Construct validity in psychological tests. *Psychology Bulletin, 52*, 281–302.

Dixon, L. (1999). Dual diagnosis of substance abuse in schizophrenia: Prevalence and impact on outcomes. *Schizophrenia Research, 35*, S93–S100. https://doi.org/10.1016/S0920-9964(98)00161-3

Eaton, N. R., Bringmann, L. F., Elmer, T., Fried, E. I., Forbes, M. K., Greene, A. L., Krueger, R. F., Kotov, R., McGorry, P. D., Mei, C., & Waszczuk, M. A. (2023). A review of approaches and models in psychopathology conceptualization research. *Nature Reviews Psychology, 2*(10), 622–636. https://doi.org/10.1038/s44159-023-00218-4

Epskamp, S., Borsboom, D., & Fried, E. I. (2018). Estimating psychological networks and their accuracy: A tutorial paper. *Behavior Research Methods, 50*(1), 195–212. https://doi.org/10.3758/s13428-017-0862-1

First, M. B. (2005). Clinical utility: A prerequisite for the adoption of a dimensional approach in DSM. *Journal of Abnormal Psychology, 114*(4), 560–564. https://doi.org/10.1037/0021-843X.114.4.560

First, M. B. (2009). Harmonisation of ICD–11 and DSM–V: Opportunities and challenges. *The British Journal of Psychiatry, 195*(5), 382–390. https://doi.org/10.1192/bjp.bp.108.060822

First, M. B. (2010). Clinical utility in the revision of the Diagnostic and Statistical Manual of Mental Disorders (DSM). *Professional Psychology: Research and Practice, 41*(6), 465–473. https://doi.org/10.1037/a0021511

First, M. B., Pincus, H. A., Levine, J. B., Williams, J. B. W., Ustun, B., & Peele, R. (2004). Clinical utility as a criterion for revising psychiatric diagnoses. *American Journal of Psychiatry, 161*(6), 946–954. https://doi.org/10.1176/appi.ajp.161.6.946

Forbes, M. K., Wright, A. G. C., Markon, K. E., & Krueger, R. F. (2021). Quantifying the reliability and replicability of psychopathology network characteristics. *Multivariate Behavioral Research, 56*(2), 224–242. https://doi.org/10.1080/00273171.2019.1616526

Fried, E. I. (2020). Lack of theory building and testing impedes progress in the factor and network literature. *Psychological Inquiry, 31*(4), 271–288. https://doi.org/10.1080/1047840X.2020.1853461

Gallagher, O., Regan, E. E., & O'Reilly, G. (2024). The power threat meaning framework 5 years on—A scoping review of the emergent empirical literature. *British Journal of Psychology, 115*(3), 555–576. https://doi.org/10.1111/bjop.12702

Garcia, D. J., Skadberg, R. M., Schmidt, M., Bierma, S., Shorter, R. L., & Waugh, M. H. (2018). It's not that difficult: An interrater reliability study of the DSM–5 Section III alternative model for personality disorders. *Journal of Personality Assessment, 100*(6), 612–620. https://doi.org/10.1080/00223891.2018.1428982

Gordon, R. M., & Bornstein, R. F. (2018). Construct validity of the Psychodiagnostic Chart: A transdiagnostic measure of personality organization, personality syndromes, mental functioning, and symptomatology. *Psychoanalytic Psychology, 35*(2), 280–288. https://doi.org/10.1037/pap0000142

Gordon, R. M., & Stoffey, R. W. (2014). Operationalizing the Psychodynamic Diagnostic Manual: A preliminary study of the Psychodiagnostic Chart. *Bulletin of the Menninger Clinic, 78*(1), 1–15. https://doi.org/10.1521/bumc.2014.78.1.1

Gunderson, J. G. (2010). Commentary on "Personality traits and the classification of mental disorders: Toward a more complete integration in DSM-5 and an empirical model of psychopathology." *Personality Disorders, 1*(2), 119–122. https://doi.org/10.1037/a0019974

Haeffel, G. J., Jeronimus, B. F., Kaiser, B. N., Weaver, L. J., Soyster, P. D., Fisher, A. J., Vargas, I., Goodson, J. T., & Lu, W. (2021). Folk classification and factor rotations: Whales, sharks, and the problems with the Hierarchical Taxonomy of Psychopathology (HiTOP). *Clinical Psychological Science, 10*(2), 259–278. 21677026211002500. https://doi.org/10.1177/21677026211002500

Hansen, S. J., Christensen, S., Kongerslev, M. T., First, M. B., Widiger, T. A., Simonsen, E., & Bach, B. (2019). Mental health professionals' perceived clinical utility of the *ICD-10* vs. *ICD-11* classification of personality disorders. *Personality and Mental Health, 13*(2), 84–95. https://doi.org/10.1002/pmh.1442

Haslbeck, J. M. B., Borsboom, D., & Waldorp, L. J. (2021). Moderated network models. *Multivariate Behavioral Research, 56*(2), 256–287. https://doi.org/10.1080/00273171.2019.1677207

Hasler, G., Moergeli, H., & Schnyder, U. (2004). Outcome of psychiatric treatment: What is relevant for our patients? *Comprehensive Psychiatry, 45*(3), 199–205. https://doi.org/10.1016/j.comppsych.2004.02.001

Helmich, M. A., Schreuder, M. J., Bringmann, L. F., Riese, H., Snippe, E., & Smit, A. C. (2024). Slow down and be critical before using early warning signals in psychopathology. *Nature Reviews Psychology, 3*(11), 767–780. https://doi.org/10.1038/s44159-024-00369-y

Hopwood, C. J. (2018). A framework for treating DSM-5 alternative model for personality disorder features. *Personality and Mental Health, 12*(2), 107–125. https://doi.org/10.1002/pmh.1414

Hopwood, C. J., Bagby, R. M., Gralnick, T., Ro, E., Ruggero, C., Mullins-Sweatt, S., Kotov, R., Bach, B., Cicero, D. C., Krueger, R. F., Patrick, C. J., Chmielewski, M., DeYoung, C. G., Docherty, A. R., Eaton, N. R., Forbush, K. T., Ivanova, M. Y., Latzman, R. D., Pincus, A. L., . . . Zimmermann, J. (2020). Integrating psychotherapy with the hierarchical taxonomy of psychopathology (HiTOP). *Journal of Psychotherapy Integration, 30*(4), 477–497. https://doi.org/10.1037/int0000156

Insel, T., Cuthbert, B., Garvey, M., Heinssen, R., Pine, D. S., Quinn, K., Sanislow, C., & Wang, P. (2010). Research domain criteria (RDoC): Toward a new classification framework for research on mental disorders. *The American Journal of Psychiatry, 167*(7), 748–751. https://doi.org/10.1176/appi.ajp.2010.09091379

Johnson, J. C. S., Byrne, G. J., & Pelecanos, A. M. (2022). The prevalence of subthreshold psychiatric symptoms and associations with alcohol and substance use disorders: From a nationally representative survey of 36,309 adults. *BMC Psychiatry, 22*(1), 270. https://doi.org/10.1186/s12888-022-03834-1

Johnstone, L., & Boyle, M. (2018). The power threat meaning framework: An alternative nondiagnostic conceptual system. *Journal of Humanistic Psychology, 65*(4), 800–817. https://doi.org/10.1177/0022167818793289

Jonas, K. G., Stanton, K., Simms, L. J., Mullins-Sweatt, S., Gillett, D., Dainer, E., Nelson, B. D., Cohn, J. R., Guillot, S. T., Kotov, R., Cicero, D. C., & Ruggero, C. (2022). *HiTOP Digital Assessment and Tracker (HiTOP-DAT) Manual.* https://doi.org/10.17605/OSF.IO/8HNGD

Kamphuis, J. H., Noordhof, A., & Hopwood, C. J. (2021). When and how assessment matters: An update on the Treatment Utility of Clinical Assessment (TUCA). *Psychological Assessment, 33*(2), 122–132. https://doi.org/10.1037/pas0000966

Kessler, R. C., Chiu, W. T., Demler, O., Merikangas, K. R., & Walters, E. E. (2005). Prevalence, severity, and comorbidity of 12-month DSM-IV disorders in the National Comorbidity Survey Replication. *Archives of General Psychiatry, 62*(6), 617–627. https://doi.org/10.1001/archpsyc.62.6.617

Kingdon, D. G., & Turkington, D. (2022). *Cognitive-behavioral therapy of schizophrenia.* Psychology Press. https://doi.org/10.4324/9781003210528

Kirmayer, L. J., & Ryder, A. G. (2016). Culture and psychopathology. *Current Opinion in Psychology, 8*, 143–148. https://doi.org/10.1016/j.copsyc.2015.10.020

Kotov, R., Krueger, R. F., Watson, D., Achenbach, T. M., Althoff, R. R., Bagby, R. M., Brown, T. A., Carpenter, W. T., Caspi, A., Clark, L. A., Eaton, N. R., Forbes, M. K., Forbush, K. T., Goldberg, D., Hasin, D., Hyman, S. E., Ivanova, M. Y., Lynam, D. R., Markon, K., . . . Zimmerman, M. (2017). The Hierarchical Taxonomy of Psychopathology (HiTOP): A dimensional alternative to traditional nosologies. *Journal of Abnormal Psychology, 126*(4), 454–477. https://doi.org/10.1037/abn0000258

Kotov, R., Krueger, R. F., Watson, D., Cicero, D. C., Conway, C. C., DeYoung, C. G., Eaton, N. R., Forbes, M. K., Hallquist, M. N., Latzman, R. D., Mullins-Sweatt, S. N., Ruggero, C. J., Simms, L. J., Waldman, I. D., Waszczuk, M. A., & Wright, A. G. C. (2021). The Hierarchical Taxonomy of Psychopathology (HiTOP): A quantitative nosology based on consensus of evidence. *Annual Review of Clinical Psychology, 17*, 83–108. https://doi.org/10.1146/annurev-clinpsy-081219-093304

Kotov, R., Perlman, G., Gámez, W., & Watson, D. (2015). The structure and short-term stability of the emotional disorders: A dimensional approach. *Psychological Medicine, 45*(8), 1687–1698.

Kroenke, K., Spitzer, R. L., & Williams, J. B. W. (2002). The PHQ-15: Validity of a new measure for evaluating the severity of somatic symptoms. *Psychosomatic Medicine, 64*(2), 258–266. https://doi.org/10.1097/00006842-200203000-00008

Krueger, R. F., Derringer, J., Markon, K. E., Watson, D., & Skodol, A. E. (2012). Initial construction of a maladaptive personality trait model and inventory for DSM-5. *Psychological Medicine, 42*(9), 1879–1890. https://doi.org/10.1017/s0033291711002674

Krueger, R. F., Eaton, N. R., Clark, L. A., Watson, D., Markon, K. E., Derringer, J., Skodol, A., & Livesley, W. J. (2011). Deriving an empirical structure of personality pathology for DSM-5. *Journal of Personality Disorders, 25*(2), 170–191. https://doi.org/10.1521/pedi.2011.25.2.170

Krueger, R. F., Markon, K. E., Patrick, C. J., Benning, S. D., & Kramer, M. D. (2007). Linking antisocial behavior, substance use, and personality: An integrative quantitative model of the adult externalizing spectrum. *Journal of Abnormal Psychology, 116*, 645–666. https://doi.org/2007-17062-001 [pii] 10.1037/0021-843X.116.4.645

Lahey, B. B. (2021). *Dimensions of psychological problems: Replacing diagnostic categories with a more science-based and less stigmatizing alternative.* Oxford University Press.

Lahey B. B, Applegate B., Chronis A. M., Jones H. A., Williams S. H., Loney J., & Waldman, I. D. (2008) Psychometric characteristics of a measure of emotional dispositions developed to test a developmental propensity model of conduct disorder. *Journal of Clinical Child and Adolescent Psychology, 37*(4),794–807. doi: 10.1080/15374410802359635.

Lengel, G. J., & Mullins-Sweatt, S. N. (2017). The importance and acceptability of general and maladaptive personality trait computerized assessment feedback. *Psychological Assessment, 29*(1), 1–12. https://doi.org/10.1037/pas0000321

Lingiardi, V., & McWilliams, N. (2017). *Psychodynamic Diagnostic Manual: Second Edition: PDM-2* (2nd). The Guilford Press. https://www.guilford.com/books/Psychodynamic-Diagnostic-Manual/Lingiardi-McWilliams/9781462530540

Livesley, W. J., & Jackson, D. N. (2002). *Dimensional Assessment of Personality Pathology-Basic Questionnaire (DAPP-BQ).* Sigma Press.

Loevinger, J. (1957). Objective tests as instruments of psychological theory. *Psychological Reports, 3*(3), 635–694. https://doi.org/10.2466/pr0.1957.3.3.635

Lowe, J. R., & Widiger, T. A. (2009). Clinicians' judgments of clinical utility: A comparison of the DSM-IV with dimensional models of general personality. *Journal of Personality Disorders, 23*(3), 211–229. https://doi.org/10.1521/pedi.2009.23.3.211

McCabe, G. A., & Widiger, T. A. (2020). A comprehensive comparison of the ICD-11 and DSM–5 section III personality disorder models. *Psychological Assessment, 32*(1), 72–84. https://doi.org/10.1037/pas0000772

McGorry, P. D. (2019). The quest for clinical utility and construct validity in psychiatric diagnosis. In I. B. Hickie & P. D. McGorry (Eds.), *Clinical staging in psychiatry: Making diagnosis work for research and treatment* (pp. 278–283). Cambridge University Press. https://doi.org/10.1017/9781139839518.014

McGorry, P. D., Hickie, I. B., Yung, A. R., Pantelis, C., & Jackson, H. J. (2006). Clinical staging of psychiatric disorders: A heuristic framework for choosing earlier, safer and more effective interventions. *Australian & New Zealand Journal of Psychiatry, 40*(8), 616–622. https://doi.org/10.1080/j.1440-1614.2006.01860.x

McWilliams, N., Grenyer, B. F. S., & Shedler, J. (2018). Personality in PDM-2: Controversial issues. *Psychoanalytic Psychology, 35*(3), 299–305. https://doi.org/10.1037/pap0000198

Milinkovic, M. S., & Tiliopoulos, N. (2020). A systematic review of the clinical utility of the DSM–5 section III alternative model of personality disorder. *Personality Disorders: Theory, Research, and Treatment, 11*(6), 377–397. https://doi.org/10.1037/per0000408

Morey, L. C. (1991). *The Personality Assessment Inventory professional manual.* Psychological Assessment Resources.

Morey, L. C. (2017). Development and initial evaluation of a self-report form of the DSM-5 Level of Personality Functioning Scale. *Psychological Assessment, 29*(10), 1302–1308. https://doi.org/10.1037/pas0000450

Morey, L. C. (2018). Application of the DSM-5 Level of Personality Functioning Scale by Lay Raters. *Journal of Personality Disorders, 32*(5), 709–720. https://doi.org/10.1521/pedi_2017_31_305

Morey, L. C., Berghuis, H., Bender, D. S., Verheul, R., Krueger, R. F., & Skodol, A. E. (2011). Toward a model for assessing level of personality functioning in DSM–5, Part II: Empirical articulation of a core dimension of personality pathology. *Journal of Personality Assessment*, *93*(4), 347–353. https://doi.org/10.1080/00223891.2011.577853

Morey, L. C. & Hopwood, C. J. (2020). Brief report: Expert preferences for categorical, dimensional, and mixed/hybrid approaches to personality disorder diagnosis. *Journal of Personality Disorders*, *34*(Supplement C), 124–131. https://doi.org/10.1521/pedi_2019_33_398. PMID: 30650000.

Morey, L. C., Skodol, A. E., & Oldham, J. M. (2014). Clinician judgments of clinical utility: A comparison of DSM-IV-TR personality disorders and the alternative model for DSM-5 personality disorders. *Journal of Abnormal Psychology*, *123*(2), 398–405. https://doi.org/10.1037/a0036481

Morrison, A. P. (2017). A manualised treatment protocol to guide delivery of evidence-based cognitive therapy for people with distressing psychosis: Learning from clinical trials. *Psychosis*, *9*(3), 271–281.

Mullins-Sweatt, S. N., Lengel, G. J., & DeShong, H. L. (2016). The importance of considering clinical utility in the construction of a diagnostic manual. *Annual Review of Clinical Psychology*, *12*(1), 133–155. https://doi.org/10.1146/annurev-clinpsy-021815-092954

Mullins-Sweatt, S. N., & Widiger, T. A. (2009). Clinical utility and DSM-V. *Psychological Assessment*, *21*(3), 302–312. https://doi.org/10.1037/a0016607

Nelson, B., McGorry, P. D., & Fernandez, A. V. (2021). Integrating clinical staging and phenomenological psychopathology to add depth, nuance, and utility to clinical phenotyping: A heuristic challenge. *The Lancet Psychiatry*, *8*(2), 162–168. https://doi.org/10.1016/S2215-0366(20)30316-3

Olbert, C. M., Gala, G. J., & Tupler, L. A. (2014). Quantifying heterogeneity attributable to polythetic diagnostic criteria: Theoretical framework and empirical application. *Journal of Abnormal Psychology*, *123*(2), 452–462.

Olthof, M., Hasselman, F., & Lichtwarck-Aschoff, A. (2020). Complexity in psychological self-ratings: Implications for research and practice. *BMC Medicine*, *18*(1), 317. https://doi.org/10.1186/s12916-020-01727-2

Oltmanns, J. R., & Widiger, T. A. (2018). A self-report measure for the ICD-11 dimensional trait model proposal: The Personality inventory for ICD-11. *Psychological Assessment*, *30*(2), 154–169. https://doi.org/10.1037/pas0000459

Oltmanns, J. R., & Widiger, T. A. (2020). The five-factor personality inventory for ICD-11: A facet-level assessment of the ICD-11 trait model. *Psychological Assessment*, *32*(1), 60–71. https://doi.org/10.1037/pas0000763

Omur, D. (2023). *How is the power threat meaning framework being used by clinical psychologists in clinical practice?* Thesis, University of East London School of Psychology.

OPD Task Force. (2008). *Operationalized Psychodynamic Diagnosis OPD- 2: Manual of diagnosis and treatment planning*. Hogrefe Publishing Corp. https://www.hogrefe.com/us/shop/operationalized-psychodynamic-diagnosis-opd-2-67442.html

Piotrowski, C. (2017). The status of the Personality Assessment Inventory (PAI) in training and practice: Evidence from the emerging literature. *SIS Journal of Projective Psychology & Mental Health*, *24*(2), 83–90. Health Research Premium Collection.

Preti, E., Di Pierro, R., Costantini, G., Benzi, I. M. A., De Panfilis, C., & Madeddu, F. (2018). Using the structured interview of personality organization for DSM-5 level of personality functioning rating performed by inexperienced raters. *Journal of Personality Assessment*, *100*(6), 621–629. https://doi.org/10.1080/00223891.2018.1448985

Raskin, J. D., Maynard, D., & Gayle, M. C. (2022). Psychologist attitudes toward DSM-5 and its alternatives. *Professional Psychology: Research and Practice*, *53*(6), 553–563. https://doi.org/10.1037/pro0000480

Reed, G. M. (2010). Toward ICD-11: Improving the clinical utility of WHO's international classification of mental disorders. *Professional Psychology: Research and Practice*, *41*(6), 457–464. https://doi.org/10.1037/a0021701

Reinfeld, S., Gill, P., Cáceda, R., & Batra, J. (2023). Integrating psychiatric services in the emergency room to improve patient care by using quality improvement methods. *The Journal of Nervous and Mental Disease*, *211*(7), 550. https://doi.org/10.1097/NMD.0000000000001664

Robinaugh, D. J., Hoekstra, R. H. A., Toner, E. R., & Borsboom, D. (2020). The network approach to psychopathology: A review of the literature 2008–2018 and an agenda for future research. *Psychological Medicine, 50*(3), 353–366. https://doi.org/10.1017/S0033291719003404

Roche, M. J., Jacobson, N. C., & Phillips, J. J. (2018). Expanding the validity of the level of personality functioning scale observer report and self-report versions across psychodynamic and interpersonal paradigms. *Journal of Personality Assessment, 100*(6), 571–580. https://doi.org/10.1080/00223891.2018.1475394

Rojas, S. L., & Widiger, T. A. (2014). Convergent and discriminant validity of the five factor form. *Assessment, 21*(2), 143–157. https://doi.org/10.1177/1073191113517260

Ruggero, C. J., Kotov, R., Hopwood, C. J., First, M., Clark, L. A., Skodol, A. E., Mullins-Sweatt, S. N., Patrick, C. J., Bach, B., Cicero, D. C., Docherty, A., Simms, L. J., Bagby, R. M., Krueger, R. F., Callahan, J. L., Chmielewski, M., Conway, C. C., De Clercq, B., Dornbach-Bender, A., . . . Zimmermann, J. (2019). Integrating the Hierarchical Taxonomy of Psychopathology (HiTOP) into clinical practice. *Journal of Consulting and Clinical Psychology, 87*(12), 1069–1084. https://doi.org/10.1037/ccp0000452

Samuel, D. B., & Widiger, T. A. (2006). Clinicians' judgments of clinical utility: A comparison of the DSM-IV and five-factor models. *Journal of Abnormal Psychology, 115*(2), 298–308. https://doi.org/10.1037/0021-843X.115.2.298

Santisteban, D. A., Muir-Malcolm, J. A., Mitrani, V. B., & Szapocznik, J. (2002). Integrating the study of ethnic culture and family psychology intervention science. In *Family psychology: Science-based interventions* (pp. 331–351). American Psychological Association. https://doi.org/10.1037/10438-016

Scott, J., & Henry, C. (2017). Clinical staging models: From general medicine to mental disorders. *British Journal of Psychiatry Advances, 23*(5), 292–299. https://doi.org/10.1192/apt.bp.116.016436

Scott, J., Iorfino, F., Capon, W., Crouse, J., Nelson, B., Chanen, A. M., Dwyer, D., Conus, P., Bechdolf, A., Ratheesh, A., Raballo, A., Yung, A., Berk, M., McKenna, S., Hockey, S., Hutcheon, A., Scott, E., McGorry, P., Shah, J., & Hickie, I. B. (2024). Staging 20: Refining transdiagnostic clinical staging frameworks to enhance reliability and utility for youth mental health. *The Lancet Psychiatry, 11*(6), 461–471. https://doi.org/10.1016/S2215-0366(24)00060-9

Sellbom, M. (2019). The MMPI-2-Restructured Form (MMPI-2-RF): Assessment of personality and psychopathology in the twenty-first century. *Annual Review of Clinical Psychology, 15*, 149–177. https://doi.org/10.1146/annurev-clinpsy-050718-095701

Shedler, J., Beck, A., Fonagy, P., Gabbard, G. O., Gunderson, J., Kernberg, O., Michels, R., & Westen, D. (2010). Personality disorders in DSM-5. *American Journal of Psychiatry, 167*(9), 1026–1028. https://doi.org/10.1176/appi.ajp.2010.10050746

Shorter, E. (2008). History of psychiatry. *Current Opinion in Psychiatry, 21*(6), 593.

Simms, L. J., Goldberg, L. R., Roberts, J. E., Watson, D., Welte, J., & Rotterman, J. H. (2011). Computerized adaptive assessment of personality disorder: Introducing the CAT–PD project. *Journal of Personality Assessment, 93*(4), 380–389.

Simms, L. J., Wright, A. G. C., Cicero, D., Kotov, R., Mullins-Sweatt, S. N., Sellbom, M., Watson, D., Widiger, T. A., & Zimmermann, J. (2022). Development of Measures for the Hierarchical Taxonomy of Psychopathology (HiTOP): A collaborative scale development project. *Assessment, 29*(1), 3–16. https://doi.org/10.1177/10731911211015309

Skodol, A. E. (2012). Personality disorders in DSM-5. *Annual Review of Clinical Psychology, 8*, 317–344. https://doi.org/10.1146/annurev-clinpsy-032511-143131

Slavin-Mulford, J., Sinclair, S. J., Stein, M., Malone, J., Bello, I., & Blais, M. A. (2012). External validity of the Personality Assessment Inventory (PAI) in a clinical sample. *Journal of Personality Assessment, 94*(6), 593–600. https://doi.org/10.1080/00223891.2012.681817

Spitzer, R. L., First, M. B., Shedler, J., Westen, D., & Skodol, A. E. (2008). Clinical utility of five dimensional systems for personality diagnosis: A "Consumer Preference" study. *Journal of Nervous & Mental Disease, 196*(5), 356–374. https://doi.org/10.1097/NMD.0b013e3181710950

Spitzer, R. L., & Wakefield, J. C. (1999). DSM-IV diagnostic criterion for clinical significance: Does it help solve the false positives problem? *American Journal of Psychiatry, 156*(12), 1856–1864. https://doi.org/10.1176/ajp.156.12.1856

Stefanis, N. C., Hanssen, M., Smirnis, N. K., Avramopoulos, D. A., Evdokimidis, I. K., Stefanis, C. N., Verdoux, H., & Van Os, J. (2002). Evidence that three dimensions of psychosis have a distribution in the general population. *Psychological Medicine*, *32*(02), 347–358.

Tracy, M., Tiliopoulos, N., Sharpe, L., & Bach, B. (2021a). The clinical utility of the ICD-11 classification of personality disorders and related traits: A preliminary scoping review. *Australian & New Zealand Journal of Psychiatry*, *55*(9), 849–862. https://doi.org/10.1177/00048674211025607

Tracy, M., Tiliopoulos, N., Sharpe, L., & Bach, B. (2021b). The clinical utility of the ICD-11 classification of personality disorders and related traits: A preliminary scoping review. *Australian & New Zealand Journal of Psychiatry*, *55*(9), 849–862. https://doi.org/10.1177/00048674211025607

Tylicki, J. L., Martin-Fernandez, K. W., & Ben-Porath, Y. S. (2019). Predicting therapist ratings of treatment progress and outcomes with the MMPI-2-RF. *Journal of Clinical Psychology*, *75*(9), 1673–1683. https://doi.org/10.1002/jclp.22795

Ustun, T. B., Kostanjesek, N., Chatterji, S., Rehm, J., & World Health Organization. (2010). *Measuring health and disability: Manual for WHO Disability Assessment Schedule (WHODAS 2.0)*. World Health Organization.

Wakefield, J. C. (2016). Diagnostic issues and controversies in DSM-5: Return of the false positives problem. *Annual Review of Clinical Psychology*, *12*, 105–132. https://doi.org/10.1146/annurev-clinpsy-032814-112800

Watson, D., O'Hara, M. W., Naragon-Gainey, K., Koffel, E., Chmielewski, M., Kotov, R., Stasik, S. M., & Ruggero, C. J. (2012). Development and validation of new anxiety and bipolar symptom scales for an expanded version of the IDAS (the IDAS-II). *Assessment*, *19*(4), 399–420.

Weekers, L. C., Hutsebaut, J., De Saeger, H., & Kamphuis, J. H. (2024). Comparing the clinical utility of the alternative model for personality disorders to the Section II personality disorder model: A randomized controlled trial. *Personality Disorders: Theory, Research, and Treatment*, *15*(5). https://doi.org/10.1037/per0000651

Weekers, L. C., Hutsebaut, J., Rovers, J. M. C., & Kamphuis, J. H. (2024). Head-to-head comparison of the alternative model for personality disorders and Section II personality disorder model in terms of predicting patient outcomes 1 year later. *Personality Disorders: Theory, Research, and Treatment*, *15*(2), 101–109. https://doi.org/10.1037/per0000637

Whetter, D. (2023). *Exploring attitudes towards the power threat meaning framework and its utility*. Thesis, University of Leicester. https://doi.org/10.25392/leicester.data.24619593.v1

Wichers, M., Smit, A. C., & Snippe, E. (2020). Early warning signals based on momentary affect dynamics can expose nearby transitions in depression: A confirmatory single-subject time-series study. *Journal for Person-Oriented Research*, *6*(1), 1. https://doi.org/10.17505/jpor.2020.22042

Widiger, T. A., Frances, A. J., Pincus, H. A., Davis, W. W., & First, M. B. (1991). Toward an empirical classification for the DSM-IV. *Journal of Abnormal Psychology*, *100*(3), 280–288. https://doi.org/10.1037/0021-843X.100.3.280

Widiger, T. A., Lynam, D. R., Miller, J. D., & Oltmanns, T. F. (2012). Measures to assess maladaptive variants of the five-factor model. *Journal of Personality Assessment*, *94*(5), 450–455. https://doi.org/10.1080/00223891.2012.677887

Widiger, T. A., & Trull, T. J. (2007). Plate tectonics in the classification of personality disorder: Shifting to a dimensional model. *American Psychologist*, *62*(2), 71–83. doi: 10.1037/0003-066X.62.2.71

World Health Organization. (2019). *International statistical classification of diseases and related health problems (11th ed.)*. https://icd.who.int/.

Wright, C. V., Beattie, S. G., Galper, D. I., Church, A. S., Bufka, L. F., Brabender, V. M., & Smith, B. L. (2017). Assessment practices of professional psychologists: Results of a national survey. *Professional Psychology: Research and Practice*, *48*(2), 73–78. https://doi.org/10.1037/pro0000086

Zimmerman, M. (2021). Why hierarchical dimensional approaches to classification will fail to transform diagnosis in psychiatry. *World Psychiatry*, *20*(1), 70–71. https://doi.org/10.1002/wps.20815

Zimmermann, J., Altenstein, D., Krieger, T., Holtforth, M. G., Pretsch, J., Alexopoulos, J., Spitzer, C., Benecke, C., Krueger, R. F., Markon, K. E., & Leising, D. (2014). The structure and correlates of self-reported DSM-5 maladaptive personality traits: Findings from two German-speaking samples. *Journal of Personality Disorders*, *28*(4), 518–540. https://doi.org/10.1521/pedi_2014_28_130

APPENDIX

TABLE 21.1 Non-exhaustive List of Dimensional Measures of Psychopathology

Instrument	Format	Coverage of HiTOP	Reference
Achenbach System of Empirically Based Assessment (ASEBA) for youth	Parent-, Teacher-, Self-report	Internalizing & Disinhibited Externalizing spectra, 8 syndromes	Achenbach, T. M. & Rescorla, L. A. (2001) *Manual for the ASEBA school-age forms and profiles*. Burlington, VA: University of Vermont Research Center for Children, Youth, and Families
Achenbach System of Empirically Based Assessment (ASEBA) for adults and elderly	Informant-, Self-report	Internalizing & Disinhibited Externalizing spectra, 8 syndromes	Achenbach, T. M. & Rescorla, L. A. (2003) *Manual for the ASEBA adult forms and profiles*. Burlington, VT: University of Vermont.
Child and Adolescent Psychopathology Scale (CAPS)	Interview	Internalizing & Disinhibited Externalizing spectra, 6 syndromes	Lahey B. B, Applegate B., Chronis A. M., Jones H. A., Williams S. H., Loney J, & Waldman, I. D. (2008). Psychometric characteristics of a measure of emotional dispositions developed to test a developmental propensity model of conduct disorder. *Journal of Clinical Child and Adolescent Psychology*, *37*(4),794–807. doi: 10.1080/15374410802359635.
Externalizing Spectrum Inventory (ESI)	Self-report	Disinhibited Externalizing spectrum, 2 subfactors, 23 traits/components	Krueger, R. F., Markon, K. E., Patrick, C. J., Benning, S. D., & Kramer, M. D. (2007). Linking antisocial behavior, substance use, and personality: An integrative quantitative model of the adult externalizing spectrum. *Journal of Abnormal Psychology*, *116*, 645–666. https://doi.org/2007-17062-001 [pii] 10.1037/0021-843X.116.4.645
Inventory for Depression and Anxiety Symptoms (IDAS-II)	Self-report	Internalizing spectrum, 3 subfactors, 18 components	Watson, D., O'Hara, M. W., Naragon-Gainey, K., Koffel, E., Chmielewski, M., Kotov, R., Stasik, S. M., & Ruggero, C. J. (2012). Development and validation of new anxiety and bipolar symptom scales for an expanded version of the IDAS (the IDAS-II). *Assessment*, *19*(4), 399–420.
Interview for Mood and Anxiety Symptoms (IMAS)	Interview	Internalizing spectrum, 3 subfactors, 10 syndromes, 32 components	Kotov, R., Perlman, G., Gámez, W., & Watson, D. (2015). The structure and short-term stability of the emotional disorders: A dimensional approach. *Psychological Medicine*, *45*(8), 1687–1698.
Scale for the Assessment of Negative Symptoms (SANS) and Scale for the Assessment of Positive Symptoms (SAPS)	Interview	Thought Disorder spectrum, 2 syndromes, 4 components	Andreasen, N. C. (1982). *Scale for the assessment of positive symptoms*. University of Iowa, Department of Psychiatry. Andreasen, N. C. (1984). *Scale for the assessment of negative symptoms*. University of Iowa College of Medicine.

Schedule for Nonadaptive and Adaptive Personality, 2nd edition (SNAP-2)	Self-, informant-report	4 domains, 15 traits	Clark, L. A., Simms, L. J., Wu, K., & Casillas, A. (2014). *SNAP-2 Schedule for Nonadaptive and Adaptive Personality—Second Edition: Manual for Administration, Scoring, and Interpretation*. University of Notre Dame, Notre Dame, IN.
Personality Inventory for *DSM-5* (PID-5)	Self-, informant-report	5 domains, 25 traits	Krueger, R. F., Eaton, N. R., Clark, L. A., Watson, D., Markon, K. E., Derringer, J., Skodol, A., & Livesley, W. J. (2011). Deriving an Empirical Structure of Personality Pathology for *DSM-5*. *Journal of Personality Disorders*, *25*(2), 170–191. https://doi.org/10.1521/pedi.2011.25.2.170
Five Factor Form (FFF)	Self-, therapist- report	5 domains, 30 traits	Rojas, S. L., & Widiger, T. A. (2014). Convergent and discriminant validity of the Five Factor Form. *Assessment*, *21*(2), 143–157. https://doi.org/10.1177/1073191113517260
Five-Factor Model Personality Disorder Scales	Self-report	5 domains, 99 traits	Widiger, T. A., Lynam, D. R., Miller, J. D., & Oltmanns, T. F. (2012). Measures to Assess Maladaptive Variants of the Five-Factor Model. *Journal of Personality Assessment*, *94*(5), 450–455. https://doi.org/10.1080/00223891.2012.677887
Computerized Adaptive Test of Personality Disorder (CAT-PD)	Self-report	5 domains, 33 traits	Simms, L. J., Goldberg, L. R., Roberts, J. E., Watson, D., Welte, J., & Rotterman, J. H. (2011). Computerized adaptive assessment of personality disorder: Introducing the CAT–PD project. *Journal of Personality Assessment*, *93*(4), 380–389
Dimensional assessment of personality pathology—Basic Questionnaire (BQ)	Self-report	4 domains, 18 traits	Livesley, W. J., & Jackson, D. N. (2002). *Dimensional Assessment of Personality Pathology-Basic Questionnaire (DAPP-BQ)*. Sigma Press
Personality Assessment Inventory (PAI)	Self-report	5 spectra, 15 syndromes, 30 components/traits	Morey, L. C. (1991). *The Personality Assessment Inventory professional manual*. Psychological Assessment Resources.
Minnesota Multiphasic Personality Inventory-2 Restructured Form (MMPI-2-RF)/ Personality Psychopathology—Five (PSY-5)	Self-report	3 higher-order dimensions, 5 personality domains, 9 syndromes, 23 components/traits	Ben-Porath, Y. S., & Tellegen, A. (2020). *Minnesota Multiphasic Personality Inventory-3 (MMPI-3) Manual for administration, scoring, and interpretation*. University of Minnesota Press.

TABLE 21.2 Studies Comparing the Clinical Utility of Dimensional and Categorical Classification Systems

Authors	Year	Brief Methods	Construct Validity	Diagnostic Accuracy	Descriptive Utility	Ease of Use	Communicative Value	Treatment Planning
Bagby & Widiger	2020	A special section in Psychological Assessment introducing papers discussing the construct validity of the *ICD-11* PD model.	Briefly summarized findings from several studies indicating construct validity for the new dimensional PD organization in the *ICD-11*	N/A	N/A	N/A	N/A	N/A
Balling et al.	2023	143 practicing clinicians rated three clinical vignettes using both *HiTOP* and *DSM* systems, followed by ratings of perceived clinical utility for both systems.	N/A	*HiTOP* was rated higher than the *DSM-5*.	*HiTOP* was rated higher than the *DSM-5*.	*HiTOP* was rated higher than the *DSM-5*.	*HiTOP* was rated higher than the *DSM-5* for communicating with patients. No differences for communicating with other professionals.	*HiTOP* was rated higher than the *DSM-5*.
Bornstein & Natoli	2019	Meta-analysis of 11 studies. Inclusion criteria: (1) studies included ratings from mental health professionals and/or trainees for at least one categorical and one dimensional PD model, and (2) enough information so that effect sizes can be computed.	N/A	Dimensional models were rated higher than categorical models.	Dimensional models were rated higher than categorical models.	N/A	Dimensional models were rated higher than categorical models for communicating with patients.	Dimensional models were rated higher than categorical models.

Brown et al.	2022	124 psychologists and psychiatrists applied the *DSM-5* and *ICD-11* PD diagnostic systems to a current patient, followed by metrics on clinical utility.	N/A	N/A	The *ICD-11* was rated higher than the *DSM-5*.	The *ICD-11* was rated higher than the *DSM-5*.	The *ICD-11* was rated higher than the *DSM-5* for communicating with patients and other professionals.	The *ICD-11* was rated higher than the *DSM-5*.
Cano & Sharp	2023	Study 1: 703 undergraduate students read assessment reports that varied on two dimensions for severity (i.e., low, moderate, high) and type (dimensional, dimensional-categorical hybrid, categorical). Study 2: 154 participants with a borderline PD diagnosis and family members read assessment reports that varied by type for the second study. All participants provided ratings of clinical utility.	N/A	N/A	Participants rated the *DSM-5* Section II model similar to the *AMPD*, but higher than the dimensional *ICD-11* in ease of understanding and comprehensiveness in description.	N/A	Participants rated the *DSM-5* Section II model similar to the *AMPD*, but higher than the dimensional *ICD-11* for communicating with professionals and families.	Participants rated the *DSM-5* Section II model similar to the *AMPD*, but higher than the dimensional *ICD-11* for usefulness in seeking treatment.
Hansen et al.	2019	163 mental health professionals (primarily psychologists, nurses, and medical doctors) applied the *ICD*-10 PD types and categories or the *ICD-11* PD severity and trait domain qualifiers to a current patient, followed by metrics on clinical utility.	N/A	*ICD-11* was rated higher than the *ICD*-10.	No differences were found.	*ICD-11* was rated higher than the *ICD*-10.	*ICD-11* was rated better for communicating with patients. No differences in communicating with other professionals.	*ICD-11* was rated higher than the *ICD*-10.

(continued)

TABLE 21.2 Continued

Authors	Year	Brief Methods	Construct Validity	Diagnostic Accuracy	Descriptive Utility	Ease of Use	Communicative Value	Treatment Planning
Lowe & Widiger	2009	1,572 practicing psychologists were randomly assigned to one of three cases. Each rated their assigned case using the *DSM*-IV and one of four alternative dimensional models (i.e., FFM, TCI, MPQ, SWAP). Clinicians then provided clinical utility ratings for the model.	N/A	All dimensional models were rated higher than the *DSM-IV*. No differences were found among dimensional models.	All dimensional models were rated higher than the *DSM-IV*. No differences were found among dimensional models.	No differences were found among models.	All dimensional models were rated higher than the *DSM-IV*. No differences were found among dimensional models.	All dimensional models were rated higher than the *DSM-IV*. No differences were found among dimensional models.
Milinkovic & Tiliopoulos	2020	20 studies included in the review had an empirical design, included a clinical population, evaluated the clinical utility of the *AMPD*, and were not conducted in a nonclinical setting.		Eight of 13 studies found support for the *AMPD*'s diagnostic accuracy.		Five of 13 studies found support for the *AMPD*'s ease of use.	Eight of 20 studies found higher support for the *AMPD*.	13 of 13 studies found strong support for the *AMPD*.
Morey, Skodol, & Oldham	2014	337 mental health clinicians applied the *DSM-IV-TR* PD system and the *AMPD* to one of their patients, then rated each system for clinical utility.	N/A	The *AMPD* was rated higher than the *DSM-IV-TR*.	The *AMPD* was rated higher than the *DSM-IV-TR*.	The *DSM-IV-TR* was rated higher than the *AMPD*	The *DSM-IV-TR* was rated higher.	The *AMPD* was rated higher than the *DSM-IV-TR*.
Samuel & Widiger	2006	245 practicing psychologists read one of three case vignettes and provided *DSM-IV* and FFM ratings. Following PD ratings, participants rated each system for clinical utility.	N/A	N/A	The FFM was rated higher than the *DSM-IV*.	The FFM was rated marginally higher than the *DSM-IV*.	The FFM was rated much higher for communicating with patients, but ratings were similar for communicating with professionals.	The FFM was rated higher than the *DSM-IV*.

Spitzer et al.	2008	206 practicing psychologists and 191 psychiatrists selected one of their own patients and applied each of the Five Factor Model, Cloninger's Psychobiological Model, SWAP Prototype Matching, *DSM-IV* Prototype Matching, *DSM-IV* Criterion Counting in an assessment exercise. Ratings of clinical utility were completed after the exercise	N/A	N/A	The two prototype matching models were rated highest.	The *DSM-IV* prototype matching system was rated easiest to use.	The two prototype matching models were rated highest.	N/A
Tracy et al.	2021	8 studies were selected for the review. Longitudinal studies and studies that did not investigate the clinical utility of dimensional approaches were excluded. Studies that focused on outcome research and not clinical utility were also excluded, along with studies that focused solely on nonclinical populations.	Three of the five studies investigating construct validity found moderate to strong support for the *ICD-11*'s goodness of fit.	Two studies found very limited support for diagnostic accuracy. One study found strong support	N/A	One study found strong support for the *ICD-11*'s ease of use.	Two studies focusing on clinician perceptions found moderate to strong support for the *ICD-11* PD.	All three studies that investigated the usefulness of *ICD-11* for treatment planning found strong support.
Hansen et al.	2019	163 mental health professionals (primarily psychologists, nurses, and medical doctors) applied the *ICD-10* PD types and categories or the *ICD-11* PD severity and trait domain qualifiers to a current patient, followed by metrics on clinical utility.	N/A	*ICD-11* was rated higher than the *ICD-10*.	No differences were found.	*ICD-11* was rated higher than the *ICD-10*.	*ICD-11* was rated better for communicating with patients. No differences in communicating with other professionals.	*ICD-11* was rated higher than the *ICD-10*.

CHAPTER 22

Applicability for Dimensional Diagnosis in Underrepresented and Epistemically Excluded Populations

SIENNA R. NIELSEN, SHAYAN ASADI, AND CRAIG RODRIGUEZ-SEIJAS

Introduction

DIMENSIONAL psychiatric diagnostic systems are positioned as improving upon many of the limitations of the traditional categorical classification system. These include poor construct validity, disorder heterogeneity, artificial discontinuity between nonpathological and pathological functioning, and high prevalence of diagnostic comorbidity (Cuthbert, 2020; Kotov et al., 2017; Kotov et al., 2021; Rodriguez-Seijas et al., 2015). In addition, dimensional diagnostic systems have been positioned as more favorable for representing the psychosocial needs of individuals from marginalized populations (Eaton et al., 2021; Rodriguez-Seijas et al., 2023). In this chapter, we discuss some ways that dimensional classification models/systems are better suited for addressing the psychiatric needs of members of marginalized, underrepresented, and epistemically excluded (Settles et al., 2020) populations. When compared with categorical classification systems like the *Diagnostic and Statistical Manual of Mental Disorders* 5th Edition (DSM-5-TR; American Psychiatric Association, 2022) and the International Classification of Disorders 11th Edition (ICD-11; World Health Organization, 2019), dimensional classification systems like the Hierarchical Taxonomy of Psychopathology (HiTOP; DeYoung et al., 2023; Kotov et al., 2017; 2021; see Pham and Forbes, this volume) may be better suited for improving psychiatric diagnostic reliability and validity for all patients, with particular impact for individuals from marginalized groups. Rather than outlining the process of implementing dimensional systems in psychiatric diagnosis (for readers interested in this specific topic, see Ruggero et al., 2019), this chapter focuses on the influence of classification type on three major areas relevant to diverse and underrepresented populations: (1) clinician bias, (2) criterion bias, and (3) the formal incorporation of sociocontextual factors.

Throughout this chapter we use various terms to refer to populations that are typically not the focus of study within mainstream psychopathology theory, research, and intervention—like "marginalized" and "epistemically excluded." We define these groups as those who have been underrepresented, stigmatized, mistreated, or denied access to health-determining resources such as adequate safety, nutrition, social support, and medical care based on such social statuses and identities as race, ethnicity, sex assigned at birth, sexual orientation, and gender status. Other social variables like financial status, geographic location, language, immigration status, and physical or cognitive ability similarly impact individuals' environments with importance for psychiatric classification. Though the epistemology of psychology and psychopathology research is beyond the scope of this chapter, readers interested in the negative effects of epistemic exclusion on marginalized populations can see Settles and colleagues (2020).

In comparing classification types, we focus primarily on the DSM-5-TR as an example of categorical classification, and HiTOP as an example of dimensional classification. Though we focus on the HiTOP model, we believe that the incorporation of sociocultural context may be similarly applied to other categorical and dimensional diagnostic systems discussed throughout this Handbook. The principles that we discuss, outlining the importance of formally inculcating sociocultural context within classification systems, are not inherent to the HiTOP dimensional system. Instead, overlooking context is a feature of mainstream psychopathology epistemology.

Improving Diagnostic Reliability and Validity to Limit Effects of Clinician Bias

There is a long history of inequitable physical and mental healthcare for marginalized groups. Clinician implicit biases regarding identities such as race, ethnicity, gender, and sexual orientation have been significantly associated with lower quality healthcare, including lower quality patient-provider interactions, lower treatment adherence, and worse treatment outcomes (Ayhan et al., 2020; Hall et al., 2015. Previous scholarship using the traditional DSM categorical classification system illustrates how an individual's identities unduly influence the categorical diagnoses that will be applied to them and the treatment they receive, with worse outcomes for individuals from marginalized groups (Eubanks-Carter & Goldfried, 2006; Garb, 2021). Diagnostic bias can promote a vicious cycle in which individuals from marginalized groups could receive poorer quality psychiatric evaluation, resulting in poorer psychiatric care and worse mental and physical health outcomes, thereby perpetuating psychiatric inequity.

Poor Diagnostic Reliability Enables Clinician Bias

Clinician bias plays a greater role in diagnostic systems with poor reliability. In traditional categorical systems—like the DSM-5-TR—diagnostic criteria that are used to assign a categorical diagnosis are historically decided based on clinical expertise. This system relies on theoretical assumptions about how symptoms *should* cluster to represent an underlying psychiatric disorder, largely based on expert consensus. However, diagnostic criteria heavily overlap across diagnostic categories (Forbes et al., 2024), and the same diagnoses can manifest with different symptom combinations. The result is high comorbidity among and heterogeneity within psychiatric disorders (Pincus et al., 2004), contributing to poor reliability in psychiatric diagnosis. Thus, multiple clinicians can come to different diagnostic conclusions about the same psychiatric patient. Additionally, the same clinician could come to different diagnostic conclusions about psychiatric patients with similar symptoms but different social identities. Poor diagnostic reliability is a feature of traditional classification systems that stymies appropriate care for patients. While issues with diagnostic reliability create problems in assessment and treatment for patients of all backgrounds, they disproportionately affect members of marginalized groups (Garb, 2021).

Research on categorical classification frameworks demonstrates that patient identity characteristics influence clinician diagnostic decisions. With high comorbidity and heterogeneity in categorical diagnoses, clinicians might rely on their perceived expertise, including individually developed heuristics and assumptions, when it comes to final diagnostic decisions.

This can manifest as clinician biases impacting categorical diagnostic decision-making. For example, Eubanks-Carter and Goldfried (2006) found that psychologists were more likely to diagnose a hypothetical client with borderline personality disorder if the client were male and gay or bisexual than if the client were heterosexual, holding constant all other aspects of the patient's presentation. Similarly, Rodriguez-Seijas and colleagues (2024) found that psychologists, psychiatrists, mental health counsellors, and social workers were more likely to assign a borderline personality disorder primary diagnosis when presented identical clinical vignettes if the patient described was transgender rather than cisgender.

Other studies suggest that clinician bias may influence persistent misdiagnosis in many disorders using categorical systems such as the DSM and ICD, including under-diagnosis of autism based on sex assigned at birth (Russell et al., 2011), attention deficit/hyperactivity disorder based on race and ethnicity (Bax et al., 2019; Zablotsky & Alford, 2020), and antisocial personality disorder based on race (Mikton & Grounds, 2007). Clinician racial bias may also result in misdiagnosis of primary psychotic disorders in the presence of affective symptoms among Black patients (Gara et al., 2019; Jegarl et al., 2023). In one study exploring how behavioral dimensions related to thought disorder symptoms (i.e., speech disorganization and negative symptomatology) and schizophrenia diagnosis, racial bias was observed at the global categorical diagnostic level, such that Black participants were more likely to be diagnosed with schizophrenia despite few differences in symptomatology. Differences in speech patterns also interacted with patients' race in relation to clinicians' diagnostic decisions, such that clinicians rated Black patients' speech as more disorganized (Schwartz et al., 2019). These findings suggest that individuals' identities and their belonging to a marginalized group impacts the type of categorical diagnosis that gets assigned to them.

Higher Diagnostic Reliability and Validity Limits Effects of Clinician Bias

Dimensionally based classification systems—like the HiTOP model—have been shown to be more reliable across clinicians than are categorical measures (Eaton et al., 2013; Krueger et al., 2003; Markon et al., 2011). The greater reliability of these systems is in part due to greater construct validity. Dimensional systems offer diagnostic constructs that are both more homogenous and more representative of underlying processes of psychopathology, thereby improving both validity and reliability. In the HiTOP dimensional structure, classification relies on the co-occurrence of symptoms and other behavioral indicators to identify clinically relevant dimensions from which psychiatric disorder diagnoses can be built (i.e., more bottom-up), as opposed to the creation of behavioral indicators assumed to represent a specific categorical diagnosis (i.e., more top-down). For example, the HiTOP internalizing spectrum is a dimension encompassing symptom categories of distress and fear due to their frequent co-occurrence as observed across a multitude of studies (Kim et al., 2021; Watson et al., 2022). The dimensional structure of HiTOP assumes that shared underlying processes are responsible for frequently co-occurring symptoms. In the Research Domain Criteria (RDoC; Cuthbert & Insel, 2013), another dimensional model, this assumption of shared underlying mechanisms is even more explicit. For example, the RDoC arousal/regulatory domain organizes symptoms resulting from neurobehavioral dysfunction in regulatory mechanisms. What remains to be considered is how precisely these dimensions become translated into a practical diagnostic entity. Nonetheless, by focusing on groupings of symptoms with assumed shared underlying mechanisms, dimensional models such as HiTOP and RDoC improve construct validity and reduce issues of heterogeneity and comorbidity compared to the DSM-5. In doing so, dimensional systems also improve diagnostic reliability for all patients, which can be assumed to also impact individuals from marginalized backgrounds.

Empirical evidence also suggests that dimensional ratings of psychopathology—when compared with categorical diagnostic criterion counts—are less biased (Gordon, 2006; Rodriguez-Seijas et al., 2024; Samuel & Widiger, 2009). Clinician bias has been repeatedly indicated in categorical personality disorder diagnoses, likely due to particularly poor issues of heterogeneity and comorbidity in the diagnostic categorization of personality disorders in the DSM (Morey & Benson, 2016). In one study in which client gender in vignettes of personality disorder presentations was manipulated, clinician bias was observed for histrionic and antisocial personality disorder diagnoses when using categorical but not dimensional ratings (Samuel & Widiger, 2009). Alternative approaches to the traditional categorical diagnostic system have also demonstrated less racial bias. In another study in which client race was manipulated, clinician bias was observed for categorical diagnosis of eating disorders, but not dimensional symptom ratings (Gordon et al., 2006). In another study examining racial bias in eating disorder diagnosis, clinicians demonstrated bias in preferentially diagnosing eating disorders when presented with vignettes reflecting White and Hispanic patients compared with Black patients, despite no differences across patient racial groups in the clinicians' ratings of individual eating disorder symptoms (Gordon et al., 2006). These findings are consistent with other data demonstrating that clinician biases are most evident in the final categorical diagnostic decision. For example, ratings of diagnostic criteria and dimensional symptom assessments appear less susceptible to clinician diagnostic bias related to a patient's possession of a marginalized identity than the categorical diagnostic decision (Morey & Benson, 2016; Morey & Ochoa, 1989; Rodriguez-Seijas et al., 2024). Thus, clinician bias appears to be most impactful at the categorical diagnostic level, and less influential in a more homogenous or lower-order dimensional diagnostic assessment. By moving away from categorical diagnoses, dimensional classification systems may reduce the impact of clinician biases in diagnostic decision-making.

Understanding and Alleviating Criterion Bias

Another factor from which bias might emerge is the fundamental nature of the diagnostic classification system itself. That is, assumptions that underlie the categorical or dimensional systems—and the psychopathology categories and domains they represent—might differentially impact individuals from marginalized backgrounds, leading to disparities in how psychopathology is officially defined (i.e., criterion bias). In the traditional categorical diagnostic system, the polythetic criteria used for the adjudication of any specific diagnosis purportedly represent behavioral manifestations of a specific, unobserved diagnostic category—a latent variable. It is assumed that the behavioral indicators that represent those diagnostic categories are equally representative of the underlying latent diagnosis *for all people*. However, this might not always be the case.

For instance, some of our work highlights how indicators of the DSM-5 borderline personality disorder diagnosis are more frequently endorsed and are less reflective of underlying psychopathology dimensions among sexual and gender minority individuals when compared with cisgender heterosexual persons. The central feature of borderline personality disorder is "a pervasive pattern of instability of interpersonal relationships, self-image, and affects, and marked impulsivity" (APA, 2013, p. 663), which can be extremely distressing for patients and their social support networks. Borderline personality disorder is more frequently diagnosed among sexual (Rodriguez-Seijas et al., 2021b, 2021a) and gender (Rodriguez-Seijas, Morgan et al., 2023; Zimmerman et al., 2022) minority individuals relative to cisgender heterosexuals when examining both epidemiological data as well as data from psychiatric treatment facilities. Additionally, sexual minority individuals more frequently endorse several behaviors considered indicators of the borderline personality disorder diagnosis when compared with heterosexual individuals; sexual minority individuals often endorse these behaviors without any associated distress or impairment when compared with heterosexuals (Rodriguez-Seijas et al., 2021a).

Sexual minority individuals' endorsement of some behavioral indicators of the borderline personality disorder latent variable, however, differ in their relation to that underlying latent variable level than when the same behaviors are endorsed by heterosexual individuals. In other words, the behaviors that are used to indicate a specific diagnostic criterion might function differently among individuals from differing backgrounds. For example, impulsive sexual behavior as an indicator of the borderline personality disorder impulsivity criterion and self-injurious behaviors as indicators of the borderline personality disorder criterion of chronic suicidality demonstrate differential item functioning in relation to the borderline personality disorder diagnosis latent variable (Asadi et al., 2025). Endorsement of these behaviors among sexual minority individuals is "easier," since the endorsement of these behaviors is associated with lower levels of the underlying borderline personality disorder latent factor than the same endorsement for heterosexuals. In other words, a sexual minority individual matched with a heterosexual individual on BPD severity would indicate more impulsive sexual behavior than would the heterosexual individual, suggesting that impulsive sexual behavior might not be a comparable indicator of overall BPD severity among sexual minority versus heterosexual populations. Thus, the assumptions that behavioral indicators of traditional categorical diagnoses are universal and can be applied equally across populations is not accurate. This is what we mean when we refer to criterion bias. Because the specific behavioral indicators of any traditional categorical diagnosis might not function identically among individuals from all populations, they introduce a level of bias in the criteria and the diagnostic category itself that might contribute to observed diagnostic disparities.

The standard theory, research, and treatment of personality disorders—like borderline personality disorder—fail to critically address how the sociocultural contexts in which individuals live is related to psychiatric diagnosis (Rodriguez-Seijas, 2022; Rodriguez-Seijas, Rogers et al., 2023). The sociocultural contexts in which sexual and gender minority individuals exist might predispose them to behaviors that develop in response to these environments, are understandable and functional responses to the environment, and may or may not be associated with impairment or psychopathology. For example, investigations of heightened interpersonal problems, identity dysfunction, and disinhibition as criteria for borderline personality pathology often consider heterosexual norms of interpersonal relationships, identity functioning, and sexual behaviors that are not always consistent with norms within sexual minority communities (Eaton, 2020; Eaton et al., 2021 Rodriguez-Seijas, 2022; Rodriguez-Seijas et al., 2023a, 2023b 2024).

For instance, due to the challenges of navigating heterosexist and cisnormative environments, sexual and gender minority individuals often experience more interpersonal conflicts within complicated social networks (Harkless & Flowers, 2005; Peplau & Fingerhut, 2007), which might lead to increased incidence of behaviors associated with the borderline personality disorder criteria of unstable interpersonal relationships. It is culturally normative for sexual minority and gender minority individuals to experience fluctuations and difficulties navigating identity expression into adulthood (Goldhammer et al., 2019; Katz-Wise, 2015; Porter, 2023). An untrained or ignorant healthcare provider might confuse such normative identity experiences as indicators of the borderline personality disorder diagnosis. Sexual minority groups also may have a higher number of sexual partners compared to heterosexual individuals (Kuyper & Vanwesenbeeck, 2011). However, sexual behavior might not be as indicative of underlying borderline personality disorder as similar behavior among heterosexuals (Asadi et al., 2024). Thus, traditional categorical personality disorder diagnosis might instill bias within the assumptions that are made about how behaviors represent the underlying diagnostic category, with particular ramifications for individuals from marginalized populations.

Do dimensional classification systems alleviate the problem of criterion bias? Not entirely. Psychiatric assessments in dimensional systems are still susceptible to criterion bias in which the indicators that are selected to represent the underlying dimension(s) might not equally represent psychopathology across contexts and populations, potentially resulting in inappropriate pathologization of normative behavior among individuals from marginalized groups. For instance, in one study of a dimensional measure of maladaptive personality trait domains, we found that sexual and gender minority individuals were more inclined to endorse several indicators within the maladaptive antagonism and detachment domains. This bias at the item level was a function of group status independent of elevated personality pathology. More importantly, accounting for this non-invariance in a single item nullified observed group differences in the antagonism domain (Asadi et al., 2024).

Data-driven dimensional systems like HiTOP might be just as susceptible to criterion bias when developed without the intentional representation of sociocultural contexts, how they relate to historically marginalized groups, and the implications for behavioral indicators of the underlying dimensions being examined. Indeed, we have previously discussed this precise topic in the measurement of compulsive sexual behavior and how traditional measures conflate compulsive sexual behavior with such factors as stigma, normative differences, and concealment among sexual and gender minority individuals (Rodriguez-Seijas, Li et al., 2023). Be they traditional categorical diagnoses based on expert consensus or data-driven diagnoses based on underlying dimensions, without a deliberate focus on understanding the mental health needs of marginalized populations and without the inclusion of scholars who focus on how sociocontextual factors impact mental health, the result will be the inculcation of bias within these classification systems.

Several solutions have been proposed to reduce criterion bias in assessment (Frisby, 2024). These solutions largely emphasize the need for rigorous psychometric testing of bias in psychiatric assessment. Psychometric testing for bias may include testing for differential item functioning and measurement invariance in assessments between groups with different psychosocial experiences (Frisby, 2024). By testing for differential item functioning and measurement invariance, we can identify whether individual criteria function similarly as indicators of the same category of psychopathology across different patients. Items that do not function similarly across patients of different social identities can be removed or adapted until assessment items reflect latent psychopathology similarly across patients. Where dimensional classification models differ from traditional categorical models, however, is that their data-driven focus allows space for explicitly testing and updating the models in relation to marginalized populations and reducing criterion bias, even if this has not been a major focal area to date. We believe that traditional categorical diagnoses, often descended from expert consensus and in which changes are difficult to implement once a diagnosis becomes cemented within the DSM, might not possess this level of flexibility. This becomes particularly important as new disorders are introduced into traditional categorical classification systems. For instance, Jennings and colleagues (2022) outline how the relative ignorance of how minority stress pathways impact sexual behavior among sexual and gender minority individuals introduces bias in the estimation of the novel compulsive sexual behavior disorder within the International Classification of Disorders (ICD).

On the other hand, by virtue of being descended from a data-driven approach rather than expert consensus, the HiTOP model's internalizing, externalizing, and thought disorder dimensions have been researched and replicated in many countries, demonstrating cross-national generalizability. Further, studies using U.S. samples have explicitly investigated measurement invariance of the internalizing and externalizing factors across such sociodemographic groupings as race/ethnicity, sex assigned at birth, sexual orientation, and age (for an in-depth review of the HiTOP literature with respect to marginalized populations, see Rodriguez-Seijas, Li et al., 2023). Studies have also examined how specific behavioral indicators like those traditionally associated with borderline personality disorder (Asadi et al., 2024) and the use of alcohol and other substances during sexual activity (Rodriguez-Seijas et al., 2024) differentially relate to underlying psychopathology dimensions by virtue of marginalized status like sexual minority identity.

Because of the data-driven approach to understanding psychopathology, dimensional systems like the HiTOP model are positioned to accommodate a level of plurality that might be of particular consequence for reducing criterion bias. The HiTOP consortium possesses an explicit process for amending the model based on empirical evidence (Forbes et al., 2024) and has already demonstrated the use of this process in updating the model. For example, based on input from scholars in the substance use disorder fields, the language of the model was changed in reference to substance use from "substance abuse" to "problematic substance use." While this example might not be specifically pertinent to marginalized populations, it demonstrates the relative flexibility with which the model can be amended based on scientific evidence. Thus, a dimensional, data-driven classification system such as HiTOP might be more conducive to alleviating the potentially detrimental impact of criterion bias than is traditional categorical classification systems. To do so, however, it will be crucial to incorporate the feedback of historically excluded researchers and clinicians with lived experiences of minority cultures, toward more inclusive and informed assessment development (Rodriguez-Seijas, Li et al., 2023; Settles et al., 2020; Verona, 2022).

Representing Psychosocial Needs of Marginalized Groups

Incorporating sociocultural context in psychiatric assessment, diagnosis, and treatment is not a new idea. In 1990, the American Psychological Association (APA) provided clinicians with guidelines for treating racial and ethnic minorities, stating: "psychological service providers need a sociocultural framework to consider diversity of values, interactional styles, and cultural expectations in a systematic fashion." Since then, the APA (2017) has released a set of ten updated provider multicultural guidelines that incorporate empirical research to emphasize the influence of sociocultural context of patient experiences. For example, Guideline 5 encourages that "[Psychologists] seek to address institutional barriers and related inequities, disproportionalities, and disparities . . . as they seek to promote justice, human rights, and access to quality and equitable mental and behavioral health services" (APA, 2015, p. 14), and Guideline 6 encourages promotion of "culturally adaptive interventions and advocacy within and across systems" (APA, 2015, p. 4). Additional guidelines have been published for working with sexual minority (APA, 2012) and gender minority (APA, 2015) patients. The DSM-5-TR also includes general guidelines for considering sociocultural context in diagnosis in a separate "Culture and Psychiatric Diagnosis" section (American Psychiatric Association, 2022). Ample research suggests that a patient's sociocultural context influences psychiatric disorder etiology (Meyer, 2003; Stein et al., 2022), symptom presentation (Rao et al., 2007), and treatment preferences (Burckell & Goldfried, 2006; Cabral & Smith, 2011). Incorporating sociocultural contexts in psychotherapy adaptations can improve treatment outcomes for historically marginalized groups (Arundell et al., 2021). Understanding sociocultural influences, therefore, at multiple stages of the assessment, diagnosis, and treatment process can promote culturally informed diagnosis and treatment, facilitate clinician cultural sensitivity, and reduce psychiatric inequity.

While these guidelines provide empirical support to motivate culturally informed diagnosis and treatment, the disorder-specific approach inherent to the traditional categorical classification system creates obstacles that apply to the focus on marginalized populations. Specifically, the impact of psychosocial stressors is often transdiagnostic and associated with underlying dimensions more than specific diagnostic categories (e.g., Eaton et al., 2021; Pachankis, 2015; Rodriguez-Seijas et al., 2019). For example, childhood maltreatment experiences are better associated with dimensions of internalizing and externalizing psychopathology than specific DSM diagnoses (Keyes et al., 2012). The relation between mental health and stigma-related stressors in marginalized groups is also better represented by transdiagnostic, dimension models (Cohen et al., 2016; Rodriguez-Seijas et al., 2015). For instance, among Black Americans and Black people of Caribbean descent, the experiences of racial discrimination are better associated with the internalizing and externalizing psychopathology dimensions than any specific discrete categorical disorders (Rodriguez-Seijas et al., 2015).

Adopting a more dimensional classification approach, therefore, streamlines research, assessment, diagnosis, and treatment, particularly for marginalized populations (Eaton et al., 2021). A disorder-specific approach results in an unwieldy literature in which each sociocontextual factor's associations with a specific disorder domain is examined in a bivariate manner, resulting in dozens to potentially hundreds of research studies documenting similar results. Dimensional classification systems may be more capable of clarifying the relationships between sociocontextual factors and psychopathology, which is of particular importance for marginalized populations (Cohen et al., 2016; Keyes et al., 2012; Rodriguez-Seijas et al., 2015). Mechanisms of psychopathology, such as exposure to specific social stressors, can be more clearly linked to expressions of psychopathology in research using a dimensional framework. Indeed, research suggests that sociocontextual factors like minority stress processes overwhelmingly relate to psychiatric disorder domains by virtue of their associations with underlying dimensions. By approaching this literature from a dimensional standpoint, then, we coalesce seemingly disparate literatures on any specific disorder category by focusing on the shared liability that unites them (i.e., the underlying dimensions). Transdiagnostic, dimensional classification systems of psychopathology may then be more conducive to incorporating the impact of sociocontextual factors into their conceptualizations than are traditional categorical diagnoses.

Further, dimensional systems might also be more conducive to ongoing efforts at refining the models to better represent the psychosocial needs of individuals from marginalized backgrounds. For instance, as we've outlined previously, it would be entirely possible to chart a research program squarely focused on testing how specific behavioral indicators of psychopathology differentially relate to psychopathology dimensions based on group membership. For instance, appreciating the sociocultural contexts in which sexual and gender and ethnoracial minority individuals exist can provide testable hypotheses to examine such things as differential item functioning in specific behaviors and psychopathology domains (see Figure 22.1). This would require aligning research with specific behavioral indicators rather than the more heterogeneous and comorbid binary DSM categorical diagnoses.

Dimensional systems that focus on transdiagnostic phenomena, like the HiTOP model, may provide a better framework for conceptualizing patient mental health needs for all individuals,

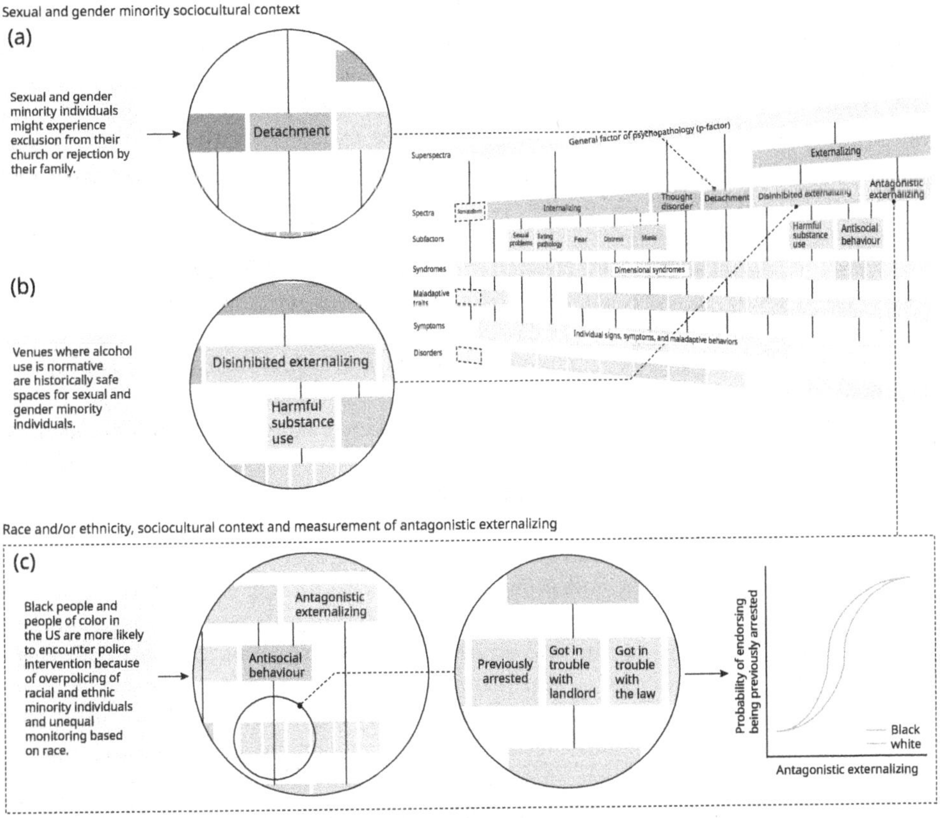

FIGURE 22.1 An illustration of how a dimensional framework can be used to test differential item functioning within the HiTOP model. Credit: Rodriguez-Seijas, C., Li, J. J., Balling, C., Brandes, C., Bernat, E., Boness, C. L., Forbes, M. K., Forbush, K. T., Joyner, K. J., Krueger, R. F., Levin-Aspenson, H. F., Michelini, G., Ro, E., Rutter, L., Stanton, K., Tackett, J. L., Waszczuk, M., & Eaton, N. R. (2023). Diversity and the Hierarchical Taxonomy of Psychopathology (HiTOP). *Nature Reviews Psychology*, 2(8), Article 8.

by providing a more reliable system for tracking symptoms and choosing effective treatments when compared with a more traditional, disorder-specific approach (Hopwood et al., 2020). Dimensional psychopathology systems may also be particularly helpful for identifying the psychosocial needs of marginalized populations (Eaton, 2020; Garb, 2021; Krueger & Bezdijan, 2009; Langwerden et al., 2021). Dimensional systems are better positioned to incorporate social contextual factors, highlighting specific experiences as mechanisms for symptom manifestation.

Reducing Treatment Inequity

Many individuals experiencing severe distress associated with any specific categorical disorder often exhibit additional symptoms (e.g., depression and anxiety symptoms often present together); comorbidity is the rule rather than the exception. In general, co-occurring symptoms might be overlooked if they are not a part of an individual's primary categorical diagnosis, with consequences for intervention impact. This becomes a magnified issue, considering how clinician bias impacts how mental healthcare providers attend to specific psychopathology signs and symptoms among individuals from marginalized populations, as discussed previously. Additional research demonstrates that clinician bias influences not only categorical diagnoses, but also important treatment decisions. For instance, clinician racial bias influences diagnosis and subsequent treatment decisions when assessing mood disorder symptoms in Black Americans compared with White Americans (Dixon et al., 2001; Jegarl et al., 2023). Similarly, clinicians are more likely to diagnose Black Americans experiencing mood disorder symptoms with a primary psychotic disorder diagnosis than White Americans (Schwartz & Blankenship, 2014). By highlighting psychotic disorder symptoms over mood disorder symptoms, Black Americans are then less likely to receive treatment for their mood disorder symptoms than White Americans (Dixon et al., 2001). Black patients in the United States receiving treatment for substance use disorders are less likely to additionally receive services for comorbid anxiety and mood symptoms compared with White patients (Hatzenbeuhler et al., 2008). These results suggest that, in the case of categorical comorbidity, relying on clinician expertise to draw final conclusions regarding final diagnoses allows for the undue influence of clinician bias on treatment decisions.

Apart from the general issue with comorbidity that differentially impacts marginalized populations, the traditional categorical system further begets a disorder-specific treatment approach. Disorder-specific treatments are protocols developed to treat a single categorical disorder, such as major depressive disorder or social anxiety disorder explicitly. However, contemporary dimensional classification systems, such as HiTOP, provide a better framework for intervention and research on treatments targeting symptom reduction across myriad categorical diagnostic domains (Hopwood et al., 2020; Kotov et al., 2017; Mullins-Sweatt et al., 2020), which may be of particular importance for marginalized populations (Eaton et al., 2021). Their focal areas are the underlying dimensions that tie specific symptoms and categorical diagnoses together. These underlying dimensions are arguably the areas of focus in dimensional models of psychopathology, as opposed to treating a specific categorical diagnosis. Treatments focusing on co-occurring symptoms rather than categorical, disorder-specific DSM diagnoses, such as the Unified Protocol for the Transdiagnostic Treatment of Emotional Disorders, have been found to be similarly effective and more widely applicable than disorder-specific protocols (Barlow et al., 2017). Treatments targeting higher-order underlying personality dimensions, such as BPD Compass (Sauer-Zavala et al., 2023), have been effective in reducing personality disorder symptoms. Thus, treatment focused at the transdiagnostic dimensional rather than disorder-specific diagnostic level may streamline clinician training and reduce clinician burden in areas with limited psychiatric treatment resources, potentially expanding effective care to historically marginalized groups.

For example, adaptations of transdiagnostic, dimensional treatments that address sociocontextual factors that are important for understanding and ameliorating psychosocial health difficulties among sexual minority individuals have shown promise in widespread amelioration of symptoms across several traditional categorical domains (Keefe et al., 2023; Pachankis, 2015; Pachankis et al., 2022). These interventions, like the ESTEEM (Effective Skills to Empower Effective Men; Burton et al., 2019) and EQuIP (Empowering Queer Identities in Psychotherapy; Scheer et al., 2023) protocols, were developed with a focus on how minority stress processes that sexual minority individuals face compromise health in a manner that transcends diagnostic boundaries (Pachankis et al., 2019; Rodriguez-Seijas et al., 2019). These types of interventions were developed to be transdiagnostic, and thereby correspond with more dimensional approaches to psychiatric classification, due to the high comorbidity of psychiatric and behavioral disorders observed among sexual minority individuals (Pachankis, 2015).

It might be tempting to conclude that by virtue of their more transdiagnostic, dimensional focus rather than disorder-specific approach, dimensional interventions are superior to traditional, diagnostic category-based interventions. However, the novelty of these interventions is not so much the dimensional psychopathology focus per se. Instead, it is in the focus on the social and contextual stressors that predispose sexual minority individuals to experience worse mental health outcomes and greater psychiatric comorbidity in which lies the true innovation of these interventions. Both disorder-specific affirming interventions and these transdiagnostic interventions for sexual minority individuals focus on the same over-arching principles. That is, their major areas of focus are the social contextual factors that predispose widespread psychiatric ill-health (i.e., examining how minority stress processes compromise health; see Rogers et al., 2022 for a review of disorder-specific and dimensional affirming interventions for sexual minority populations). Thus, while we believe that transdiagnostic dimensional intervention approaches can be particularly beneficial for marginalized communities, to date, these dimensional approaches' novelty has been through the incorporation of sociocontextual factors rather than through a formal definition of dimensional psychopathology, as we discuss throughout this Handbook.

In our view, the major advantage that dimensional models of psychopathology hold in reference to treatment outcomes when specifically focusing on marginalized populations is one of the same advantages that they hold in general: focusing treatment at the underlying dimensions that cut across traditional categorical domains streamlines treatment targets with concomitant reductions across myriad domains. As a reminder, though, this advantage of dimensional approaches with respect to treatment will be impacted by issues related to criterion bias discussed previously in this chapter. If the behavioral indicators used to index any psychopathology dimensions do not reflect those underlying dimensions appropriately, then assumptions that interventions focused on those specific dimensions are a route to reducing myriad impairing behaviors across diverse populations will be misguided. For example, the regular use of substances during sexual activity shows associations with the externalizing psychopathology dimension, reflecting problems with impulsivity, disinhibition, and sensation seeking (Rodriguez-Seijas et al., 2017). Be this the case, interventions targeting the disinhibition domain might be beneficial for reducing such a behavior. However, this association might not be the case for all populations. Indeed, the use of substances during sexual behavior—with the exception of methamphetamine—shows very little associations with these maladaptive personality domains associated with the externalizing dimension in the HiTOP model among sexual minority men (Rodriguez-Seijas et al., 2024). If a clinician assumes sex-related substance use in a gay male client is evidence of significant impulsive behavior, they might misconceptualize their patient's distress while overpathologizing potentially normative behavior. Alternatively, they might overlook how the behavior indexes a different domain. Misdiagnosis could result in inappropriate treatment for impulsive behavior or problematic substance use while ignoring other important psychopathology dimensions that might be pertinent for individuals from this population. By doing so, it also risks creating a rift in the therapeutic alliance.

One of the major advantages of dimensional classification systems, we believe, is the relative ease with which the many issues we highlight in this chapter can be researched and incorporated into a more pluralistic classification system that can better support the needs and experiences of individuals from marginalized backgrounds.

Epistemology of Categorical versus Dimensional Psychopathology Models

Arguably, psychopathology is typically theorized as an intra-individual feature of the person. This is exemplified in the field of personality disorders research, where DSM-I characterized personality disorders as resultant from some constitutional defect, with insufficient focus given to how social, contextual, and environmental factors impact these very mental health outcomes; contemporary personality disorder research continues in this intra-individual deficit framing (Rodriguez-Seijas, 2022; Rodriguez-Seijas, Rogers et al., 2023). Intersectionality theory (Bowleg, 2008; Crenshaw, 1991) focuses on understanding how social forces like power and privilege create a complex tapestry that determines differential health among populations. Psychology in general (Buchanan & Wiklund, 2020)—and clinical psychology and psychiatry specifically (Rodriguez-Seijas et al., 2024)—fails to include a focus on social and contextual factors within its remit. Psychological classification is no different.

As Settles and colleagues (2020) exhaustively document, mainstream psychology—and we argue this extends to psychopathology and classification research and development as well—excludes scholars, scholarship, and expertise that is necessary for understanding the ameliorating psychiatric disparities observed among underrepresented, marginalized, and epistemically excluded populations. By continued pushing of intersectionality theory to the scientific fringes, the field creates a cycle that not only ignores this important scholarship, but actively denigrates it. Instead, the field propagates in a manner that both reduces complex phenomena to seemingly universal elemental units and simultaneously decontextualizes theory and research as a means to assert universality of constructs. While we have espoused how we believe a dimensional approach can overcome several issues pertinent to the health of marginalized populations in the sections above, it is noteworthy that dimensional approaches inculcate these same colonial biases and practices to the detriment of diverse, underrepresented, and epistemically excluded populations.

What does this look like? Continuing with the HiTOP model as our illustration, research on the HiTOP model to date has been exclusively quantitative; focused on assumptions of universality; aimed at unearthing assumedly causal mechanisms underlying psychopathology, which we would argue reflect an assumption of intra-individual dysfunction; and exists from a consortium of scholars who largely represent dominant populations within psychological research (Rodriguez-Seijas, Li et al., 2023). These are the characteristics of mainstream psychological research described by Settles and colleagues (2020). Since our examples related to criterion bias pertain to the personality disorder classification, the DSM-5 Alternative Model of Personality Disorders (AMPD) can be used as another illustration. The AMPD is an example of a dimensional-categorical hybrid system in which theorized underlying dimensions of personality pathology are used for the provision of a categorical personality disorder diagnosis (Sharp & Miller, 2022). Thus, it represents an illustration of using a dimensional approach for the purpose of improving diagnostic classifications. This hybrid model was proposed with the intent to improve reliability in personality disorder diagnoses, and provide a conceptual framework more aligned with empirical research on the structure of personality pathology. While there are several issues related to the AMPD (see Widiger & Hines, 2022 for greater discussion of conceptual issues pertinent to the AMPD), we focus our discussion on issues relevant for marginalized populations, as we see some of these issues reflective of what we discuss with respect to dimensional classification systems like the HiTOP model as well.

Little focus within the AMPD (Rodriguez-Seijas, 2022) has been on marginalized populations. Indeed, reducing diagnostic bias has not been at the forefront of the AMPD or dimensional psychopathology models. Instead, we would assert that there is an implicit assumption that creating a more reliable and valid classification system by virtue of statistical rigor results in an inherent amelioration of the problems related to diagnostic inequity. This is the sort of assumption that is inherent to much of the mental health field, whereby a color-evasive approach (Annamma et al., 2017) is prioritized and an assumption is made that not explicitly focusing on equity will somehow alleviate inequity (Rodriguez-Seijas et al., 2024).

A color-evasive approach is one that downplays the impact of context (e.g., racism that begets race) in its remit. And this is often achieved through a reliance on dominant philosophies and approaches. It is not that any of these approaches is wrong per se, but that the exclusive reliance on these approaches without the inclusion of expertise and diverse ways of understanding mental health stymies an appropriate focus and applicability to underrepresented populations. A focus on exclusively quantitative data neglects rich mixed methods and qualitative approaches that can be essential for understanding how contexts impact behaviors and the underlying domains affiliated with them. An assumption—and perhaps search for—universality ignores the equifinality underlying behaviors. Social withdrawal, for instance, might signify the HiTOP detachment domain for many, but might be a better reflection of environmental stigma and a behavioral response that engenders safety rather than intra-individual psychopathology for sexual and gender minority individuals (see Figure 22.1). A lack of scholars with expertise in marginalized populations can impact how bias becomes instantiated in dimensional assessment measures.

In sum, while a dimensional approach like the HiTOP model holds the potential to alleviate several issues pertinent to diverse and marginalized populations, it is important to reckon with how the prevailing philosophy of that approach can inadvertently prevent this.

Breaking the Cycle of Psychiatric Inequity over Time

Over time, dimensional classification may help reduce societal stigma and clinician biases. Dimensional classification systems provide a framework normalizing that all individual experiences fall on a spectrum, which may reduce the sense of alienation from "normal" functioning that can occur with categorical diagnoses (Eaton et al., 2021; Teachman et al., 2006). Incorporating sociocultural factors into a dimensional framework of psychopathology may additionally alleviate stigma by emphasizing sociocultural mechanisms of symptom presentation, thereby removing blame from the individual. For example, our research suggests that stressful situations in daily life experienced at higher rates by marginalized groups (e.g., stress from health, work, or social issues) elicit similarly increased negative reactions regardless of individual differences in personality, shifting focus from the individual to the environment (Ringwald et al., 2024). While greater incorporation of sociocultural influences could reduce clinician bias over time in either categorical or dimensional classification systems, the dimensional system might be more conducive to highlighting concrete relationships between sociocultural factors and psychopathology domains (Cohen et al., 2016; Keyes et al., 2012; Rodriguez-Seijas et al., 2015). Given that dimensional symptom assessment may be less susceptible to clinician bias, dimensional systems in clinician training may challenge existing clinician biases. For example, dimensional models may provide a framework to understand how structural sociocultural processes—such as systemic marginalization—and daily life stressors—such as mistreatment—empirically relate to psychiatric symptom presentation and severity, development, and maintenance. Understanding the links between sociocultural processes and specific symptoms may foster clinician empathy and understanding, thereby reducing stigma and marginalization within the mental health care system. Further research is needed to assess a dimensional classification in interventions reducing clinician biases.

While we believe that dimensional classification systems improve upon many of the psychometric limitations of traditional categorical systems, we remain reserved at this time about how much dimensional models of psychopathology inherently reduce diagnostic inequity. We see dimensional diagnostic systems as holding the potential to better improve psychiatric equity and better accommodate the psychosocial needs of marginalized populations compared to categorical systems. However, the switch to a dimensional framework alone may not substantially reduce inequity. First, there are many factors contributing to psychiatric inequity, such as accessibility to mental health services (Le Cook et al., 2013; Priester et al., 2016), financial barriers to care (Alegria et al., 2022), and stigma (Gary, 2005; Hatzenbuehler, 2017). Many of these factors demand reform beyond diagnostic classification changes (Lee-Tauler et al., 2018). Additionally, fully implementing a dimensional classification system that reduces psychiatric inequity and addresses psychosocial needs of marginalized groups will require intentional research and planning across levels of provider education and patient care. Major limitations in implementations of a dimensional system currently include (1) identifying an appropriate dimensional model for widespread implementation (rather than a hybrid categorical-dimensional model), and (2) establishing a framework for incorporating dimensional social and contextual factors.

Recommendations for Incorporating Sociocontextual Factors

Although dimensional classification systems of psychopathology may be more conducive to incorporating sociocultural factors, it is also important to consider *how* we typically think about and incorporate sociocultural and contextual factors. Many of the sociocultural factors included in research on mental illness are assessed and interpreted categorically, such as a race, ethnicity, gender, sexual and gender minority status, etc. However, there are many reasons that a categorical classification system for sociocultural factors is flawed. Analogous to problems with the traditional categorical classification system for psychopathology, each marginalized category is highly heterogeneous in terms of psychosocial experiences (Bostwick et al., 2010; Lopez & Gadsden, 2017; Viruell-Fuentes et al., 2012). Further, the categorical groupings on which we often focus are not based on empirically identified distinctions (Bryant et al., 2022; Hyde, 2007). Categories do not allow for the appropriate consideration of intersectionality or the experiences emerging from multiple overlapping identities within the broader sociocultural context (Seng et al., 2012, Williams, 2019). Finally, and perhaps most important, these groupings and categories do not acknowledge the underlying processes contributing to potential differences between these groups, and therefore are not consistently associated with process-dependent outcomes (Bostwick et al., 2010; Romanelli et al., 2020; Roth, 2016).

The demographic categories that are typically of focus within psychopathology theory, research, and treatment can be better considered proxies for societal systems of power and privilege. It is these systems that produce the groupings to which we attend, not vice versa. Further, the nature of social processes will differ by specific social contexts (e.g., assumptions from a U.S. context might not generalize to individuals from other regions or countries). Capturing sociocultural processes may involve connecting development of specific symptoms to uniquely stressful experiences rather than a categorical social identity status. One example is connecting internalizing symptoms to unique sexual minority stressors, such as family rejection, rather than the category of sexual minority status in itself (Meyer, 2003). Treatments adapted for sexual minorities consider minority stress as a dimensional sociocultural influence on mental health (Burton et al., 2019). When researchers and clinicians use categorical social identity statuses as proxies for external sociocultural processes, we risk perpetuating clinician biases by over-simplifying and pathologizing the experiences of historically marginalized groups (Harawa & Ford, 2009; Roth, 2016). Failing to understand the social processes that underlie many demographic categories used by researchers holds the potential to propagate inaccurate and essentialist group narratives of deficiency (Williams, 2019). Focusing on dimensional measures of sociocultural processes rather than categorical social identities may emphasize the role of sociocultural context and reduce stigmatization of social identities (Helms, 2007).

Intersectional sociocultural processes are multifaceted and multilayered, aligning more closely with a dimensional conceptualization than a categorical one. Given that dimensional frameworks of psychopathology more reliably relate to life stressors than do categorical frameworks (Cohen et al., 2016; Eaton et al., 2021; Keyes et al., 2012; Rodriguez-Seijas et al., 2015), a dimensional diagnostic classification system may be more conducive to incorporating dimensional sociocultural influences than a categorical system. A vital future direction for dimensional systems of psychopathology is the incorporation of dimensional systems of sociocultural influences on mental illness. Without the intentional acknowledgement and incorporation of dimensional sociocultural processes, dimensional systems of psychopathology remain susceptible to clinician biases and pathologization of minority patient experiences.

Conclusion

Psychiatric inequity is a long-standing public health issue that will require a reform across myriad aspects of the mental healthcare system. The diagnostic classification system plays a role in psychiatric inequity, particularly in the frequency and subsequent effects of diagnostic inequity. Some of the factors contributing to diagnostic inequities include effects of clinician biases on assessment and treatment, criterion bias in how we conceptualize indicators of psychopathology and the extent to which this generalizes across populations, poor incorporation of sociocultural influences in etiological conceptualizations of psychopathology, and an underlying philosophy that ignores these factors. A dimensional classification system—such as the HiTOP model—that conceptualizes symptom elevation and functional impairment along a spectrum might provide a framework more conducive to incorporating sociocultural influences and reducing bias, stigma, and psychiatric inequities over time when compared with traditional categorical diagnostic systems. The general advantages of dimensional systems, including improved reliability and validity in diagnoses, may reduce the effect of clinician bias on diagnostic and treatment decisions, thereby improving psychiatric care for marginalized populations. However, specific and explicit focus on encoding the impact of sociocultural contextual factors is still needed to ensure that dimensional classification systems appropriately extend to diverse, underrepresented, and marginalized populations. Continued critical psychometric investigation of dimensional assessments and incorporation of dimensional sociocultural influences are essential for the intentional reduction of psychiatric inequity in dimensional classification systems.

References

Alegría, M., Zhen-Duan, J., O'Malley, I. S., & DiMarzio, K. (2022). A new agenda for optimizing investments in community mental health and reducing disparities. *American Journal of Psychiatry*, *179*(6), 402–416.

American Psychological Association (2012). Guidelines for psychological practice with lesbian, gay, and bisexual clients. *The American Psychologist*, *67*(1), 10.

American Psychological Association (2015). Guidelines for psychological practice with transgender and gender nonconforming people. *American Psychologist*, *70*(9), 832–864.

American Psychiatric Association. (2022). *Diagnostic and statistical manual of mental disorders* (5th ed., text rev.).

Annamma, S. A., Jackson, D. D., & Morrison, D. (2017). Conceptualizing color-evasiveness: Using dis/ability critical race theory to expand a color-blind racial ideology in education and society. *Race Ethnicity and Education, 20*(2), 147–162. https://doi.org/10.1080/13613324.2016.1248837

Arundell, L. L., Barnett, P., Buckman, J. E., Saunders, R., & Pilling, S. (2021). The effectiveness of adapted psychological interventions for people from ethnic minority groups: A systematic review and conceptual typology. *Clinical Psychology Review, 88*, 102063.

Asadi, S., Cunningham, T. J., Morgan, T. A., Zimmerman, M., & Rodriguez-Seijas, C. (2024). Examining measurement invariance in the personality inventory for DSM-5 brief form across sexual and gender minority status. *Assessment, 31*(3), 678–697. https://doi.org/10.1177/10731911231176449

Asadi, S., Suzuki, T., & Rodriguez-Seijas, C. (2025). Investigating differential item functioning among borderline personality disorder diagnostic criteria and internalizing/externalizing domains based on sexual orientation. *Journal of Psychopathology and Clinical Science, 134*(1), 97.

Ayhan, C. H. B., Bilgin, H., Uluman, O. T., Sukut, O., Yilmaz, S., & Buzlu, S. (2020). A systematic review of the discrimination against sexual and gender minority in health care settings. *International Journal of Health Services, 50*(1), 44–61.

Barlow, D. H., Farchione, T. J., Bullis, J. R., Gallagher, M. W., Murray-Latin, H., Sauer-Zavala, S., . . . & Cassiello-Robbins, C. (2017). The unified protocol for transdiagnostic treatment of emotional disorders compared with diagnosis-specific protocols for anxiety disorders: A randomized clinical trial. *JAMA psychiatry, 74*(9), 875–884.

Bax, A. C., Bard, D. E., Cuffe, S. P., McKeown, R. E., & Wolraich, M. L. (2019). The association between race/ethnicity and socioeconomic factors and the diagnosis and treatment of children with attention-deficit hyperactivity disorder. *Journal of Developmental & Behavioral Pediatrics, 40*(2), 81–91

Bostwick, W. B., Boyd, C. J., Hughes, T. L., & McCabe, S. E. (2010). Dimensions of sexual orientation and the prevalence of mood and anxiety disorders in the United States. *American Journal of Public Health, 100*(3), 468–475.

Bowleg, L. (2008). When Black + lesbian + woman ≠ Black lesbian woman: The methodological challenges of qualitative and quantitative intersectionality research. *Sex Roles, 59*(5), 312–325. https://doi.org/10.1007/s11199-008-9400-z

Bryant, B. E., Jordan, A., & Clark, U. S. (2022). Race as a social construct in psychiatry research and practice. *JAMA Psychiatry, 79*(2), 93–94.

Buchanan, N. T., & Wiklund, L. O. (2020). Why clinical science must change or die: Integrating intersectionality and social justice. *Women & Therapy, 43*(3–4), 309–329. https://doi.org/10.1080/02703149.2020.1729470

Burckell, L. A., & Goldfried, M. R. (2006). Therapist qualities preferred by sexual-minority individuals. *Psychotherapy: Theory, Research, Practice, Training, 43*(1), 32.

Burton, C. L., Wang, K., & Pachankis, J. E. (2019). Psychotherapy for the spectrum of sexual minority stress: Application and technique of the ESTEEM treatment model. *Cognitive and Behavioral Practice, 26*(2), 285–299.

Cabral, R. R., & Smith, T. B. (2011). Racial/ethnic matching of clients and therapists in mental health services: A meta-analytic review of preferences, perceptions, and outcomes. *Journal of Counseling Psychology, 58*(4), 537.

Cohen J. M., Feinstein B. A., Rodriguez-Seijas C., Taylor C. B., Newman M. G. (2016). Rejection sensitivity as a transdiagnostic risk factor for internalizing psychopathology among gay and bisexual men. *Psychology of Sexual Orientation and Gender Diversity, 3*(3), 259–264. https://doi.org/10.1037/sgd0000170

Crenshaw, K. (1991). Demarginalizing the intersection of race and sex: A Black feminist critique of antidiscrimination doctrine, feminist theory, and antiracist politics [1989]. In *Feminist legal theory*. Routledge.

Cuthbert, B. N. (2020). The role of RDoC in future classification of mental disorders. *Dialogues in Clinical Neuroscience, 22*(1), 81–85.

Cuthbert, B. N., & Insel, T. R. (2013). Toward the future of psychiatric diagnosis: The seven pillars of RDoC. *BMC Medicine, 11*, 1–8.

DeYoung, C. G., & Tiberius, V. (2023). Value fulfillment from a cybernetic perspective: A new psychological theory of well-being. *Personality and Social Psychology Review*, *27*(1), 3–27.

Dixon, L., Green-Paden, L., Delahanty, J., Lucksted, A., Postrado, L., & Hall, J. (2001). Variables associated with disparities in treatment of patients with schizophrenia and comorbid mood and anxiety disorders. *Psychiatric Services*, *52*(9), 1216–1222.

Eaton, N. R. (2020). Measurement and mental health disparities: Psychopathology classification and identity assessment. *Personality and Mental Health*, *14*(1), 76–87.

Eaton, N. R., Keyes, K. M., Krueger, R. F., Balsis, S., Skodol, A. E., Markon, K. E. et al. (2021). An invariant dimensional liability model of gender differences in mental disorder prevalence: Evidence from a national sample. *Journal of Abnormal Psychology*, *121*, 282–288.

Eaton, N. R., Keyes, K. M., Krueger, R. F., Noordhof, A., Skodol, A. E., Markon, K. E. et al. (2013) Ethnicity and psychiatric comorbidity in a national sample: Evidence for latent comorbidity factor invariance and connections with disorder prevalence. *Social Psychiatry and Psychiatric Epidemiology*, *48*, 701–710.

Eubanks-Carter, C., & Goldfried, M. R. (2006). The impact of client sexual orientation and gender on clinical judgments and diagnosis of borderline personality disorder. *Journal of Clinical Psychology*, *62*(6), 751–770.

Forbes, M. K., Ringwald, W. R., Allen, T., Cicero, D. C., Clark, L. A., DeYoung, C. G., Eaton, N., Kotov, R., Krueger, R. F., Latzman, R. D., Martin, E. A., Naragon-Gainey, K., Ruggero, C. J., Waldman, I. D., Brandes, C., Fried, E. I., Goghari, V. M., Hankin, B., Sperry, S. Stanton, K., . . . & Wright, A. G. (2024). Principles and procedures for revising the hierarchical taxonomy of psychopathology. *Journal of Psychopathology and Clinical Science*, *133*(1), 4.

Frisby, M. B. (2024). Critical quantitative literacy: An educational foundation for critical quantitative research. *AERA Open*, *10*, 23328584241228223.

Gara, M. A., Minsky, S., Silverstein, S. M., Miskimen, T., & Strakowski, S. M. (2019). A naturalistic study of racial disparities in diagnoses at an outpatient behavioral health clinic. *Psychiatric Services*, *70*(2), 130–134.

Garb, H. N. (2021). Race bias and gender bias in the diagnosis of psychological disorders. *Clinical Psychology Review*, *90*, 102087.

Gary, F. A. (2005). Stigma: Barrier to mental health care among ethnic minorities. *Issues in Mental Health Nursing*, *26*(10), 979–999.

Goldhammer, H., Crall, C., & Keuroghlian, A. S. (2019). Distinguishing and addressing gender minority stress and borderline personality symptoms. *Harvard Review of Psychiatry*, *27*(5), 317–325. https://doi.org/10.1097/HRP.0000000000000234

Gordon, K. H., Brattole, M. M., Wingate, L. R., & Joiner Jr., T. E. (2006). The impact of client race on clinician detection of eating disorders. *Behavior Therapy*, *37*(4), 319–325.

Hall, W. J., Chapman, M. V., Lee, K. M., Merino, Y. M., Thomas, T. W., Payne, B. K., Eng E., Day, S. H., & Coyne-Beasley, T. (2015). Implicit racial/ethnic bias among health care professionals and its influence on health care outcomes: A systematic review. *American Journal of Public Health*, *105*(12), e60–e76.

Harawa, N. T., & Ford, C. L. (2009). The foundation of modern racial categories and implications for research on black/white disparities in health. *Ethnicity & Disease*, *19*(2), 209–217.

Harkless, L. E., & Fowers, B. J. (2005). Similarities and differences in relational boundaries among heterosexuals, gay men, and lesbians. *Psychology of Women Quarterly*, *29*(2), 167–176.

Hatzenbuehler, M. L. (2017). Advancing research on structural stigma and sexual orientation disparities in mental health among youth. *Journal of Clinical Child & Adolescent Psychology*, *46*(3), 463–475.

Helms, J. E. (2007). Some better practices for measuring racial and ethnic identity constructs. *Journal of Counseling Psychology*, *54*(3), 235.

Hopwood, C. J., Bagby, R. M., Gralnick, T., Ro, E., Ruggero, C., Mullins-Sweatt, S., Kotov, R. Bach, B., Cicero, D. C., Krueger, R. F., Patrick, C. J., Chmielewski, M., DeYoung, C. G., Docherty, A. R., Eaton, N. R., Forbush, K. T., Ivanova, M. Y., Latzman, R. D., Pincus, A. L., . . . & Zimmermann, J. (2020). Integrating psychotherapy with the hierarchical taxonomy of psychopathology (HiTOP). *Journal of Psychotherapy Integration*, *30*(4), 477.

Hyde, J. S. (2007). New directions in the study of gender similarities and differences. *Current Directions in Psychological Science, 16*(5), 259–263.

Jegarl, A. M., Jegede, O., Isom, J., Ciarleglio, N., & Black, C. (2023). Psychotic misdiagnosis of racially minoritized patients: A case-based ethics, equity, and educational exploration. *Harvard Review of Psychiatry, 31*(1), 28–36.

Jennings, T. L., Gleason, N., & Kraus, S. W. (2022). Assessment of compulsive sexual behavior disorder among lesbian, gay, bisexual, transgender, and queer clients: Commentary to the debate: "Behavioral addictions in the ICD-11." *Journal of Behavioral Addictions, 11*(2), 216–221.

Katz-Wise, S. L. (2015). Sexual fluidity in young adult women and men: Associations with sexual orientation and sexual identity development. *Psychology & Sexuality, 6*(2), 189–208.

Keefe, J. R., Rodriguez-Seijas, C., Jackson, S. D., Bränström, R., Harkness, A., Safren, S. A., Hatzenbuehler, M. L., & Pachankis, J. E. (2023). Moderators of LGBQ-affirmative cognitive behavioral therapy: ESTEEM is especially effective among Black and Latino sexual minority men. *Journal of Consulting and Clinical Psychology, 91*(3), 150–164. https://doi.org/10.1037/ccp0000799.supp

Keyes, K. M., Eaton, N. R., Krueger, R. F., McLaughlin, K. A., Wall, M. M., Grant, B. F., & Hasin, D. S. (2012). Childhood maltreatment and the structure of common psychiatric disorders. *The British Journal of Psychiatry, 200*(2), 107–115.

Kim, H., Turiano, N. A., Forbes, M. K., Kotov, R., Krueger, R. F., Eaton, N. R., & HiTOP Utility Workgroup. (2021). Internalizing psychopathology and all-cause mortality: A comparison of transdiagnostic vs. diagnosis-based risk prediction. *World Psychiatry, 20*(2), 276–282.

Kotov, R., Krueger, R. F., Watson, D., Achenbach, T. M., Althoff, R. R., Bagby, R. M., Brown, T. A., Carpenter, W. T., Caspi, A., Clark, L. A., Eaton, N. R., Forbes, M. K., Forbush, K. T., Goldberg, D. Hasin, D., Hyman, S. E., Ivanova, M. Y., Lynam, D. R., Markon, K., . . . & Zimmerman, M. (2017). The Hierarchical Taxonomy of Psychopathology (HiTOP): A dimensional alternative to traditional nosologies. *Journal of Abnormal Psychology, 126*(4), 454.

Kotov, R., Krueger, R. F., Watson, D., Cicero, D. C., Conway, C. C., DeYoung, C. G., Eaton, N. R., Forbes, M. K., Hallquist, M. N., Latzman, R. D., Mullins-Sweatt, S. N., Ruggero, C. J., Simms, L. J., Waldman, I. D., Waszczuk, M. A., & Wright, A. G. (2021). The Hierarchical Taxonomy of Psychopathology (HiTOP): A quantitative nosology based on consensus of evidence. *Annual Review of Clinical Psychology, 17*, 83–108.

Krueger, R. F., & Bezdjian, S. (2009). Enhancing research and treatment of mental disorders with dimensional concepts: Toward DSM-V and ICD-11. *World Psychiatry, 8*(1), 3.

Krueger, R. F., Chentsova-Dutton, Y. E., Markon, K. E., Goldberg, D. (2003). A cross-cultural study of the structure of comorbidity among common psychopathological syndromes in the general health care setting. *Journal of Abnormal Psychology, 112*, 437–47.

Kuyper, L., & Vanwesenbeeck, I. (2011). Examining sexual health differences between lesbian, gay, bisexual, and heterosexual adults: The role of sociodemographics, sexual behavior characteristics, and minority stress. *Journal of Sex Research, 48*(2–3), 263–274.

Langwerden, R. J., Thompson, M. G., & Wagner, E. F. (2021). Multidimensional conceptualization of identity and psychopathology: Assessing mental health disparities from an intersectional and dimensional framework. *Personality and Mental Health, 15*(4), 293–308.

Lê Cook, B., Doksum, T., Chen, C. N., Carle, A., & Alegría, M. (2013). The role of provider supply and organization in reducing racial/ethnic disparities in mental health care in the US. *Social Science & Medicine, 84*, 102–109.

Lee-Tauler, S. Y., Eun, J., Corbett, D., & Collins, P. Y. (2018). A systematic review of interventions to improve initiation of mental health care among racial-ethnic minority groups. *Psychiatric Services, 69*(6), 628–647.

López, N., & Gadsden, V. L. (2017). Health inequities, social determinants, and intersectionality. In Charlee Alexander, Velma McBride Murry, Kimber Bogard (Eds.), *Perspectives on health equity and social determinants of health* (pp. 1–10). National Academies Press.

Markon, K. E., Chmielewski, M., & Miller, C. J. (2011). The reliability and validity of discrete and continuous measures of psychopathology: A quantitative review. *Psychological Bulletin, 137*(5), 856.

Meyer, I. H. (2003). Prejudice, social stress, and mental health in lesbian, gay, and bisexual populations: Conceptual issues and research evidence. *Psychological Bulletin*, *129*(5), 674.

Mikton, C., & Grounds, A. (2007). Cross-cultural clinical judgment bias in personality disorder diagnosis by forensic psychiatrists in the UK: A case-vignette study. *Journal of Personality Disorders*, *21*(4), 400–417.

Morey, L. C., & Ochoa, E. S. (1989). An investigation of adherence to diagnostic criteria: Clinical diagnosis of the DSM-III personality disorders. *Journal of Personality Disorders*, *3*(3), 180–192.

Morey, L. C., & Benson, K. T. (2016). An investigation of adherence to diagnostic criteria, revisited: Clinical diagnosis of the DSM-IV/DSM-5 Section II personality disorders. *Journal of Personality Disorders*, *30*(1), 130–144.

Mullins-Sweatt, S. N., Hopwood, C. J., Chmielewski, M., Meyer, N. A., Min, J., Helle, A. C., & Walgren, M. D. (2020). Treatment of personality pathology through the lens of the hierarchical taxonomy of psychopathology: Developing a research agenda. *Personality and Mental Health*, *14*(1), 123–141. https://doi.org/10.1002/pmh.1464

Pachankis, J. E. (2015). A transdiagnostic minority stress treatment approach for gay and bisexual men's syndemic health conditions. *Archives of Sexual Behavior*, *44*(7), 1843–1860. https://doi.org/10.1007/s10508-015-0480-x

Pachankis, J. E., Harkness, A., Maciejewski, K. R., Behari, K., Clark, K. A., McConocha, E., Winston, R., Adeyinka, O., Reynolds, J., Bränström, R., Esserman, D. A., Hatzenbuehler, M. L., & Safren, S. A. (2022). LGBQ-affirmative cognitive-behavioral therapy for young gay and bisexual men's mental and sexual health: A three-arm randomized controlled trial. *Journal of Consulting and Clinical Psychology*, *90*(6), 459–477. https://doi.org/10.1037/ccp0000724

Peplau, L. A., & Fingerhut, A. W. (2007). The close relationships of lesbians and gay men. *Annual Review of Psychology*, *58*, 405–424.

Pincus, H. A., Tew Jr., J. D., & First, M. B. (2004). Psychiatric comorbidity: Is more less? *World Psychiatry*, *3*(1), 18.

Porter, H. (2023). It's not my sense of self that's unstable, it's the world's sense of me: The harms of the construct of 'personality disorders' towards transgender communities. *Journal of Psychosocial Studies*, *16*(2), 135–148. https://doi.org/10.1332/147867321X16862340840414

Priester, M. A., Browne, T., Iachini, A., Clone, S., DeHart, D., & Seay, K. D. (2016). Treatment access barriers and disparities among individuals with co-occurring mental health and substance use disorders: An integrative literature review. *Journal of Substance Abuse Treatment*, *61*, 47–59.

Rao, D., Young, M., & Raguram, R. (2007). Culture, somatization, and psychological distress: Symptom presentation in South Indian patients from a public psychiatric hospital. *Psychopathology*, *40*(5), 349–355.

Ringwald, W. R., Nielsen, S. R., Mostajabi, J., Vize, C. E., van den Berg, T., Manuck, S. B., Marsland, A. L., & Wright, A. G. (2024). Characterizing stress processes by linking big five personality states, traits, and day-to-day stressors. *Journal of Research in Personality*, *110*, 104487.

Rodriguez-Seijas, C. (2022). Sociocultural context and the DSM–5 alternative model of personality disorder: Comment on Widiger and Hines (2022). *Personality Disorders: Theory, Research, and Treatment*, *13*(4), 356–359. https://doi.org/10.1037/per0000535

Rodriguez-Seijas, C., Arfer, K. B., Thompson Jr, R. G., Hasin, D. S., & Eaton, N. R. (2017). Sex-related substance use and the externalizing spectrum. *Drug and Alcohol Dependence*, *174*, 39–46.

Rodriguez-Seijas, C., Burton, C. L., & Pachankis, J. E. (2019). Transdiagnostic approaches to improve sexual minority individuals' co-occurring mental, behavioral, and sexual health. In J. E. Pachankis & S. A. Safren (Eds.), *Handbook of evidence-based mental health practice with sexual and gender inorities* (pp. 457–476). Oxford University Press.

Rodriguez-Seijas C., Eaton N. R., Krueger R. F. (2015). How transdiagnostic factors of personality and psychopathology can inform clinical assessment and intervention. *Journal of Personality Assessment*, *97*(5), 425–435. https://doi.org/10.1080/00223891.2015.1055752

Rodriguez-Seijas, C., Eaton, N. R., & Pachankis, J. E. (2019). Prevalence of psychiatric disorders at the intersection of race and sexual orientation: Results from the National Epidemiologic Survey of Alcohol and Related Conditions-III. *Journal of Consulting and Clinical Psychology*, *87*(4), 321.

Rodriguez-Seijas, C., Li, J. J., Balling, C., Brandes, C., Bernat, E., Boness, C. L., Forbes, M. K., Forbush, K. T., Joyner, K. J., Krueger, R. F., Levin-Aspenson, H. F., Michelini, G., Ro, E., Rutter, L., Stanton, K., Tackett, J. L., Waszczuk, M., & Eaton, N. R. (2023). Diversity and the Hierarchical Taxonomy of Psychopathology (HiTOP). *Nature Reviews Psychology*, *2*(8), 483–495. https://doi.org/10.1038/s44159-023-00200-0

Rodriguez-Seijas, C., McClendon, J., Wendt, D. C., Novacek, D. M., Ebalu, T., Hallion, L., Hassan, N. Y., Huson, K., Spielmans, G. I., Folk, J. B., Khazem, L. R., Neblett, E. W., Cunningham, T. J., Hampton-Anderson, J., Steinman, S. A., Hamilton, J. L., & Mekawi, Y. (2024). The next generation of clinical science: Moving toward antiracism. *Clinical Psychological Science*, *12*(3), 526–546.

Rodriguez-Seijas, C., Morgan, T. A., & Zimmerman, M. (2021a). A population-based examination of criterion-level disparities in the diagnosis of borderline personality disorder among sexual minority adults. *Assessment*, *28*(4), 1097–1109. https://doi.org/10.1177/1073191121991922

Rodriguez-Seijas, C., Morgan, T. A., & Zimmerman, M. (2021b). Is there a bias in the diagnosis of borderline personality disorder among lesbian, gay, and bisexual patients? *Assessment*, *28*(3), 724–738. https://doi.org/10.1177/1073191120961833

Rodriguez-Seijas, C., Morgan, T. A., & Zimmerman, M. (2023). Transgender and gender diverse patients are diagnosed with borderline personality disorder more frequently than cisgender patients regardless of personality pathology. *Transgender Health*, *9*(6), 554–565. https://doi.org/10.1089/trgh.2023.0062

Rodriguez-Seijas, C., Rogers, B. G., & Asadi, S. (2023). Personality disorders research and social decontextualization: What it means to be a minoritized human. *Personality Disorders: Theory, Research, and Treatment*, *14*(1), 29–38. https://doi.org/10.1037/per0000600

Rodriguez-Seijas, C., Rogers, B. G., Harkness, A., Safren, S. A., & Pachankis, J. E. (2024). ParTy 'n' Play: Associations between sex-related substance use and the disinhibited externalizing spectrum among gay and bisexual men. *Clinical Psychological Science*, *12*(1), 83–97. https://doi.org/10.1177/21677026231158062

Rogers, B. G., Harkness, A., & Rodriguez-Seijas, C. (2022). 9.07—Sexual minority mental health. In G. J. G. Asmundson (Ed.), *Comprehensive clinical psychology (2nd ed.)* (pp. 96–112). Elsevier. https://doi.org/10.1016/B978-0-12-818697-8.00146-1

Roth, W. D. (2016). The multiple dimensions of race. *Ethnic and Racial Studies*, *39*(8), 1310–1338.

Romanelli, M., Xiao, Y., & Lindsey, M. A. (2020). Sexual identity–behavior profiles and suicide outcomes among heterosexual, lesbian, and gay sexually active adolescents. *Suicide and Life-Threatening Behavior*, *50*(4), 921–933.

Ruggero, C. J., Kotov, R., Hopwood, C. J., First, M., Clark, L. A., Skodol, A. E., Mullins-Sweatt, S. N., Patrick, C. J., Bach, B., Cicero, D. C., Docherty, A., Simms, L. J., Bagby, R. M., Krueger, R. F., Callahan, J. L., Chmielewski, M., Conway, C. C., De Clercq, B. Dornbach-Bender, A., Eaton, N. R., . . . & Zimmermann, J. (2019). Integrating the Hierarchical Taxonomy of Psychopathology (HiTOP) into clinical practice. *Journal of Consulting and Clinical Psychology*, *87*(12), 1069.

Russell, G., Steer, C., & Golding, J. (2011). Social and demographic factors that influence the diagnosis of autistic spectrum disorders. *Social Psychiatry and Psychiatric Epidemiology*, *46*, 1283–1293.

Samuel, D. B., & Widiger, T. A. (2009). Comparative gender biases in models of personality disorder. *Personality and Mental Health*, *3*(1), 12–25.

Sauer-Zavala, S., Southward, M. W., Fruhbauerova, M., Semcho, S. A., Stumpp, N. E., Hood, C. O., Smith, M., Elhusseini, S., & Cravens, L. (2023). BPD compass: A randomized controlled trial of a short-term, personality-based treatment for borderline personality disorder. *Personality Disorders: Theory, Research, and Treatment*, *14*(5), 534.

Scheer, J. R., Clark, K. A., McConocha, E., Wang, K., & Pachankis, J. E. (2023). Toward cognitive-behavioral therapy for sexual minority women: Voices from stakeholders and community members. *Cognitive and Behavioral Practice*, *30*(3), 471–494.

Schwartz, R. C., & Blankenship, D. M. (2014). Racial disparities in psychotic disorder diagnosis: A review of empirical literature. *World Journal of Psychiatry*, *4*(4), 133.

Schwartz, E. K., Docherty, N. M., Najolia, G. M., & Cohen, A. S. (2019). Exploring the racial diagnostic bias of schizophrenia using behavioral and clinical-based measures. *Journal of Abnormal Psychology, 128*(3), 263–271. https://doi.org/10.1037/abn0000409

Seng, J. S., Lopez, W. D., Sperlich, M., Hamama, L., & Meldrum, C. D. R. (2012). Marginalized identities, discrimination burden, and mental health: Empirical exploration of an interpersonal-level approach to modeling intersectionality. *Social Science & Medicine, 75*(12), 2437–2445.

Settles, I. H., Warner, L. R., Buchanan, N. T., & Jones, M. K. (2020). Understanding psychology's resistance to intersectionality theory using a framework of epistemic exclusion and invisibility. *Journal of Social Issues, 76*(4), 796–813. https://doi.org/10.1111/josi.12403

Sharp, C., & Miller, J. D. (2022). Ten-year retrospective on the DSM-5 alternative model of personality disorder: Seeing the forest for the trees. *Personality Disorders: Theory, Research, and Treatment, 13*(4), 301. https://doi.org/10.1037/per0000595

Stein, C. R., Sheridan, M. A., Copeland, W. E., Machlin, L. S., Carpenter, K. L., & Egger, H. L. (2022). Association of adversity with psychopathology in early childhood: Dimensional and cumulative approaches. *Depression and Anxiety, 39*(6), 524–535.

Teachman, B. A., Wilson, J. G., & Komarovskaya, I. (2006). Implicit and explicit stigma of mental illness in diagnosed and healthy samples. *Journal of Social and Clinical Psychology, 25*(1), 75–95.

Verona, E. (2022). Assessment of HiTOP constructs across the population: A commentary on the HiTOP measure development project. *Assessment, 29*(1), 88–92. https://doi.org/10.1177/10731911211048240

Viruell-Fuentes, E. A., Miranda, P. Y., & Abdulrahim, S. (2012). More than culture: structural racism, intersectionality theory, and immigrant health. *Social Science & Medicine, 75*(12), 2099–2106.

Watson, D., Forbes, M. K., Levin-Aspenson, H. F., Ruggero, C. J., Kotelnikova, Y., Khoo, S., Bagby, R. M., Sunderland, M. Patalay, P., & Kotov, R. (2022). The development of preliminary HiTOP internalizing spectrum scales. *Assessment, 29*(1), 17–33.

Widiger, T. A., & Hines, A. (2022). The *Diagnostic and statistical manual of mental disorders, Fifth Edition* alternative model of personality disorder. *Personality Disorders: Theory, Research, and Treatment, 13*(4), 347–355. https://doi.org/10.1037/per0000524

Williams, D. T. (2019). A call to focus on racial domination and oppression: A response to "Racial and ethnic inequality in poverty and affluence, 1959–2015". *Population Research and Policy Review, 38*(5), 655–663.

World Health Organization. (2019). *International statistical classification of diseases and related health problems* (11th ed.). World Health Organization.

Zablotsky, B., & Alford, J. M. (2020). Racial and ethnic differences in the prevalence of attention-deficit/hyperactivity disorder and learning disabilities among US children aged 3–17 years. NCHS Data Brief. No. 358. *National Center for Health Statistics.*

Zimmerman, M., Benjamin, I., & Rodriguez-Seijas, C. (2022). Psychiatric diagnoses among transgender and gender diverse patients compared with cisgender patients. *Journal of Clinical Psychiatry, 83*(6), 43020.

CHAPTER 23

Prospects for a Consensual Dimensional Model of Psychopathology

CHRISTOPHER J. HOPWOOD

Introduction

I was asked to "evaluate the prospects for rapprochement among disciples of different dimensional traditions and explore research programs that could quantitatively synthesize various dimensional frameworks." I structured this task into three parts. The first part is distinguishing major approaches to dimensional diagnosis. The second part is comparing these approaches in terms of their approach to dimensional diagnosis, across three possible and increasingly strict definitions of the word "dimensional." The third part is articulating how these models could be quantitatively synthesized, in the context of underlying value differences and a general lack of knowledge about psychopathology that make consensual integration challenging and, in some ways, perhaps even undesirable.

Four Paradigms

There are many specific models of mental health problems. These models vary along different axes and levels of complexity, such that there is considerable variability and debate within major traditions. The editors offered the DSM-5 Alternative Model of Personality Disorders (AMPD), psychodynamic, interpersonal, Research Domain Criteria (RDoC), network, and Hierarchical Taxonomy of Psychopathology (HiTOP) approaches as examples. Many people would organize these and other perspectives in different ways. My strategy was to use the concept of paradigms (Kuhn, 1962; Loevinger, 1987; Wiggins, 2003) to distinguish different approaches. Paradigms can be differentiated by the kind of information that is prioritized when thinking about mental health problems, the primary methods used to sort mental health data, social networks, and the goals underlying these differences (Table 23.1). Key to the idea of paradigms and the theme of this chapter is that, because of different underlying epistemologies, paradigms evaluate evidence differently, and this complicates direct comparison or quantitative synthesis.

Medical Paradigm

Although this is a progressive volume written in the spirit, which moves me as well, that the field should leave the traditional approaches in the past, it is important to acknowledge that we are not there yet. The medical model (Aftab, this volume) has been the primary organizer of psychiatric taxonomy since the publication of the third edition of the *Diagnostic and Statistical*

Manual of Mental Disorders (DSM) in 1980, and it continues to be. In this model, mental health symptoms are arranged into polythetic categories that describe ostensibly different groups of people. "Polythetic" means that a diagnosis requires some subset of all possible symptoms. For instance, there are nine possible symptoms of major depressive disorder, and a patient must have five of them to be diagnosed. This model prioritizes the problems patients present with and attempts to fit those problems into categories of disease. The primary data source is the kinds of problems that people present with, as interpreted by the clinician, and the underlying cause is generally assumed to be some kind of biological dysfunction, or at least a biologically mediated response to some kind of environmental stressor. Given the roots of this model in medicine, it is implicit that the psychiatrist is most capable of assessing symptoms and determining diagnoses.

The medical model was built upon the clinical tradition of rich description within psychiatry (Blashfield, 2012; Zachar et al., 2014). Emil Kraepelin (1905) is often given credit for this tradition, although there are certain ways in which the modern medical model deviates from Kraepelin's approach (Engstrom & Kendler, 2015). Kraepelin, a physician, published several editions of a very influential taxonomy in which mental disorders were organized based on shared features and the patient's history, similar in certain ways to the DSM. However, in the early to mid-20th century, when European and American psychiatry was the most dominant force in mental health research and practice, psychoanalysis was the dominant paradigm in psychiatry (Klerman, 1990). Diagnostic manuals such as the DSM existed but were relatively unimportant, and diagnosis was typically based on psychodynamic models, of which there were many, none of which were particularly influential on psychodynamic or other kinds of practice (Kendler et al., 2010). Generally speaking, diagnosis was unreliable and inconsistent (Beck, 1962), because systems were not well-coordinated (Blum, 1978), assessment approaches were not well validated (Horwitz, 2014), and diagnoses were based on highly inferential phenomena that were difficult to assess (Spitzer, 2001). In the late 1970s, a relatively small group of politically influential psychiatrists published several persuasive papers (Feighner et al., 1972; Robins & Guze, 1970) on a new approach to taxonomy that ultimately framed the DSM-III and came to be known as the (neo-Kraepelinian) medical model. These authors argued that the legitimacy of diagnoses should be based on five specific criteria: reliable description of features, "lab studies" (potentially including psychometric tests) consistent with this description, the establishment of boundaries from other conditions, follow-up studies to rule out other causes of symptoms, and family studies to establish relatedness. These are the foundational principles of diagnosis in the DSM-III, IV, and 5, as well as corresponding editions of the International Classification of Diseases (ICD). It must have been as exciting to be a part of the medical paradigm revolution that was generating a new and more evidence-based approach to diagnosis then as it is to be a part of the dimensional paradigm revolution now (Klerman, 1978).

Despite multiple problems discussed in the following paragraphs, the medical model is currently sustained by the inertia exerted by the diagnostic manuals and ancillary institutions. People with mental health problems throughout the world are given diagnostic codes based on the DSM/ICD. Likewise, legal, funding, and other institutions tend to view psychopathology through the lens of the medical model, as do most laypeople. The medical model has also organized intervention research for the last several decades. For example, the approach that is generally given most weight involves randomizing people with the same diagnosis to different treatments. The dominance of the randomized controlled trial (RCT) as an intervention research method illustrates the political power of an accepted paradigm. In fact, the underlying assumptions of medical models of psychopathology actually do not align that well with major theoretical models of psychotherapy. For instance, the roots of cognitive behavioral therapy (CBT) lie in a behavioral tradition that is highly skeptical of abstract latent constructs such as mental disorders (Koerner et al., 1996; Skinner, 1963). Yet CBT became the dominant approach to psychotherapy in the medical model era by adopting the medical model approach to diagnosis and applying the RCT method to test and advance its approach to treatment (Baker et al., 2008).

One strength of the medical model is that it offers a practical and useful way to classify patients (Haeffel et al., 2022). Its standardization and familiarity has value for communication across disciplines, between researchers and clinicians, between clinicians and patients, and between the mental health community and the general public. It aligns relatively well with the norms and practices in medicine more generally and provides a structure for organizing mental health institutions, treatments, and the like. A case can also be made that the existing evidence for the clinical utility of potential alternatives is insufficient to justify the massive effort that would be required in transforming psychiatric taxonomy away from the medical model (First, 2005).

However, there are also good reasons for its waning popularity. It generally has not led to better models of etiology (Cuthbert & Insel, 2013). The practical hope of symptom descriptive models was that distinguishing diagnoses on the one hand and classes of intervention (e.g., different pharmaceuticals or combinations of cognitive-behavioral techniques) on the other would lead to effective matching algorithms (Auerbach & Childress, 1987; Millon, 1983). If successful, psychiatric diagnoses could indicate a specific treatment most likely to be effective for a specific and diagnostically homogeneous group of people. Reasonable people can disagree about how much progress this approach has made (Beutler et al., 2012; Miller et al., 2013), but no reasonable person can say that the promise was fulfilled or that psychiatric categories provide a specific way to determine the form of intervention that is most likely to be useful for a particular patient (Leichsenring et al., 2022).

Moreover, specific practical and conceptual problems have been identified that have largely been the inspiration for other approaches. For instance, it is now well established that there are undesirably high levels of comorbidity (when the same person has multiple diagnoses; Brown et al., 2001) and heterogeneity (when two people with the same diagnosis are symptomatically different from one another; Allsopp et al., 2019). Decades of research show that neither psychometric nor biological evidence conform well to the DSM taxonomy, and this evidence represents exhibit A in the case for psychometric and biological paradigms, respectively, as described in the next sections. Concerns have also been expressed about process, and in particular the prioritization of committee-based decisions to determine taxonomy, the relative representation of medicine and psychiatry on these committees, and the openness and responsiveness of this system to evidence (Krueger et al., 2014).

Psychometric Paradigm

Psychometric models prioritize evidence about the between-person co-variance structure of mental health problems (i.e., how symptoms or disorders correlate with one another across people) to generate a psychiatric taxonomy. The theoretical basis for these models comes from the construct validation approach to test development, as articulated in a series of foundational papers in the middle of the 20th century (Campbell & Fiske, 1959; Cronbach & Meehl, 1955; Loevinger, 1957). The construct validation approach asserts that the best way to learn about a construct is to generate a method for assessing that construct, so that psychometric research on the assessment tool essentially equates to theoretical tests of the construct itself (Loevinger, 1957). There are three steps to developing and studying an assessment method/theoretical model. The first is to connect the content of the measure to the theoretical content of the measure. In the case of psychopathology, the content is all of the problems that

TABLE 23.1 Four Paradigms of Psychopathology

Paradigm	Medical	Psychometric	Biological	Psychodynamic
Examplar	DSM / ICD	HiTOP	RDoC	PDM/OPD
Primary Data Source	Clinician assessments of patient presenting problems	Patient report of problems on standardized measures	Neurophysiological assessments	Clinical interviews and the therapeutic process
Primary Taxonomic Strategy	Arrangement of symptoms into disorders based on clinical description	Arrangement of symptoms into dimensions based on factor analysis	Alignment of symptoms with underlying biological processes	Arrangement of symptoms based on psychoanalytic theory
Social Network	Applied psychiatrists	Quantitative psychologists	Biologically oriented scientists and practictioners	Psychoanalytic clinicians
Underlying Goal	Distinguish putatively homogeneous groups with similar mental health problems	Identify the underlying structure of mental health problems	Understand how the body and brain mediate mental health problems	Understand the meaning of peoples' mental health problems

Note. DSM = Diagnostic and Statistical Manual of Mental Disorders. ICD = International Classification of Diseases. HiTOP = Hierarchical Taxonomy of Psychopathology. RDoC = Research Domain Criteria. PDM = Psychodynamic Diagnostic Manual. OPD = Operationalized Psychodynamic Diagnosis.

mental health patients might present with, which most people within the psychometric tradition are willing to roughly operationalize as all of the symptoms in the DSM. The second is to examine the internal validity of this content. Internal validity includes the reliability of individual constructs and the structure of those constructs in relation to one another. Based on other assumptions common in this paradigm (e.g., that these symptoms reflect features of latent dimensions; see Borsboom and Cramer [2013] for an alternative perspective), co-variance (e.g., factor) analysis is the main procedure for examining the structure of psychopathology symptoms. Co-variance analysis is a broad term that includes a range of specific techniques, all of which have in common the derivation of latent dimensions based on co-variance patterns within a set of indicators. The third step is to examine external validity, or how identified dimensions are related to other phenomena, like treatment utilization, suicide risk, the effectiveness of different kinds of treatments, etc. Both medical and psychometric perspectives basically agree about the content (symptoms or features) of psychopathology, and external validity proceeds, in either case, from the way this content is structured. The core difference is in the approach to structuring the content, and the model that eventuates therefrom.

Example models/measures from this tradition are criterion B of the AMPD as measured by the Personality Inventory for DSM-5 (Krueger et al., 2012), various measures of the five-factor (McCrae & John, 1992) and interpersonal circumplex models (Gifford & O'Connor, 1987), and HiTOP (Kotov et al., 2017). Although based to a somewhat lesser degree on co-variance analysis per se, popular clinical instruments like the MMPI (Sellbom et al., 2021) and PAI (Ruiz et al., 2018) are also congenial with this model. Other chapters in this volume illustrate some of these models in detail. There are naturally important differences among each of these specific schemes, but for the purposes of this chapter I will focus on what they have in common. All of them prioritize verbally mediated data (structured interviews and especially questionnaires), all of them assume and/or conclude from evidence that variation in psychopathology can be organized into latent dimensions, and all of them prioritize analyses of individual differences, typically in cross-sectional data, via psychometric techniques as a way to determine the structure of these dimensions. In this chapter, I will focus on HiTOP as the most prominent current representation of the psychometric paradigm (this model is described in detail by Pham and Forbes, this volume).

The psychometric approach represents perhaps the most likely candidate to succeed the medical model as a paradigm for psychopathology taxonomy. It is already the dominant paradigm for research and clinical assessment within clinical and personality psychology, the discipline from which it came. Its success owes in part to political dynamics and momentum, such as the increasing influence of the HiTOP consortium (Eaton et al., 2023), but also to specific strengths. One strength is the fact that different models and measures consistently converge on a very similar hierarchical framework. While slight differences may emerge depending on item or person sampling, and convergence tends to be stronger for broad than narrow dimensions, the specific dimensions of psychometric models of psychopathology are fairly robust across interview, self-report, and informant-reported data (Boudreaux et al., 2019; Ringwald et al., 2023; Wright et al., 2013); clinical and non-clinical samples (Bagby et al., 2002);, and measures designed to assess general psychopathology, normal range personality, and personality disorders (Markon et al., 2005; Wright & Simms, 2015). There is also greater alignment with biological models of psychopathology than is the case for the medical models (Latzman et al., 2021). This level of convergence across methods supports the validity of the dimensions that constitute models like HiTOP, and particularly dimensions at the broader levels of the hierarchy.

A hierarchical model of dimensions also solves problems in the medical model (Ruggero et al., 2019). For instance, it provides a straightforward explanation for comorbidity: people would be expected to have more than one diagnosis if they have elevated levels on a broad trait that explains the co-variation among diagnostic categories. One example is that depression and anxiety can be thought of as facets of a broader internalizing or neuroticism domain, and thus people with high levels of neuroticism would be expected to be both depressed and anxious. A hierarchical model moreover provides a coherent way to conceptualize heterogeneity, in that two individuals with the same primary problems may differ from one another on other features within the model. For instance, a person with post-traumatic stress symptoms who is personologically detached and withdrawn would be expected to present differently than a person with post-traumatic stress symptoms who is extraverted and enthusiastic.

In terms of process, the argument has been made that HiTOP is more empirically based, politically transparent, and responsive to evidence than the medical model. A direct comparison of the criteria for modifying the model (Forbes et al., 2024) as well as the political processes through which decisions are made, supports this argument. Whereas judgments about DSM diagnoses and diagnostic criteria are made by committees organized by an editor and judged by the board of trustees of the American Psychiatric Association, HiTOP has a more egalitarian and evidence-based process for updating the model (Forbes et al., 2024). However, this may be a function of the relative age of these two systems; it is often the case that newer philosophical or political movements are more idealistic, transparent, and egalitarian than older ones. It is also not the case that the medical model or any of the other paradigms discussed here are not evidence-based, although the kinds of evidence that are prioritized and how they influence decisions varies.

The ultimate success of the HiTOP model for practice likely hinges most directly on its ability to tangibly improve public mental health, relative to the medical model. There is some evidence that major dimensions of psychopathology help clinicians make more reliable prognostic predictions than medical model categories (Waszczuk et al., 2022). On the other hand, there is also limited evidence that clinicians who use psychometric as opposed to medical models to organize assessment data achieve better clinical outcomes (Weekers et al., 2024). Other questions are also important but have received relatively little research attention. Would more effective treatment matching algorithms be identified if they were based on dimensional models, and could a psychometric model of psychopathology dimensions help facilitate more personalized care? Would courts make fairer decisions? Would the public save money because of the greater efficiency and effectiveness of the mental health system? Would people with mental health problems be less stigmatized? These are complex questions for reasons that go beyond the classification system being used, but ultimately an improved classification system should lead to better practical outcomes like these. Although it is reasonable to bet, given its other strengths, that a model of psychopathology based on co-variance structure will be more clinically useful than one based on the medical model, evidence to that effect is not yet strong, and the clinical utility of the psychometric approaches, relative to the medical model, remains an important topic for research (Su et al., this volume).

Biological Paradigm

The premise of biological models is that understanding the underlying biological structures and processes that are involved in both normal range and maladaptive behavior is necessary for generating a valid model of psychopathology. This premise rests on an understanding of psychopathology in terms of mediating bodily processes. The primary data sources for this approach are physiological and in particular neuroscientific, and the methods used to examine these data depend heavily on the type of variables involved.

At the time it was being formulated in the 1970s, the medical model that inspired the DSM-III was considered biological, insofar as the hope was that effectively grouping patients based on descriptive characteristics would make it more likely that underlying biological etiologies would be identified (Feighner et al., 1972). However, neuroscientific evidence accumulated since that time showed that the DSM categories do not map well onto the central nervous and other bodily systems (Casey et al., 2013). Moreover, understanding of neuroscience has become significantly more nuanced. For instance, the search for specific genes as causes for common disorders is largely over (Smoller et al., 2019), and it is now widely appreciated that psychosocial factors can also cause mental health symptoms, even if such symptoms are mediated by biological processes (Lilienfeld & Pinto, 2015).

As a result of both advances in neuroscience and the limitations of the medical model, the United States National Institutes of Mental Health developed the Research Domain Criteria (RDoC), a model of individual differences in psychopathology explicitly based on neurobiological systems (Insel et al., 2010). Although there are different biological models of psychopathology (Buchsbaum & Haier, 1983; Fowles, 1993; Thomas & Sharp, 2019), I will focus here on RDoC as the most prominent representative of the biological paradigm.

Rather than being based on symptom descriptions, the starting point for RDoC are the neural systems that are responsible for implementing the primary behavioral functions that are mediated by the brain (Cuthbert & Insel, 2013). RDoC is organized around five overall systems: negative valence (e.g., fear), positive valence (e.g., approach), cognitive (e.g., attention), social (e.g., attachment), and arousal (e.g., sleep/wake). Each system is parsed into both different subsystems and different levels of analysis ranging from self-reported attitudes and behaviors to genes.

The relative correspondence between the RDoC systems and the dimensions identified via factor analyses of symptoms is striking and suggests some possibility for integrating the biological and psychometric perspectives (Harkness, Reynolds, & Lilienfeld, 2014; Michelini et al., 2021). However, whereas the relative clinical utility of psychometric and medical models is debatable, a common criticism of biological models is that they are not sufficiently developed to be applied in everyday clinical diagnosis (Cuthbert, 2020). Indeed, many mental health treatments are psychosocial in nature and pharmacological interventions are organized primarily around descriptive symptoms. Moreover, the utility of biological assessment approaches for most common mental health problems is not well established, and the reliability of such approaches is often weak (Lilienfeld & Pinto, 2015). Indeed, RDoC does not aspire to provide a practical system for diagnosis, although it hopes to generate a more solid basis for future diagnostic systems (Insel, 2009).

Psychodynamic Paradigm

The psychodynamic paradigm is arguably the most heterogeneous of the four listed here. There is wide variability in terms of data source, presumed mechanisms of development, personality, and psychopathology (Barber & Solomonov, 2016; Greenberg & Mitchell, 1983), treatment technique (Connolly et al., 2008), and the relative importance placed upon empirical research (Bornstein, 2005) and psychiatric diagnosis (Bornstein, 2001). What all psychodynamic approaches share is an interest in making sense out of psychological data that do not appear to make sense (Loevinger, 1966). This tradition traces back to Freud, who realized that his extensive neuropsychological training was not all that useful in treating his patients, whereas the talking cure he developed with Breuer (Breuer & Freud, 1895), in which meaning is discovered in the thoughts and verbal content that initially seem meaningless, was. This perspective is also present in all of the major approaches to psychodynamic psychotherapy, in which some process of understanding and reflecting the patient's relationships with the therapist, themselves, and their attachment relationships in order to help the patient develop greater insight about themselves is considered a core mechanism (Fonagy et al., 2005).

Models within the psychodynamic paradigm share certain assumptions that guide its approach to taxonomy. These assumptions include that people are not often aware of why they do the things that they do; that problems repeat across contexts and time in a way that is patterned and thus predictable; that problems often arise as an attempted resolution among different motivations with one another and/or the constraints of reality; that attachment relationships play a particularly important role in generating, maintaining, and alleviating mental health problems; and that developmental processes are critical for understanding a person's mental functioning. Given the emphasis on factors that are outside of the patient's awareness, self-report questionnaires or symptom-based interviews are typically not regarded as sufficient for diagnosis. Rather, the dynamics of a person's mental health problems emerge in peoples' interactions, such as the way they respond to stress (i.e., defense mechanisms), the way they understand and behave in their relationships (i.e., object relations), and in the consistency and valence of their sense of self (i.e., identity). As such, a relatively intensive interaction with a trained professional who can both elicit and perceive such dynamics is thought to be required for accurate case conceptualization and diagnosis.

However, this can be facilitated by a standardized and structured model of diagnostic constructs. Two prominent contemporary models are the Psychodynamic Diagnostic Manual (PDM; PDM Task Force, 2006), developed in the United States; and the Operationalized

Psychodynamic Diagnostic (OPD; OPD Task Force, 2008), developed in Germany. There are significant differences in the way the PDM and OPD approach diagnosis, but I will focus here on what these models have in common.

First, they distinguish a general maturation dimension from specific kinds of problems (as does the Alternative Model of Personality Disorders in the DSM-5). From a psychodynamic perspective, the main driver of the potential to have mental health problems, in general, has to do with psychological maturation. To the degree that people develop increasingly sophisticated ways to manage stress, a clearer and more realistic sense of themselves, prosocial attitudes and goals, and more mature, empathic, and mutually satisfying relations with others, they are more likely to adapt to a range of circumstances and less likely to experience psychological problems (Kernberg, 1967; Loevinger, 1983; Sharp & Wall, 2021). This dimension has been given various labels, including ego development, personality organization, level of personality functioning (in the AMPD), structural integration (in the OPD), and profile of mental functioning (in the PDM). Its importance for diagnosis is that the lower a person's level, the more difficulties they will have adapting to life, in general. Its connection to psychometric and medical models is that the lower a person's level of personality functioning, the more disorders (medical model) or the less adaptive across all pathology dimensions (psychometric model) the person is likely to be.

Distinct from this general dimension of maturity and adaptation versus psychiatric severity are specific patterns of behavior, thoughts, internal conflicts, and patterns of defense. This is where differences in the PDM and OPD are most apparent. In the PDM, there are five levels: (1) experience of illness (subjective report of presenting problems), (2) interpersonal relations, (3) motivational conflicts, (4) structure (the dimension described in the previous paragraph), and (5) mental and somatic disorders (which correspond to ICD categories). In the PDM, there are three levels: (1) personality patterns and disorders (which correspond roughly to DSM personality disorder categories), (2) profile of mental functioning, and (3) symptom patterns (which correspond roughly to DSM disorder categories).

The sustained prevalence of practitioners throughout the world who use psychodynamic approaches in their work speaks to the perceived clinical utility of this paradigm. Although psychotherapy research suggests that psychodynamic approaches are not generally superior or inferior to other forms of psychotherapy (Cuijpers et al., 2021; Steinert et al., 2017), the psychodynamic paradigm connects diagnosis to psychotherapeutic practice more closely than do any of the other paradigms listed above.

Summary

Many hybrid models reflect elements of each of these classes. There are also theoretical models that attempt to integrate each of these perspectives (e.g., Contemporary Integrative Interpersonal Theory; see Pincus et al., this volume). But for the purposes of this chapter, moving forward with these imperfect categories should be at least somewhat useful for a discussion of how different approaches can be synthesized.

Three Meanings of the Word "Dimension"

Paradigmatic synthesis is complicated by the use of the word "dimension" to mean at least three different things in the psychopathology literature (Hopwood et al., 2023). In this section, I will distinguish these three meanings from one another and then compare each of the four paradigms described above in terms of these three different meanings. The three meanings of dimensions that I will distinguish are continuous, unidimensional, and hierarchical.

Continuous

By continuous, I mean that indicators of a psychopathology construct can be added up as a symptom count to indicate severity, rather than cut at some point in the distribution to indicate the difference between people who have versus people who do not have a disorder. There is relatively convincing evidence that all psychopathology constructs, as they are typically measured and defined, have continuous distributions (Haslam et al., 2012). There is strong evidence that treating them as continua improves reliability and validity, whereas dichotomizing mental health constructs loses information (Markon et al., 2011). For these reasons, it should be uncontroversial that there is value in treating mental health constructs as continua across paradigms. At the same time, there can be a practical reality that a patient must either be given or not given a diagnosis in many contexts, such as for determining eligibility for certain services or communication with thirdparty payers. Thus, there is often a clinical necessity of applying a categorical decision to a dimension. Different paradigms take different approaches to this issue.

The medical model paradigm consists almost exclusively of non-continuous categorical diagnoses. It is possible to think of these diagnoses as symptom counts, and thus continua, but manuals like the DSM or ICD use standard cut scores to indicate the presence or absence of diagnosis. The fact that these cut scores are taken seriously (insofar as they are used to represent the difference between having or not having a medical condition) likely contributes to the reification of psychiatric disorders, in the form of the beliefs like people either "have" or "don't have" depression (Hyman, 2010). These cut scores also impact the findings from epidemiological research designed to calculate the rates of disorders in a population, which in turn affects public perception, funding allocation, perceptions of diagnostic increases or decreases over time, and other important consequences (Gould et al., 1981). This is despite the fact that cut scores in the DSM were largely based on the very questionable standard of matching prevalence rates observed via unstandardized diagnoses (Spitzer et al., 1990). Thus, the relative lack of appreciation or assertion within the medical model paradigm that diagnostic thresholds are practical solutions rather than ontological realities is problematic.

Empirical evidence that psychological problems are distributed continuously is embedded into the psychometric and biological formulations of mental health. These paradigms have the opposite problem as the medical model, in that generating a clinically useful model would require establishing cut scores for diagnosis, in the absence of empirical evidence about where that cut score should lie.

Psychodynamic approaches vary in their treatment of this issue. The general severity dimension (personality functioning in the AMPD, structure in the OPD, and mental functioning in the PDM) is understood as a continuous albeit complex dimension, such that patients can be placed into specific levels of severity within a single continuum. However, different types of problems are generally treated as categories, either via prototype diagnosis (e.g., PDM personality patterns and disorders) or as imported from the DSM or ICD (Table 23.2).

Unidimensional

By unidimensional, I mean that there is psychometric evidence that all indicators of a continuous dimension are also indicators of an underlying construct. Here we can see important differences between the different paradigms.

Many medical model diagnoses are largely not unidimensional. Psychometric research shows that common diagnoses such as depression (van Loo et al., 2012), schizophrenia (Smith,

TABLE 23.2 Approach of Four Psychopathology Paradigms to Three Meanings of Dimensionality

	Continuous	Unidimensional	Hierarchical
Medical	Disorders are categorical, but could be treated as symptom counts	Many disorders are not unidimensional	Symptoms are grouped into disorders that are grouped chapters based on clinical presentation and tradition
Psychometric	Dimensions are continuous	Dimensions are unidimensional	Dimensions are organized into a hierarchy based on evidence of co-variation
Biological	Dimensions are continuous	Psychometric evidence about dimensionality is given less weight than neuropsychological evidence	Dimensions are organized into a hierarchy based on biological level of analysis
Psychodynamic	Dimensions are continuous but can be combined into prototypical diagnostic categories	Unidimensionality of dimensions is often not well-established or considered important	Dimensions are organized into a hierarchy based on psychological level of analysis

Mar, & Turoff, 1998) and borderline personality disorder (Sanislow et al., 2002) have multiple factors. However, unidimensionality does not appear to be a particularly important criterion in establishing the symptoms of disorders, which are driven more by clinical tradition than psychometric evidence, per se. Moreover, it is common for very similar indicators to be treated as symptoms of more than one disorder (Forbes et al., 2023), which is not something you would do if you believed each construct in your system represents a single, coherent, and distinct dimension.

In contrast, the psychometric paradigm takes unidimensionality quite seriously. The unidimensionality of a given scale is typically tested in a latent variable model before its external validity is examined, and indeed one of the most common metrics of reliability has to do with the degree to which the items conform to a unidimensional model (Revelle & Condon, 2019). There is a complexity to this concept, in that psychometric models can be hierarchical, such that broad traits are parsed into narrower traits. In this sense, unidimensional refers to the co-variance of indicators at successive levels; for instance, single items might be considered the indicators with respect to narrow dimensions, whereas sets of narrow dimensions can serve as the indicators of broader dimensions. This is discussed in more detail in describing the third meaning of dimension below.

In the biological approach, coherence is sought between a particular psychological function and different levels of biological structures and processes. For instance, the fear construct within the negative valence system of the RDoC framework describes fear as a unidimensional construct across different levels of analysis. It is possible that factor analyses of the indicators of fear at each of these different levels of analysis may produce different results, and RDoC is not prescriptive regarding how exactly each level of analysis should be measured or the degree to which measures should be supported by evidence of unidimensionality. Thus, it is possible that RDoC measures may not be dimensional in the sense that a given measure or set of measures of certain RDoC constructs may not meet psychometric standards of unidimensionality.

The psychodynamic approach is also not as concerned with this property of dimensions as is the psychometric approach. Psychodynamic measures are often evaluated for their unidimensionality (Cierpka et al., 2007; Taubner et al., 2013), however, psychodynamic taxonomists have proposed prototype approaches to diagnosis that mix different dimensions together (Westen et al., 2006), and these approaches have strongly influenced the PDM. In the psychodynamic approach, coherence emerges not from a model of between-person co-variance among constructs as in the psychometric paradigm, but within individuals via formulations that integrate different levels of analysis, internal conflicts, etc. It is less important that these indicators form unidimensional dimensions in nomothetic group data than that they can be used to describe the important features of unique individuals in a way that clinicians find useful (Westen et al., 2006). The validity of this assumption for clinical prediction and other activities remains an open question (Eaton et al., 2011; Yalch et al., 2012), but this difference in perspective explains why it may be less important to a psychodynamic clinician that a measure is unidimensional than that its score conveys information of interest.

Hierarchical

The most restrictive definition of dimensional is that dimensional models can be organized into a framework in which distinct (unidimensional) constructs can be distinguished from one another based on their patterns of associations. The only paradigm whose models are expected to meet this criterion is the psychometric. In the HiTOP structure, different constructs within the factor level are empirically distinct from one another, meaning that if a factor analysis were conducted on the indicators at the subfactor level, separate factors would be identified that would correspond to the factors. For instance, the subfactors sexual problems, eating problems, fear, distress, and mania are all considered indicators of the internalizing factor (with mania cross-loading on the thought disorder factor).

However, each of the other paradigms can be considered hierarchical in a different way and based on different criteria. The medical model is hierarchical in the sense that symptoms cluster into disorders and these disorders in turn cluster into chapters. In some cases, there are subsets of symptoms within a certain disorder and subsets of disorders within a certain chapter. Psychodynamic taxonomies are similar, in the sense that there are hierarchies (symptoms are understood within broader constructs involving internal conflicts and personality organization). However, in both cases this organization is based on committee reviews of various kinds of evidence (as well as psychological theory in the case of psychodynamic approaches), rather than on strict psychometric evidence. The biological model is hierarchical in the sense that broad systems are understood to have subsystems, such as the fear, anxiety, sustained threat, loss, and frustrative nonreward subsystems of the negative valence system. However, again, this hierarchy is based on a range of considerations (https://www.nimh.nih.gov/research/research-funded-by-nimh/rdoc/positive-valence-systems-workshop-proceedings) and not strictly on how verbally mediated measures of these dimensional constructs are related to one another.

This third meaning of dimension is important because it highlights important differences between the paradigms. When a person from within the psychometric perspective argues for "dimensional models of psychopathology," they very likely mean that the psychopathology taxonomy should be composed of unidimensional continuous variables whose organization is based on patterns of co-variance and discrimination within a comprehensive hierarchical factor model. None of the other paradigms would produce models that qualify as "dimensional" from this perspective, but that is in part because they do not aspire to. This raises interesting questions about what it would mean to synthesize different models, and the degree to which models from one paradigm ought to be evaluated based on the criteria valued by a different paradigm.

Synthesis?

I was asked to specifically indicate how a quantitative synthesis between these different approaches might be achieved, toward an integrative dimensional system. The challenge with synthesis traces back to the fact that paradigms are not fully commensurable, meaning that they do not place equal weight on the same kinds of evidence. Testing differences between these approaches in a way that is faithful to the epistemology of each is possible in certain ways. For instance, it would be possible to randomize clinicians to receive either DSM diagnoses, HiTOP profiles, RDoC profiles, or PDM diagnoses, and test whether treatments in one condition are more effective than treatments in others. But many differences cannot be directly tested, because they are based on different values and assumptions about what counts as the most important kind of evidence.

There is some trans-paradigmatic evidence regarding dimensional diagnosis. For instance, all paradigms should acknowledge that mental health problems are almost always distributed continuously. They should also agree that treating them that way confers greater reliability and validity, and thus assessment data should preserve the relative differences in severity that distinguishes patients across diagnostic constructs to the extent possible. Finally, they should all agree that there remains the practical problem of deciding whether a person should receive a diagnosis or not, and that there are not good empirical solutions to this problem.

However, beyond this, there is a risk that the assumptions of a paradigm that happens to enjoy popularity in one particular historical moment imposes its epistemology, through political force, onto other paradigms. For instance, as the influence of the psychometric model ascends, it is fair to ask whether all perspectives should agree that all their constructs must be organized, via psychometric methods, into hierarchies of increasingly narrow dimensions. The biological perspective might take a principled position that the diagnostic hierarchy should be based on the kinds of biological processes that mediate behavior, and that when a factor is identified in psychometric data that does not map well onto brain systems, it should be considered a methodological artifact. The psychodynamic perspective might argue that there is an important qualitative difference among different kinds of concepts (e.g., level of personality functioning and specific constellations of defense) that would be lost if they were all measured and evaluated in the same way, as is done in psychometric models (Hopwood, 2025).

A Pessimistic and an Optimistic View

So where do we go from here? There is a pessimistic and an optimistic way of thinking about prospects for quantitative synthesis.

The pessimistic way of looking at things can be illustrated with an example. Suppose we knew nothing about medical problems, and we wanted to generate a taxonomy. Patients would complain about certain kinds of symptoms: bellyaches, toothaches, sleepiness, insomnia, etc. A statistician could collect information from all the patients in a population and generate a model of how they co-vary, in a manner very similar to the psychometric approach described in this chapter. Biomedical researchers would examine the bodies of the patients, to try to figure out what part of the body was affected and generate mechanistic theories of disease.

They would generate a taxonomy based on anatomy and physiology, in a manner like the biological approach described here. Clinicians would observe their patients closely, in the hopes of building a knowledge base about what kinds of causes tend to be implicated and what kinds of interventions tend to help, and generate a taxonomy based on these perceived functional relationships, like the psychodynamic approach. While the world waited for these different approaches to make progress, a practical contingent would simply list all the problems that people seem to have and try to group them into bins as best they can to develop a useful means of communication, similar to the medical model approach.

It is difficult to imagine that these four approaches would generate the same taxonomy. Why should a factor analysis of symptoms reveal differences among the nervous, vascular, and endocrine systems? Why should experience of what kinds of interventions work correspond to the major domains of a psychometric model? Why should a better understanding of how the organs work tell us much about what it is like to be sick? This view is pessimistic in the sense that there is no clear path to an integrative model. Moreover, natural and institutional incentives for tribalism and against dialectical thinking would inhibit the kinds of multimethod, transdisciplinary approaches that would be necessary to progress toward a consensual dimensional model. Back to the current question of psychopathology: even if these incentives could be overcome, synthesis is a very hard problem, given how much is unknown about the nature and causes of mental health problems.

But there is also a more optimistic medical analogy for this problem (Karamanou et al., 2016). There was a time, beginning roughly 3,500 years ago, when doctors observed that patients who reported swelling appendages and significant swings in mood and energy would often die soon after. They also noticed around that time that such patients often had sweet urine, as evidenced by its smell, taste, or attractiveness to ants. This led to the hypothesis that manipulating the diet could be helpful. With this knowledge about both which symptoms tended to correlate and some clues about the functions of those systems, anatomists were eventually able to isolate the processing of sugars in the liver as the locus of the problem in the 19th century. This led to insulin-based treatments for diabetes that saved lives beginning in the 20th century, and a world in which individuals with diabetes can live normal and healthy lives.

In other words, it was the combination of clustering patients with common problems (as emphasized by the medical model paradigm), the statistical understanding of how patient-reported symptoms co-vary (as emphasized by the psychometric paradigm), the clinician's understanding of the functions of those symptoms (as emphasized by the psychodynamic paradigm), and the biologist's understanding of the underlying mechanisms of those symptoms (as emphasized by the biological paradigm) that led to a valid diagnosis and effective treatment. One can imagine a similar path in mental health, with the major caveat being that whereas a focal cause can be isolated in diabetes, most mental health problems are likely multiply determined, which adds considerable complexity.

Empirical Synthesis in the Short Term

In any case, the path to theoretical integration is likely very long and winding: it took 3,400 years for diabetes to be understood, which in certain ways is an easier problem. In the meantime, there are some practical opportunities to synthesize different approaches toward a more consensual dimensional model at a small scale. In fact, there is active evidence of integration in the literature. For instance, the DSM-5 AMPD assimilates concepts from three paradigms (Mulay et al., 2018). Criterion A of the AMPD is a personality functioning construct with roots in the psychodynamic paradigm, whereas criterion B is a trait model from the psychometric paradigm. AMPD diagnosis furthermore combines both criteria to enable the diagnosis of types from the medical model tradition. Proponents of various paradigms regularly express an interest or conduct studies in the direction of paradigmatic synthesis (e.g., Harkness et al., 2014; Remmers et al., 2023; Rice & Hoffman, 2014).

The psychometric paradigm has features that lend itself particularly well to integration. On the one hand, it is generic and descriptive, and thus can accommodate different theoretical models about the reasons for observed patterns of co-variance between different phenotypes. On the other hand, it is built upon a clear and straightforward methodological strategy that lends itself well to the testing of different hypotheses. As one example, there is some level of correspondence between the higher order dimensions of RDoC and HiTOP (Michelini et al., 2024). Concerted efforts to test empirical connections between neurophysiological processes and psychometric dimensions are promising (Latzmann et al., 2021), although there are also reasons to be cautious in interpreting findings in this area (Hyatt et al., 2022).

The psychometric paradigm also provides a structure for innovation, development, and incorporation of new concepts. For instance, one potential limitation of all paradigms of psychopathology is that they rest upon research conducted primarily by privileged citizens of Western cultures. This raises questions about the generalizability of the models to other cultures and regions of the world, such as between people living in Western cultures where most research is conducted and people living in the majority world where research is underrepresented. The psychometric paradigm has developed techniques to examine the degree to which constructs mean the same thing across groups, cultures, time, etc. (Schmitt & Kuljanin, 2008). These techniques can be used to examine the generalizability of certain mental health constructs or the overall structure. Thus far, evidence for generalizability of higher order dimensions is promising (Rodriguez-Seijas et al., 2023).

Another example is the integration of dynamic processes. As a framework for describing the cross-sectional co-variance structure of mental health problems, HiTOP and other psychometric models do not directly account for how people change over time, how different problems co-vary over time, or potential idiographic patterns in which within-person patterns of co-variance do not generalize across people. However, they do provide a principled structure for conceptualizing the variables that one would measure to try to understand these kinds of dynamic processes (Conway et al., 2023; Hopwood et al., 2015), and a considerable body of knowledge has accumulated based on a psychometric measurement structure about how people develop (e.g., Bleidorn et al., 2022). Nevertheless, it is possible that this structure would need to be modified to account for certain longitudinal dynamics. For instance, it could be that patterns observed in between-person data may not hold in general or for all people in within-person data (Beckmann et al., 2010). It may also be that such patterns are most useful to consider at different levels of analysis, such as the symptom or indicator level emphasized in network models (Bringmann, 2021). The general point is, by parsing phenotypes in a principled way based on between-person co-variance, psychometric models enable a coherent and standardized starting point for studies on how people and their mental health problems change over time.

Challenges and Opportunities in Ideological Diversity

At the same time, practical challenges interfere with this kind of integrative impulse in general, and in leaning too hard into one paradigm in particular. It is a fact of science that robust knowledge takes a long time. Until robust and integrative knowledge is available, different paradigms will continue to move forward with at least somewhat incommensurate assumptions, each contributing their part, but often isolated in important ways from one another.

Differences in the assumptions, norms, values, and social networks across paradigms tend to give rise to political dynamics that further fetter integration. The medical model revolution happened because a minority perspective gained cache in the academic journals and supplanted the psychodynamic paradigm's role in the DSM. The psychometric and biological paradigms are currently gaining momentum, and the psychometric paradigm is currently putting itself forward as a viable alternative for the diagnostic manuals (Kotov et al., 2017). The psychodynamic model, once dominant, has been kicked around but it survives, nonetheless. Throughout this history, the role of political factors in how diagnosis is formulated has been, at times, at least as strong as evidence (Hopwood et al., 2018; Zachar et al., 2016). There are significant incentives for people to push one ideology or another (Kuhn, 1962), and perhaps scientific advantages as well (Feyerabend, 1975; Markon, 2013). Thus, it is likely that different paradigms will continue to gain and lose popularity and influence over time based on political dynamics until a principled and integrative framework is achieved.

My own view in this context is that all psychopathologists ought to be working toward a diagnostic scheme that is more evidence-based and clinically useful than the current one. However, a full synthesis is not going to be possible anytime soon, and a synthesis that forces diverse perspectives to adopt the ideological assumptions of a single hegemonic paradigm would be counterproductive.

Diagnostic Manuals

This leaves the practical problem of what to do about diagnostic manuals. Given the tension between ideological plurality in psychopathology science and the necessity of coherence and certainty in a diagnostic manual, it is not possible for a diagnostic manual to accurately reflect the full, messy, and uncertain state of research at the time it is published. In that sense, manuals are decoupled somewhat from evidence, at least as some people view it, and their organizing principles are likely to conflict with certain assumptions and values in the scientific community. That said, manuals should be signposts of the best available knowledge at the time they are written, and they play an important role in organizing mental health research and practice. A case can be made on those grounds that manuals ought to be guided by the paradigm that the largest plurality of scientists agrees has the most evidence and clinical utility at the time they are published. At this time, I, along with many others, would argue that the psychometric paradigm is best suited to offer such a model, because it solves many of the practical problems of the current medical model paradigm such as comorbidity and heterogeneity, it is more amenable to clinical practice than models from the biological paradigm, it is arguably more evidence based and more popular among a wider range of mental health researchers than the psychodynamic paradigm, and it is less likely to be viewed negatively by clinicians of other popular theoretical persuasions.

Practically speaking, the current state of knowledge and political momentum portends a reorganization of diagnostic phenotypes based on something like HiTOP (with the caveat that some forms of psychopathology are not yet included within HiTOP specifically). At the same time, to the extent that features of other perspectives could supplement this approach in a way that improves it, all the better. For example, cut scores on dimensions could be based on those from the medical model, arbitrary as they are, to preserve continuity of rates. When possible, evidence about biological (and psychosocial) etiology could be used to better understand psychometrically generated constructs, and in some cases perhaps even to arrange constructs differently based on etiological as opposed to psychometric evidence. Considerations like level of maturation, unconscious dynamics, and internal conflicts could be incorporated in principled ways to texture diagnostic constructs as well, as has been done in the AMPD. This temporary solution is not final or even particularly satisfying, but it is probably the best we can do on the long road toward paradigmatic integration, until some other paradigm convinces the field that it is in a stronger position to guide clinical diagnosis.

Ironic Aside about Categories, Dimensions, and Utility

Like me, the editors of this book are on record as advocates of psychometric models of diagnosis, and the conceit of this book is that you should be as well. Yet when the editors asked me to distinguish different approaches, I sorted them into categories, knowing full well that these paradigms could be parsed in terms of profiles of dimensions (e.g., how much psychometric vs. other kinds of data are important, the value of clinical expertise, the importance of etiology vs. description, etc.). These paradigm categories are not valid any more than psychiatric disorder categories are. Different authors would not have used the same categories or labels, there is significant heterogeneity within each category, and there is significant overlap across categories.

An underappreciated skill in the psychological literature, in which logrolling is incentivized by personal and institutional rewards, is keeping seemingly incompatible things in our heads at the same time. Dialectics stimulate progress in mental health and in science (Hegel, 1969). Even as we are encouraged to transition to dimensional models of psychopathology, we can acknowledge that invalid categories can be useful. It might be interesting for readers to think about how they would have organized this chapter in terms of the dimensions that describe differences among the four paradigms I have described, and whether that would have made it better. I submit that it was better to use admittedly flawed categories in this case.

Conclusion

In this chapter, I distinguished medical model, psychometric, biological, and psychodynamic paradigms of psychopathology, and compared each of them in terms of the degree to which they are dimensional across three different meanings of that term (continuous, unidimensional, and hierarchical). I then used the interface of these four paradigms and three meanings of dimension to evaluate prospects for a consensual dimensional model of psychopathology. I concluded that synthesis will take a very long time. In the short term, the psychometric paradigm should overtake the medical model paradigm as the dominant approach to classifying mental health problems, because it rests on a firmer body of evidence. But there are reasonable concerns about models based on co-variance analysis in terms of clinical utility and incommensurable epistemology, and some of these concerns can be addressed by complementing it with features of other paradigms.

References

Allsopp, K., Read, J., Corcoran, R., & Kinderman, P. (2019). Heterogeneity in psychiatric diagnostic classification. *Psychiatry Rresearch*, *279*, 15–22.

Auerbach, A. H., & Childress, A. R. (1987). The value of DSM-III for psychotherapy: A feasibility study. *The Journal of Nervous and Mental Disease*, *175*(3), 138–142.

Bagby, R. M., Ryder, A. G., Ben-Dat, D., Bacchiochi, J., & Parker, J. D. (2002). Validation of the dimensional factor structure of the Personality Psychopathology Five in clinical and nonclinical samples. *Journal of Personality Disorders*, *16*(4), 304–316.

Baker, T. B., McFall, R. M., & Shoham, V. (2008). Current status and future prospects of clinical psychology: Toward a scientifically principled approach to mental and behavioral health care. *Psychological Science in the Public Interest*, *9*(2), 67–103.
Barber, J. P., & Solomonov, N. (2016). Psychodynamic theories. In J. C. Norcross, G. R. VandenBos, D. K. Freedheim, & B. O. Olatunji (Eds.), *APA handbook of clinical psychology: Theory and research* (pp. 53–77). American Psychological Association.
Beck, A. T. (1962). Reliability of psychiatric diagnoses: 1. A critique of systematic studies. *American Journal of Psychiatry*, *119*(3), 210–216.
Beckmann, N., Wood, R. E., & Minbashian, A. (2010). It depends how you look at it: On the relationship between neuroticism and conscientiousness at the within-and the between-person levels of analysis. *Journal of Research in Personality*, *44*(5), 593–601.
Beutler, L. E., Forrester, B., Gallagher-Thompson, D., Thompson, L., & Tomlins, J. B. (2012). Common, specific, and treatment fit variables in psychotherapy outcome. *Journal of Psychotherapy Integration*, *22*(3), 255–281.
Blashfield, R. K. (2012). *The classification of psychopathology: Neo-Kraepelinian and quantitative approaches*. Springer.
Bleidorn, W., Schwaba, T., Zheng, A., Hopwood, C. J., Sosa, S. S., Roberts, B. W., & Briley, D. A. (2022). Personality stability and change: A meta-analysis of longitudinal studies. *Psychological Bulletin*, *148*(7–8), 588–619.
Blum, J. D. (1978). On changes in psychiatric diagnosis over time. *American Psychologist*, *33*(11), 1017–1031.
Borsboom, D., & Cramer, A. O. (2013). Network analysis: An integrative approach to the structure of psychopathology. *Annual Review of Clinical Psychology*, *9*, 91–121.
Bornstein, R. F. (2001). The impending death of psychoanalysis. *Psychoanalytic Psychology*, *18*(1), 3–20.
Bornstein, R. F. (2005). Reconnecting psychoanalysis to mainstream psychology: Challenges and opportunities. *Psychoanalytic Psychology*, *22*(3), 323–340.
Boudreaux, M. J., South, S. C., & Oltmanns, T. F. (2019). Symptom-level analysis of *DSM–IV/DSM–5* personality pathology in later life: Hierarchical structure and predictive validity across self- and informant ratings. *Journal of Abnormal Psychology*, *128*(5), 365–384.
Breuer, J. & Freud, S., (1895/2007). *Studien über Hysterie*. Fischer.
Bringmann, L. F. (2021). Person-specific networks in psychopathology: Past, present, and future. *Current Opinion in Psychology*, *41*, 59–64.
Brown, T. A., Campbell, L. A., Lehman, C. L., Grisham, J. R., & Mancill, R. B. (2001). Current and lifetime comorbidity of the *DSM-IV* anxiety and mood disorders in a large clinical sample. *Journal of Abnormal Psychology*, *110*(4), 585–599.
Buchsbaum, M. S., & Haier, R. J. (1983). Psychopathology: Biological approaches. *Annual Review of Psychology*, *34*(1), 401–430.
Campbell, D. T., & Fiske, D. W. (1959). Convergent and discriminant validation by the multitrait-multimethod matrix. *Psychological Bulletin*, *56*(2), 81–105.
Casey, B. J., Craddock, N., Cuthbert, B. N., Hyman, S. E., Lee, F. S., & Ressler, K. J. (2013). DSM-5 and RDoC: Progress in psychiatry research? *Nature Reviews Neuroscience*, *14*(11), 810–814.
Cierpka, M., Grande, T., Rudolf, G., Von Der Tann, M., & Stasch, M. (2007). The operationalized psychodynamic diagnostics system: Clinical relevance, reliability and validity. *Psychopathology*, *40*(4), 209–220.
Connolly Gibbons, M. B., Crits-Christoph, P., & Hearon, B. (2008). The empirical status of psychodynamic therapies. *Annual Review of Clinical Psychology*, *4*, 93–108.
Conway, C. C., Kotov, R., Krueger, R. F., & Caspi, A. (2023). Translating the hierarchical taxonomy of psychopathology (HiTOP) from potential to practice: Ten research questions. *American Psychologist*, *78*(7), 873–885.
Cronbach, L. J., & Meehl, P. E. (1955). Construct validity in psychological tests. *Psychological Bulletin*, *52*(4), 281–302.
Cuijpers, P., Quero, S., Noma, H., Ciharova, M., Miguel, C., Karyotaki, E., Cipriani, A., Cristea, I. A., & Furukawa, T. A. (2021). Psychotherapies for depression: A network meta-analysis covering efficacy, acceptability and long-term outcomes of all main treatment types. *World Psychiatry*, *20*(2), 283–293.

Cuthbert, B. N. (2020). The role of RDoC in future classification of mental disorders. *Dialogues in Clinical Neuroscience*, *22*(1), 81–85.

Cuthbert, B. N., & Insel, T. R. (2013). Toward the future of psychiatric diagnosis: The seven pillars of RDoC. *BMC Medicine*, *11*(1), 126.

Eaton, N. R., Bringmann, L. F., Elmer, T., Fried, E. I., Forbes, M. K., Greene, A. L., Krueger, R. F., Kotov, R., McGorry, P. D., Mei, C., & Waszczuk, M. A. (2023). A review of approaches and models in psychopathology conceptualization research. *Nature Reviews Psychology*, *2*(10), 622–636.

Eaton, N. R., Krueger, R. F., South, S. C., Simms, L. J., & Clark, L. A. (2011). Contrasting prototypes and dimensions in the classification of personality pathology: Evidence that dimensions, but not prototypes, are robust. *Psychological Medicine*, *41*(6), 1151–1163.

Engstrom, E. J., & Kendler, K. S. (2015). Emil Kraepelin: Icon and reality. *American Journal of Psychiatry*, *172*(12), 1190–1196.

Feighner, J. P., Robins, E., Guze, S. B., Woodruff, R. A., Winokur, G., & Munoz, R. (1972). Diagnostic criteria for use in psychiatric research. *Archives of General Psychiatry*, *26*(1), 57–63.

Feyerabend, P. (1975). *Against method*. New Left Books.

First, M. B. (2005). Clinical utility: A prerequisite for the adoption of a dimensional approach in *DSM*. *Journal of Abnormal Psychology*, *114*(4), 560–564.

Fonagy, P., Roth, A., & Higgitt, A. (2005). Psychodynamic psychotherapies: Evidence-based practice and clinical wisdom. *Bulletin of the Menninger Clinic*, *69*(1), 1–58.

Forbes, M. K., Baillie, A. J., Batterham, P., Calear, A., Kotov, R., Krueger, R. F., Markon, K. E., Mewton, L., Pellicano, L., Roberts, M., & Clark, L. A. (2023). Reconstructing psychopathology: A data-driven reorganization of the symptoms in DSM-5. https://osf.io/preprints/psyarxiv/7um9a

Forbes, M. K., Ringwald, W. R., Allen, T., Cicero, D. C., Clark, L. A., DeYoung, C. G., Eaton, N., Kotov, R., Krueger, R. F., Latzman, R. D., Martin, E. A., Naragon-Gainey, K., Ruggero, C. J., Waldman, I. D., Brandes, C., Fried, E. I., Goghari, V. M., Hankin, B., Sperry, S., . . . & Wright, A. G. C. (2024). Principles and procedures for revising the hierarchical taxonomy of psychopathology. *Journal of Psychopathology and Clinical Science*, *133*(1), 4–19.

Fowles, D. C. (1993). Biological variables in psychopathology: A psychobiological perspective. In *Comprehensive handbook of psychopathology* (pp. 85–104).Springer US.

Gifford, R., & O'Connor, B. (1987). The interpersonal circumplex as a behavior map. *Journal of Personality and Social Psychology*, *52*(5), 1019–1026.

Greenberg, J. R., & Mitchell, S. A. (1983). *Object relations in psychoanalytic theory*. Harvard University Press.

Gould, M. S., Wunsch-Hitzig, R., & Dohrenwend, B. (1981). Estimating the prevalence of childhood psychopathology: A critical review. *Journal of the American Academy of Child Psychiatry*, *20*(3), 462–476.

Haeffel, G. J., Jeronimus, B. F., Kaiser, B. N., Weaver, L., Jo Soyster, P. D., Fisher, A. J., Vargas, I., Goodson, J. T., Lu, W. (2022). Folk classification and factor rotations: Whales, sharks, and the problems with the hierarchical taxonomy of psychopathology (HiTOP). *Clinical Psychological Science*, *10*(2), 259–278.

Harkness, A. R., Reynolds, S. M., & Lilienfeld, S. O. (2014). A review of systems for psychology and psychiatry: Adaptive systems, personality psychopathology five (PSY–5), and the DSM–5. *Journal of Personality Assessment*, *96*(2), 121–139.

Haslam, N., Holland, E., & Kuppens, P. (2012). Categories versus dimensions in personality and psychopathology: A quantitative review of taxometric research. *Psychological Medicine*, *42*(5), 903–920.

Hegel, G. W. F. (1969). *Hegel's science of logic* (A.V. Miller, Trans.). Humanities Press.

Hopwood, C. J. (2025). Personality functioning, problems in living, and personality traits. *Journal of Personality Assessment*, *107*(2), 143–158.

Hopwood, C. J., Kotov, R., Krueger, R. F., Watson, D., Widiger, T. A., Althoff, R. R., . . . & Zimmermann, J. (2018). The time has come for dimensional personality disorder diagnosis. *Personality and Mental Health*, *12*(1), 82–86.

Hopwood, C. J., Morey, L. C., & Markon, K. E. (2023). What is a psychopathology dimension? *Clinical Psychology Review*, *106*, 102356.

Hopwood, C. J., Zimmermann, J., Pincus, A. L., & Krueger, R. F. (2015). Connecting personality structure and dynamics: Towards a more evidence-based and clinically useful diagnostic scheme. *Journal of Personality Disorders, 29*(4), 431–448.

Horwitz, A. V. (2014). DSM-I and DSM-II. *The encyclopedia of clinical psychology*, 1–6.

Hyatt, C. S., Sharpe, B. M., Owens, M. M., Listyg, B. S., Carter, N. T., Lynam, D. R., & Miller, J. D. (2022). Searching high and low for meaningful and replicable morphometric correlates of personality. *Journal of Personality and Social Psychology, 123*(2), 463–480.

Hyman, S. E. (2010). The diagnosis of mental disorders: The problem of reification. *Annual Review of Clinical Psychology, 6*, 155–179.

Insel, T. R. (2009). Translating scientific opportunity into public health impact: A strategic plan for research on mental illness. *Archives of General Psychiatry, 66*(2), 128–133.

Insel, T., Cuthbert, B., Garvey, M., Heinssen, R., Pine, D. S., Quinn, K., Sanislow, C., & Wang, P. (2010). Research domain criteria (RDoC): Toward a new classification framework for research on mental disorders. *American Journal of Psychiatry, 167*(7), 748–751.

Karamanou, M., Protogerou, A., Tsoucalas, G., Androutsos, G., & Poulakou-Rebelakou, E. (2016). Milestones in the history of diabetes mellitus: The main contributors. *World Journal of Diabetes, 7*(1), 1–7.

Kendler, K. S., Muñoz, R. A., & Murphy, G. (2010). The development of the Feighner criteria: A historical perspective. *American Journal of Psychiatry, 167*(2), 134–142.

Kernberg, O. (1967). Borderline personality organization. *Journal of the American Psychoanalytic Association, 15*(3), 641–685.

Klerman, G. L. (1978). The evolution of a scientific nosology. In J. C. Shershow (Ed.), *Schizophrenia: Science and practice* (pp. 99–121). Harvard University Press.

Klerman, G. L. (1990). Paradigm shifts in USA psychiatric epidemiology since World War II. *Social Psychiatry and Psychiatric Epidemiology, 25*(1), 27–32.

Koerner, K., Kohlenberg, R. J., & Parker, C. R. (1996). Diagnosis of personality disorder: A radical behavioral alternative. *Journal of Consulting and Clinical Psychology, 64*(6), 1169–1176.

Kotov, R., Krueger, R. F., Watson, D., Achenbach, T. M., Althoff, R. R., Bagby, R. M., Brown, T. A., Carpenter, W. T., Caspi, A., Clark, L. A., Eaton, N. R., Forbes, M. K., Forbush, K. T., Goldberg, D., Hasin, D., Hyman, S. E., Ivanova, M. Y., Lynam, D. R., Markon, K., . . . & Zimmerman, M. (2017). The Hierarchical Taxonomy of Psychopathology (HiTOP): A dimensional alternative to traditional nosologies. *Journal of Abnormal Psychology, 126*(4), 454–477.

Kraepelin, E. (1905). *Die Königliche Psychiatrische Klinik in München*. Barth.

Krueger, R. F., Derringer, J., Markon, K. E., Watson, D., & Skodol, A. E. (2012). Initial construction of a maladaptive personality trait model and inventory for DSM-5. *Psychological Medicine, 42*(9), 1879–1890.

Krueger, R. F., Hopwood, C. J., Wright, A. G. C., & Markon, K. E. (2014). *DSM-5* and the path toward empirically based and clinically useful conceptualization of personality and psychopathology. *Clinical Psychology: Science and Practice, 21*(3), 245–261.

Kuhn, T.S. (1962). *The structure of scientific revolutions*. University of Chicago Press.

Latzman, R. D., Krueger, R. F., DeYoung, C. G., & Michelini, G. (2021). Connecting quantitatively derived personality–psychopathology models and neuroscience. *Personality Neuroscience, 4*, e4.

Leichsenring, F., Steinert, C., Rabung, S., & Ioannidis, J. P. (2022). The efficacy of psychotherapies and pharmacotherapies for mental disorders in adults: An umbrella review and meta-analytic evaluation of recent meta-analyses. *World Psychiatry, 21*(1), 133–145.

Lilienfeld, S. O., & Pinto, M. D. (2015). Risky tests of etiological models in psychopathology research: The need for meta-methodology. *Psychological Inquiry, 26*(3), 253–258.

Loevinger, J. (1957). Objective tests as instruments of psychological theory. *Psychological Reports, 3*(3), 635–694.

Loevinger, J. (1966). Three principles for a psychoanalytic psychology. *Journal of Abnormal Psychology, 71*(6), 432–443.

Loevinger, J. (1983). On ego development and the structure of personality. *Developmental Review, 3*(3), 339–350.

Loevinger, J. (1987). *Paradigms of personality.* WH Freeman/Times Books/Henry Holt & Co.
Markon, K. E. (2013). Wake up and smile, or how I learned to stop worrying and love epistemological pluralism: Commentary on "A postmortem and future look at the personality disorders in DSM-5."
Markon, K. E., Chmielewski, M., & Miller, C. J. (2011). The reliability and validity of discrete and continuous measures of psychopathology: A quantitative review. *Psychological Bulletin, 137*(5), 856–879.
Markon, K. E., Krueger, R. F., & Watson, D. (2005). Delineating the structure of normal and abnormal personality: An integrative hierarchical approach. *Journal of Personality and Social Psychology, 88*(1), 139–157.
McCrae, R. R., & John, O. P. (1992). An introduction to the five-factor model and its applications. *Journal of Personality, 60*(2), 175–215.
Michelini, G., Carlisi, C. O., Eaton, N. R., Elison, J. T., Haltigan, J. D., Kotov, R., . . . & Wilson, S. (2024). Where do neurodevelopmental conditions fit in transdiagnostic psychiatric frameworks? Incorporating a new neurodevelopmental spectrum. *World Psychiatry, 23*(3), 333–357.
Michelini, G., Palumbo, I. M., DeYoung, C. G., Latzman, R. D., & Kotov, R. (2021). Linking RDoC and HiTOP: A new interface for advancing psychiatric nosology and neuroscience. *Clinical Psychology Review, 86*, 102025.
Miller, S. D., Hubble, M. A., Chow, D. L., & Seidel, J. A. (2013). The outcome of psychotherapy: Yesterday, today, and tomorrow. *Psychotherapy, 50*(1), 88–97.
Millon, T. (1983). The DSM-III: An insider's perspective. *American Psychologist, 38*(7), 804–814.
Mulay, A. L., Cain, N. M., Waugh, M. H., Hopwood, C. J., Adler, J. M., Garcia, D. J., Kurtz, J. E., Lenger, K. A., & Skadberg, R. (2018). Personality constructs and paradigms in the alternative DSM-5 model of personality disorder. *Journal of Personality Assessment, 100*(6), 593–602.
OPD Force. (2008). *Operationalized psychodynamic diagnosis OPD-2: Manual of diagnosis and treatment planning.* Hogrefe Publishing GmbH.
PDM Task Force. (2006). *Psychodynamic diagnostic manual.* Alliance of Psychoanalytic Organizations.
Remmers, C., Wester, R., Repnik, L. G., Plumbohm, M., Unger, S., & Jauk, E. (2023). Psychodynamic theory meets HiTOP: The nomological network between motivational conflicts and dimensions of the hierarchical taxonomy of psychopathology (HiTOP). *Journal of Research in Personality, 106*, 104418.
Revelle, W., & Condon, D. M. (2019). Reliability from α to ω: A tutorial. *Psychological Assessment, 31*(12), 1395–1411.
Rice, T. R., & Hoffman, L. (2014). Defense mechanisms and implicit emotion regulation: A comparison of a psychodynamic construct with one from contemporary neuroscience. *Journal of the American Psychoanalytic Association, 62*(4), 693–708.
Ringwald, W. R., Forbes, M. K., & Wright, A. G. (2023). Meta-analysis of structural evidence for the Hierarchical Taxonomy of Psychopathology (HiTOP) model. *Psychological Medicine, 53*(2), 533–546.
Robins, E., & Guze, S. B. (1970). Establishment of diagnostic validity in psychiatric illness: Its application to schizophrenia. *American Journal of Psychiatry, 126*(7), 983–987.
Rodriguez-Seijas, C., Li, J. J., Balling, C., Brandes, C., Bernat, E., Boness, C. L., . . . & Eaton, N. R. (2023). Diversity and the Hierarchical Taxonomy of Psychopathology (HiTOP). *Nature Reviews Psychology*, 1–13.
Ruggero, C. J., Kotov, R., Hopwood, C. J., First, M., Clark, L. A., Skodol, A. E., Mullins-Sweatt, S. N., Patrick, C. J., Bach, B., Cicero, D. C., Docherty, A., Simms, L. J., Bagby, R. M., Krueger, R. F., Callahan, J. L., Chmielewski, M., Conway, C. C., De Clercq, B., Dornbach-Bender, A., . . . & Zimmermann, J. (2019). Integrating the Hierarchical Taxonomy of Psychopathology (HiTOP) into clinical practice. *Journal of Consulting and Clinical Psychology, 87*(12), 1069–1084.
Ruiz, M. A., Hopwood, C. J., Edens, J. F., Morey, L. C., & Cox, J. (2018). Initial development of pathological personality trait domain measures using the Personality Assessment Inventory (PAI). *Personality Disorders: Theory, Research, and Treatment, 9*(6), 564–573.
Sanislow, C. A., Grilo, C. M., Morey, L. C., Bender, D. S., Skodol, A. E., Gunderson, J. G., Shea, M. T., Stout, R. L., Zanarini, M. C., & McGlashan, T. H. (2002). Confirmatory factor analysis of DSM-IV criteria for borderline personality disorder: Findings from the collaborative longitudinal personality disorders study. *American Journal of Psychiatry, 159*(2), 284–290.

Schmitt, N., & Kuljanin, G. (2008). Measurement invariance: Review of practice and implications. *Human Resource Management Review, 18*(4), 210–222.

Sellbom, M., Kremyar, A. J., & Wygant, D. B. (2021). Mapping MMPI-3 scales onto the hierarchical taxonomy of psychopathology. *Psychological Assessment, 33*(12), 1153–1168.

Sharp, C., & Wall, K. (2021). DSM-5 level of personality functioning: Refocusing personality disorder on what it means to be human. *Annual Review of Clinical Psychology, 17*, 313–337.

Skinner, B. F. (1963). Behaviorism at Fifty: The rapid growth of a scientific analysis of behavior calls for a restatement of the philosophy of psychology. *Science, 140*(3570), 951–958.

Smith, D. A., Mar, C. M., & Turoff, B. K. (1998). The structure of schizophrenic symptoms: A meta-analytic confirmatory factor analysis. *Schizophrenia Research, 31*(1), 57–70.

Smoller, J. W., Andreassen, O. A., Edenberg, H. J., Faraone, S. V., Glatt, S. J., & Kendler, K. S. (2019). Psychiatric genetics and the structure of psychopathology. *Molecular Psychiatry, 24*(3), 409–420.

Spitzer, R. L. (2001). Values and assumptions in the development of DSM-III and DSM-III-R: An insider's perspective and a belated response to Sadler, Hulgus, and Agich's "On values in recent American psychiatric classification." *The Journal of Nervous and Mental Disease, 189*(6), 351–359.

Spitzer, R. L., Davies, M., & Barkley, R. A. (1990). The DSM-III-R field trial of disruptive behavior disorders. *Journal of the American Academy of Child & Adolescent Psychiatry, 29*(5), 690–697.

Steinert, C., Munder, T., Rabung, S., Hoyer, J., & Leichsenring, F. (2017). Psychodynamic therapy: As efficacious as other empirically supported treatments? A meta-analysis testing equivalence of outcomes. *American Journal of Psychiatry, 174*(10), 943–953.

Taubner, S., Hörz, S., Fischer-Kern, M., Doering, S., Buchheim, A., & Zimmermann, J. (2013). Internal structure of the Reflective Functioning Scale. *Psychological Assessment, 25*(1), 127–135.

Thomas, J. G., & Sharp, P. B. (2019). Mechanistic science: A new approach to comprehensive psychopathology research that relates psychological and biological phenomena. *Clinical Psychological Science, 7*(2), 196–215.

Van Loo, H. M., De Jonge, P., Romeijn, J. W., Kessler, R. C., & Schoevers, R. A. (2012). Data-driven subtypes of major depressive disorder: A systematic review. *BMC Medicine, 10*, 1–12.

Waszczuk, M. A., Hopwood, C. J., Luft, B. J., Morey, L. C., Perlman, G., Ruggero, C. J., Skodol, A. E., & Kotov, R. (2022). The prognostic utility of personality traits versus past psychiatric diagnoses: Predicting future mental health and functioning. *Clinical Psychological Science, 10*(4), 734–751.

Weekers, L. C., Hutsebaut, J., De Saeger, H., & Kamphuis, J. H. (2024). Comparing the clinical utility of the alternative model for personality disorders to the Section II personality disorder model: A randomized controlled trial. *Personality Disorders: Theory, Research, and Treatment, 15*(5), 386.

Westen, D., Shedler, J., & Bradley, R. (2006). A prototype approach to personality disorder diagnosis. *American Journal of Psychiatry, 163*(5), 846–856.

Wiggins, J. S. (2003). *Paradigms of personality assessment*. Guilford Press.

Wright, A. G., Krueger, R. F., Hobbs, M. J., Markon, K. E., Eaton, N. R., & Slade, T. (2013). The structure of psychopathology: Toward an expanded quantitative empirical model. *Journal of Abnormal Psychology, 122*(1), 281–294.

Wright, A. G., & Simms, L. J. (2015). A metastructural model of mental disorders and pathological personality traits. *Psychological Medicine, 45*(11), 2309–2319.

Yalch, M. M., Thomas, K. M., & Hopwood, C. J. (2012). The validity of trait, symptom and prototype approaches for describing borderline and antisocial personality disorders. *Personality and Mental Health, 6*(3), 207–216.

Zachar, P., Krueger, R. F., & Kendler, K. S. (2016). Personality disorder in DSM-5: An oral history. *Psychological Medicine, 46*(1), 1–10.

Zachar, P., Stoyanov, D. S., Aragona, M., & Jablensky, A. (2014). *Alternative perspectives validation*. Oxford University Press.

INDEX

For the benefit of digital users, indexed terms that span two pages (e.g., 52–53) may, on occasion, appear on only one of those pages.

Note: Tables and figures are indicated by an italic *t* and *f* following the page number.